Bone Metastases from Prostate Cancer

Francesco Bertoldo • Francesco Boccardo
Emilio Bombardieri • Laura Evangelista
Riccardo Valdagni
Editors

Bone Metastases from Prostate Cancer

Biology, Diagnosis and Management

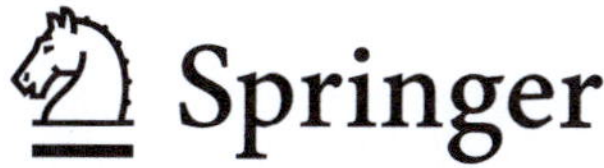

Editors
Francesco Bertoldo
University of Verona
Director of Metabolic Bone Diseases and Osteoncology Unit, Internal Medicine Department of Medicine
Verona
Italy

Francesco Boccardo
IRCCS AOU San Martino-IST National Cancer Research Institute
Department of Internal Medicine and Medical specialties (DIMI), School of Medical and Pharmacological Sciences, University of Genoa, Academic Unit of Medical Oncology, Department of Oncology (DIPOE)
Genova
Italy

Emilio Bombardieri
Humanitas Gavazzeni Clinic
Clinical Scientific Director
Department of Nuclear Medicine
Bergamo
Italy

Laura Evangelista
Veneto Institute of Oncology
IOV - IRCCS
Nuclear Medicine and Molecular Imaging Unit
Padova
Italy

Riccardo Valdagni
Radiation Oncology 1 and Prostate Cancer Program, Fondazione IRCCS Istituto Nazionale dei Tumori
Department of Oncology and Hemato-oncology, Università di Milano
Milano
Italy

ISBN 978-3-319-42326-5 ISBN 978-3-319-42327-2 (eBook)
DOI 10.1007/978-3-319-42327-2

Library of Congress Control Number: 2016957630

Printed on acid-free paper

This Springer imprint is published by Springer Nature
The registered company is Springer International Publishing AG Switzerland
The registered company address is Gewerbestrasse 11, 6330 Cham, Switzerland

Foreword

Would you like to know everything that there is to know about bone metastases from prostate cancer? Prostate cancer is the second most diagnosed malignancy and the sixth cause of cancer-related death worldwide and is one of the cancers that most frequently metastasizes to the bone. Would you like to be knowledgeable about all of the new imaging techniques and treatments available for bone metastases? This textbook is not only on bone metastases but is an up-to-date review on everything the clinician needs to know about prostate cancer.

This book was conceived with the intention to emphasize bone pathology and metastases, critical to prostate cancer. You will learn about the complex histology, high heterogeneity, and bone matrix-derived factors. Each chapter is thorough, well written, and up to date. There is a section devoted to markers of bone turnover in bone metastasis and new markers. Many chapters contain beautiful illustrations and images of bone metastases. You will learn about non-osteoclastic bone, bone resorption mediated by metalloproteases, periostin, bone sialoprotein, osteopontin, and other emerging markers. You will acquire the ability to compare new markers with "classic" bone markers.

You are invited to improve your knowledge of bone homing and metastasis, the result of a multistep process that requires an interaction between tumor cells and the bone microenvironment that starts with tumor malignant progression and invasion through the extracellular matrix and leads to bone metastases. You will gain knowledge about the role of epithelial-mesenchymal plasticity in bone homing, the role of chemokines and their receptors, and the role of microRNAs. You will also understand the many signaling pathways implicated in the development of prostate cancer bone metastases.

There is an increasing need for validated, reliable circulating tumor markers. PSA is discussed in great detail and the clinical settings, in which it is most useful, with an exhaustive summary of recommendations as to its predictive use in staging, and detection of recurrence.

You will learn about the different methodologies in detecting circulating tumor cells (CTCs). CTCs can provide valuable information about disease heterogeneity, clonal evolution, disease progression, and response and development of resistance to therapies such as novel AR-directed treatments.

Conventional imaging methods are inadequate for the assessment of changes in bone metastases in response to various treatments. PET with various targeted radiotracers is required. There are several chapters devoted to distinguishing among the different imaging methodologies: ^{99m}Tc-biphosphonates planar scintigraphy or SPECT/CT, ^{18}F-FDG PET, ^{18}F- NaF PET/CT, ^{11}C/^{18}F choline PET/CT, and ^{68}Ga-PSMA PET/CT. You will learn about the different sensitivities and insensitivities of these modalities in identifying disease and capturing degrees of biological response and the challenges such as flare phenomenon. PSMA-based PET imaging agents fall into three categories. Consider also the auspicious performance of ^{18}F-FACBC, ^{68}Ga-PSMA PET/CT for investigating prostate cancer patients with biochemical recurrence.

Radiation therapy techniques are continually evolving, not only for treating the prostate. Careful attention is paid to new techniques for the palliation of bone metastases. There is an excellent summary of randomized trials comparing single versus multiple fractions in the palliative setting, data on stereotaxic irradiation for oligometastatic disease, and much more.

This book discusses classic hormonal therapy, first-generation antiandrogens, and novel second-generation antiandrogens. You will learn about AR splice variants, such as AR-V7 and AR567e, and their predictive and prognostic value. The cross-resistance between abiraterone and enzalutamide are important topics.

Chemotherapy with docetaxel and cabazitaxel plays an important role in patients with prostate cancer. The trials that have further investigated these agents in CRPC are reviewed. You will learn about Radium-223 that can not only decrease symptomatic skeletal events but also increases survival.

A hot topic in CRPC is molecular profiling. Studies have shown that around 90% of mCRPC patients harbor clinically actionable molecular alterations and 23% harbor DNA repair pathway aberrations that may respond to PARP inhibitors or platinum. The clinical trials in hormone-sensitive prostate cancer are also reviewed in great detail, as is the treatment of oligometastatic disease with radiation or surgery.

Nociceptive and neuropathic pain, pain assessment, pain syndromes in prostate cancer bone pain, and treatment of cancer-induced bone pain are extensively reviewed as well as simultaneous palliative care.

The economic impact of prostate cancer bone metastases and skeletal-related events is also explored. This book concludes with discussions on the importance of a multidisciplinary team approach to prostate cancer and the importance and benefits of well-organized prostate cancer units.

This textbook is a must for anyone who is interested in prostate cancer. It is well written, up to date, and highly relevant.

Cora N. Sternberg, MD, FACP

Preface

Skeletal metastases affect more than 80% of men with metastatic prostate cancer, and they are the main cause for patients' poor quality of life, morbidity, and mortality. In the recent years, there was a tremendous improvement in the options of treatment for patients with metastatic prostate cancer. New hormonal, cytotoxic, immunotherapeutic drugs and new therapeutic radiation-based strategies have been developed. These approaches achieved very important results also in terms of overall survival and appear to be suitable for a large number of patients with metastatic prostate cancer, either those affected by hormone-naïve prostate cancer (HNPC) or those affected by castration-resistant prostate cancer (CRPC). One could say that while in the past the majority of patients, especially those affected by CRPC, were candidate only to best supportive care, at present most of them can afford upon different treatment choices able to impact favorably both with their life expectancy and their quality of life as well as upon novel therapeutic options and new combination strategies which promise to further improve patient outcomes.

In view of the increasing interest and number of scientific contributions in this area, we have conceived the idea to invite a number of distinguished colleagues to summarize the state of the art and to examine the new perspectives from their different points of view on the most important topics related to bone metastases in prostate cancer, starting from the physiopathological background of bone metastatization and the biological mechanisms involved in bone remodeling and in skeletal homing of cancer cells, which are the premises to a rational approach to the disease. Markers of these phenomena are described and analyzed in view of their clinical applications in everyday clinical practice. A special focus was given to the putative role of circulating cancer cells, circulating markers of bone metabolism, and markers of prostatic cancer. The metabolic relevance of the mechanisms involved in bone metastatization is also described in the perspective of the technological advancements of metabolic imaging that visualizes bone metastases through new radiopharmaceuticals capable to target bone changes caused by metastasis or directly prostate cancer cells. New modalities of metabolic imaging, such as ^{18}F-fluoride, ^{18}F/^{11}C-choline, and ^{18}F-FDG positron emission tomography (PET)/computed tomography (CT), are reported, including the most recent experimental tracers like ^{68}Ga-prostate specific membrane antigen (^{68}Ga-PSMA). In the radiological area, the contribution of the multimodality magnetic resonance imaging (MRI) in improving the accuracy of CT has been critically discussed, also in terms of availability of this technique and relative costs. As a logical consequence of an adequate diagnosis and staging, attention was moved to the available treatment options for patients with prostate cancer bone metastases (hormonal therapy, chemotherapy, chemotherapy associated with hormonal manipulations, bone targeted drugs, surgery, external beam therapy, and radio-metabolic therapy). The evaluation of treatment response in bone metastatic prostate cancer is one of the key points addressed in the textbook due to the limits of currently available tools, namely, radiology and nuclear medicine imaging. The putative advantages of one or more techniques over the others have been specifically analyzed. The putative role in implementing the definition of tumor response at the bone level by the dosage of markers of bone turnover and of prostate-specific antigen (PSA) has been also considered. The performances and limitations of the criteria adopted in the most important clinical trials and which are currently recommended by the Guidelines of the Scientific Societies have also been critically reviewed. A look at other issues that are strictly correlated with the management of the patients affected by bone metastases has been provided. The abovementioned issues include bone pain palliation and prevention of major adverse skeletal events as well as the social and economic impact of bone metastases, which intuitively is not limited to the costs more directly related to patient care. The necessity of addressing this increasingly important health problem through a multidisciplinary team of clinicians able to intercept all the patient needs and to provide an appropriate answer to all of them has also been addressed, with the hope that this model could become standard for the majority of the centers involved in the management of prostate cancer. Our ambition, as editors of this volume, was to provide the readers with a complete but clear-cut information about the most relevant results achieved in the different areas concerning the topic as well as a look at the researches that are still going on and that promise to further change the course of the disease and of its management. Let's hope we have reached the scope, thanks to the efforts of the authors who have accepted to actively provide their contributions and to the editor staff who trusted in this task and whose help and assistance was essential to complete it.

Francesco Bertoldo
Francesco Boccardo
Emilio Bombardieri
Laura Evangelista
Riccardo Valdagni

Contents

1 Biology and Pathophysiology of Bone Metastasis in Prostate Cancer

Francesco Bertoldo

1.1 Distribution and Preferential Site of Bone Metastasis in Prostate Cancer Patients

Several studies have attempted to correlate the extent of skeletal metastatic involvement, the number of bone metastases (BMTs) identified by bone scintigraphy or the distribution of BMTs (axial vs appendicular) with survival in patients with advanced prostate cancer (PC) [1, 2]. The number of BMTs has recently been evaluated as a prognostic predictor [3]. Patients with metastatic castration-resistant PC with a higher number of BMTs had a shorter progression-free survival (PFS) and overall survival (OS; hazard ratio 2.0; 95 % confidence interval 1.7–2.4). Patients with 1–4 BMTs have much better PFS and OS than those with 5–20 BMTs [4]. It should, however, be taken into account that among the predictors of prognosis, coexisting non-osseous metastatic disease is an important determinant of prognosis in patients with BMTs [5, 6].

It is well known that a BMT most commonly affects the axial skeleton and that patients with BMT confined to the vertebrae have a better prognosis. Several studies have shown that the distribution and sites of predilection were similar in PC and breast cancer, with the ribs, spine and ilium reported to be those for BMT. However, recent data have shown that in early stages of breast cancer and PC the distribution in the thoracic skeleton is higher for the former than for the latter. In PC the distribution is 80 % in the spine and pelvis. In the advanced stages and in cases of extensive BMT, it seems that there are no differences in skeletal distribution between breast and PC, with a high frequency of BMT to the ribs and sternum in patients with PC as well [7, 8]. Interestingly, BMT is rarely observed in the mid-distal bones of the extremities, unlike that reported in a few other studies [9].

F. Bertoldo, MD
Metabolic Bone Diseases and Osteo-oncology Unit, Internal Medicine Department of Medicine, University of Verona, Verona, Italy
e-mail: francesco.bertoldo@univr.it

1.2 Pathology of Bone Metastasis from Prostate Cancer

Prostate cancer BMT is usually defined as "osteoblastic" by conventional radiographs. However, recent studies have shown a high heterogeneity of lesions, with synchronous osteolysis in BMT of PC, even when the overall character seems to be blastic [10]. Histomorphometric studies have shown that blastic lesions are mixed in nature, with increased activity of both osteoblasts and osteoclasts [11]. In bone biopsies of prostate BMT, an increase in the osteoid surface and osteoid volume and an elevation in the mineral

F. Bertoldo et al. (eds.), *Bone Metastases from Prostate Cancer*,
DOI 10.1007/978-3-319-42327-2_1

apposition rate, demonstrating an accelerated state of bone formation, have been demonstrated. It was interesting to note that the new bone was formed in the marrow spaces and not adjacent to the bone surface; that is, the bone may form de novo in the marrow without the requirement of pre-existing bone resorption. Spindle-shaped cells or flat cells were seen lining woven osteoid and entrapped as osteocytes in the woven bone [12]. Surprisingly, well-differentiated osteoblasts, defined as cuboidal cells with basophilic cytoplasm lining the osteoid, were rarely observed on the woven bone, but they were observed in areas of bone repair secondary to bone necrosis. The osteoid is not fully mineralised and woven bone is formed, which has a low level of mineral density and a poorly organised lamellar bone. Furthermore, trabecular bone in metastatic lesions showed an increase in connectivity and surface irregularity, suggesting that strong effects of bone resorption and bone formation might occur in osteoblastic BMT [13]. In "osteoblastic" metastases osteoclasts were observed in the usual focal pattern on the surface of woven or lamellar bone or osteoid, and on the eroded surface area the number of osteoclasts was found to have greater than normal values [12]. Despite the osteoblastic nature of BMT, approximately half of 101 biopsies of BMT in bisphosphonate-naive PC patients were osteopaenic and half were osteodense, and this pattern was also reproduced in individual patients [12]. The undermineralised woven bone and the osteopaenic/osteolytic component of BMT may contribute to the histological frailty observed in the skeleton in PC patients, even in dense metastatic lesions (Fig. 1.1).

Bone metastases in castration-resistant PC patients were characterised according to expression levels of steroidogenic enzyme and androgen receptor splice variants. It was found that increased tumour expression of steroidogenic enzymes in individual patients is associated with advanced tumour stage. Interestingly, there are distinct subgroups of CRPC patients with BMTs expressing high levels of AKR1C3 (that convert circulating dehydroepiandrosterone and androstenedione (synthesised in the adrenals) into 5-androstenediol and testosterone) or expressing high levels of ligand binding domain (LBD)-truncated, constitutively active androgen receptor splice variants (AR-Vs). The possible clinical relevance of this is that patients with high AKR1C3 expression and low AR-V expression may show a good response to treatment with abiraterone acetate (Cyp17 inhibition) and/or would benefit from drugs targeting AKR1C3, whereas patients with a high expression of constitutively active AR-Vs will probably not respond to abiraterone acetate or to any therapy targeting androgen synthesis or the LBD of the AR [14].

1.3 Pathophysiology of Bone Metastasis

1.3.1 Pathophysiological Heterogeneity

The osteoblastic lesion is a very complex multistep process that is not fully understood in detail. It is the result of releasing osteoblast-promoting factors such as bone morphogenetic protein (BMP), Wnt family ligand, endothelin-1 and PDGF from PC cells and of a closed interaction with bone matrix, stroma cells and bone cells. Another characteristic of BMT from PC is the biological and pathophysiological heterogeneity. The high level of heterogeneity of the BMTs in PC from the pathological point of view reflects the great complexity of the biology and molecular regulation that underlie their pathophysiology. Lytic and blastic metastases share many molecular mechanisms that give an account of similar therapeutic outcome treating them with bone-modifying agents such as zoledronic acid and denosumab. The complexity of the bone response in PC invasion is underscored by the variety of soluble factors, signalling pathways and transcriptional regulators involved. The abnormal bone response is further promoted by the potential for osteomimicry of the tumour cells signalling in a paracrine fashion within the bone environment and an autocrine signalling cascade of the bone cells themselves. These interactions between the PC cells and bone cells often yield a predominantly osteoblastic response. However,

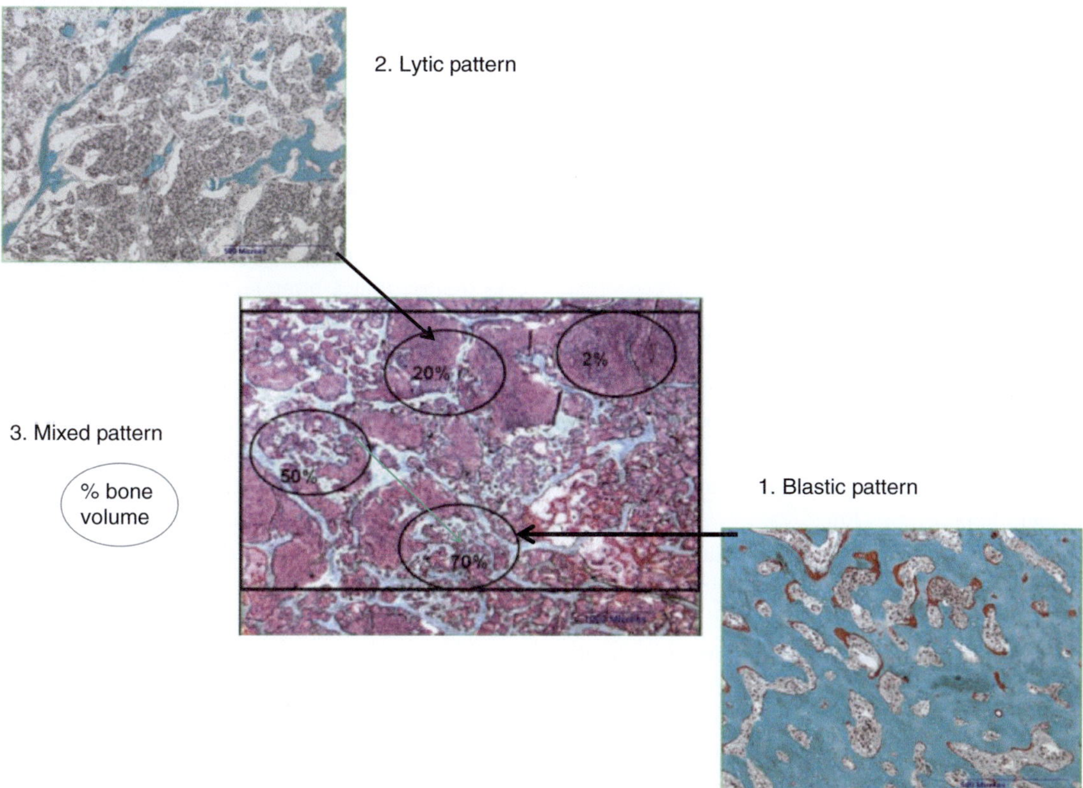

Fig. 1.1 Histopathology of bone metastasis (BMT) from prostate cancer (PC). In the same patient, BMTs are heterogeneous, with predominantly blastic (*1*) and predominantly lytic metastases (*2*). Furthermore, as shown in the histopathological sections in the same specimen of a single metastasis, there is an alternation of predominantly lytic and blastic area (mixed pattern) (*3*): 2–20 % Bone volume: predominantly lytic area; 50–70 % bone volume: predominantly blastic area (Modified from Roudier et al. [12]). *Green* bone, *red* osteoid, *grey/pink* tumour stroma

the formation of osteoblastic bone is also often associated with a significant osteolytic component, leading to a mixed, woven bone response in the same patient at different metastatic sites.

Bone remodelling proteins and transcripts in human specimens of PC BMTs were analysed in detail [15]. The main bone remodelling proteins that were recognised were assessed in lytic and blastic BMTs: BMP-2, BMP-7, dickkopf-related protein 1 (DKK-1), receptor tyrosine-protein kinase erbB-3 (ErbB3), endothelin-1 (ET-1), NEL-like protein 1 (NELL-1), tumour necrosis factor receptor superfamily 11B (OPG), phosphoglycerate kinase 1 (PGK1), sclerostin, substance P, a putative osteoblastic factor EMI domain-containing protein 1 (Emu1) and two putative osteolytic factors, matrix metalloproteinase-12 (MMP-12) and secreted frizzled-related protein 1 (SFRP1). Interestingly, many of these proteins and transcripts were equally expressed in lytic and blastic BMTs, such as BMP-2, BMP-7, DKK-1 and sclerostin. Instead, expression of some of these, such as OPG, Emu1, PGK1 and substance P, was higher in prevalent blastic lesions than in lytic lesions, but not the transcripts. OPG, PGK1 and substance P have been proven to inhibit osteoclastogenesis and induce osteoblastic differentiation. Emu1 has been shown to be prevalent in the epithelium during embryonic development and it has been hypothesised that Emu1 in PC aids adhesion The single proteins are probably not the unique drivers for conditioning the evolution towards a blastic phenotype of the metastasis, and a possible explanation for the characteristic "predominantly osteoblastic phenotype" is that PC expresses a disproportionate number of pro-osteoblastic and pro-osteolytic factors and the relative prevalence of the former will determine the pathological aspect of the lesion [15, 16].

1.3.2 The Role of Osteoclasts in Blastic and Mixed Bone Metastases

Independently from the phenotype of the lesion, osteoclasts, mainly in the first phases of BMT development, are principally responsible for the initiation, development and clinical consequences such as pain, fracture and hypercalcemia of the evident bone lesion (Fig. 1.2).

Osteoclasts have two pivotal functions in the development of bone lesions: they reabsorb the bone, creating the necessary space for the penetration and development of metastasis into the bone, and they enrich, as a direct consequence of the bone matrix breakdown, the bone micro-environment of a plethora of growth factors and tumour-seeking factors that sustain the proliferation of the cancer cells, which is essential during the first phases of metastasis. These mechanisms are the basis of the "seed and soil" concept, where the bone micro-environment factors represent the fertile ground (the soil) and the "seed" represents cancer cell growth.

Physiologically, bone resorption and bone formation in skeletal remodelling are almost always tightly coupled. The bone resorption by osteoclasts is regulated by the RANK/RANKL/OPG axis, where osteoblasts expressing RANKL induce recruitment, differentiation and activation of osteoclasts, binding and activating of RANK, and conversely expressing OPG, the RANKL decoy receptor, and osteoblasts inhibit the excess osteoclastogenesis. The ratio RANKL/OPG in bone micro-environment drives the equilibrium between bone formation and resorption.

Expression of RANKL by stromal cells/osteoblasts and osteocytes is regulated by cytokines and paracrine hormones that stimulate bone resorption [17] such as interleukin-1 (IL-1), IL-6, IL-11, IL-17, prostaglandin E2 (PGE2), parathyroid hormone (PTH) and parathyroid hormone-related peptide (PTHrP), which stimulate osteoblasts or their progenitors to express RANKL and/or to downregulate the expression of OPG [18]. Recently, the role of osteocytes through the Wnt/DKK-1 and sclerostin pathway has been elucidated (Fig. 1.2) [19].

The tumour cells co-opting the normal process that regulates bone resorption interfere with the balance of the RANKL/RANK/OPG axis. The tumour/bone interface is replete with factors that stimulate bone resorption directly produced by tumour cells themselves, by macrophages and T cells associated with metastasis or by stromal cells influenced by metastasising cells. PTHrP, IL-8 and PGE2 have been shown to increase expression of RANKL and downregulate OPG expression either in vitro in the osteoblast/tumour cell coculture or in vivo using the BMT model [17–20].

Parathyroid hormone-related peptide is not physiologically present in the circulation, but it has been found to be widely distributed in most fetal and adult tissues [21], suggesting that it might act in an autocrine/paracrine manner. This peptide plays an important role in regulating many tissues including cancer tissue [22]. PTHrP is expressed by many types of cancer cells, such as breast cancer and PC, and has been proposed as an antigen for cancer immunotherapy [23–26]. PTHrP, as PTH in physiology, stimulates osteoblasts expressing PTHR1 receptor to express RANKL, which activates osteoclasts [27]. Interestingly, it has been found that T cells also express PTHR1 and are activated by PTH and PTHrP [28, 29], contributing to osteoclast activation via RANKL. It has been demonstrated that in mice bone resorption may be prevented by the immunosuppressor abatacept, a CTLA4-Ig preventing T-cell activation [30].

In addition to PTHrP, IL-8 plays an important role in the activation of osteoclasts. IL-8 is the human homologue to murine MIP-2 belonging to the family of chemokine CXC and is constitutively produced by osteoblasts [31]. IL-8 is overexpressed in the breast cancer cell line [32], and it is believed that it acts before PTHrP in the early stages of

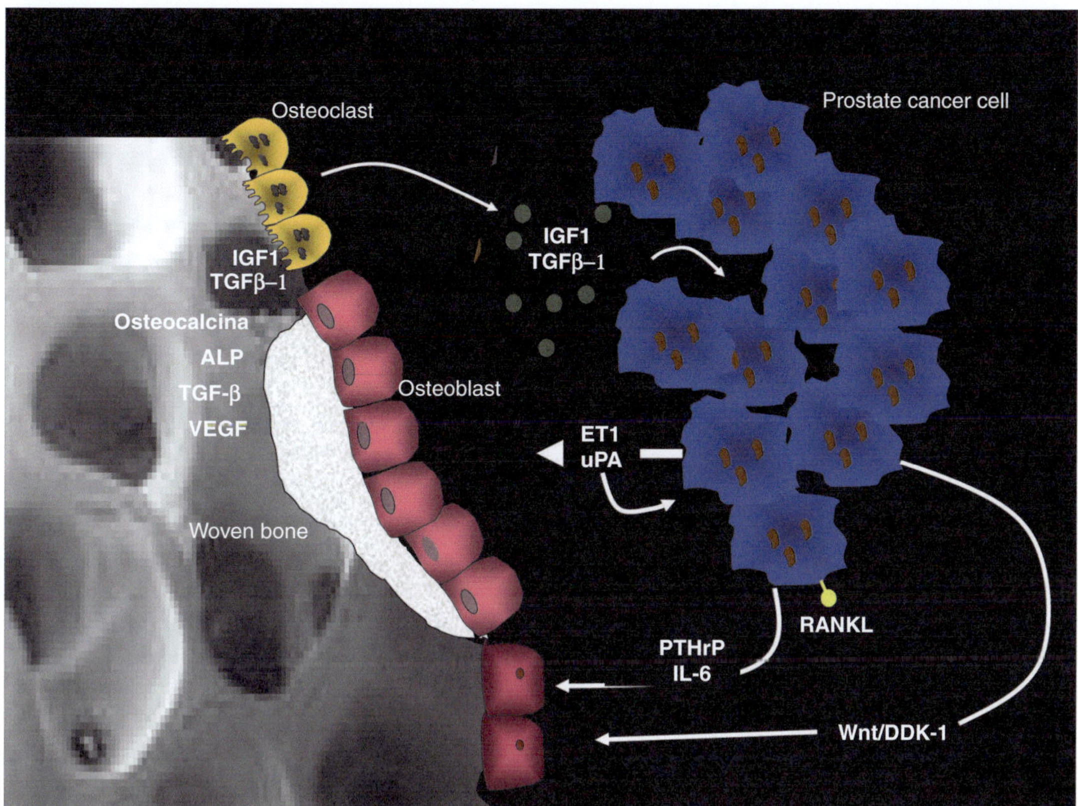

Fig. 1.2 Physiopathology of blastic bone metastasis (BMT). Osteoclasts (*yellow cells*) reabsorbing bone facilitate the expansion of PC metastasis and make available in the bone microenvironment factors promoting penetration and growth of metastasis (TGF beta, osteopontin, FGF, PDGF, VEGF, IGF-1 and IGF-1 are described in detail in the text). In turn, PC cells express cytokines (RANKL, DKK-1 and hormone such as PTHrP) that maintain osteoclast activity and cytokine and factors such as uPA and ET-1, inducing osteoblast bone formation. In the micro-environment of a BMT site, the high bone turnover is characterised by the alternation of osteoclast (lytic) areas and osteoblastic (woven bone) areas, resulting in a disorganised and frail bone structure

breast cancer metastasis stimulating osteoclasts via RANKL [32, 33] and then initiating the vicious cycle that maintains osteolysis in cancer metastasis. It has been suggested that IL-8 might also directly stimulate osteoclasts [33], increase angiogenesis and suppress osteoblast activity [34, 35].

Cancer cells in BMT produce many factors that activate T cells, as discussed above. T cells of patients with breast, prostate and lung cancer support osteoclastogenesis by secreting TNF alpha and expressing RANKL. In addition, T cells suppress the osteoprotegerin action secreting TRAIL (TNF-related apoptosis-inducing ligand), therefore inhibiting the anti-osteoclastogenic effect of osteoprotegerin [36]. In turn, cancer cells produce many factors such as PTHrP, IL-7 and IL-,8 which could recruit or activate T cells with the consequence of further stimulating osteoclastic bone resorption. These mechanisms contribute to the imbalance towards the osteolytic phenotype of the bone lesion.

Studies using RANKL inhibitors have shown the almost complete dependence of tumour-mediated osteoclastogenesis on RANKL. Treatment of mice with OPG-Fc prevented the progression of osteolysis induced by the breast cancer cell line MDA-MB-231 [37]. RANKL inhibition has been shown to prevent the implantation and development of osteolytic lesions in the PC3 cell line in animals [38, 39].

The efficacy of RANKL inhibition was also demonstrated in mixed BMTs in animals, where OPG-Fc blocked the establishment and progression of bone lesions [40, 41]. Recent data indicate that cathepsin G activity at the tumour–bone interface plays an important role in tumour-induced osteolysis and suggest that cathepsin G might be a potentially novel therapeutic target in the treatment of BMT. In a mouse model that mimics osteolytic changes associated with breast cancer-induced BMTs, it has recently been demonstrated that cathepsin G, cooperating with MMP9 and MMP13, is able to cut the extracellular domain of RANKL, generating active soluble RANKL, which is critical for widespread differentiation and activation of osteoclast precursors [42].

Furthermore, some RANKL-independent ways for osteoclast activation in BMT have been found. Some cancer cells, such as PC and breast cancer, may express RANKL and directly activate osteoclasts [43, 44]. Breast cancer cells, myeloma cells and other cancer cells could directly activate osteoclasts in the early stages of BMT via IL-8 production and via MIP-1, a member of the CXC chemokine family that is naturally secreted by osteoblasts and is primarily associated with cell adhesion and migration. It is chemotactic for monocytes and monocyte-like cells, including osteoclast precursors. It directly stimulates osteoclast formation and differentiation in a dose-dependent manner, through the receptors CCR1 and CCR5 expressed by osteoclasts. Moreover, neutralising antibody against MIP-1 blocks MIP-1-induced osteoclast activation [45, 46].

1.3.3 The Role of Osteoblasts in Blastic and Mixed Bone Metastases

In blastic metastases the number and activity of osteoblasts are amplified. Osteoblast differentiates from bone marrow mesenchymal stem cells. A variety of factors contribute to osteoblast formation, including insulin-like growth factor, endothelin-1, BMPs and sclerostin and Wnt proteins (Fig. 1.2) [47, 48].

1.3.4 Endothelin-1

Production of endothelin-1 (ET-1) from PC cells has proven to induce a blastic metastasis promoting osteoblast differentiation and activity. ET-1 is a small vasoconstrictive peptide that plays a key role in vascular homeostasis. ET-1 promotes osteoblast function by binding to ET receptor subtype A (ET_A). The activation of receptor ET_A stimulates phosphate transport and is important for the initiation of bone matrix calcification. ET-1 also increases osteoblast proliferation and inhibits osteoclast formation and motility, and recently it has been suggested that these actions might be indirect and mediated through the Wnt/DKK-1 pathway, inhibiting DKK-1 [49–51]. ET-1 can also enhance the mitogenic effect of other growth factors, such as insulin-like growth factor 1 (IGF-1), platelet-derived growth factor (PDGF) and epidermal growth factor (EGF) [52]. Furthermore, ET-1 has been found to be elevated in androgen-resistant advanced PC. However, there are some doubts with regard to the pivotal role of ET-1 in osteoblastic lesions from PC, because a clinical trial with atrasentan, a selective ET receptor antagonist, produced a modest effect on metastatic PC [53].

1.3.5 Bone Morphogenetic Proteins

The expression of several BMPs has been detected in BMTs from PC. BMPs seem to have a crucial role in contributing to osteoblastic phenotype of BMT in PC. BMPs are members of TGF-beta family and are known to be involved in cancer cell migration. In PC tissues, the expression of BMP-7 was higher in metastatic bone than in normal tissue.

The BMPs are not only expressed by osteoblasts and stored in the bone matrix, but are also actively expressed from PC cells. The osteoblastic effects of BMPs are confirmed by the expression of noggin (an antagonist of BMPs) in PC cell lines. A recent study suggests that BMP-4 signalling inducing apoptosis and Smad-mediated gene expression can be repressed by IGF-1 by activating mTOR signalling in prostate epithelial cells

(NRP-152), suggesting a crosstalk between BMP and IGF signalling. It has been recently demonstrated that BMP-7 secreted from bone stromal cells induces reversible senescence in prostate cancer stem-like cells (CSCs) by activating p38 mitogen-activated protein kinase and increasing expression of the cell cycle inhibitor, p21, and the metastasis suppressor gene, NDRG1 (N-myc downstream-regulated gene 1). This effect of BMP-7 depended on BMPR2 (BMP receptor 2), and BMPR2 expression correlated inversely with recurrence and BMT in PC patients. Importantly, this effect was reversible upon withdrawal of BMP-7 [54]. Recently, it has been shown that using CaP/bone stromal cell line coculture models, one possible mechanism underlying the castration resistance induced by BMTs involves BMP-6 induction by bone stroma-derived WNT5A. BMP-6, in turn, permits CaP cells to proliferate in the absence of androgens [55].

1.3.6 Wnt/DKK-1 Pathway

Canonical Wnt proteins bind at the cell surface at a co-receptor consisting of frizzled (FZD) and low-density lipoprotein receptor-related protein 5/6 (LRP5/LRP6). The activation of the canonical pathway signal results in the stabilisation and accumulation of beta-catenin, which upon translocation into the nucleus serves as co-factor for the T-cell factor family of transcription factors [56]. Canonical Wnt signalling directly controls multiple steps of osteoblast development, regulating the fate of mesenchymal precursors by determining the commitment to a chondroblastic or osteoblastic lineage [48, 57]. Furthermore, the Wnt, indirectly dependent on the activation of beta-catenin, suppresses osteoclast recruitment and activity via osteoprotegerin (OPG). In fact, OPG is a Wnt-responsive target gene and was found to be reduced in beta-catenin knock-out osteoblasts and upregulated in cells with hyperactive Wnt signalling [48, 57]. Interestingly, a reciprocal regulation of RANKL by Wnt was observed in osteoblasts where enhanced Wnt signalling led to increased RANKL expression and vice versa [58].

The canonical Wnt pathway is regulated by a large number of antagonists, including the DKK family and secreted frizzled-related proteins (SFRPs). DKK-1 is present in mature osteoblast/osteocytes, suggesting that the Wnt/DKK-1 balance might regulate bone homeostasis [59]. DDK-1 binds the Wnt co-receptors LRP5 and LRP6 and blocks canonical Wnt signalling [60]. In the presence of DKK-1, osteoblast differentiation is impaired and Wnt-mediated suppression of osteoclast differentiation via osteoprotegerin is blocked, resulting in a dysregulation of RANKL/osteoprotegerin expression with increased osteoclast activity [61].

Direct evidence that canonical Wnt signalling participates with Wnt antagonists in adult bone biology modulating bone remodelling is also of great interest in understanding bone metastasis development and the phenotype of the single metastasis. The Wnt signal has recently been found to be expressed in PC and in multiple myeloma [62, 63]. Interestingly, in early stage of PC BMT, it has been supposed that an "osteolytic phase" driven by an overexpression of DKK-1 favours tumour establishment within the bone [47] and a molecular switch with suppression of DKK-1 signal mediates the transition to an osteoblastic phase of BMT [47]. Overexpression of DKK-1 in prostate C4-2B cells changes a mixed osteolytic–osteoblastic phenotype to an osteolytic phenotype. The equilibrium between Wnt and DKK-1 expression could dictate the phenotype of BMTs and may speculatively explain the heterogeneity of histological aspects of BMTs found in individual patients or the shift from osteoblastic to osteolytic aspects in the single metastasis. Other studies suggest that non-canonical Wnt signalling also stimulates osteoblast differentiation, through BMP-dependent and BMP-independent signalling pathways [64].

1.3.7 VEGF

Vascular endothelial growth factor, as in breast cancer BMT, has been shown to be upregulated in PC and is associated with clinical stage, Gleason score, progression and survival [65, 66]. It has been recently demonstrated that osteocytes are also critical mediators in the bone metastatic niche, not only through soluble factors and cell contact but also via tumour-generated pressure [67].

1.3.8 Role of Mineralised Bone Matrix Resorption in the Vicious Cycle of Lytic Metastasis

The mineralised bone tissue contributes actively to the development and overgrowth of the metastases themselves. Bone breakdown by osteoclasts releases a variety of growth factors previously stored in proactive form by osteoblasts during the bone formation phase and physiologically destined for bone remodelling modulation and bone response to bone inflammation or trauma healing [68]. It is well known that the bone matrix represents a mine of growth factors (such as pro-cytokines); chemotactic and adhesive factors for bone cells and cancer cells, such as TGFβ, PDGF, BMPs, FGFs, IGF-1 and IGF-2; and bone matrix proteins such as osteopontin, osteocalcin, osteonectin and bone sialoprotein [69]. Interestingly, many of these factors may also be expressed actively in breast cancer and PC.

The concentration of these molecules in the micro-environment of the bone remodelling site is a critical regulator of cellular proliferation, differentiation, extracellular matrix deposition and mineralisation, is responsible for the coupling between bone resorption and bone formation and serves as survival and growth factors for cancer cells. Furthermore, physical factor such as tumour-generated pressure acting on osteocytes and factors generated during osteoclast activity, such as low oxygen content, acid pH and high extracellular calcium concentration, are combined to sustain the favourable vicious cycle of tumour growth [67, 70].

1.3.9 TGFβ

Of the growth factors stored in the bone matrix, TGFβ is not the most abundant, but has been well-studied, particularly in cancer bone disease. TGFβ binds to a heterodimeric receptor and can activate either the canonical Smad signalling pathway or Smad-independent pathways [71]. TGFβ, of all the factors delivered from bone matrix, is the major stimulator of cancer cells to express PTHrP, which is expressed in many osteolytic cancer cell lines, and its expression is higher in BMTs than in non-skeletal metastases. As a consequence of the increased PTHrP expression via TGFβ, more osteoclasts reabsorb more of the bone matrix, expanding the lytic bone lesion and increasing locally the concentration of TGFβ and other growth factors. TGFβ, as discussed above, stimulates COX-2 expression in osteoblasts, in bone marrow cells and in breast cancer cells. COX-2 expression in breast cancer cells correlates with the secretion of IL-8 and IL-11, which may induce osteoclastogenesis either via RANKL or independently of RANKL respectively. TGFβ is also reported to act on the tumour cells to induce the production of VEGF and connective tissue growth factors (CTGF) [72]. Runx2 gene expression, regulating the expression of osteopontin and metalloproteases MMP-9 and MMP-13, which are involved in bone resorption and osteoclast recruitment, may be modulated by TGFβ both in cancer cells and in osteoblasts.

1.3.10 IGF-1

The insulin-like growth factors 1 and 2 are among the most abundant non-collagen proteins in mineralised bone. Both IGFs act in cancer and in metastases promoting angiogenesis and inducing cell proliferation and cancer invasion. IGF-1 released from bone by osteoclast bone resorption binds to the type I IGF receptor (IGF-IR) on cancer cell membrane and induces the transcription factor NF-kB, which in turn stimulates target gene transcription, stimulating cancer cell proliferation and chemotaxis and inhibiting apoptosis, leading to BMTs. IGFs promote osteoblasts to increase bone matrix apposition and decrease collagen degradation [73]. IGF-1 is upregulated in PC metastases to the bone and contributes to cancer cell proliferation and chemotaxis. In clinical studies, levels of IGF also correlate with cancer progression, as high levels of IGF-1 are associated with a Gleason score 7. The protein level of IGFs and IGF-binding proteins (IGFBPs), which serve as carrier proteins for IGFs, could be mediated by proteolysis of IGFBPs. Indeed, hydrolysing IGFBPs by urokinase-type plasminogen activator (uPA) increases IGF levels and stimulates osteoblast proliferation. The cleavage of IGFBP-3 by PSA also increases IGF-1 expression, rendering IGF-1 available to bind to its receptor and stimulate osteoblast proliferation [74].

Over expression of uPA has been shown in PC cells, and uPA seems to increase metastasis to the bone. uPA is associated with an aggressive disease phenotype, progression and metastasis to the bone and can be used as a factor in the prognosis and progression of PC [75]. The cleavage of IGFBP-3 by PSA also increases IGF-1 expression, rendering IGF-1 available to bind to its receptor and stimulate osteoblast proliferation. In PC biopsies of BMTs, IGF-IR is increased. Neutralising antibodies against human IGF-1 or mouse or human IGF-2 decreases the development of bone lesions in a prostate xenograft model. Currently, taking all data together, the complex role of IGFs in BMTs phatophysiology has not yet fully elucidated [76].

Finally, it is relevant that many bone matrix-derived factors, including TGFβ, PDGF and BMPs, have the ability to induce the epithelial–mesenchymal transition of cancer cells, which greatly enhances their malignant phenotype, and therefore implicates them in the activation of dormant tumour cells [77].

References

1. Crawford ED, Eisenberger MA, McLeod DG, Spaulding JT, Benson R, Dorr FA, Blumenstein BA, Davis MA, Goodman PJ (1989) A controlled trial of leuprolide with and without flutamide in prostatic carcinoma. N Engl J Med 321(7):419–424
2. Soloway MS, Hardeman SW, Hickey D, Raymond J, Todd B, Soloway S, Moinuddin M (1988) Stratification of patients with metastatic prostate cancer based on extent of disease on initial bone scan. Cancer 61(1): 195–202
3. Vargas HA, Wassberg C, Fox JJ, Wibmer A, Goldman DA, Kuk D, Gonen M, Larson SM, Morris MJ, Scher HI, Hricak H (2014) Bone metastases in castration-resistant prostate cancer: associations between morphologic CT patterns, glycolytic activity, and androgen receptor expression on PET and overall survival. Radiology 271(1):220–229
4. Tait C, Moore D, Hodgson C, Brown M, Morris T, Growcott J, Malone M, Hughes A, Renehan A, Clarke NW, Dive C (2014) Quantification of skeletal metastases in castrate-resistant prostate cancer predicts progression-free and overall survival. BJU Int 114(6b):E70–E73
5. Pond GR, Sonpavde G, de Wit R, Eisenberger MA, Tannock IF, Armstrong AJ (2014) The prognostic importance of metastatic site in men with metastatic castration-resistant prostate cancer. Eur Urol 65(1): 3–6
6. Ost P, Decaestecker K, Lambert B, Fonteyne V, Delrue L, Lumen N, Ameye F, De Meerleer G (2014) Prognostic factors influencing prostate cancer-specific survival in non-castrate patients with metastatic prostate cancer. Prostate 74(3):297–305
7. Wang CY, Wu GY, Shen MJ, Cui KW, Shen Y (2013) Comparison of distribution characteristics of metastatic bone lesions between breast and prostate carcinomas. Oncol Lett 5(1):391–397
8. Kakhki VR, Anvari K, Sadeghi R, Mahmoudian AS, Torabian-Kakhki M (2013) Pattern and distribution of bone metastases in common malignant tumors. Nucl Med Rev Cent East Eur 16(2):66–69
9. Conti G, La Torre G, Cicalese V, Micheletti G, Ludovico MG, Vestita GD, Cottonaro G, Introini C, Cecchi M (2008) Prostate cancer metastases to bone: observational study for the evaluation of clinical presentation, course and treatment patterns. Presentation of the METAURO protocol and of patient baseline features. Arch Ital Urol Androl 80(2):59–64
10. Goltzman D (1997) Mechanisms of the development of osteoblastic metastases. Cancer 80(8 Suppl): 1581–1587
11. Clarke NW, McClure J, George NJ (1991) Morphometric evidence for bone resorption and replacement in prostate cancer. Br J Urol 68(1):74–80
12. Roudier MP, Morrissey C, True LD, Higano CS, Vessella RL, Ott SM (2008) Histopathological assessment of prostate cancer bone osteoblastic metastases. J Urol 180(3):1154–1160
13. Sone T, Tamada T, Jo Y, Miyoshi H, Fukunaga M (2004) Analysis of three-dimensional microarchitecture and degree of mineralization in bone metastases from prostate cancer using synchrotron microcomputed tomography. Bone 35(2):432–438
14. Jernberg E, Thysell E, Bovinder Ylitalo E, Rudolfsson S, Crnalic S, Widmark A, Bergh A, Wikström P (2013) Characterization of prostate cancer bone metastases according to expression levels of steroidogenic enzymes and androgen receptor splice variants. PLoS One 8(11):e77407. doi:10.1371/journal.pone.0077407
15. Larson SR, Zhang X, Dumpit R, Coleman I, Lakely B, Roudier M, Higano CS, True LD, Lange PH,

Montgomery B, Corey E, Nelson PS, Vessella RL, Morrissey C (2013) Characterization of osteoblastic and osteolytic proteins in prostate cancer bone metastases. Prostate 73(9):932–940

16. Fang J, Xu Q (2015) Differences of osteoblastic bone metastases and osteolytic bone metastases in clinical features and molecular characteristics. Clin Transl Oncol 17(3):173–179
17. Martin TJ (2004) Paracrine regulation of osteoclast formation and activity: milestones in discovery. J Muscoloskelet Neuronal Interact 4:243–253
18. Ohshiba T, Miyaura C, Inada M et al (2003) Role of RANKL induced osteoclast formation and MMP dependent matrix degradation in bone destruction by breast cancer metastasis. Br J Cancer 88: 1318–1326
19. Dallas SL, Prideaux M, Bonewald LF (2013) The osteocyte: an endocrine cell … more. Endocr Rev 34(5):658–690
20. Kitazawa S, Kitazawa R (2002) RANK ligand is a prerequisite for cancer associated osteolytic lesions. J Pathol 198:228–236
21. Strewler GI (2000) Mechanisms of disease: the physiology of parathyroid hormone related protein. N Engl J Med 342:177–185
22. Falzon M, Du P (2000) Enhanced growth of MCF-7 breast cancer cells overexpressing parathyroid hormone related peptide. Endocrinology 141:1882–1892
23. Vargas SJ, Gillespie MT, Powell GJ et al (1992) Localization of parathyroid hormone-related protein mRA expression in metastatic lesions by in situ hybridization. J Bone Miner Res 7:971–980
24. Kohno N, Kitazawa S, Fukase M et al (1994) The expression of parathyroid hormone related protein in human breast cancer with skeletal metastases. Surg Today 24:215–220
25. Arima Y, Matsueda S, Yano H et al (2005) Parathyroid hormone related protein as a common target molecule in specific immunotherapy for a wide variety of tumour types. Int J Oncol 27:981–988
26. Yao A, Harada A, Matsueda S et al (2005) New epitope peptides derived from parathyroid hormone related protein which have the capacity to induce prostate cancer reactive cytotoxic T-lymphocytes in HLA-A2* prostate cancer patients. Prostate 62:233–242
27. Karaptis AC, Goltzman D (2000) PTH PTHrP effects on the skeleton. Rev Endocr Metab Disord 1:331–341
28. Yamamoto I, Bringhurst FR, Potts JT et al (1988) Properties of parathyroid hormone receptors on circulating bovine lymphocytes. J Bone Miner Res 3:289–295
29. Atkinson MJ, Hesch RD, Cade C et al (1987) Parathyroid hormone stimulation of mitosis in rat thymic lymphocytes is independent of cyclic AMP. J Bone Miner Res 2:303–309
30. Wu X, Qian W, Ryan M et al (2005) Continuous PTH treatment causes bone loss through upregulated T cell localization to the bone surfaces. J Bone Miner Res 20(Suppl 1):S14
31. Graves DT, Jiang Y, Valente AJ (1999) The expression of monocyte chemoattractant protein 1 and other chemokines by osteoblasts. Front Biosci 4:571–580
32. Bendre M, Gaddy-Kurten D, Foote-Mon T et al (2006) Expression of interleukin 8 and not parathyroid hormone related protein by human breast cancer cells correlates with bone metastasis in vivo. Cancer Res 66:2250–2256
33. Bendre M, Montague D, Peery T et al (2003) Interleukin 8 stimulation of osteoclastogenesis and bone resorption is a mechanism for the increased osteolysis of metastatic bone disease. Bone 33:28–37
34. Guise TA, Chirgwin JM (2003) Transforming growth factor beta in osteolytic breast cancer bone metastases. Clin Orthop Relat Res 4155:532–538
35. Dovio A, Sartori ML, Masera RG et al (2004) Effects of physiological concentration of steroid hormones and interleukin 11 on basal and stimulated production of interleukin 8 by human osteoblast like cells with different functional profiles. Clin Exp Rheumatol 22:79–84
36. Founier P, Chirgwin JM, Guise T (2006) New insights into the role of T cells in the vicious cycle of bone metastases. Curr Opin Rheumatol 18(4):396–404
37. Kostenuik PJ, Bolon B, Morony S et al (2004) Gene therapy with human recombinant osteoprotegerin reverses established osteopenia in ovariectomized mice. Bone 34(4):656–64
38. Whang PG, Schwarz EM, Gamradt SC et al (2005) The effects of RANK blockade and osteoclast depletion in a model of pure osteoblastic prostate cancer metastasis in bone. J Orthop Res 23:1475–1483
39. Miller R, Jones J, Tometsko M et al (2005) Antituomour efficacy of the RANK ligand inhibitor OPG-Fc in the MDA-231 breast cancer and PC3 prostate cancer experimental osteolytic metastases models. J Bone Miner Res 20(Suppl 1):S117
40. Yonou H, Kanomata N, Goya M et al (2003) Osteprotegerin/osteoclastogenesis inhibitory factor decreases human prostate cancer burden in human adult bone implanted into nonobese diabetic/sever combined immunodeficient mice. Cancer Res 63:2096–2102
41. Zhang J, Dai J, Qi Y et al (2001) Osteoprotegerin inhibits prostate cancer induced osteoclastogenesis and prevents prostate tumour growth in the bone. J Clin Invest 107:1235–1244
42. Wilson TJ, Nannuru KC, Futakuchi M, Sadanandam A, Singh RK (2008) Cathepsin G enhances mammary tumor-induced osteolysis by generating soluble receptor activator of nuclear factor-kappaB ligand. Cancer Res 68(14):5803–5811
43. Brown J, Corey E, Lee Z et al (2001) Osteoprotegerin and rank ligand expression in prostate cancer. Urology 57:611–616
44. Farrugia AN, Atkins GJ, To L et al (2003) Receptor activator of nuclear factor kappaB ligand expression by human myeloma cells mediates osteoclast for-

mation in vitro and correlates with bone destruction in vivo. Cancer Res 63:5438–5445
45. Terpos E, Dimopoulos MA (2005) Myeloma bone disease: pathophysiology and management. Ann Oncol 16:1223–1231
46. Choi SJ, Oba Y, Gazitt Y et al (2001) Antisense inhibition of macrophage inflammatory protein 1 alpha blocks bone destruction in a model of myeloma bone disease. J Clin Invest 108:1833–1841
47. Hall CL, Keller ET (2006) The role of Wnts in bone metastases. Cancer Metastasis Rev 25:551–558
48. Hall CL, Kang S, Macdougald OA et al (2006) Role of Wnts in prostate cancer bone metastases. J Cell Biochem 97:661–672
49. Clines GA, Mohammad KS, Bao Y, Stephens OW, Suva LJ, Shaughnessy JD Jr, Fox JW, Chirgwin JM, Guise TA (2007) Dickkopf homolog 1 mediates endothelin-1-stimulated new bone formation. Mol Endocrinol 21(2):486–498
50. Chiao JW, Moonga BS, Yang YM, Kancherla R, Mittelman A, Wu-Wong JR, Ahmed T (2000) Endothelin-1 from prostate cancer cells is enhanced by bone contact which blocks osteoclastic bone resorption. Br J Cancer 83:360–365
51. Yin JJ, Mohammad KS, Kakonen SM, Harris S, Wu-Wong JR, Wessale JL, Padley RJ, Garrett IR, Chirgwin JM, Guise TA (2003) A causal role for endothelin-1 in the pathogenesis of osteoblastic bone metastases. Proc Natl Acad Sci U S A 100:10954–10959
52. Nelson JB, Chan-Tack K, Hedican SP, Magnuson SR, Opgenorth TJ, Bova GS, Simons JW (1996) Endothelin-1 production and decreased endothelin B receptor expression in advanced prostate cancer. Cancer Res 56:663–668
53. Russo A, Bronte G, Rizzo S, Fanale D, Di Gaudio F, Gebbia N, Bazan V (2010) Anti- endothelin drugs in solid tumors. Expert Opin Emerg Drugs 15:27–40
54. Kobayashi A, Okuda H, Xing F, Pandey PR, Watabe M, Hirota S, Pai SK, Liu W, Fukuda K, Chambers C, Wilber A, Watabe K (2011) Bone morphogenetic protein 7 in dormancy and metastasis of prostate cancer stem-like cells in bone. J Exp Med 208(13): 2641–2655
55. Lee GT, Kang DI, Ha Y-S, Jung YS, Chung J, Min K, Kim TH, Moon KH, Chung JM, Lee DH, Kim W-J, Kim IY (2014) Prostate cancer bone metastases acquire resistance to androgen deprivation via WNT5A-mediated BMP-6 induction. Br J Cancer 110(6):1634–1644
56. Van de WM, Cavallo R, Dooijes D et al (1997) Armadillo coactivates transcription driven by the product of the Drosophila segment polarity gene dTCF. Cell 88:789–799
57. Day TF, Guo X, Garrett-Beal L et al (2005) Wnt/β-catenin signalling in mesenchymal progenitors controls osteoblast and chondrocyte differentiation during vertebrate skeletogenesis. Dev Cell 8:739–750
58. Glass DA, Bialek P, Ahn JD et al (2005) Canonical Wnt signalling in differentiated osteoblasts controls osteoclast differentiation. Dev Cell 8:751–764
59. Zhang Y, Wang Y, Li X et al (2004) The LRP 5 high-bone-mass G171V mutation disrupts LRP5 interaction with Mesd. Mol Cell Biol 24:4677–4684
60. Bafico A, Liu G, Yaniv A et al (2001) Novel mechanism of Wnt signalling inhibition mediated by Dikkopf 1 interaction with LRP6/Arrow. Nat Cell Biol 3:683–686
61. MacDonald BT, Joiner D, Oyserman S et al (2007) Bone mass is inversely proportional to DKK1 levels in mice. Bone 41:331–339
62. Pearse R (2006) Wnt antagonism in multiple myeloma: a potential cause of uncoupled bone remodelling. Clin Cancer Res 12(Suppl 20):6274S–6278S
63. Rosol TJ, Tannehill-Gregg SH, Corn S et al (2004) Animal models of bone metastasis. Cancer Treat Res 118:47–81
64. Dai J, Hall CL, Escara-Wilke J, Mizokami A, Keller JM, Keller ET (2008) Prostate cancer induces bone metastasis through Wnt-induced bone morphogenetic protein-dependent and independent mechanisms. Cancer Res 68:5785–5794
65. Rahim F, Hajizamani S, Mortaz E, Ahmadzadeh A, Shahjahani M, Shahrabi S, Saki N (2014) Molecular regulation of bone marrow metastasis in prostate and breast cancer. Bone Marrow Res 2014:405920
66. Roberts E, Cossigny DA, Quan GM (2013) The role of vascular endothelial growth factor in metastatic prostate cancer to the skeleton. Prostate Cancer 2013:418340
67. Sottnik JL, Dai J, Zhang H, Campbell B, Keller ET (2015) Tumor-induced pressure in the bone microenvironment causes osteocytes to promote the growth of prostate cancer bone metastases. Cancer Res 75(11):1–8
68. Monolagas SC, Jilka RL (1995) Bone marrow, cytokines and bone remodelling. N Engl J Med 332:305–311
69. Dallas SL, Rosser JL, Mundy GR et al (2002) Proteolysis of latent tranforming growth factor beta binding protein1 by osteoclasts. A cellular mechanism for release of TGF beta from bone matrix. J Biol Chem 277:21352–21360
70. Liao J, Schneider A, Datta NS, McCauley LK (2006) Extracellular calcium as a candidate mediator of prostate cancer skeletal metastasis. Cancer Res 66(18):9065–9073
71. Javelaud D, Alexaki VI, Dennler S, Mohammad KS, Guise TA, Mauviel A (2011) TGF-β/SMAD/GLI2 signaling axis in cancer progression and metastasis. Cancer Res 71(17):5606–5610
72. Wakefield LM, Hill CS (2013) Beyond TGFβ: roles of other TGFβ superfamily members in cancer. Nat Rev Cancer 13(5):328–341
73. Lee HL, Pienta KJ, Kim WJ, Cooper CR (2003) The effect of bone-associated growth factors and cytokines on the growth of prostate cancer cells derived

from soft tissue versus bone metastases in vitro. Int J Oncol 22(4):921–926
74. Bogdanos J, Karamanolakis D, Tenta R, Tsintavis A, Milathianakis C, Mitsiades C, Koutsilieris M (2003) Endocrine/paracrine/autocrine survival factor activity of bone microenvironment participates in the development of androgen ablation and chemotherapy refractoriness of prostate cancer metastasis in skeleton. Endocr Relat Cancer 10(2):279–289
75. Wang N, Docherty FE, Brown HK, Reeves KJ, Fowles AC, Ottewell PD, Dear TN, Holen I, Croucher PI, Eaton CL (2014) Prostate cancer cells preferentially home to osteoblast-rich areas in the early stages of bone metastasis: evidence from in vivo models. J Bone Miner Res 29(12):2688–2696
76. Rubin J, Fan X, Rahnert J et al (2006) IGF1 secretion by prostate carcinoma cell does not alter tumor bone cell interactions in vitro or in vivo. Prostate 66:789–800
77. Morrison CD, Parvani JG, Schiemann WP (2013) The relevance of the TGF-β Paradox to EMT-MET programs. Cancer Lett 341(1):30–40

Markers of Bone Turnover in Bone Metastasis from Prostate Cancer

2

Francesco Bertoldo

Bone homeostasis is achieved through a continuous remodelling process on the bone surface of the balanced resorption of old bone by osteoclasts and the formation of new bone by osteoblasts. Local and systemic growth factors regulate the differentiation and activity of the osteoclasts and osteoblasts (and osteocytes). Maintenance and repair of normal bone result in the release of enzymes, peptides and mineral components that have been characterised as serum and urinary biochemical markers of bone remodelling [1]. High bone turnover in cancer patients is crucial for all the steps of bone metastatic disease, from the homing of circulating cancer cells into the bone (premetastatic niche) to the complication of bone metastasis (BMT) (skeletally related events [SREs]). Therefore, elevated bone turnover marker could predict bone metastasis, risk of bone progression and risk of SREs, potentially becoming a potent prognostic predictor (Fig. 2.1). For this reason, biochemical markers of bone remodelling are potentially an ideal tool for evaluating changes in bone turnover, such as those associated with malignant bone lesions and response to treatment. Osteoclast and osteoblast activity (and probably that of cancer cells) is associated with the release of distinct biochemical markers that are amenable to non-invasive measurements of the blood or urine.

Breakdown products of type I collagen by osteolysis as cross-linked collagen peptides (the amino (N)- and carboxy (C) terminal cross-linked telopeptide of type I collagen, NTX and CTX, respectively), and the terminal peptides that are cleaved from procollagen before its integration into new bone matrix (e.g. procollagen type I N-terminal and C-terminal peptides, or P1NP and P1CP), can provide meaningful insights into the ongoing effects of tumour growth on bone turnover (Fig. 2.2). Bone-specific alkaline phosphatase (bone ALP) concentrations in serum reflect the ongoing rate of osteogenesis [2]. The International Osteoporosis Foundation and the International Federation of Clinical Chemistry and Laboratory Medicine recommend that a marker of bone formation (serum procollagen type I N propeptide) and a marker of bone resorption (serum C-terminal telopeptide of type I collagen) be used as reference analytes for bone turnover markers in clinical studies [2] (Fig. 2.3). Nowadays, a number of bone markers can be determined using enzyme immunological procedures (enzyme-linked immunosorbant assay) by means of a commercial kit that can be easily adapted to laboratory automated machines to achieve greater analytical reliability during determination compared with manual methods [3]. Although a great deal of the data in the literature are obtained on markers analysed

F. Bertoldo, MD
Metabolic Bone Diseases and Osteo-oncology Unit, Internal Medicine, Department of Medicine, University of Verona, Verona, Italy
e-mail: francesco.bertoldo@univr.it

F. Bertoldo et al. (eds.), *Bone Metastases from Prostate Cancer*,
DOI 10.1007/978-3-319-42327-2_2

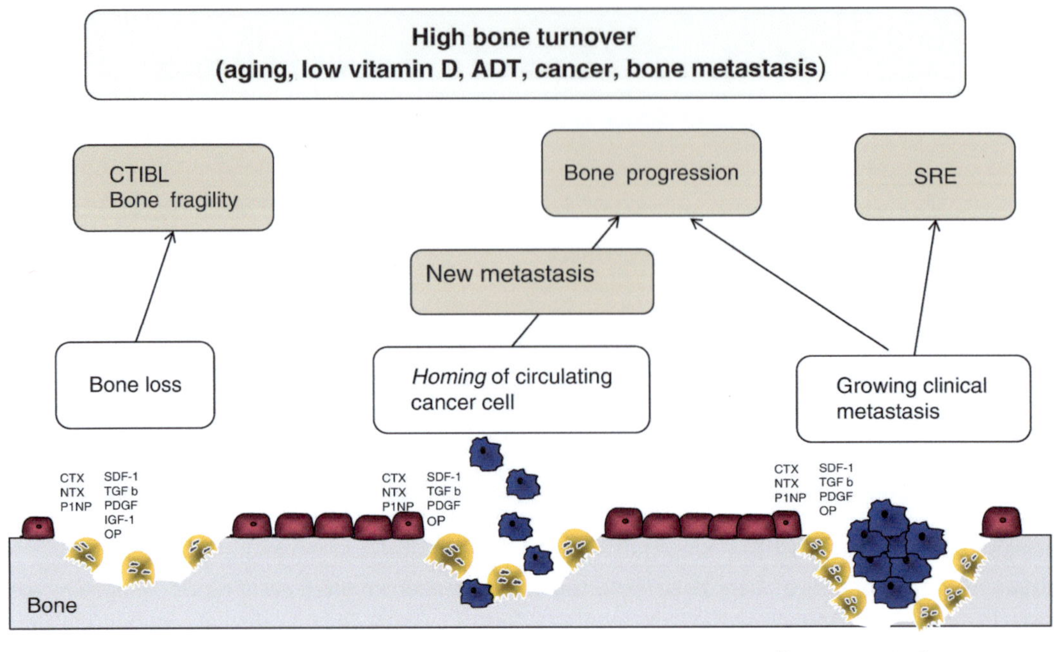

Fig. 2.1 Bone turnover is usually very high in prostate cancer (PC) patients for many reasons (aging, vitamin D deficiency, androgen deprivation therapy, or abiraterone or enzalutamide, cytokines released from primary cancer and for metastatic cancer cells activating the bone microenvironment). High bone turnover increases the rate of bone loss and impairs bone quality, increasing the risk of fragility fractures. Consensually, high bone turnover promotes the homing of circulating cancer cells and the promotion of the so-called osteoblastic premetastatic niche. A clinically evident bone metastasis (BMT) develops and grows due to the effect of growth factors released from bone matrix breakdown. The increase in size of the BMT into a frail bone finally increases the risk of an SRE. In a patient with PC bone disease, all these steps are present at the same time as a continuum in the skeleton. *ADT* androgen deprivation therapy, *CTIBL* cancer treatment-induced bone loss, *SRE* skeletal related event (fracture, pain, cord compression, orthopaedic surgery, radiotherapy), *yellow cell* osteoclast, *red cell* osteoblast, *blue cell* PC cell

from urine samples (i.e. NTX), analysis of makers of bone turnover on serum and plasma are recommended because of lower inter- and intraindividual variability [2]. Standardised assays are available for many bone turnover markers and normal or reference ranges for several markers have been established. As the normal range changes with age and sex, selection of appropriate reference values is critical for data interpretation [2, 4]. In systemic metabolic bone diseases, such as osteoporosis, primary hyperparathyroidism and osteomalacia, biochemical markers reflect ongoing rates of bone resorption and formation in the body as a whole. Therefore, bone marker assessments in "focal" diseases, such as Paget disease or BMT, do not provide information specific to individual lesion sites. Moreover, changes in bone marker levels are tissue specific (bone) and not disease specific and are associated with an imbalance in skeletal metabolism independently of the underlying cause [1, 5]. In cancer patients, bone turnover markers may be very high for many concomitant causes, such as age, vitamin D deficiency, adjuvant hormone therapy and BMT, but it is impossible to distinguish the contributions of the different components that elevate the marker levels in the serum and urine (Figs. 2.1 and 2.3). For example, NTX levels were similar in PC patients on androgen deprivation therapy with and without BMT. Furthermore differences between bone resorption markers and bone formation markers were not found in patients with BMT from different cancers [6, 7]. In an attempt to differentiate the source of the marker (BMT vs non-metastatic

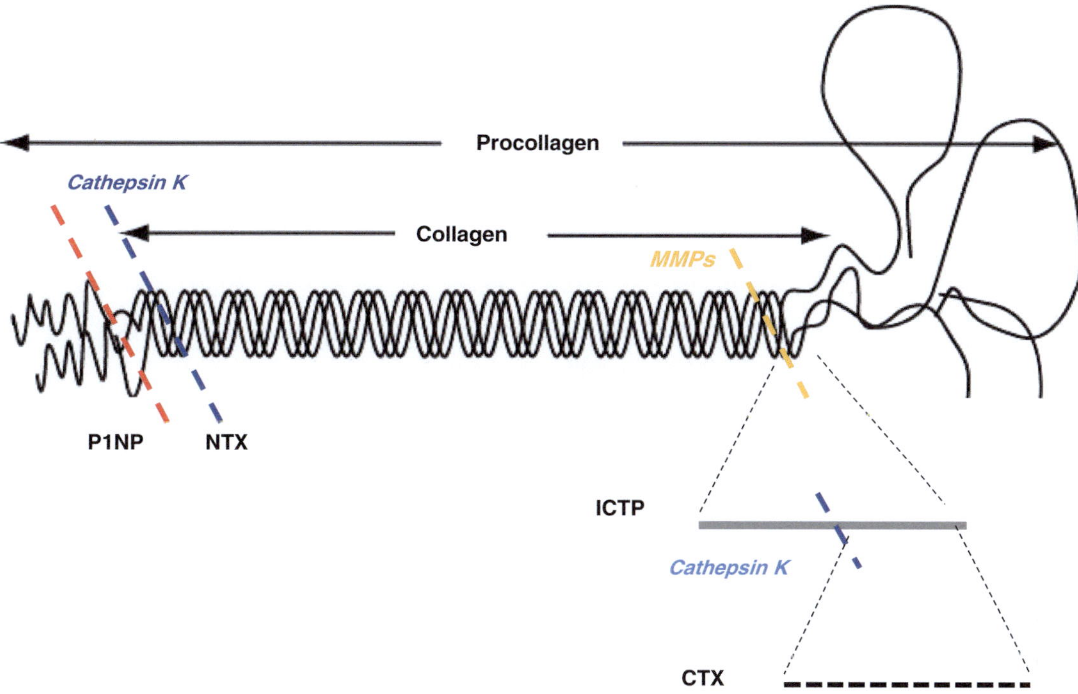

Fig. 2.2 Schematic representation of the amino-terminal propeptide procollagen type 1 (*P1NP*), N-terminal cross-linking telopeptide collagen type 1 (*NTX*), and C-terminal cross-linking telopeptide collagen type 1 (*CTX*). P1NP epitope is used as a marker of bone formation. NTX, CTX and ICTP epitopes are used as markers of bone resorption on type I collagen. CTX epitope is constituted by an eight-amino acid sequence on the C-telopeptide of a1. The cross-linked carboxy-terminal telopeptide collagen type 1 (*ICTP*) epitope is a larger conformational epitope including at least two telopeptides and the first phenylalanine of the phenylalanine-rich region. It is a product of metalloprotease breakdown of collagen type 1. As shown in the figure, cathepsin K degrades the ICTP epitope whereas it generates CTX

skeletal), the non-isomerised form of CTX and type I collagen breakdown products generated by matrix metalloprotease (ICTP), apparently more specific for BMT breakdown, have been evaluated (Fig. 2.2) [8].

The clinical utility of bone markers as diagnostic indicators of bone metastatic disease and as prognostic indicators has been extensively examined. Several studies have revealed an association between bone turnover marker and the presence or progression of skeletal metastases from prostate cancer (PC) [9, 11, 12]. In these studies the formation marker and resorption markers are elevated in the case of typical osteoblastic osseous metastasis expressing a disrupted balance between bone formation and resorption. P1NP, bone sialoprotein (BSP), and osteoprotegerin (OPG) showed more significant differences between PC patients with and without BMT. BSP is not a typical bone marker and works as a general tumour marker [13]. In addition to being elevated in PC patients with BMT, OPG correlates with the extent of osseous metastasis. Furthermore, in association with RANKL, it may predict recurrence after radical prostatectomy [14–16]. P1NP as bone ALP correlates with the extent of osseous changes (bone scan index). Bone ALP had the highest diagnosis accuracy (72 % sensitivity, 88 % specificity) and P1NP the greatest diagnostic specificity (92 %) [11]. Recently, the elevated alkaline velocity was found to be an independent predictor of OS and BMT-free survival in patients with CRPC [17]. On the other hand, recent data do not confirm the diagnostic performance of P1NP. Current consensus is that

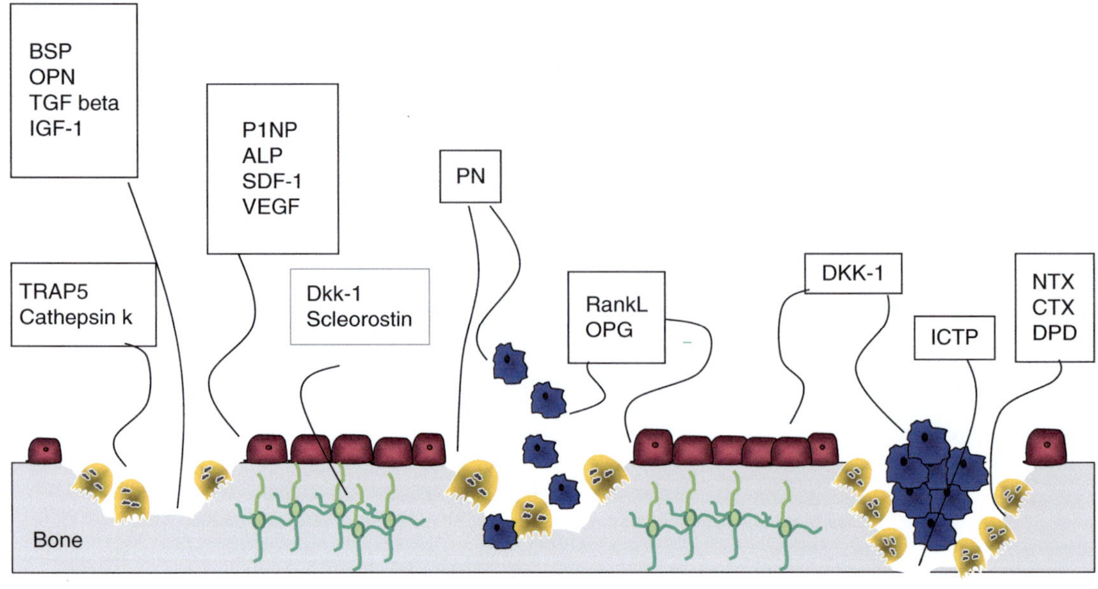

Fig. 2.3 Schematic representation of the origin of peptides used as markers of bone formation and reabsorption of bone by osteoblasts, osteoclasts, osteocytes and cancer cells. NTX and CTX derived from bone breakdown by osteoclasts through cathepsin K, ICTP mainly by cancer cell bone breakdown through metalloproteases. Cathepsin K and TRAP5 are expressed from osteoclasts during their osteolytic activity. Periostin (*PN*) is stored by osteoblasts during bone formation, but released during osteoclast activity. It is also expressed directly from cancer cells. P1NP and alkaline phosphatase (*ALP*) expressed from osteoblasts are used as markers of bone formation. Osteoblasts also express vascular endothelial growth factor (*VEGF*) and chemokine (*SDF-1*), RANKL and osteoprotegerin (*OPG*). DKK-1 and sclerostin are expressed by osteocytes, osteoblasts and PC cells. Bone sialoprotein (*BSP*), osteopontin (*OPN*), transforming growth factor-1 (*TGF-β*) and insulin-like growth factor-1 (*IGF-1*) are released from bone matrix during osteoclastic (and cancer) bone reabsorption (see text for details)

the diagnostic sensitivity and/or specificity of bone markers for the presence of BMT or the prognostic role of bone lesion progression are not sufficient to utilise the results to diagnose BMT [18]. The mean values of the areas under the ROC curve from several studies were 0.81, 0.80 and 0.77 for P1NP, bone ALP and ICTP suggesting that these markers might have diagnostic values in interaction with safely defined reference thresholds or during their course [5, 10, 19]. Data on the use of bone markers as predictors for SRE and survival are quite encouraging [18, 20]. Retrospective analyses of data from phase III trials of zoledronic acid in patients with CRPC and BMT showed that both baseline and on-study elevation in bone marker levels, specifically NTX, were associated with increased risks of SRE, disease progression and death [18, 21–23]. A high baseline level of urinary NTX (above 180 nmol/mmol creatinine) was associated with a more than 2.5-fold increase in the risk of death (RR 2.58, 95 % CI 1.92–3.47) compared with low baseline levels of NTX (<55 nmol/mmol creatinine) [18, 22]. Also, baseline bone ALP was associated with a 4 % increase in the risk of death and SRE per 200 IU/L increase. Elevated bone ALP levels at baseline were associated with a shorter time to the first on-study SRE and a shorter time to the first pathological fracture. The cumulative incidence of SRE over a 1-year period was nearly doubled (50.7 % vs 26.5 %) among patients with elevated versus normal baseline bone ALP [23]. Adequate suppression of NTX and bone ALP levels during treatment (zoledronic acid plus docetaxel vs docetaxel alone) was associated with longer survival time, and similar results have been confirmed by others [23, 24].

Recently, bone ALP velocity (>6.3 IU/L/year) was found to be an independent predictor of overall survival in CRPC. A fivefold increase in death was observed among CRPC patients with rapid bone ALP velocity (OR 5.11, 95 % CI 2.24–11.67) [17]. Other more recent bone markers have been found to be associated with prognosis in PC patients. P1NP and ICTP were associated with survival after 15 months of zoledronic acid therapy [25]. Baseline and 3 months after, zoledronic acid P1NP and CTX predict survival and (only P1NP) risk of SRE [26]. The association of CTX or NTX with P1NP confirmed the prognostic role of these bone markers [27].

The data summarised above suggest that bone turnover markers might be useful to optimise the use of bone-targeted therapy for metastatic bone disease. Promoting lifelong therapy contradictory with the paucity of data regarding the usefulness and the safety (osteonecrosis of jaw and atypical hip fractures) of treatment durations with bone-modifying agents beyond 2—3 years. The serial measurement of BTMs could be a strategy in tailoring the therapy regimen and could help the decision on the optimal duration of antiresorptive therapy, which could allow treatment frequency to be reduced and even theoretically removed for periods in the context of optimal bone metabolism control [28]. In summary, at present, the potential for the clinical use of markers of bone turnover for diagnosis, prognosis and monitoring therapy in cancer patients with BMT remains unfulfilled and the routine use of these markers cannot yet be recommended. As stated in consensus publications, there is a need for harmonisation, standardisation and common reference ranges [18, 29, 30] although a recent position paper solicited their introduction into a clinical setting [28].

2.1 New Bone Markers

2.1.1 ICTP

ICTP, which reflects non-osteoclastic bone resorption mediated by metalloproteases (MMPs), is liberated to the bloodstream during pathological conditions. Serum ICTP is relatively insensitive to changes in bone remodelling mediated by normal osteoclastic activity.

In a retrospective analysis of four bone markers (NTX-l, ICTP, total ALP, and TRAP5b) in breast cancer patients with and without BMTs, only ICTP and TRAP5b were significantly higher in those patients with BMTs compared with those without (visceral metastases or no metastases). The ICTP and TRAP5b levels were also related to the number of BMTs on the other hand [31]. Furthermore in another study in breast cancer patients comparing a cohort with and without BMTs, ICTP was the marker with higher sensitivity (65 %), and it had similar specificity to bone ALP (91 vs 92 % for bone ALP) [32].

In a prospective cohort study, three bone markers (NTX-l, ICTP, and bone ALP) were tested in 123 patients with various metastatic cancers, 26 of which were extraosseous only (45 bone-only and 52 bone plus visceral). NTX-l and ICTP, but not bone ALP, were associated with bone disease progression. Moreover, NTX-l had the highest sensitivity (70 %), specificity (80 %), positive (72 %), and negative (79 %) predictive values for bone disease progression in the set of markers analysed (for an increase X30% from baseline). Curiously, when assessing ICTP, not only did it increase in the context of bone and extraskeletal progression, but it also did not decrease with bisphosphonate (BP) therapy [9]. This led the authors to speculate that ICTP could represent a bone collagen product derived from an osteoclast-independent mechanism of bone degradation (MMP-1 action on bone collagen) and therefore not influenced by BP therapy (Fig. 2.3).

2.2 Periostin

Periostin is a highly conserved matricellular protein that shares close homology with the insect cell adhesion molecule fasciclin 1. Periostin is expressed in a broad range of tissues, including the skeleton, where it serves both as a structural molecule of the bone matrix and as a signalling molecule through integrin receptors and Wnt-beta-catenin pathways, stimulating osteoblast function and bone formation. The development of periostin-null mice has allowed the crucial role of periostin in dentinogenesis and osteogenesis to be elucidated, in addition to the skeletal response to mechanical loading and parathyroid hormone. Periostin binding to the integrins activates the Akt/PKB- and FAK-mediated signalling pathways, leading to increased cell survival, angiogenesis, invasion, metastasis, and, importantly, epithelial–mesenchymal transition of carcinoma cells [33]. In situ RNA hybridisation in biopsies of breast cancer metastases showed that the periostin gene was highly expressed in the stromal cells immediately surrounding the tumour but not within the breast cancer cells themselves [34]. Although periostin is highly expressed in various types of human cancers, its function is still unclear. In mice the administration of PN1-Ab, a neutralising antibody of periostin, significantly inhibited the growth of primary tumours and metastatic tumours, associated with the prevention of bone destruction, resulting in increased survival of mice. In addition, in vitro, PN1-Ab significantly inhibited the proliferation, migration, and invasion of 4T1 mouse breast cancer cells, which produced periostin [35]. Nude mice were inoculated with human MDA-B02 breast cancer cells. Mouse-derived periostin was markedly overexpressed (eightfold) in metastatic legs compared with non-inoculated mice. Serum periostin levels were also markedly increased in metastatic mice and correlated with in situ expression levels. Immunostaining showed that periostin is derived from the surrounding stromal cells of BMT. It was suggested that periostin might be a biochemical marker of the early stromal response associated with breast cancer BMT formation [36]. The use of circulating periostin as a potential clinical biomarker has been explored in different non-skeletal conditions. These include cancers and, more specifically in the metastasis process, respiratory diseases such as asthma, kidney failure, renal injury, and cardiac infarction. A study including breast cancer and small cell lung cancer patients showed that serum periostin levels were elevated in breast cancer patients presenting with BMTs compared with similar breast cancer patients with no evidence of BMT. No correlation was found between the serum periostin level and any other prognostic factors, such as clinical stage and lymph node metastasis in breast cancer [37]. In postmenopausal osteoporosis, serum levels have been shown to predict the risk of fracture—more specifically non-vertebral—independently of bone mineral density. Because of its preferential localisation in cortical bone and periosteal tissue, it may be speculated that serum periostin might be a marker of cortical bone metabolism, although additional studies are clearly needed (Fig. 2.3) [36].

2.3 Bone Sialoprotein and Osteopontin

Small integrin-binding ligand N-linked glycoproteins (SIBLINGs), a family of five integrin-binding glycophosphoproteins, including osteopontin (OPN) and bone sialoprotein (BSP), are an emerging group of proteins used by cancer cells to facilitate expansion [38].

High levels of OPN and BSP expression could enhance the affinity of metastasis of cancer cells to the bone. However, the value of OPN and BSP in predicting BM and survival in NPC has not been elucidated. It has been suggested that OPN is overexpressed and associated with tumour progression in various cancers, including breast cancer and PC [39, 40].

SIBLING expression in different osteotropic cancers may be useful for establishing the risk of BMT in cancer patients. For example, increased expression of BSP in many osteotropic cancers, including PC, may predict BMT in this cancer [41].

Studies examining BSP levels in primary breast cancer tissue suggest that elevated levels of this SIBLING might be prognostic for shorter survival and correlate with the development of BMT [42]. Similarly, elevated levels of BSP in the blood correlate with, and may be predictive of, BMT in several osteotropic malignancies, including the breast, lung, prostate, and multiple myeloma [43].

Serum BSP levels in PC increase only in the later stages of the disease, calling into question the prognostic value of BSP in PC [13, 44]. Some authors consider BSP and OPN to be general tumour markers rather than exclusive bone markers, as serum levels also increase in localised PC, and currently BSP and OPN are seen as bone markers with ambivalence (Fig. 2.3) [5, 44].

2.4 Sclerostin and DKK-1

Among the potential markers, dickoppf-1 (DKK-1) and sclerostin have shown interesting evidence, as they have been found to be elevated in different cancer types, including PC. Sclerostin and dickkopf-1 (DKK-1) are specific inhibitors of Wnt signalling and are also considered as bone remodelling markers. Sclerostin is produced by osteocytes, whereas DKK-1 is produced by osteoblasts and by a variety of different cells in several tissues, including cancer cells. Both sclerostin and DKK-1 are secreted into the circulation, and serum levels reflect the inhibition of bone formation. Wnt proteins physiologically induce the differentiation and maturation of osteoblasts, and the secretion of Wnt proteins was shown to increase bone formation in osteoblastic metastases [45]. DKK-1 is a negative regulator of bone formation by antagonising the Wnt pathway, and it is also involved in the proliferation of stem cells and tumorigenic processes. The expression of DKK-1 in PC samples is conflicting, because literature data report either an increase or a non-significant change in PCa samples. Sclerostin is a related cysteine-rich glycoprotein that is predominantly secreted by osteocytes. Sclerostin interaction with LRP5/LRP6 leads to complex formation with Kremen and subsequent degradation, therefore leading to inhibition of Wnt signalling. Given the central role played by Wnt proteins within bone biology, the involvement of Wnts and Wnt inhibitors in PC-induced osteoblastic metastases has been extensively investigated. Interestingly, gene and protein expression in BMT specimens from PC patients showed that sclerostin and DKK-1 were not significantly different in osteoblastic and osteolytic metastases [46]. There are conflicting results on the levels of DKK-1 in PC patients with or without BMTs [47, 48]. Cumulative data suggest that the balance between Wnt and Wnt inhibitors might determine the osteogenic nature of PCa skeletal metastases and that DKK-1 may serve as a molecular switch between osteolytic and osteoblastic aspects of PCa BMTs. The use of DKK-1 and sclerostin as markers of bone turnover in a clinical setting seems rather premature (Fig. 2.3).

2.5 Other Emerging Markers of Bone Metastatic Disease from Prostate Cancer

New biomarkers, in combination with traditional markers of bone turnover, could help to improve the strategy for managing bone metastatic disease. Recently, xMAP multiplex technology has been developed, enabling the simultaneous measurement of large numbers of circulating biomarkers in a small sample volume.

In a recent study, nine new bone markers were tested by a commercially available multiplex Human Cancer/Metastasis Biomarker Panel [49]. Dickkopf-related protein 1 (DKK-1), growth differentiation factor 15 (GDF15), neuron-specific enolase (NSE), osteoprotegerin (OPG), osteonectin, periostin, tartrate-resistant acid phosphatase (TRAP5), tumour necrosis factor-related weak inducer of apoptosis (TWEAK), and chitinase-3-like protein 1 (YKL40) were tested in patients with BMTs from prostate, breast, lung and pancreatic cancer and compared with carboxy-terminal telopeptide (CTX) and procollagen type 1 *N*-terminal propeptide (PINP). Among the nine new markers of BMT, only GFD15, TRAP5, TWEAK, and YKLO40 showed a promising profile.

Growth differentiation factor 15 (GDF15) is a divergent member of the transforming growth factor-β (TGF-β) superfamily, also known as macrophage inhibitory cytokine-1 (MIC-1), prostate-derived factor (PDF), placental TGF-β (PTGF-β), placental bone morphogenetic protein, and nonsteroidal anti-inflammatory drug-activated gene-1 (NAG-1). GDF15 expression level is usually low in resting cells, but may be substantially increased following a response to diverse cellular stress signals, such as hypoxia, inflammation, short-wavelength light exposure, acute tissue injury and during cancer progression. The deregulation of GDF15 expression has been associated with diverse human disease development and cancer progression. The GDF15 level was increased in the serum of patients with various cancers, including melanoma, oral squamous cell carcinoma, and gastrointestinal, colorectal, pancreatic, prostate, breast, and cervical epithelial cancers. GFD15 resulted in higher levels in patients with BMT than in controls. DF15 may play an anti-tumoral role during the early stages of cancer, but, conversely, it can promote invasiveness and metastatic behaviour at advanced stages, and is involved in the epithelial-mesenchymal transition in tumours [50]. The roles of GDF15 in modulating osteoclast differentiation and in therapy for BMTs from PC have recently been identified [51].

Westhrin et al. described the role of GDF15 in osteoclast differentiation and showed an association between high serum GDF15 level and bone disease in multiple myeloma [52].

A further promising marker for BMT in the multiplex panel is TRAP5. This is one of the most abundant enzymes in osteoclasts and is a well-known marker of osteoclast activity and bone resorption. Elevated TRAP levels are found in many benign metabolic bone diseases such as Paget disease, haemodialysis, primary hyperparathyroidism, and metastatic malignancies involving bone resorption, multiple myeloma and bilateral ovariectomy [53]. TRAP has been found to be elevated in patients with BMTs compared with patients with no BMTs, in patients without treatment (denosumab) compared with the control group, and in patients with extensive BMTs [54, 55]. Recently, TRACP-5b, pyridinoline cross-linked carboxy-terminal telopeptide of type I collagen (1CTP), N-terminal cross-linking telopeptides of type I collagen (NTX), and bone-specific alkaline phosphatase (BAP) were measured in breast cancer patients with BMTs treated with zoledronic acid or denosumab. Although bone-modifying agents reduced the baseline levels of TRACP-5b, NTX, and BAP significantly, the reduction patterns differed. TRACP-5b appears to affect levels most quickly and sensitively, possibly because of its direct link to the number and activity of osteoclasts [56].

Tumour necrosis factor-related weak inducer of apoptosis is a member of the TNF ligand superfamily and is also a multifunctional soluble cytokine. TWEAK mRNA and protein have mainly been detected in endothelial cells, activated monocytes and T cells, macrophages, and dendritic cells. The multiple biological effects of TWEAK are mediated by binding to its cognate receptor Fn14 and include cell death, apoptosis, inflammation, angiogenesis, and cell proliferation. For these characteristics, TWEAK is an established key player in the pathogenesis of inflammatory diseases. Serum levels of TWEAK were found to be higher in patients with solid tumour and bone metastatic disease compared with patients without metastases in the bones. TWEAK plays a role in the progression of multiple myeloma and may facilitate bone destruction and solid tumour spread into bones [57].

Finally, higher serum levels of YKL4O (chitinase-3-like protein 1) were found in the bone metastasis groups compared with the controls. YKL4O is secreted by chondrocytes, synovial cells and macrophages and is suspected to play a role in remodelling or degradation of the extracellular matrix [58]. YKL4O has been found to be related to testosterone tissue levels in nipple aspiration fluid of patients with breast cancer and in breast cancer cell lines [59]. It plays a role in inflammation and tissue remodelling in several human diseases. YKL4O is described as being associated with a poor outcome of metastatic PC and non-small cell lung cancer (NSCLC) and a marker for early death in PC. Thus, it could serve as a new prognostic biomarker in patients [60].

Interestingly, when these new markers were compared with "classic" bone markers, such as CTX and PINP, the best marker of BMTs was PINP, whereas the five novel markers surprisingly performed better than CTX [49].

References

1. Fohr B, Dunstan CR, Seibel MJ (2003) Clinical review 165: markers of bone remodeling in metastatic bone disease. J Clin Endocrinol Metab 88(11):5059–5075
2. Vasikaran S, Eastell R, Bruyère O, Foldes AJ, Garnero P, Griesmacher A, McClung M, Morris HA, Silverman S, Trenti T, Wahl DA, Cooper C, Kanis JA, IOF-IFCC Bone Marker Standards Working Group (2011) Markers of bone turnover for the prediction of fracture risk and monitoring of osteoporosis treat-

ment: a need for international reference standards. Osteoporos Int 22(2):391–420

3. Schafer AL, Vittinghoff E, Ramachandran R, Mahmoudi N, Bauer DC (2010) Laboratory reproducibility of biochemical markers of bone turnover in clinical practice. Osteoporos Int 21(3):439–445
4. Coleman R, Brown J, Terpos E, Lipton A, Smith MR, Cook R, Major P (2008) Bone markers and their prognostic value in metastatic bone disease: clinical evidence and future directions. Cancer Treat Rev 34(7):629–639
5. Jung K, Lein M (2014) Bone turnover markers in serum and urine as diagnostic, prognostic and monitoring biomarkers of bone metastasis. Biochim Biophys Acta 1846(2):425–438
6. Michaelson MD, Marujo RM, Smith MR (2004) Contribution of androgen deprivation therapy to elevated osteoclast activity in men with metastatic prostate cancer. Clin Cancer Res 10(8):2705–2708
7. Garnero P, Buchs N, Zekri J, Rizzoli R, Coleman RE, Delmas PD (2000) Markers of bone turnover for the management of patients with bone metastases from prostate cancer. Br J Cancer 82(4):858–864
8. Garnero P, Ferreras M, Karsdal MA, Nicamhlaoibh R, Risteli J, Borel O, Qvist P, Delmas PD, Foged NT, Delaissé JM (2003) The type I collagen fragments ICTP and CTX reveal distinct enzymatic pathways of bone collagen degradation. J Bone Miner Res 18(5):859–867
9. Costa L, Demers LM, Gouveia-Oliveira A, Schaller J, Costa EB, de Moura MC, Lipton A (2002) Prospective evaluation of the peptide-bound collagen type I cross-links N-telopeptide and C-telopeptide in predicting bone metastases status. J Clin Oncol 20(3):850–856
10. Koizumi M, Yonese J, Fukui I, Ogata E (2001) The serum level of the amino-terminal propeptide of type I procollagen is a sensitive marker for prostate cancer metastasis to bone. BJU Int 87(4):348–351
11. Zafeirakis AG, Papatheodorou GA, Limouris GS (2010) Clinical and imaging correlations of bone turnover markers in prostate cancer patients with bone only metastases. Nucl Med Commun 31(3):249–253
12. Koopmans N, de Jong IJ, Breeuwsma AJ, van der Veer E (2007) Serum bone turnover markers (PINP and ICTP) for the early detection of bone metastases in patients with prostate cancer: a longitudinal approach. J Urol 178(3 Pt 1):849–853
13. Fedarko NS, Jain A, Karadag A, Van Eman MR, Fisher LW (2001) Elevated serum bone sialoprotein and osteopontin in colon, breast, prostate, and lung cancer. Clin Cancer Res 7(12):4060–4066
14. Brown JM, Vessella RL, Kostenuik PJ, Dunstan CR, Lange PH, Corey E (2001) Serum osteoprotegerin levels are increased in patients with advanced prostate cancer. Clin Cancer Res 7(10):2977–2983
15. Mountzios G, Terpos E, Syrigos K, Papadimitriou C, Papadopoulos G, Bamias A, Mavrikakis M, Dimopoulos MA (2010) Markers of bone remodeling and skeletal morbidity in patients with solid tumors metastatic to the skeleton receiving the biphosphonate zoledronic acid. Transl Res 155(5):247–255
16. Todenhöfer T, Hennenlotter J, Leidenberger P, Wald A, Hohneder A, Kühs U, Mischinger J, Aufderklamm S, Gakis G, Blumenstock G, Stenzl A, Schwentner C (2014) Serum receptor activator of nuclear factor kB ligand (RANKL) levels predict biochemical recurrence in patients undergoing radical prostatectomy. BJU Int 113(1):152–159
17. Metwalli AR, Rosner IL, Cullen J, Chen Y, Brand T, Brassell SA, Lesperance J, Porter C, Sterbis J, McLeod DG (2014) Elevated alkaline phosphatase velocity strongly predicts overall survival and the risk of bone metastases in castrate-resistant prostate cancer. Urol Oncol 32(6):761–768
18. Coleman R, Costa L, Saad F, Cook R, Hadji P, Terpos E, Garnero P, Brown J, Body JJ, Smith M, Lee KA, Major P, Dimopoulos M, Lipton A (2011) Consensus on the utility of bone markers in the malignant bone disease setting. Crit Rev Oncol Hematol 80(3):411–432
19. Kamiya N, Suzuki H, Yano M, Endo T, Takano M, Komaru A, Kawamura K, Sekita N, Imamoto T, Ichikawa T (2010) Implications of serum bone turnover markers in prostate cancer patients with bone metastasis. Urology 75(6):1446–1451
20. Saad F, Eastham JA, Smith MR (2012) Biochemical markers of bone turnover and clinical outcomes in men with prostate cancer. Urol Oncol 30(4):369–378
21. Coleman RE, Major P, Lipton A, Brown JE, Lee KA, Smith M, Saad F, Zheng M, Hei YJ, Seaman J, Cook RJ (2005) Predictive value of bone resorption and formation markers in cancer patients with bone metastases receiving the bisphosphonate zoledronic acid. Clin Oncol 23(22):4925–4935
22. Cook RJ, Coleman R, Brown J, Lipton A, Major P, Hei YJ, Saad F, Smith MR (2006) Markers of bone metabolism and survival in men with hormone-refractory metastatic prostate cancer. Clin Cancer Res 12(11 Pt 1):3361–3367.99–100
23. Smith MR, Cook RJ, Coleman R, Brown J, Lipton A, Major P, Hei YJ, Saad F (2007) Predictors of skeletal complications in men with hormone-refractory metastatic prostate cancer. Urology 70(2):315–319
24. Som A, Tu SM, Liu J, Wang X, Qiao W, Logothetis C, Corn PG (2012) Response in bone turnover markers during therapy predicts overall survival in patients with metastatic prostate cancer: analysis of three clinical trials. Br J Cancer 107(9):1547–1553
25. Jung K, Miller K, Wirth M, Albrecht M, Lein M (2011) Bone turnover markers as predictors of mortality risk in prostate cancer patients with bone metastases following treatment with zoledronic acid. Eur Urol 59(4):604–129
26. Alcaraz A, González-López R, Morote J, de la Piedra C, Meseguer C, Esteban E, Climent M, González-Gragera B, Alvarez-Ossorio JL, Chirivella I, Mellado B, Lara PC, Vázquez F, Contreras JA, Carles J, Murias A, Calderero V, Comet-Batlle J, González-Del Alba A, León-Mateos L, Mañas A, Segarra J, Lassa A, González-Enguita C, Méndez MJ, Samper P, Unda M, Mahillo-Fernández I, Bellmunt J; TUGAMO GROUP (2013) Biochemical markers of bone turn-

over and clinical outcome in patients with renal cell and bladder carcinoma with bone metastases following treatment with zoledronic acid: the TUGAMO study. Br J Cancer 109(1):121–30
27. Brasso K, Christensen IJ, Johansen JS, Teisner B, Garnero P, Price PA, Iversen P (2006) Prognostic value of PINP, bone alkaline phosphatase, CTX-I, and YKL-40 in patients with metastatic prostate carcinoma. Prostate 66(5):503–513
28. Coleman R, Body JJ, Aapro M et al (2014) Bone health in cancer patients: ESMO Clinical Practice guidelines. Ann Oncol 25:1–14. doi:10.1093/annonc/mdu103
29. Bauer D, Krege J, Lane N, Leary E, Libanati C, Miller P, Myers G, Silverman S, Vesper HW, Lee D, Payette M, Randall S (2012) National Bone Health Alliance Bone Turnover Marker Project: current practices and the need for US harmonization, standardization, and common reference ranges. Osteoporos Int 23(10):2425–2433
30. Cavalier E, Bergmann P, Bruyère O, Delanaye P, Durnez A, Devogelaer JP, Ferrari SL, Gielen E, Goemaere S, Kaufman JM, Toukap AN, Reginster JY, Rousseau AF, Rozenberg S, Scheen AJ, Body JJ (2016) The role of biochemical of bone turnover markers in osteoporosis and metabolic bone disease: a consensus paper of the Belgian Bone Club. Osteoporos Int 27(7):2181–2195
31. Wada N, Fujisaki M, Ishii S, Ikeda T, Kitajima M (2001) Evaluation of bone metabolic markers in breast cancer with bone metastasis. Breast Cancer 8:131–137
32. Ulrich U, Rhiem K, Schmolling J, Flaskamp C, Paffenholz I, Salzer H et al (2001) Cross-linked type Icollagen C- and N-telopeptides in women with bone metastases from breast cancer. Arch Gynecol Obstet 264:186–190
33. Morra L, Moch H (2011) Periostin expression and epithelial-mesenchymal transition in cancer: a review and an update. Virchows Arch 459(5):465–475
34. Sasaki H, Yu CY, Dai M, Tam C, Loda M, Auclair D, Chen LB, Elias A (2003) Elevated serum periostin levels in patients with bone metastases from breast but not lung cancer. Breast Cancer Res Treat 77(3):245–252
35. Kyutoku M, Taniyama Y, Katsuragi N, Shimizu H, Kunugiza Y, Iekushi K, Koibuchi N, Sanada F, Oshita Y, Morishita R (2011) Role of periostin in cancer progression and metastasis: inhibition of breast cancer progression and metastasis by anti-periostin antibody in a murine model. Int J Mol Med 28(2):181–186
36. Contié S, Voorzanger-Rousselot N, Litvin J, Clézardin P, Garnero P (2011) Increased expression and serum levels of the stromal cell-secreted protein periostin in breast cancer bone metastases. Int J Cancer 128(2):352–360
37. Bonnet N, Garnero P, Ferrari S (2015) Periostin action in bone. Mol Cell Endocrinol. pii: S0303-7207(15)30170-2. doi:10.1016/j.mce.2015.12.014
38. Kruger TE, Miller AH, Godwin AK, Wang J (2014) Bone sialoprotein and osteopontin in bone metastasis of osteotropic cancers. Crit Rev Oncol Hematol 89(2):330–341
39. Carlinfante G, Vassiliou D, Svensson O et al (2003) Differential expression of osteopontin and bone sialoprotein in bone metastasis of breast and prostate carcinoma. Clin Exp Metastasis 20:437–444
40. Khodavirdi AC, Song Z, Yang S et al (2006) Increased expression of osteopontin contributes to the progression of prostate cancer. Cancer Res 66:883–888
41. Waltregny D, Bellahcene A, Van Riet I, Fisher LW, Young M, Fernandez P et al (1998) Prognostic value of bone sialoprotein expression in clinically localized human prostate cancer. J Natl Cancer Inst 90:1000–1008
42. Bellahcene A, Kroll M, Liebens F, Castronovo V (1996) Bone sialoprotein expression in primary human breast is associated with bone metastases development. J Bone Miner Res 11:665–670
43. Uccello M, Malaguarnera G, Vacante M, Motta M (2011) Serum bone sialoprotein levels and bone metastases. J Cancer Res Ther 7:115–119
44. Jain A, McKnight DA, Fisher LW, Humphreys EB, Mangold LA, Partin AW et al (2009) Small integrin-binding proteins as serum markers for prostate cancer detection. Clin Cancer Res 15:5199–5207
45. Ferreira A, Alho I, Casimiro S, Costa L (2015) Bone remodeling markers and bone metastases: from cancer research to clinical implications. Bonekey Rep 4:668
46. Larson SR, Zhang X, Dumpit R, Coleman I, Lakely B, Roudier M, Higano CS, True LD, Lange PH, Montgomery B, Corey E, Nelson PS, Vessella RL, Morrissey C (2013) Characterization of osteoblastic and osteolytic proteins in prostate cancer bone metastases. Prostate 73(9):932–940
47. D'Amelio P, Roato I, Oderda M, Soria F, Zitella A, Ferracini R, Mengozzi G, Gontero P, Isaia GC (2014) DKK-1 in prostate cancer diagnosis and follow up. BMC Clin Pathol 14(1):11
48. Roato I, D'Amelio P, Gorassini E, Grimaldi A, Bonello L, Fiori C, Delsedime L, Tizzani A, De Libero A, Isaia G, Ferracini R (2008) Osteoclasts are active in bone forming metastases of prostate cancer patients. PLoS One 3(11):e3627
49. Windrichova J, Fuchsova R, Kucera R, Topolcan O, Fiala O, Finek J, Slipkova D, Karlikova M, Svobodova J (2016) Testing of a novel cancer metastatic multiplex panel for the detection of bone-metastatic disease – a pilot study. Anticancer Res 36(4):1973–1978
50. Li C, Wang J, Kong J, Tang J, Wu Y, Xu E, Zhang H, Lai M (2016) GDF15 promotes EMT and metastasis in colorectal cancer. Oncotarget 7(1):860–872
51. Vanhara P, Hampl A, Kozubik A, Soucek K (2012) Growth/differentiation factor-15: prostate-cancer suppressor or promoter? Prostate Cancer Prostatic Dis 15:320–328

52. Westhrin M, Moen SH, Holien T, Mylin AK, Heickendorff L, Olsen OE, Sundan A, Turesson I, Gimsing P, Waage A, Standal T (2015) Growth differentiation factor 15 (GDF15) promotes osteoclast differentiation and inhibits osteoblast differentiation and high serum GDF15 levels are associated with multiple myeloma bone disease. Haematologica 100:e511–e514
53. Halleen JM, Tiitinen SL, Ylipahkala H, Fagerlund KM, Vaananen HK (2006) Tartrate-resistant acid phosphatase 5b (TRACP5b) as a marker of bone resorption. Clin Lab 52:499–509
54. Sarvari BK, Sankara Mahadev D, Rupa S, Mastan SA (2015) Detection of bone metastases in breast cancer (BC) patients by serum tartrate-resistant acid phosphatase 5b (TRACP 5b), a bone resorption marker and serum alkaline phosphatase (ALP), a bone formation marker, in lieu of whole-body skeletal scintigraphy with technetium99m MDP. Indian J Clin Biochem 30:66–71
55. Tang C, Liu Y, Qin H, Li X, Guo W, Li J, Wang W, Qu L, Hu H, Xu C, Zheng L, Huang Y, Liu B, Gao H, Halleen JM, Liu X (2013) Clinical significance of serum BAP, TRACP 5b and ICTP as bone metabolic markers for bone metastasis screening in lung cancer patients. Clin Chim Acta 426:102–107
56. Nishimukai A, Higuchi T, Ozawa H, Yanai A, Miyagawa Y, Murase K, Imamura M, Takatsuka Y, Miyoshi Y (2016) Different patterns of change in bone turnover markers during treatment with bone-modifying agents for breast cancer patients with bone metastases. Breast Cancer. doi:10.1007/s12282-016-0695-2
57. Mehta RS, Chong DQ, Song M, Meyerhardt JA, Ng K, Nishihara R, Qian Z, Morikawa T, Wu K, Giovannucci EL, Fuchs CS, Ogino S, Chan AT (2015) Association between plasma levels of macrophage inhibitory cytokine-1 before diagnosis of colorectal cancer and mortality. Gastroenterology 149:614–622
58. Volck B, Price PA, Johansen JS, Sorensen O, Benfield TL, Nielsen HJ, Calafat J, Borregaard N (1998) YKL40, a mammalian member of the chitinase family, is a matrix protein of specific granules in human neutrophils. Proc Assoc Am Physicians 110:351–360
59. Shidfar A, Fatokun T, Ivancic D, Chatterton RT, Khan SA, Wang J (2016) Protein biomarkers for breast cancer risk are specifically correlated with local steroid hormones in nipple aspirate fluid. Horm Cancer 7(4):252–259
60. Thom I, Andritzky B, Schuch G, Burkholder I, Edler L, Johansen JS, Bokemeyer C, Schumacher U, Laack E (2010) Elevated pretreatment serum concentration of YKL40 — an independent prognostic biomarker for poor survival in patients with metastatic nonsmall cell lung cancer. Cancer 116:4114–4121

Bone Homing and Metastasis

3

Matteo Santoni, Antonio Lopez-Beltran, Marina Scarpelli, Roberta Mazzucchelli, Rossana Berardi, Liang Cheng, and Rodolfo Montironi

3.1 Introduction

Bone metastasization is a frequent event for a variety of cancer cells, including breast, prostate, lung, and thyroid tumors. In these diseases, the rate of bone involvement can overcome 70 %, for a total of more than 350,000 patients/year died in the United States with bone metastasis (BMs) [1, 2].

Bone homing is the result of a multistep process that requires a straight interaction between tumor cells and bone microenvironment that starts with tumor malignant progression and invasion through the extracellular matrix (ECM) and leads to bone metastasization [3]. This event presents several similarities with the homing of hematopoietic stem cells (HSCs) [4] and requires the acquisition of migratory properties by tumor cells through a physiological process named epithelial mesenchymal transition (EMT) in which polarized epithelial cells gain mesenchymal, fibroblast-like properties and show altered cell–cell and cell–matrix interactions and increased motility [5].

Homing of tumor cells to the bone may present as both an early and late event. Indeed, several tumors including renal cell carcinoma can develop bone metastases even more than 10 years after the resection of the primary tumor [6, 7]. This may be partially explained by the presence of disseminated tumor cells (DTCs) homing to the bone marrow and entering a dormant phase to evade apoptosis and successively switch to a proliferative and aggressive phenotype [8].

Prostate cancer (PCa) is one of the cancers that more frequently metastasize to the bone (Figs. 3.1 and 3.2). Approximately 70 % of patients undergoing radical prostatectomy (RP) show DTCs in their bone marrow at time of surgery, which are independent predictors of tumor recurrence [9]. The prognostic significance of this metastatic site has been recently investigated in a meta-analysis led by Halabi and colleagues analyzing individual patient data from 8,820 men with metastatic castration-resistant prostate cancer (mCRPCa) treated with docetaxel from nine

M. Santoni • R. Berardi
Medical Oncology, Università Politecnica delle Marche, Azienda Ospedaliero-Universitaria Ospedali Riuniti Umberto I, GM Lancisi, G Salesi, Ancona, Italy

A. Lopez-Beltran
Department of Surgery, Cordoba University Medical School, Cordoba, Spain

M. Scarpelli • R. Mazzucchelli • R. Montironi (✉)
Section of Pathological Anatomy, Polytechnic University of the Marche Region, School of Medicine, United Hospitals, Via Conca 71, Torrette, Ancona I–60126, Italy
e-mail: r.montironi@univpm.it

L. Cheng
Department of Pathology and Laboratory Medicine, Indiana University School of Medicine, Indianapolis, IN, USA

F. Bertoldo et al. (eds.), *Bone Metastases from Prostate Cancer*,
DOI 10.1007/978-3-319-42327-2_3

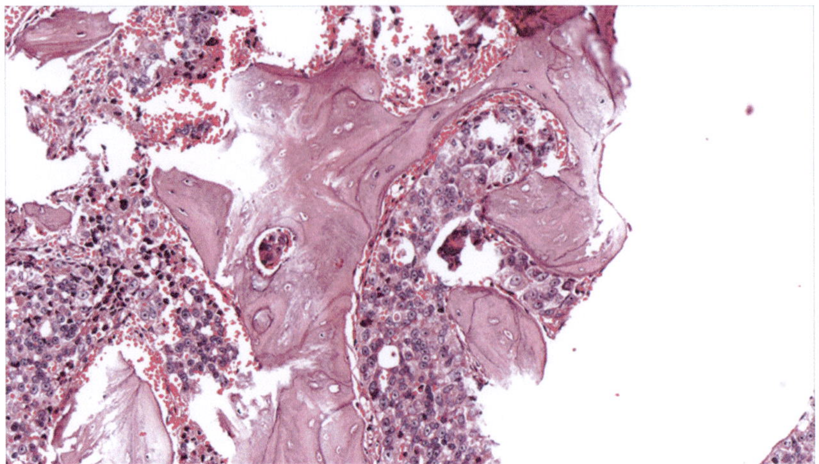

Fig. 3.1 Bone metastasis of high-grade prostate cancer

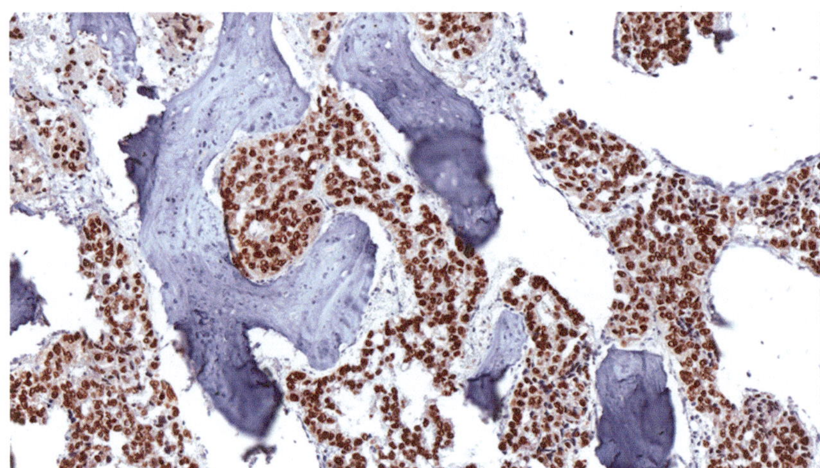

Fig. 3.2 Bone metastasis of prostate cancer. The neoplastic cells are immunostained with antibody against prostein

phase III trials [10]. In this analysis, the authors showed that over 70 % of enrolled patients presented the bone with or without lymph node metastases. In addition, the presence of bone metastases, as well as of nonvisceral involvement, was associated with decreased lethality as compared to lung and liver metastases [10].

Understanding the mechanisms by which PCa cells migrate into the bone will represent a major step forward for the early detection of bone involvement in patients with PCa and for the design of agents specifically targeting bone homing and preventing this phenomenon.

In this chapter, we describe the main mechanisms involved in PCa bone homing and metastasis.

3.2 Homing of PCa Cells to the Bone: The Role of Cellular Plasticity

The biological scenario underlying bone homing has not been completely clarified and includes a huge variety of mechanisms. Among them, the selective pressure exerted by bone microenvironment seems to majorly contribute to tumor cell homing [11, 12]. Indeed, it has been shown that the frequency of mitochondrial DNA mutations is significantly higher in BMs compared to both soft tissue metastases and the primary tumor [11]. Otherwise, the contribution of osteoclasts does not seem to be relevant in the initiation phase of PCa bone metastasization [12].

Cellular plasticity is the ability of differentiated cells of deviating to other cell types when exposed to different conditions. Through this phenomenon, differentiated cells can acquire cancer stem cell (CSC) properties under specific oncogenic insults, leading to aberrant cell reprogramming and, as a consequence, to a series of diseases including cancer [13]. Indeed, CSC status and EMT and mesenchymal-epithelial transition (MET) are interconnected reversible dynamic processes that facilitate cells to adapt to stimuli from altered microenvironments [14]. In breast cancer, CSCs have been shown to reversibly switch from mesenchymal-like to epithelial-like states. Bone colonization from breast CSCs can induce the co-expression of mesenchymal and epithelial markers and the transition from a $CD44^+/CD24^-$ to a $CD44^-/CD24^+$ phenotype [15, 16], thus underlining the complexity of tumor cell bone homing and stem cell trafficking.

At present, data on the role of cellular plasticity in bone homing and development of BMs from PCa are still inconclusive [17]. Thus, while several studies have observed that the interaction between androgen refractory PCa cell lines and bone stromal cells led to the acquisition of a mesenchymal phenotype via EMT characterized by a switch from E- to N-cadherin expression [14, 18], the study published by Josson et al. has reported increased E-cadherin expression as a result of a similar interaction [19].

Cellular plasticity may be the result of physiological stimuli and induced by therapeutic agents. Hypoxia seems to majorly contribute to the promotion of cellular plasticity [20], and E-cadherin is implicated in the regulation of the response of cancer cells to hypoxia by inducing the expression of hypoxia-inducible factor-1α (HIF-1α) [21]. On the other hand, the selective pressure exerted by androgen-deprivation therapy (ADT) may give rise to CSCs as well as EMT and neuroendocrine (NE) differentiation, which are associated with PCa growth, metastasis, and resistance to therapies [22, 23].

Based on these data, several strategies are emerging to modulate the contribution of bone microenvironment in patients with PCa. Among them, abiraterone acetate seems to represent an effective strategy in this context. Food and Drug Administration (FDA) approved this drug in combination with prednisone on April 2011 for metastatic castration-resistant PCa following docetaxel and on December 2012 for metastatic castration-resistant PCa before chemotherapy. In 2015, Santini and his group have first revealed that abiraterone acetate can affect the differentiation and activity of osteoclasts by inhibiting marker genes including TRAP, cathepsin K, and metalloproteinase-9 (MMP-9) [24]. Moreover, abiraterone acetate can promote osteoblast differentiation and the deposition of bone matrix through the upregulation of specific genes such as ALP and osteocalcin [24]. However, the role of abiraterone acetate in modulating bone homing has not been clarified so far and seems to merit further investigations.

3.3 Epithelial-Mesenchymal Plasticity in Bone Homing

During embryonic morphogenesis, epithelial cells exhibit enormous plasticity and transit into a mesenchymal state by activating the EMT process. Through this program, epithelial cells lose their junctions and produce vimentin filaments, thus enhancing their ability to migrate and invade during developmental morphogenesis [25, 26] (Fig. 3.3). During EMT, E-cadherin gene transcriptional repression, promoter methylation, and protein phosphorylation and degradation have been observed [27, 28]. On the other hand, N-cadherin, fibronectin, and cell surface proteins CD44 [29] and integrin β6 [30].

The expression of EMT and its reversal MET are fundamental processes for the development and progression of genitourinary tumors [31–34]. In PCa, the functional cross talk between EMT and castration resistance, which is crucial during prostate carcinogenesis, is mediated by the Twist1/AR signaling axis and promoted by the activity of transforming growth factor-β (TGF-β) [35].

TGF-β upregulates a variety of genes, such as prostate transmembrane protein, androgen induced 1 (PMEPA1), that is a regulator of TGF-β and correlates with tumor aggressiveness and

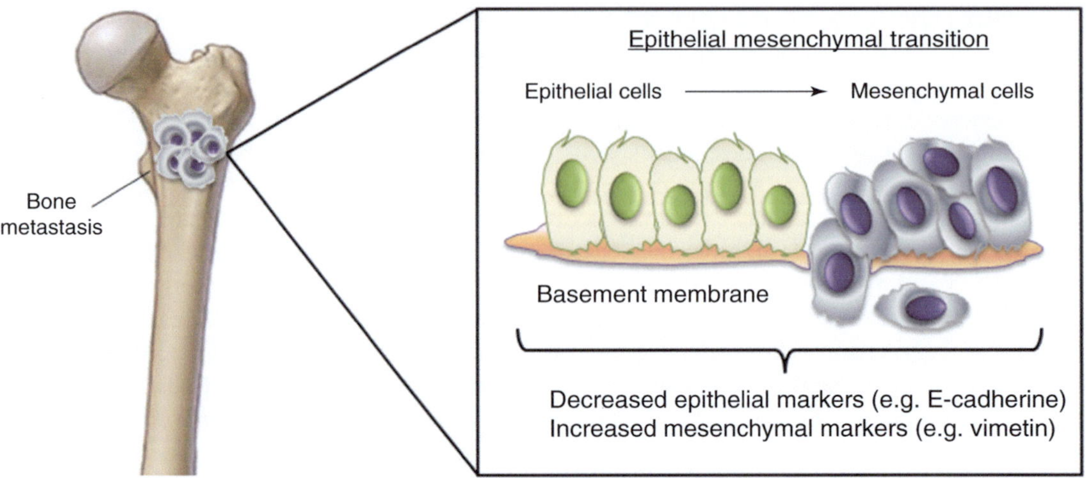

Fig. 3.3 Epithelial-mesenchymal transition (EMT) in prostate bone metastases (BMs)

BMs [36]. Interestingly, the knockdown of PMEPA1 has been associated with increased pro-metastatic gene expression and bone homing in PCa mouse models [36].

Furthermore, TGF-β expression resulted increased in BMs compared to visceral PCa metastases in a series of 149 visceral and BMs from 62 patients with castration-resistant PCa [37]. In this study, nuclear Twist, Slug, and Zeb1 localization and an EMT-like phenotype were present only in a small subset of castration-resistant PCa BMs [37].

E-cadherin is involved in maintaining the pluripotent and self-renewal ability of prostate CSCs [28, 38, 39]. Interestingly, E-cadherin loss, which is crucial for the acquisition of PCa migratory properties and bone homing, is associated with activated androgen receptor (AR) [40] and correlates with PCa progression and Gleason score [41], while increased N-cadherin has been reported to predict clinical recurrence in PCa patients following RP [42], thus representing a potential therapeutic target in castration-resistant PCa [43].

3.4 The Role of Chemokines and Their Receptors

Chemokines are a superfamily of low-molecular-weight proteins including inducers and inhibitors of angiogenesis. The altered balance between these stimuli can lead to chronic inflammatory diseases, as well as to tumor initiation and spreading [44].

The chemokine family includes CXC ligand 1 (CXCL1) to CXCL16. These ligands interact with the CXC chemokine receptors (CXCR1–CXCR5), members of the rhodopsin-like seven-transmembrane G protein-coupled receptor family, to exert their activity [45, 46].

Several studies demonstrated that chemokines and their receptors are implicated in chemotaxis of cancer cells toward bone and the lymph nodes. Among CXCRs, CXCR4 has been shown to play an essential role for both normal prostate tissue and PCa development and progression. CXCR4 binds to CXCL12/SDF-1, which is implicated in the maintenance of leukocyte trafficking during homeostasis. In PCa, SDF-1 supports the invasion of PCa cell lines through basement membranes, which is conversely inhibited by anti-CXCR4 antibodies [47].

It is interesting to note that PCa cell androgen-mediated motility seems to be dependent on functional CXCR4/CXCR7 heterodimers [48]. Moreover, prostate CSCs expressing CXCR4 compete with HSCs for bone marrow niches. Blocking CXCR4-dependent bone homing, the formation of BMs is suppressed [49]. It should be noted that the expression of CXCR4 is low in BMs, suggesting that this receptor may be essential for bone homing but not for distant tumor growth [50]. The potential role of CXCR4 as a potential therapeutic target is also sustained by the evidence that Plerixafor, a CXCR4 inhibitor, seems to be effective in PCa xenograft mouse models [51]. Furthermore, homing may be also prevented by agents such as pertussis toxin, which inhibits G proteins, and chelerythrine chloride, which inhibits protein kinase C.

3.5 The Role of MicroRNAs

Regarding the role played by microRNAs (miRNAs) in the control of PCa metastases, they are involved in regulating the complex metastatic cascade at multiple levels. Fu and his group have compared the expressions of four miRNAs (miR-335, miR-543, miR-196, and miR-19a) between primary PCa and BMs [52]. By using reverse transcription-quantitative polymerase chain reaction, they showed that the four miRNAs were significantly downregulated in BMs compared to PCa. Additionally, miR-335 and miR-543 downregulation was confirmed in 20 paired primary tumors and BMs [52]. Exogenous miR-335 and miR-543 significantly reduced the expression level of endothelial nitric oxide synthase (eNOS) and markedly affected the migratory and invasive properties of PCa cells in vitro [52].

It has been shown that loss of miR-15 and miR-16, together with increased miR-21 expression, promotes PCa metastasization and bone homing [53]. In the same view, dysregulation of the epidermal growth factor receptor (EGFR) signaling pathway seems to sustain PCa bone homing by constraining the tumor-suppressive role of miR-1 and promoting the oncogenic activation of Twist1 [54].

Furthermore, Wang et al. revealed that miR-573 expression is significantly higher in primary PCa compared to metastases [55]. They showed that miR-573 inhibited PCa cell migration and invasion as well as TGF-β1-induced EMT in vitro and lung metastases in vivo. In addition, miR-573 modulates the activation of *fibroblast growth factor receptor 1* (*FGFR1*) gene in response to fibroblast growth factor 2 (FGF2) and, together with GATA3 (which directly increases miR-573 expression), regulates EMT contribution to bone homing and metastasis [55]. Interestingly, the downregulation of miR-573 is associated with higher Gleason score and cancer-related mortality [55].

3.6 The Role of Other Molecules and Signaling Pathways

Several other signaling pathways are implicated in the development of PCa BMs. Among them, receptor activator of nuclear factor kappa-B (RANK)/RANK-ligand(L) axis [56] and wingless-type (WNT) signaling pathway/Dickkopf WNT signaling pathway inhibitor 1 (Dkk1) [57] constitutes two of the most promising targets for interfering with bone homing in PCa patients. RANKL is a transmembrane signaling receptor expressed on the surface of osteoclast precursors and binds to RANK to mediate osteoclast-induced bone remodeling that is fundamental to create a favorable bone environment for PCa cells [58]. Similarly, runt-related transcription factor 2 (RUNX2), which is a crucial factor for osteoblast differentiation [59], contributes to bone formation and homing of cancer cells.

As for cyclin A1 (CCNA1), Miftakhova et al. showed that the expression of this protein results in increased in the lymph node, lung, and BMs and was associated with aromatase (CYP19A1), a key enzyme in the regulation of the balance between androgens and estrogens [60]. In an in vitro model of high ALDH activity in PCa, both CCNA1 and CYP19A1 promoted local bone marrow-releasing factors, including AR, estrogen, and MMP9 and provided a suitable microenvironment that sustained metastatic growth of PCa cells in the bone marrow [60].

Concerning insulin-like growth factor (IGF)-1 and IGF-2, which are two of the most abundant nonstructural proteins in the bone matrix [61], they seem to contribute to cancer cell migration to the bone, as well as to the adhesion with the bone marrow stromal cells [62]. Among other proteins, CD26/dipeptidyl peptidase IV (DPPIV) is a membrane-bound extracellular peptidase cleaving the chemokine SDF-1α at its position two proline. CD26/DPPIV triggers PCa metastasis to the bone marrow and is involved in stem cell homing and mobilization [63].

Finally, also low pH in bone microenvironment [64] and altered calcium levels [65] can promote skeletal metastasis formation

Conclusions

The management of PCa patients with BMs represents a major challenge for medical oncologists due to the considerable morbidity associated with skeletal-related events (SREs), such as bone pain, hypercalcemia, pathologic fractures, and the compression of the spinal cord. The cooperative reciprocal interactions among heterogeneous compartments including PCa cells, osteoblasts, and osteoclasts in the bone microenvironment promote tumor cell homing and metastasis, thus representing a promising future therapeutic and diagnostic target for these patients.

Recent technical advances have provided the opportunity to investigate the complexity of biological systems at the single-cell level. On this scenario, modulating tumour environmental conditions and characterizing genes associated with bone spreading will be key issues for cancer research in future years. This will be crucial for the identification of prognostic or predictive biomarkers for the early detection of metastatic disease, for the assessment of tumor response to therapy and to guide treatment decisions, and potentially for the prevention BM formation in patients with PCa [66].

In conclusion, significant progresses have been made in our knowledge of the complex mechanisms underlying bone homing in PCa. However, the route to a complete comprehension of this process and toward the design of effective and personalized strategies for PCa patients with BMs seems still so far away.

References

1. Coleman RE (2006) Clinical features of metastatic bone disease and risk of skeletal morbidity. Clin Cancer Res 12(20 Pt 2):6243s–6249s
2. Mundy GR (2002) Metastasis to bone: causes, consequences and therapeutic opportunities. Nat Rev Cancer 2(8):584–593
3. Mishra A, Shiozawa Y, Pienta KJ, Taichman RS (2011) Homing of cancer cells to the bone. Cancer Microenviron 4(3):221–235
4. Wilson A, Trumpp A (2006) Bone-marrow haematopoietic-stem-cell niches. Nat Rev Immunol 6(2):93–106
5. Pietilä M, Ivaska J, Mani SA (2016) Whom to blame for metastasis, the epithelial-mesenchymal transition or the tumor microenvironment? Cancer Lett. pii: S0304-3835(16)00005-7
6. Santoni M, Conti A, Porta C, Procopio G, Sternberg CN, Basso U, De Giorgi U, Bracarda S, Rizzo M, Ortega C, Massari F, Iacovelli R, Derosa L, Masini C, Milella M, Di Lorenzo G, Atzori F, Pagano M, Buti S, De Vivo R, Mosca A, Rossi M, Paglino C, Verzoni E, Cerbone L, Muzzonigro G, Falconi M, Montironi R, Burattini L, Santini D, Cascinu S (2014) Sunitinib, pazopanib or sorafenib for the treatment of patients with late-relapsing (>5 years) metastatic renal cell carcinoma. J Urol 193(1):41–47, pii: S0022-5347(14)03958-5
7. Santoni M, Conti A, Procopio G, Porta C, Ibrahim T, Barni S, Guida FM, Fontana A, Berruti A, Berardi R, Massari F, Vincenzi B, Ortega C, Ottaviani D, Carteni G, Lanzetta G, De Lisi D, Silvestris N, Satolli MA, Collovà E, Russo A, Badalamenti G, Luzi Fedeli S, Tanca FM, Adamo V, Maiello E, Sabbatini R, Felici A, Cinieri S, Montironi R, Bracarda S, Tonini G, Cascinu S, Santini D (2015) Bone metastases in patients with metastatic renal cell carcinoma: are they always associated with poor prognosis? J Exp Clin Cancer Res 34:10
8. Townson JL, Chambers AF (2006) Dormancy of solitary metastatic cells. Cell Cycle 5(16):1744–1750
9. Morgan TM et al (2009) Disseminated tumor cells in prostate cancer patients after radical prostatectomy and without evidence of disease predicts biochemical recurrence. Clin Cancer Res 15(2):677–683
10. Halabi S, Kelly WK, Ma H, Zhou H, Solomon NC, Fizazi K, Tangen CM, Rosenthal M, Petrylak DP, Hussain M, Vogelzang NJ, Thompson IM, Chi KN, de Bono J, Armstrong AJ, Eisenberger MA, Fandi A, Li S, Araujo JC, Logothetis CJ, Quinn DI, Morris MJ, Higano CS, Tannock IF, Small EJ (2016) Meta-analysis evaluating the impact of site of metastasis on overall survival in men with castration-resistant prostate cancer. J Clin Oncol 34(14):1652–1659, pii: JCO657270
11. Arnold RS, Fedewa SA, Goodman M, Osunkoya AO, Kissick HT, Morrissey C et al (2015) Bone metastasis in prostate cancer: recurring mitochondrial DNA mutation reveals selective pressure exerted by the bone microenvironment. Bone 78:81–86
12. Zalucha JL, Jung Y, Joseph J, Wang J, Berry JE, Shiozawa Y et al (2015) The role of osteoclasts in early dissemination of prostate cancer tumor cells. J Cancer Stem Cell Res 3. pii: e1005
13. Vicente-Dueñas C, Gutiérrez de Diego J, Rodríguez FD, Jiménez R, Cobaleda C (2009) The role of cellular plasticity in cancer development. Curr Med Chem 16(28):3676–3685

14. Xu J, Wang R, Xie ZH, Odero-Marah V, Pathak S, Multani A et al (2006) Prostate cancer metastasis: role of the host microenvironment in promoting epithelial to mesenchymal transition and increased bone and adrenal gland metastasis. Prostate 66(15):1664–1673
15. Liu S, Cong Y, Wang D et al (2014) Breast cancer stem cells transition between epithelial and mesenchymal states reflective of their normal counterparts. Stem Cell Reports 2(1):78–91
16. D'Amico L, Patanè S, Grange C et al (2013) Primary breast cancer stem-like cells metastasise to bone, switch phenotype and acquire a bone tropism signature. Br J Cancer 108(12):2525–2536
17. Jadaan DY, Jadaan MM, McCabe JP (2015) Cellular plasticity in prostate cancer bone metastasis. Prostate Cancer 651580. doi:10.1155/2015/651580
18. Zhau HE, Odero-Marah V, Lue H-W et al (2008) Epithelial to mesenchymal transition (EMT) in human prostate cancer: lessons learned from ARCaP model. Clin Exp Metastasis 25(6):601–610
19. Josson S, Sharp S, Sung S-Y et al (2010) Tumor-stromal interactions influence radiation sensitivity in epithelial-versus mesenchymal-like prostate cancer cells. J Oncol 2010:10. doi:10.1155/2010/232831.232831
20. Conley SJ, Gheordunescu E, Kakarala P et al (2012) Antiangiogenic agents increase breast cancer stem cells via the generation of tumor hypoxia. Proc Natl Acad Sci U S A 109(8):2784–2789
21. Chu K, Boley KM, Moraes R, Barsky SH, Robertson FM (2013) The paradox of E-cadherin: role in response to hypoxia in the tumor microenvironment and regulation of energy metabolism. Oncotarget 4(3):446–462
22. Bishop JL, Davies A, Ketola K, Zoubeidi A (2015) Regulation of tumor cell plasticity by the androgen receptor in prostate cancer. EndocrRelat Cancer 22(3):R165–R182
23. Santoni M, Conti A, Burattini L, Berardi R, Scarpelli M, Cheng L et al (2014) Neuroendocrine differentiation in prostate cancer: novel morphological insights and future therapeutic perspectives. Biochim Biophys Acta 1846(2):630–637
24. Iuliani M, Pantano F, Buttigliero C, Fioramonti M, Bertaglia V, Vincenzi B et al (2015) Biological and clinical effects of abiraterone on anti-resorptive and anabolic activity in bone microenvironment. Oncotarget 6(14):12520–12528
25. Boyer B, Thiery JP (1993) Epithelium-mesenchyme interconversion as example of epithelial plasticity. APMIS 101:257–268
26. Hay ED (1995) An overview of epithelio–mesenchymal transformation. Acta Anat (Basel) 154:8–20
27. Batlle E, Sancho E, Franci C, Dominguez D, Monfar M, Baulida J, Garcia De Herreros A (2000) The transcription factor snail is a repressor of E-cadherin gene expression in epithelial tumour cells. Nat Cell Biol 2:84–89
28. Graff JR, Herman JG, Lapidus RG, Chopra H, Xu R, Jarrard DF, Isaacs WB, Pitha PM, Davidson NE, Baylin SB (1995) E-cadherin expression is silenced by DNA hypermethylation in human breast and prostate carcinomas. Cancer Res 55:5195–5199
29. Kuo YC, Su CH, Liu CY, Chen TH, Chen CP, Wang HS (2009) Transforming growth factor-β induces CD44 cleavage that promotes migration of MDA-MB-435s cells through the up-regulation of membrane type 1-matrix metalloproteinase. Int J Cancer 124:2568–2576
30. Bates RC, Bellovin DI, Brown C, Maynard E, Wu B, Kawakatsu H, Sheppard D, Oettgen P, Mercurio AM (2005) Transcriptional activation of integrin β6 during the epithelial–mesenchymal transition defines a novel prognostic indicator of aggressive colon carcinoma. J Clin Invest 115:339–347
31. Montironi R, Santoni M, Scarpelli M, Piva F, Lopez-Beltran A, Cheng L, Briganti A, Montorsi F (2015) Re: epithelial-to-mesenchymal transition in renal neoplasms. Eur Urol 68(4):736–737
32. Piva F, Giulietti M, Santoni M, Occhipinti G, Scarpelli M, Lopez-Beltran A, Cheng L, Principato G, Montironi R (2016) Epithelial to mesenchymal transition in renal cell carcinoma: implications for cancer therapy. Mol Diagn Ther 20(2):111–117
33. Chaffer CL, Brennan JP, Slavin JL, Blick T, Thompson EW, Williams ED (2006) Mesenchymal-to-epithelial transition facilitates bladder cancer metastasis: role of fibroblast growth factor receptor-2. Cancer Res 66(23):11271–11278
34. Bae KM, Parker NN, Dai Y, Vieweg J, Siemann DW (2011) E-cadherin plasticity in prostate cancer stem cell invasion. Am J Cancer Res 1(1):71–84
35. Shiota M, Itsumi M, Takeuchi A, Imada K, Yokomizo A, Kuruma H, Inokuchi J, Tatsugami K, Uchiumi T, Oda Y, Naito S (2015) Crosstalk between epithelial-mesenchymal transition and castration resistance mediated by Twist1/AR signaling in prostate cancer. Endocr Relat Cancer 22(6):889–900
36. Fournier PG, Juárez P, Jiang G, Clines GA, Niewolna M, Kim HS et al (2015) The TGF-β signaling regulator PMEPA1 suppresses prostate cancer metastases to bone. Cancer Cell 27(6):809–821
37. Haider M, Zhang X, Coleman I, Ericson N, True LD, Lam HM, Brown LG, Ketchanji M, Nghiem B, Lakely B, Coleman R, Montgomery B, Lange PH, Roudier M, Higano CS, Bielas JH, Nelson PS, Vessella RL, Morrissey C (2016) Epithelial mesenchymal-like transition occurs in a subset of cells in castration resistant prostate cancer bone metastases. Clin Exp Metastasis 33(3):239–248
38. Bae K-M, Su Z, Frye C et al (2010) Expression of pluripotent stem cell reprogramming factors by prostate tumor initiating cells. J Urol 183(5):2045–2053
39. Celià-Terrassa T, Meca-Cortés Ó, Mateo F et al (2012) Epithelial-mesenchymal transition can suppress major attributes of human epithelial tumor-initiating cells. J Clin Invest 122(5):1849–1868
40. Liu YN, Liu Y, Lee HJ et al (2008) Activated androgen receptor downregulates E-cadherin gene expression and promotes tumor metastasis. Mol Cell Biol 28: 7096–7108

41. Makrilia N, Kollias A, Manolopoulos L et al (2009) Cell adhesion molecules: role and clinical significance in cancer. Cancer Invest 27:1023–1037
42. Gravdal K, Halvorsen OJ, Haukaas SA et al (2007) A switch from E-cadherin to N-cadherin expression indicates epithelial to mesenchymal transition and is of strong and independent importance for the progress of prostate cancer. Clin Cancer Res 13:7003–7011
43. Tanaka H, Kono E, Tran CP et al (2010) Monoclonal antibody targeting of N-cadherin inhibits prostate cancer growth, metastasis and castration resistance. Nat Med 16:1414–1420
44. Santoni M, Bracarda S, Nabissi M, Massari F, Conti A, Bria E, Tortora G, Santoni G, Cascinu S (2014) CXC and CC chemokines as angiogenic modulators in non-haematological tumors. Biomed Res Int 2014:768758
45. Luster AD (1998) Chemokines–chemotactic cytokines that mediate inflammation. N Engl J Med 338:436–445
46. Murphy PM (1994) The molecular biology of leukocyte chemoattractant receptors. Annu Rev Immunol 12:593–633
47. Taichman RS et al (2002) Use of the stromal cell-derived factor-1/CXCR4 pathway in prostate cancer metastasis to bone. Cancer Res 62(6):1832–1837
48. Hsiao JJ, Ng BH, Smits MM, Wang J, Jasavala RJ, Martinez HD et al (2015) Androgen receptor and chemokine receptors 4 and 7 form a signaling axis to regulate CXCL12-dependent cellular motility. BMC Cancer 15:204
49. Shiozawa Y, Pedersen EA, Havens AM, Jung Y, Mishra A, Joseph J et al (2011) Human prostate cancer metastases target the hematopoietic stem cell niche to establish footholds in mouse bone marrow. J Clin Invest 121(4):1298–1312
50. Eaton CL, Colombel M, van der Pluijm G, Cecchini M, Wetterwald A, Lippitt J et al (2010) Evaluation of the frequency of putative prostate cancer stem cells in primary and metastatic prostate cancer. Prostate 70(8):875–882
51. Domanska UM, Timmer-Bosscha H, Nagengast WB, Oude Munnink TH, Kruizinga RC, Ananias HJ et al (2012) CXCR4 inhibition with AMD3100 sensitizes prostate cancer to docetaxel chemotherapy. Neoplasia 14:709–718
52. Fu Q, Liu X, Liu Y, Yang J, Lv G, Dong S (2015) MicroRNA-335 and −543 suppress bone metastasis in prostate cancer via targeting endothelial nitric oxide synthase. Int J Mol Med 36(5):1417–1425
53. Bonci D, Coppola V, Patrizii M, Addario A, Cannistraci A, Francescangeli F et al (2015) A microRNA code for prostate cancer metastasis. Oncogene. doi:10.1038/onc.2015.176
54. Chang YS, Chen WY, Yin JJ, Sheppard-Tillman H, Huang J, Liu YN (2015) EGF receptor promotes prostate cancer bone metastasis by downregulating miR-1 and activating TWIST1. Cancer Res 75(15): 3077–3086
55. Wang L, Song G, Tan W, Qi M, Zhang L, Chan J, Yu J, Han J, Han B (2015) MiR-573 inhibits prostate cancer metastasis by regulating epithelial-mesenchymal transition. Oncotarget 6(34):35978–35990
56. Li X, Liu Y, Wu B, Dong Z, Wang Y, Lu J et al (2014) Potential role of the OPG/RANK/RANKL axis in prostate cancer invasion and bone metastasis. Oncol Rep 32(6):2605–2611
57. Hall CL, Kang S, MacDougald OA, Keller ET (2006) Role of Wnts in prostate cancer bone metastases. J Cell Biochem 97(4):661–672
58. Lacey DL, Timms E, Tan HL, Kelley MJ, Dunstan CR, Burgess T, Elliott R, Colombero A, Elliott G, Scully S, Hsu H, Sullivan J, Hawkins N, Davy E, Capparelli C, Eli A, Qian YX, Kaufman S, Sarosi I, Shalhoub V, Senaldi G, Guo J, Delaney J, Boyle WJ (1998) Osteoprotegerin ligand is a cytokine that regulates osteoclast differentiation and activation. Cell 93(2):165–176
59. Miller J et al (2002) The core-binding factor beta subunit is required for bone formation and hematopoietic maturation. Nat Genet 32(4):645–649
60. Miftakhova R, Hedblom A, Semenas J, Robinson BD, Simoulis A, Malm J, Rizvanov A, David Heery D, Mongan NP, Maitland NJ, Allegrucci C, Persson JL (2016) Cyclin A1 and P450 aromatase promote metastatic homing and growth of stem-like prostate cancer cells in the bone marrow. Cancer Res 76(8):2453–2464, pii: canres.2340.2015
61. Hauschka PV et al (1986) Growth factors in bone matrix. Isolation of multiple types by affinity chromatography on heparin-Sepharose. J Biol Chem 261(27):12665–12674
62. Golen CM et al (2006) Insulin-such as growth factor-I receptor expression regulates neuroblastoma metastasis to bone. Cancer Res 66(13):6570–6578
63. Christopherson KW 2nd, Hangoc G, Broxmeyer HE (2002) Cell surface peptidase CD26/dipeptidylpeptidase IV regulates CXCL12/stromal cell-derived factor-1 alpha-mediated chemotaxis of human cord blood CD34+ progenitor cells. J Immunol 169(12): 7000–7008
64. Webb SD, Sherratt JA, Fish RG (1999) Alterations in proteolytic activity at low pH and its association with invasion: a theoretical model. Clin Exp Metastasis 17(5):397–407
65. Sanders JL et al (2001) Ca(2+)-sensing receptor expression and PTHrP secretion in PC-3 human prostate cancer cells. Am J Physiol Endocrinol Metab 281(6):1267–1274
66. Cho WJ, Oliveira DS, Najy AJ, Mainetti LE, Aoun HD, Cher ML, Heath E, Kim HR, Bonfil RD (2016) Gene expression analysis of bone metastasis and circulating tumor cells from metastatic castrate-resistant prostate cancer patients. J Transl Med 14(1):72

Markers of Prostate Cancer: The Role of Circulating Tumor Markers in the Management of Bone Metastases

4

Massimo Gion, Chiara Trevisiol, Giulia Rainato, and Aline S.C. Fabricio

The present chapter concerns the role of circulating tumor markers in the management of bone metastases in patients with prostate cancer. We first discuss the contemporary notion of tumor markers from a general point of view. We focus on some specific characteristics of prostate-specific antigen (PSA), showing why it is the sole circulating tumor marker presently recommended in the follow-up of patients – with or without metastases – treated with curative intents for a primary prostate cancer. The role of PSA in the different clinical settings in which the marker may be used is then discussed. The position of the most recent clinical practice guidelines is examined, and recommendations concerning PSA are presented and discussed with reference to key clinical scenarios. We considered the initial assessment of the risk of developing bone metastases, the early detection of relapse during the follow-up, and the management of the relapse; this latter issue is discussed considering separately patients with biochemical relapse and those with manifest clinical metastases.

M. Gion (✉) • A.S.C. Fabricio
Centro Regionale Specializzato e Programma Regionale Biomarcatori, Azienda ULSS 12 Veneziana, Venice, Italy
e-mail: massimo.gion@ulss12.ve.it

C. Trevisiol • G. Rainato
Istituto Oncologico Veneto IOV – IRCCS, Padova, Italy

4.1 Contemporary Notion of "Tumor Marker"

According to a recent definition, a cancer biomarker is "A characteristic that is objectively measured and evaluated as an indicator of normal biological processes, pathogenic processes, or pharmacologic responses to a therapeutic intervention" [1]. This definition has been tailored in order to adapt biomarkers to both the traditional areas of utilization and the emerging needs related to the development and the early validation of new anticancer agents. As such, this is a broad definition which encompasses a wide variety of different indicators, such as soluble circulating biomarkers, prognostic and predictive tissue biomarkers, imaging-related biomarkers, as well as clinical signs or symptoms, which are per se "biomarker" of the response to some of the available molecular targeted antigens [1].

The present chapter focuses on a subset of biomarkers, represented by soluble, proteinaceous molecules measurable in body fluids, traditionally referred to as "tumor markers".

In order to facilitate the appropriate use of tumor markers in clinical practice, it is crucial to be aware of some limitations that after over four decades of research and clinical applications have appeared to be inherent to tumor markers [2]. First, the conventional term "tumor marker" is currently considered misleading, because the so-called tumor markers are not "tumor specific."

F. Bertoldo et al. (eds.), *Bone Metastases from Prostate Cancer*,
DOI 10.1007/978-3-319-42327-2_4

In fact a variety of conditions may affect the actual level of the markers in the bloodstream, encompassing the production and the release from the tumor (when present), the production and release of the marker by normal tissues, the presence of cross-reacting substances, the dilution in bloodstream, metabolism, and excretion. Therefore, circulating levels of so-called tumor markers are the sum of several variables, including (when present) malignancy. Physiological conditions and lifestyle patterns, diseases other than cancer, and iatrogenic artifacts may interfere with the production and release of markers from healthy tissues, thus causing false-positive results. Therefore, it is presently well established that tumor markers have a poor diagnostic specificity for the tumor and – with the exception of few circumstances – they are not useful in the differential diagnosis of a malignancy. Second, tumor marker circulating levels are directly related to tumor bulk: the larger the tumor, the higher the detectable concentration of the marker in the bloodstream. A consequence of this is that the level of the marker is expected to be low in a patient with a minimal tumor mass; therefore, tumor markers present poor diagnostic sensitivity in the early detection of malignancies.

Third, a point of weakness of tumor markers as diagnostic tools is their poor tumor-type specificity. For instance, many different tissues may produce and release carcinoembryonic antigen, alpha-fetoprotein, as well as the carbohydrate antigens CA125, CA19.9, and CA15.3. Thus, low positive levels of these markers are poorly informative in the clinical practice.

Remarkably, the above-mentioned limitations – poor diagnostic sensitivity and specificity and poor tumor-type specificity – have different implications in different clinical scenarios, depending on the prevalence of the malignancy. A marker may be ineffective if used for the diagnosis of a malignancy in asymptomatic subjects or in patients with indeterminate symptoms, since false-positive results are expected to be much more numerous than true-positive ones, thus leading to a very low-positive predictive value. Conversely, the same tumor marker could be effective if used in the follow-up of an operated patient with intermediate-high risk of relapse. In fact, in this latter scenario, the true-positive results are expected to be prevalent on false-positive ones, thus leading to a higher positive predictive value [3]. The same marker would be very effective to monitor the response to therapy in patients with metastatic disease, since changes in the marker levels during the treatment are almost certainly related to the response – or no response – of the malignancy to the therapy.

> In summary, diagnostic performance of circulating tumor markers depends on the clinical setting in which they are applied. Hence, the clinical usefulness of tumor markers is strictly related to the appropriateness of their use. A marker inappropriately requested may be useless at best, whereas a marker requested in the right patient, for the right clinical question and in the right scenario, may have a pivotal role in clinical decision making.

4.2 Prostate-Specific Antigen: A Singular Tumor Marker

Prostate-specific antigen (PSA), also referred to as kallikrein-3, is a glycoprotein member of the kallikrein peptidase family, produced and released by prostate glandular epithelium. PSA has been extensively studied, and is currently used as a tumor marker in patients with suspicious or diagnosed prostate cancer. PSA presents two valuable features that may be considered almost exclusive in the landscape of the available circulating tumor markers. First, PSA has an absolute specificity for a single type of tissue, that is, prostate glandular epithelium; second, PSA is expressed and released by the majority of prostate cancers; only a limited number of prostate cancers express low PSA levels or do not express PSA at all, but this occurs almost exclusively in undifferentiated tumors [4].

While these features are of no special value when PSA is used for the diagnosis of a suspicious prostate cancer, they are indeed crucial in a patient followed up after a diagnosis of prostate cancer. In fact, the absolute tissue specificity of PSA is of no help in the diagnostic phase of prostate cancer. In a subject with an intact prostate gland, any increase of circulating PSA may be due to a plethora of causes other than cancer, because of the lack of tumor specificity of the marker. From the point of view of laboratory medicine, PSA is the ideal organ-specific marker, such as aspartate transferase for liver disease, but it is much more specific. In view of this, PSA is considered a very effective marker to monitor benign prostatic hyperplasia and to predict its major complications [5]. On the other hand, this is the major shortcoming of PSA as a diagnostic tool for prostate cancer. Not surprisingly, over the past two decades, the awareness of the ineffectiveness of PSA to detect prostate cancer prompted extensive research on PSA derivatives (i.e., PSA density, PSA velocity), PSA isoforms (i.e., free PSA, conjugated PSA, proPSA) [7], and novel biomarkers belonging to different molecular families (i.e., PCA-3, TMPRSS2-ERG gene fusions) [8]. Conversely, when patients diagnosed with prostate cancer have been treated, PSA *becomes* cancer specific. If the patient is radically treated with curative intent, prostate gland is either completely removed by surgery or biologically shut down by radiotherapy. Therefore, PSA must become undetectable after prostatectomy or reach stable, very low, nadir values after radiotherapy. Under these clinical circumstances, any increase of PSA values is cancer specific, since no other healthy or benign tissue exists in the body that is capable of producing and releasing detectable PSA amounts.

The second valuable feature of PSA concerns the homogeneity of its production by prostate cancer. Many other malignancies present a low rate of positivity of tumor marker in the early phase of metastatic outspread. For instance, in early phases of relapse, the positivity rate of CA15.3 in patients with breast cancer is approximately 50–60 % and that of CEA in colorectal cancer 60–80 %; moreover, both makers show specificity values lower that 70–80. On the contrary, almost all patients with relapsing prostate cancer exhibit a PSA increase. Distant metastases have been shown to occur very rarely also in patients with undetectable PSA, but this occurs almost exclusively in undifferentiated tumors [4]. The almost unique behavior of PSA is due to both the high rate of prostate malignancies producing PSA and the entire absence of "noise" that might mislead the PSA assay result. For instance, CA15.3 and CEA have a baseline level due to the production of the marker by diverse tissues, and small increases due to tumor progression may remain masked within the baseline "noise" level. On the contrary, any value of detectable PSA is a signal of the tumor. Therefore, PSA is extremely useful in monitoring patients radically treated for prostate cancer since no false-positive results may occur and even a very small amount of marker may indicate the relapse. Not surprisingly, the research in this scenario has mainly pursued the refinement of PSA-based decision criteria and the integration of PSA with other clinical and pathological information.

In summary, in patients radically cured for prostate cancer, PSA presents the characteristics of the ideal tumor markers that are, absolute diagnostic specificity, very high diagnostic sensitivity, minimal invasiveness, widespread availability, high reproducibility, and low cost.

4.3 Clinical Settings in Which PSA May Be Used in the Decision Process

PSA has been extensively studied, in association with other clinical and pathological variables, as a predictive marker of disease outcome in patients diagnosed with prostate cancer. The scenarios in which PSA has been evaluated are: (i) the prediction of outcomes in newly diagnosed patients before any therapeutic intervention, (ii)

Table 4.1 Catalog of prostate cancer predictive tools

Clinical question	No. of tools concerning the clinical question	No. of tool that considered PSA	No. of tools subjected to validation
Prediction of the presence of prostate cancer in the initial biopsy setting	12	12	5
Prediction of the presence of prostate cancer in other than an initial biopsy setting (repeat biopsy)	14	14	6
Prediction of pathologic stage in men who underwent radical prostatectomy for clinically localized prostate cancer	29	29	22
Preoperative prediction of biochemical recurrence in men who underwent radical prostatectomy	9	9	6
Postoperative prediction of biochemical recurrence in men who underwent radical prostatectomy	8	6	5
Pretreatment prediction of biochemical recurrence in men treated with radiotherapy	10	10	5
Prediction of metastasis and survival	17	16	13
Prediction of life expectancy	4	2	2
Prediction of specific pathological features or biochemical recurrence after radical prostatectomy for clinically localized prostate cancer based on novel variables	6	6	6

Modified from Ref. [15]

the prediction of clinical relapse after the radical treatment of primary prostate cancer, and (iii) the prediction of survival in patients with bone metastases. These scenarios are complex and outcomes of interest differ within the same scenario [9, 10]. In fact, the prediction of outcome in newly diagnosed patients encompasses the prediction of pathological stage, the assessment of risk of bone metastases, and assessment of life expectancy. Likewise, the prediction of clinical relapse concerns patients with biochemical recurrence after either radical prostatectomy or curative radiotherapy as well as patients without evidence of metastases receiving androgen-deprivation therapy (ADT) or those become castration-resistant while on ADT.

Accurate estimates of the probability of diverse risks are crucial in the decision process. Given the complexity of the disease, when choices have to be taken on the individual-patient basis, both subjective and objective variables may bias clinicians' estimates of risks. For that reason, many predictive models have been developed with the scope of improving accuracy and reproducibility of estimates. A variety of predictive tools have been proposed, including risk groupings, probability tables, nomograms, artificial neural networks (ANNs), and classification and regression tree (CART) analyses. Their complexity ranges from group classification based on a limited number of parameters, such as the D'Amico risk criterion [11] or the University of California, San Francisco Cancer of the Prostate Risk Assessment (CAPRA) [12], to more complex "Kattan-type" nomograms [13] or Partin probability tables [14]. A published catalog of prostate cancer predictive tools identified 109 prediction tools, 68 of which have been validated, to be applied in a variety of clinical scenarios, as summarized in Table 4.1 [15].

While approximately half of the tools have been developed to predict either the result of biopsy or pathological stage, 54 tools were focused on the prediction of outcomes after the treatment of primary tumor in newly diagnosed patients. The majority of them (49/54) included PSA and 68.5 % underwent either internal or external validation, while only a limited number of tools (6/109) considered novel variables [15]. Notably, these tools have been tested and validated in thousands of patients.

In summary, PSA has been extensively studied in all the clinical conditions that may occur from the treatment with curative intent of the primary prostate cancer to the development and the treatment of the bone. Many diagnostic tools integrating PSA with other clinical and pathological information have been developed to facilitate unbiased clinical decisions

4.4 The Position of Clinical Practice Guidelines

From the above findings, it could be argued that evidence should be adequate to provide clinicians with established recommendations for the clinical practice.

We therefore examined available guidelines in order to search for established recommendations concerning the use of PSA for either the prediction or management of metastatic prostate cancer. In the context of a broader project aimed at updating the synopsis of existing recommendations on tumor markers in solid tumors [16], we set up a search strategy and explored the following databases: Pubmed-Medline, National Guideline Clearinghouse (NGC) and GIN library; we also interrogated 11 websites of scientific societies producing guidelines and 61 websites of medical scientific societies [16]. The search was conducted in the last 5 years and sorted 96 documents identified as guidelines concerning prostate cancer, which were further examined and selected on the basis of the methodological quality and rate of utilization by clinicians in Italy. The methodological quality was evaluated according to inclusion criteria set by National Guideline Clearinghouse, and documents were selected if the clinical practice guideline was based on a systematic review and a description of the search strategy was reported. Widely used guidelines were considered also when methodology was not fully compliant with above mentioned criteria. A total of 35 guidelines concerning prostate cancer were eventually selected. The recommendations concerning the use of PSA in the different clinical settings were extracted and synoptically presented.

4.5 PSA as Risk Predictor in Newly Diagnosed Patients Before Any Therapeutic Intervention

In this clinical setting, PSA may provide information on both long-term outcomes – such as biochemical recurrence, clinical recurrence, and survival – and the risk that occult bone metastases may be already present at the time of first diagnosis. Table 4.2 summarizes the recommendations of the examined guidelines.

Six clinical practice guidelines recommend the use of PSA to categorize patients into risk groups [17–22]; all of them recommend to use the D'Amico risk criterion [11], in which PSA is used in association with Gleason score and clinical stage. More complex algorithms are mentioned by some guidelines [21, 24–26], but no specific approaches are suggested in the recommendations other than the D'Amico risk criterion.

Five clinical practice guidelines consider the risk of metastatic spread in newly diagnosed patients with apparently locoregional disease and conclude that bone scan positivity is expected to be extremely low (<1 %) in low-risk patients with PSA values ≤10 ng/mL [18, 21–24]. As a result, all the five examined guidelines state that imaging staging (CT and bone scan) should be considered in patients with a PSA level >20 ng/mL prior to treatment.

In summary, PSA determination is recommended in newly diagnosed patients before any therapeutic intervention and the result considered in association with clinical stage and biopsy Gleason score to predict the risk of recurrence.

A value of PSA >10 or >20 ng/mL is *per se* a predictor of intermediate or high risk, respectively.

Bone scan should be performed with a PSA > 20 ng/mL.

Table 4.2 Summary of recommendation(s) on PSA as risk predictor in the pretreatment staging of prostate cancer

Organization	Summary of recommendation(s)	PSA risk criteria
Cancer Care Ontario (2010) [17]	PSA is used as risk stratification to plan treatment type	Low risk: PSA ≤10 ng/mL *and* a biopsy Gleason score of 6 or less *and* clinical stage T1c or T2a Intermediate risk: PSA >10 to 20 ng/mL *or* a biopsy Gleason score of 7 *or* clinical stage T2b High risk: PSA >20 ng/mL *or* a biopsy Gleason score of 8 to 10 *or* clinical stage T2c
American Urological Association (2011) [18]	PSA in association with Gleason score and clinical stage is used as risk stratification to discuss with the patient the choice of therapy options Radiographic staging (CT and bone scan) is recommended for patients with or a PSA level >20 ng/mL prior to treatment	
European Society of Medical Oncology (2013) [19]	Localized disease should be classified as low, intermediate, or high risk as a guide to staging and therapy	
National Institute for Health and Care Excellence (2014) [20]	PSA, Gleason score, and clinical stage are predictive factors for risk groups	
European Association of Urology (2015) [21]	PSA in association with Gleason score and clinical stage is used to determine risk groups for biochemical recurrence of localized and locally advanced prostate cancer Bone scan positivity rate is extremely low (<1 %) in low-risk patients (≤10 ng/mL)	
National Comprehensive Cancer Network (2015) [22]	PSA, Gleason score, and clinical stage are predictive factors for risk groups Bone scan if any of these: T1 and PSA >20, T2 and PSA >10 mL	
Groupe Européen de Curiethérapie-European SocieTy for Radiotherapy and Oncology (2013) [23]	Isotope bone scan should be considered for all patients with a PSA > 20 ng/mL	PSA > 20 ng/mL
American Urological Association (2013) [24]	Routine use of a bone scan is not required for staging asymptomatic men with clinically localized prostate cancer when their PSA level is equal to or less than 20.0 ng/mL Computed tomography or magnetic resonance imaging scans may be considered for the staging of men with high-risk, clinically localized prostate cancer when the PSA is greater than 20.0 ng/mL or when locally advanced or when the Gleason score is greater than or equal to 8	PSA > 20 ng/mL

4.6 PSA for the Detection of Recurrence and Assessment of Adverse Outcomes After the Treatment of the Primary Tumor

The natural history of prostate cancer is characteristically long, and recurrence may occur years after the treatment of the primary tumor with curative intent. In the long term, a significant percentage of patients – from 11 to 40 % according to different studies – will eventually develop recurrent disease [27–29]. Bone metastases represent the predominant site of distant recurrence in patients with prostate cancer, occurring in a high percentage of patients as unique site of metastatic spread [30].

Given its excellent characteristics of sensitivity and specificity, PSA is the tool of choice for the routine monitoring of patients with prostate cancer treated with curative intent, in order to detect early disease recurrence. However, just thanks to its elevated sensitivity, PSA may become detectable years before the occurrence of clinical signs of disease progression. The occurrence of detectable PSA values in many patients, without overt signs of regional or distant progressive disease after initial therapy with curative intent, leads to identify a new clinical scenario, labeled as *biochemical recurrence* or *PSA recurrence*. It has been estimated that approximately 35–50 % of patients will experience a PSA recurrence within 10 years after radical prostatectomy or radiation therapy [31]. The time between PSA recurrence and the occurrence metastatic disease is variable and in general extended, with a reported median time of 8 years [32]. Frequently androgen deprivation therapy (ADT) is prescribed before metastases appear, and many patients with PSA recurrence after primary therapy receive ADT [33–35]. Men developing PSA progression while receiving ADT are considered castration-resistant prostate cancer (CRPC), and those cases in which metastases are undetectable by imaging are labeled as nonmetastatic CRPC (M0-CRPC). It has been reported that approximately 10–20 % of patients, without evidence of metastases and treated with ADT, will eventually develop CRPC within approximately 5 years [33]. CRPC is a further step in the progression of prostate cancer toward clinically evident disseminated disease; 33 % of CRPC patients have been shown to develop bone metastases within 2 years [33], and different studies report a median survival from CRPC diagnosis ranging from 9 to 30 months [36].

The follow-up after the treatment of the primary tumor with curative intent is a manifold scenario in which variations of clinical conditions over time induce different clinical questions. The key point is to offer appropriate treatment options to each individual patients, weighing the benefit of supplying potential life prolonging therapies to patients with aggressive prostate cancer and the risk of over-treating men with indolent disease.

During this long-lasting time period after radical treatment of primary prostate cancer, the questions facing both the clinician and patient are as follows: When PSA reliably indicates the biochemical recurrence? Which is the risk of clinical progression after the biochemical recurrence in patients either on ADT or in the CRPC phase?

4.6.1 PSA as Indicator of Biochemical Recurrence

All examined guidelines recommend to offer to patients periodical PSA determinations to detect disease recurrence. The detection of biochemical relapse after prostatectomy is a relatively simple issue, and clinical practice guidelines agree that any rise in PSA to detectable levels after radical prostatectomy indicates a biochemical relapse. Also, the value of 0.2 ng/mL is unanimously considered the cutoff value to indicate a PSA relapse. Notably, a confirmatory PSA determination is recommended by most guidelines (Table 4.3).

The definition of biochemical recurrence following radiation therapy is more difficult because radiotherapy, differently from radical prostatectomy, does not remove all PSA-producing cells at once. The average half-life of serum PSA after radiation therapy has been reported to be 1.9 months [39], and the achievement of PSA nadir value may require up to 3 years [21, 40]. Consensus was initially reached by the American Society of Therapeutic Radiology and Oncology on the definition of treatment failure after external beam radiation therapy with or without hormonal therapy as a rise by 2 ng/mL or more above the nadir PSA [41], and this criterion is presently adopted by clinical practice guidelines (Table 4.3).

An emerging issue is the risk of anxiety and depression that may arise in patients with biochemical recurrence or even in men undergoing long-term PSA monitoring. Two guidelines [38, 42] explicitly recommend to periodically assess for anxiety or depression the patients in follow-up after treatment of primary tumor with curative intent using specific tools.

Additional criteria have been developed to define relapsing CRPC while on ADT therapy and are reported by some clinical practice guidelines (Table 4.4).

All guidelines agree on the clinical meaning of a rise of PSA, as well as on the value of 2 ng/mL to consider a possible occurrence of CRPC. Three out of four guidelines recommend that castrate levels of circulating testosterone are a requisite to interpret rising PSA in ADT patients [21, 24, 44]. Conversely, the recommendations

Table 4.3 Summary of recommendation(s) on PSA criteria to define biochemical relapse

Organization	PSA criteria to define biochemical relapse
Alberta Health Services (2013) [37]	After radical prostatectomy: any rise in PSA After radiation therapy (with or without hormonal therapy): rise by 2 ng/mL (mcg/L) or more above the nadir PSA (defined as the lowest PSA achieved).
American Society of Clinical Oncology (2014) [38]	Detectable or increasing PSA value after surgery that is 0.2 ng/ mL, with a second confirmatory level 0.2 ng/mL
European Association of Urology (2015) [21]	After radical prostatectomy, recurrent cancer may be defined by two consecutive PSA values of>0.2 ng/mL After radiation therapy, a rising PSA level over 2 ng/mL above the nadir PSA is the most reliable sign of recurrent disease
American Urological Association-American Society for Radiation Oncology (2013) [39]	PSA value after surgery that is≥0.2 ng/mL with a second confirmatory level≥0.2 ng/mL Some modalities (e.g., bone scan) are extremely low in patients with PSA values below 10 ng/mL
National Comprehensive Cancer Network (2015) [22]	Detectable PSA that increases on 2 or more determinations (PSA recurrence)

Table 4.4 PSA and definition of relapsing prostate cancer after castration

Organization	Criteria to identify CRPC
European Association of Urology (2015) [21]	PSA level greater than 2 ng/mL
	Three consecutive rises of PSA, 1 week apart, resulting in two 50 % increases over the nadir
	Castrate level of testosterone (less than 50 ng/ mL or 1.7 nmol/L)
American Urological Association (2013) [24]	PSA level greater than 2 ng/mL
	Rise has to be at least 25 % over nadir and the rise has to be confirmed by a second PSA at least 3 weeks later
	Castrate levels of testosterone (less than 50 ng/ mL or 1.7 nmol/L)
Spanish Oncology Genitourinary Group (2012) [43]	PSA level greater than 2 ng/mL above the nadir
	Three consecutive PSA rises (1 week apart) resulting in two increases of 25 % above the nadir
Advanced Prostate Cancer Consensus Conference (2015) [44]	A rising PSA confirmed by a second value 3 or more weeks later
	Castrate levels of testosterone (less than 50 ng/ mL or 1.7 nmol/L)

differ in part as concerns the rate of increase of PSA (50 % or 25 %) to be considered to establish the progression. However, the differences of suggested PSA increases do not influence the actual value of the marker in the detection of CRPC.

In summary, PSA is a very effective tool for the early detection of relapse during both the follow-up after radical prostatectomy or radiation therapy and ADT administration.

PSA-based decision criteria are well established and easy to use.

4.6.2 PSA as Risk Predictor of Clinical Progression and Adverse Outcome After the Treatment of the Primary Tumor

The risk of biochemical recurrence may be assessed both before and soon after the radical prostatectomy. The position of the scientific community – expressed in clinical practice guidelines – on the role of PSA as a risk predictor in the pretreatment staging of prostate cancer has been mentioned above (see Table 4.2). Various authors have also proposed post-intervention risk assessment based on pathological findings, in

Table 4.5 Summary of recommendation(s) on PSA as risk predictor

Organization	Criteria to predict the risk of clinical relapse
Alberta Health Services (2013) [37]	PSA relapse within 12 months of surgery is a strong predictor of adverse long-term outcome PSADT appears to have prognostic power
European Association of Urology (2015) [21]	After radical prostatectomy, high risk: PSADT < 3 months or time to PSA-recurrence < 3 years. Low risk: PSADT > 12 months and PSA recurrence > 3 years following surgery After radiation therapy, high risk: PSADT < 3 months and PSA recurrence < 3 years. Low risk: PSADT > 15 months and PSA recurrence > 3 years
National Comprehensive Cancer Network (2015) [22]	PSADT >= 10 vs < 10 months as decision criteria

addition to clinical information and pre-intervention PSA level. Several variables have been considered by different studies, including surgical Gleason score, surgical margin status, extracapsular extension, lymph node invasion, and seminal vesicle invasion. In spite of increased available information, the reported predictive accuracies of risk assessment for biochemical recurrence do not differ significantly between postoperative (from 76 to 90 %) and preoperative (form 77 to 94 %) [15].

When the biochemical recurrence occurs during the follow-up, the evaluation of the risk of clinical recurrence is pivotal to take proper clinical choices. The scenario of rising PSA without evidence of metastases concerns both ADT naive patients in follow-up after the treatment of the primary tumor and patients which have developed a M0-CRPC while on ADT.

Beside clinical and therapeutic issues, several PSA-related variables potentially associated to outcomes of interest have been evaluated, including time of PSA failure, trigger PSA, PSA doubling time (PSADT), and PSA velocity. Identified guidelines concerning this issue (Table 4.5) recommend to consider PSADT and time to PSA relapse from surgery. Two guidelines recommending PSADT suggest, however, different cutoff points [21, 22].

Both PSA and PSAD have been shown to be the only significant parameters to predict the risk of a positive bone scan also in M0-CRPC [33, 45, 46]. PSA and PSADT have also been reported to be strong predictors for the length of life and prostate cancer-specific mortality [45].

However, cutoff points of PSADT reported in the literature are variable, presumably depending at least in part on both the mixed patient series examined (i.e., followed-up after prostatectomy after radiation therapy or both) and the considered scenario (i.e., ADT naive patients, M0-CRPC). Accordingly, Freeland et al. have recently commented that "the exact risk threshold that should prompt imaging should be left to the discretion of the patient and treating physician" [45]. In fact, the association between PSADT and disease progression or prostate cancer-specific mortality is almost certainly represented by a continuous relationship, with shorter PSADT values being associated to a high risk for prostate cancer-specific mortality and longer ones being associated to a lower risk. The Prostate-Specific Antigen Working Group Guidelines on PSADT have established that men with a PSADT of less than 3 months are at extremely high risk for adverse clinical outcomes and men with a slow PSADT (more than 15 months) have an extremely low risk of death from prostate cancer [47]. However, the panel recognized that no best threshold is known for patients with an intermediate PSADT of 3–15 months, which unfortunately represent the majority of patients with biochemical relapse [47].

A major shortcoming affecting PSADT reliability is the complexity of standardization of its calculation. In general, PSADT is calculated by the natural log of 2 divided by the slope of the linear regression line of log of the PSA over time [46]. However, it has been shown that the comparability of results obtained in different studies may be affected by several variables, including methods of calculating (log-slope method or two-point method), calculation interval (two consecutive increases of PSA level, each greater than 25 % of the nadir value or nadir value), data acquisition (PSA assay type, minimum PSA increase, sampling frequency), and data analysis (either nadir subtraction or not) [48]. In addition, it has been reported that 33 % of cancers may not follow first-order kinetics in their growth [49]. Therefore, even if PSADT calculation was perfectly standardized, PSADT should not be evaluable by the reported equation, and the values of PSADT could be misleading in a third of the patients [49].

In summary, PSADT is an effective predictor of risk of recurrence, bone metastases, and prostate cancer-specific mortality. However, caution is requested to properly use PSADT in clinical practice, and the clinician must be aware of the following shortcomings: (i) PSADT is very informative in its extreme values (very fast and very slow), while its association with clinical outcomes is less stringent in its intermediate values range, and (ii) calculation is not easy, nor standardized.

4.7 PSA as a Test to Monitor Response to Treatment of Bone Metastases

Almost all identified guidelines recommend to include PSA and testosterone in the periodical evaluation of metastatic patients during hormonal treatment and suggest a timing ranging from 3 to 6 months after the initiation of treatment [21, 22, 24, 26, 42, 49, 50].

In general, as long as PSA remains at the nadir value achieved with the treatment, the probability of progression is low, and the use of routine bone scans of other imaging techniques is not justified [24, 36].

During the administration of several types of systemic therapies, a confirmed PSA decline of >50 % is reported as PSA benefit [24, 26]. However, this criterion is not presented as a recommendation, but it is reported in the guidelines within the discussion regarding the comparison of different therapeutic regimens. Therefore, it can be assumed that further investigation is needed to establish PSA-based surrogate criteria of response or failure to systemic therapies of metastatic prostate cancer.

In summary, regular determinations of PSA are recommended in the monitoring of systemic treatment of prostate cancer patients with bone metastases. In general, if PSA remains at the lowest value achieved with the treatment, the probability of progression is low.

4.8 Concluding Remarks

PSA is a very effective tumor marker when it is used in the follow-up of patients previously treated with curative intent for primary prostate cancer. Due to the absence of tissues producing PSA other than prostate gland, the diagnostic specificity of an increasing PSA value is almost absolute after radical prostatectomy and radiation therapy. Sensitivity is also very high, because of the absence of biochemical noise in the bloodstream due to PSA from other sources. For these reasons PSA is the sole tumor marker presently recommended in the management of patients after radical treatment of primary prostate cancer.

The early detection of biochemical relapse represents a clinical quandary, due to both the long natural history of prostate cancer and the relative prevalence of patients' indolent disease from one side and the occurrence of aggressive disease in some patients form the other side. After biochemical relapse, PSA-based criteria are used to identify aggressive tumors from indolent ones and to tailor clinical decisions on the individual patient. PSADT is the most effective PSA-based criteria to predict the risk of bone metastases and survival. Very high and very low PSADTs are in fact very predictive. However, the best threshold for patients with intermediate values has not yet defined. Likewise PSA-based decision criteria of response or failure to systemic treatment of bone metastases are still pragmatic. Therefore further research is needed to optimize and standardize some of the most promising and clinically crucial PSA-based decision criteria.

References

1. Khleif SN, Doroshow JH, Hait WN (2010) AACR-FDA-NCI Cancer Biomarkers Collaborative AACR-FDA-NCI Cancer Biomarkers Collaborative consensus report: advancing the use of biomarkers in cancer drug development. Clin Cancer Res 16(13): 3299–3318
2. Diamandis EP (2014) Present and future of cancer biomarkers. Clin Chem Lab Med 52(6):791–794
3. Akobeng AK (2007) Understanding diagnostic tests 2: likelihood ratios, pre- and post-test probabilities and their use in clinical practice. Acta Paediatr 96(4):487–491
4. Sandblom G, Ladjevardi S, Garmo H, Varenhorst E (2008) The impact of prostate-specific antigen level at diagnosis on the relative survival of 28,531 men with localized carcinoma of the prostate. Cancer 112(4): 813–819
5. Roehrborn CG, McConnell J, Bonilla J, Rosenblatt S, Hudson PB, Malek GH, Schellhammer PF, Bruskewitz R, Matsumoto AM, Harrison LH, Fuselier HA, Walsh P, Roy J, Andriole G, Resnick M, Waldstreicher J (2000) Serum prostate specific antigen is a strong predictor of future prostate growth in men with benign prostatic hyperplasia. PROSCAR long-term efficacy and safety study. J Urol 163(1):13–20.
6. Lepor A, Catalona WJ, Loeb S (2016) The prostate health index: its utility in prostate cancer detection. v Urol Clin North Am 43(1):1–6
7. Yang Z, Yu L, Wang Z (2016) PCA3 and TMPRSS2-ERG gene fusions as diagnostic biomarkers for prostate cancer. Chin J Cancer Res 28(1):65–71
8. Freedland SJ, Moul JW (2007) Prostate specific antigen recurrence after definitive therapy. J Urol 177: 1985–1991
9. Briganti A, Suardi N, Gallina A, Abdollah F, Novara G, Ficarra V, Montorsi F (2014) Predicting the risk of bone metastasis in prostate cancer. Cancer Treat Rev 40:3–11
10. D'Amico AV, Whittington R, Malkowicz SB, Schultz D, Blank K, Broderick GA, Tomaszewski JE, Renshaw AA, Kaplan I, Beard CJ, Wein A (1998) Biochemical outcome after radical prostatectomy, external beam radiation therapy, or interstitial radiation therapy for clinically localized prostate cancer. JAMA 280:969–974
11. Cooperberg MR, Pasta DJ, Elkin EP, Litwin MS, Latini DM, Du Chane J, Carroll PR (2005) The University of California, San Francisco Cancer of the Prostate Risk Assessment score: a straightforward and reliable preoperative predictor of disease recurrence after radical prostatectomy. J Urol 173:1938–1942
12. Kattan MW, Eastham JA, Stapleton AM, Wheeler TM, Scardino PT (1998) A preoperative nomogram for disease recurrence following radical prostatectomy for prostate cancer. J Natl Cancer Inst 90(10): 766–771
13. Partin AW, Kattan MW, Subong EN, Walsh PC, Wojno KJ, Oesterling JE, Scardino PT, Pearson JD (1997) Combination of prostate-specific antigen, clinical stage, and Gleason score to predict pathological stage of localized prostate cancer. A multi-institutional update. JAMA 277:1445–1451
14. Shariat SF, Karakiewicz PI, Roehrborn CG, Kattan MW (2008) An updated catalog of prostate cancer predictive tools. Cancer 113:3075–3099
15. Gion M, Trevisiol C, Pregno S, Fabricio ASC (2010) Guida all'uso clinico dei biomarcatori in oncologia. Biomedia, Milano
16. Chin JL, Srigley J, Mayhew LA, Rumble RB, Crossley C, Hunter A, Fleshner N, Bora B, McLeod R, McNair S, Langer B, Evans A (2010) Guideline for optimization of surgical and pathological quality performance for radical prostatectomy in prostate cancer management: evidentiary base. Can Urol Assoc J 4(1):13–25
17. Thompson I, Thrasher JB, Aus G, Burnett AL, Canby-Hagino ED, Cookson MS, D'Amico AV, Dmochowski RR, Eton DT, Forman JD, Goldenberg SL, Hernandez J, Higano CS, Kraus SR, Moul JW, Tangen CM; AUA Prostate Cancer Clinical Guideline Update Panel (2007) Guideline for the management of clinically localized prostate cancer: 2007 update. J Urol 177(6):2106–2131
18. Horwich A, Parker C, de Reijke T, Kataja V; ESMO Guidelines Working Group (2013) Prostate cancer: ESMO Clinical Practice Guidelines for diagnosis, treatment and follow-up. Ann Oncol 24(Suppl6):vi106–114
19. National Collaborating Centre for Cancer (2014) Prostate cancer: diagnosis and treatment. National Institute for Health and Care Excellence, London
20. Mottet N, Bellmunt J, Briers E, van den Bergh RCN, Bolla M, van Casteren NJ, Cornford P, Culine S, Joniau S, Lam T, Mason MD, Matveev V, van der Poel H, van der Kwast TH, Rouvière O, Wiegel T (2015) Guidelines on prostate cancer. European Association of Urology, Arnhem
21. National Comprehensive Cancer Network (NCCN) (2015) Clinical practice guidelines in oncology. Prostate cancer. Washington, PA: National Comprehensive Cancer Network
22. Hoskin PJ, Colombo A, Henry A, Niehoff P, Paulsen Hellebust T, Siebert FA, Kovacs G (2013) GEC/ESTRO recommendations on high dose rate afterloading brachytherapy for localised prostate cancer: an update. Radiother Oncol 107(3):325–332
23. Greene KL, Albertsen PC, Babaian RJ, Carter HB, Gann PH, Han M, Kuban DA, Sartor AO, Stanford JL, Zietman A, Carroll P; American Urological Association (2013) Prostate specific antigen best

practice statement: 2009 update. J Urol 189(1 Suppl):S2–S11
24. Alberta Provincial Genitourinary Tumour Team (2013) Prostate cancer. Cancer Control Alberta, Edmonton
25. Associazione Italiana di Oncologia Medica (2014) Linee guida carcinoma della prostata. AIOM, Milano
26. Banefelt J, Liede A, Mesterton J, Stålhammar J, Hernandez RK, Sobocki P, Persson BE (2014) Survival and clinical metastases among prostate cancer patients treated with androgen deprivation therapy in Sweden. Cancer Epidemiol 38:442–447
27. Norgaard M, Jensen AO, Jacobsen JB, Cetin K, Fryzek JP, Sorensen HT (2010) Skeletal related events, bone metastasis and survival of prostate cancer: a population based cohort study in Denmark (1999–2007). J Urol 184:162–167
28. Nguyen-Nielsen M, Liede A, Maegbaek ML, Borre M, Harving N, Hernandez RK, Toft Sørensen H, Ehrenstein V (2015) Survival and PSA-markers for mortality and metastasis in nonmetastatic prostate cancer treated with androgen deprivation therapy. Cancer Epidemiol 39:623–632
29. Hess KR, Varadhachary GR, Taylor SH et al (2006) Metastatic patterns in adenocarcinoma. Cancer 106:1624–1633
30. Freedland SJ, Humphreys EB, Mangold LA, Eisenberger M, Dorey FJ, Walsh PC, Partin AW (2005) Risk of prostate cancer-specific mortality following biochemical recurrence after radical prostatectomy. JAMA 294:433–439
31. Pound CR, Partin AW, Eisenberger MA et al (1999) Natural history of progression after PSA elevation following radical prostatectomy. JAMA 281:1591–1597
32. Crawford ED, Stone NN, Yu EY, Koo PJ, Freedland SJ, Slovin SF, Gomella LG, Berger ER, Keane TE, Sieber P, Shore ND, Petrylak DP; Prostate Cancer Radiographic Assessments for Detection of Advanced Recurrence (RADAR) Group (2014) Challenges and recommendations for early identification of metastatic disease in prostate cancer. Urology 83:664–669
33. Kawakami J, Cowan JE, Elkin EP, Latini DM, DuChane J, Carroll PR et al (2006) Androgen-deprivation therapy as primary treatment for localized prostate cancer: data from Cancer of the Prostate Strategic Urologic Research Endeavor (CaPSURE). Cancer 106(8):1708–1714
34. Sharifi N, Gulley JL, Dahut WL (2005) Androgen deprivation therapy for prostate cancer. JAMA 294(2):238–244
35. Kirby M, Hirst C, Crawford ED (2011) Characterising the castration resistant prostate cancer population: a systematic review. Int J Clin Pract 65:1180–1192
36. Zagars GK, Pollack A (1993) The fall and rise of prostate-specific antigen. Kinetics of serum prostate-specific antigen levels after radiation therapy for prostate cancer. Cancer 72:832–834
37. Freedland SJ, Rumble RB, Finelli A, Chen RC, Slovin S, Stein MN, Mendelson DS, Wackett C, Sandler HM (2014) Adjuvant and salvage radiotherapy after prostatectomy: American Society of Clinical Oncology clinical practice guideline endorsement. J Clin Oncol 32(34):3892–3898
38. Thompson IM, Valicenti RK, Albertsen P, Davis BJ, Goldenberg SL, Hahn C, Klein E, Michalski J, Roach M, Sartor O, Wolf JS Jr, Faraday MM (2013) Adjuvant and salvage radiotherapy after prostatectomy: AUA/ASTRO Guideline. J Urol 190(2):441–449
39. Izawa JI, Klotz L, Siemens DR, Kassouf W, So A, Jordan J, Chetner M, Iansavichene AE (2011) Prostate cancer screening: Canadian guidelines 2011. Can Urol Assoc J 5(4):235–240
40. Roach M 3rd, Hanks G, Thames H Jr, Schellhammer P, Shipley WU, Sokol GH, Sandler H (2006) Defining biochemical failure following radiotherapy with or without hormonal therapy in men with clinically localized prostate cancer: recommendations of the RTOG-ASTRO Phoenix Consensus Conference. Int J Radiat Oncol Biol Phys 65(4):965–974
41. Skolarus TA, Wolf AM, Erb NL, Brooks DD, Rivers BM, Underwood W 3rd, Salner AL, Zelefsky MJ, Aragon-Ching JB, Slovin SF, Wittmann DA, Hoyt MA, Sinibaldi VJ, Chodak G, Pratt-Chapman ML, Cowens-Alvarado RL (2014) American Cancer Society prostate cancer survivorship care guidelines. CA Cancer J Clin 64(4):225–249
42. Climent MA, Piulats JM, Sánchez-Hernández A, Arranz JÁ, Cassinello J, García-Donas J, González del Alba A, León-Mateos L, Mellado B, Méndez-Vidal MJ, Pérez-Valderrama B; Spanish Oncology Genitourinary Group (2012) Recommendations from the Spanish Oncology Genitourinary Group for the treatment of patients with metastatic castration-resistant prostate cancer. Crit Rev Oncol Hematol 83(3):341–352
43. Gillessen S, Omlin A, Attard G, de Bono JS, Efstathiou E, Fizazi K, Halabi S, Nelson PS, Sartor O, Smith MR, Soule HR, Akaza H, Beer TM, Beltran H, Chinnaiyan AM, Daugaard G, Davis ID, De Santis M, Drake CG, Eeles RA, Fanti S, Gleave ME, Heidenreich A, Hussain M, James ND, Lecouvet FE, Logothetis CJ, Mastris K, Nilsson S, Oh WK, Olmos D, Padhani AR, Parker C, Rubin MA, Schalken JA, Scher HI, Sella A, Shore ND, Small EJ, Sternberg CN, Suzuki H, Sweeney CJ, Tannock IF, Tombal B (2015) Management of patients with advanced prostate cancer: recommendations of the St Gallen Advanced Prostate Cancer Consensus Conference (APCCC) 2015. Ann Oncol 26(8):1589–1604
44. Freedland SJ, Howard LE, Hanyok BT, Kadiyala VK, Kuang JY, Whitney CA, Wilks FR, Kane CJ, Terris MK, Amling CL, Cooperberg MR, Aronson WJ, Moreira DM (2016) Validation of a bone scan positivity risk table in non-metastatic castration-resistant prostate cancer. BJU Int
45. Moreira DM, Howard LE, Sourbeer KN et al (2015) Predicting bone scan positivity in non-metastatic castration-resistant prostate cancer. Prostate Cancer Prostatic Dis 18:333–337
46. Arlen PM, Bianco F, Dahut WL, D'Amico A, Figg WD, Freedland SJ, Gulley JL, Kantoff PW, Kattan

MW, Lee A, Regan MM, Sartor O (2008) Prostate specific antigen working group guidelines on prostate specific antigen doubling time. J Urol 179: 2181–2186

47. Daskivich TJ, Regan MM, Oh WK (2006) Prostate specific antigen doubling time calculation: not as easy as 1, 2, 4. J Urol 176:1927–1937
48. Scher HI, Eisenberger M, D'Amico AV, Halabi S, Small EJ, Morris M, Kattan MW, Roach M, Kantoff P, Pienta KJ, Carducci MA, Agus D, Slovin SF, Heller G, Kelly WK, Lange PH, Petrylak D, Berg W, Higano C, Wilding G, Moul JW, Partin AN, Logothetis C, Soule HR (2004) Eligibility and outcomes reporting guidelines for clinical trials for patients in the state of a rising prostate-specific antigen: recommendations from the Prostate-Specific Antigen Working Group. J Clin Oncol 22(3):537–556
49. Basch E, Loblaw DA, Oliver TK, Carducci M, Chen RC, Frame JN, Garrels K, Hotte S, Kattan MW, Raghavan D, Saad F, Taplin ME, Walker-Dilks C, Williams J, Winquist E, Bennett CL, Wootton T, Rumble RB, Dusetzina SB, Virgo KS (2014) Systemic therapy in men with metastatic castration-resistant prostate cancer: American Society of Clinical Oncology and Cancer Care Ontario clinical practice guideline. J Clin Oncol 32(30):3436–3448
50. Cookson MS, Lowrance WT, Murad MH, Kibel AS; American Urological Association (2015) Castration-resistant prostate cancer: AUA guideline amendment. J Urol 193(2):491–499

Circulating Tumor Cells (CTCs) and Metastatic Prostate Cancer (mPCa)

5

Elisabetta Rossi and Rita Zamarchi

5.1 CTCs as Prognostic and Predictive Biomarker

The process by which we are finally able to license any clinical-pathological parameter as a biomarker passes through some mandatory steps, namely, analytical validity, clinical validity and, hopefully, clinical utility [1].

In particular, the clinical validity defines a test that is clinically usable [1], on the basis of reliability, accuracy, and needed sensitivity and on specific and predictive value for impacting patient care. On the other hand, with clinical utility, we refer to the ability of a test to be used into the medical practice, because of an improved benefit or reduction in cost beyond the best available test.

CTCs could affect the clinical utility in PCa in different manner:

1. From changing treatment decision (stopping a therapy that does not work or on the contrary, continuing a therapy beneficial for patients)
2. Improving tolerability of a systemic regimen
3. Improving survival (improving treatment selection and reduction in toxicity)
4. Improving cost-effectiveness (with reduction of ineffective drug explosion time) [2]

In European countries, during the last decade, the 5-year relative survival percentages for PCa steadily increased from 73.4 % in 1999–2001 to 83.4 % in 2005–2007 [3]. This encouraging result is undoubtable due to the extensive use of PSA screening and the radical prostatectomy, despite the other side of the coin being that the number needed to treat to prevent one death at 18 years of follow-up was eight men [4], a relevant rate of overdiagnosis and overtreatment.

However, due to the nonnegligible risk of the incidence of distant metastases over the next 18 years after the first diagnosis (a cumulative incidence of 26.1 % in the radical prostatectomy group and of 38.3 % in the watchful waiting group, respectively) [4], the need to improve our capacity to stratify PCa patients according their risk of disease recurrence remains high.

This is particularly relevant for a public, universalistic health system like the European one. Indeed, because of the expected increase of life expectancy and incidence of PCa, we can expect that the disease's economic burden in Europe will also increase substantially. It is estimated that the total economic costs of PCa in Europe exceed € 8.43 billion [5], with a high proportion of the costs of PCa care occurring in the first year after

E. Rossi (✉)
Department of Surgery, Oncology and Gastroenterology, Oncology Section, University of Padova, Padova, Italy
e-mail: elisabetta.rossi@unipd.it

R. Zamarchi
Immunology and Molecular Oncology Unit, IOV-IRCCS, Padova, Italy
e-mail: rita.zamarchi@unipd.it

F. Bertoldo et al. (eds.), *Bone Metastases from Prostate Cancer*,
DOI 10.1007/978-3-319-42327-2_5

diagnosis. In European countries with available data (UK, Germany, France, Italy, Spain, the Netherlands), this amounted to € 106.7–179.0 million for all PCa patients diagnosed in 2006.

The first analytically and clinically validated CTC detection platform was the CellSearch® system. In a first published clinical study, the platform was tested in patients ($n=964$) from different cancers and in 324 healthy donors or benign disease samples. In 123 patients (188 samples) affected by metastatic prostate cancer, 77 samples showed more than 5 CTCs/7.5 ml of peripheral blood. Based on the absence of CTCs in healthy controls, a high specificity (>99 %) using a cutoff of a single CTC was observed [6]. In mPCa the number of CTCs detected per 7.5 mL of whole blood can range widely depending on the context.

Speaking about PCa, Moreno et al. firstly reported in 2001 that CTC levels can be quantified in the circulation of these patients and that the change of the numbers of CTCs correlates with disease progression with no diurnal variations [7]. In 2007, Danila and colleagues reported that the number of CTCs before therapy provides unique information relative to prognosis and that the shedding of cells into the circulation represents an intrinsic property of the tumor, based on the extent of the disease [8].

In 2008, the results of the first important trial that studied the association of CTC count with overall survival (OS) in castration-resistant prostate cancer (CRPC) (IMMC-38, NCT00133900) were published. In this trial, 276 patients affected by CRPC were prospectively evaluated; the CTC counting was performed at diagnosis and after initiation of treatment with cytotoxic chemotherapy. This study demonstrated that an unfavorable CTC level, defined as a value equal or higher than 5 cells/7.5 mL, was associated with a shorter median overall survival at all predefined time points (6.7–9.5 months vs. 19.6–20.7 months; HR, 3.6–6.5; $P<0.0001$) [9].

At baseline, 57 % of patients had an unfavorable CTC count with a decreased median survival of 11.5 months; this finding was significantly lower when compared with 21.7 months for patients with a favorable CTC count (defined as CTC level lower than 5 cells/7.5 mL). Patients converting from unfavorable CTC level at baseline to favorable CTC count after treatment had a corresponding improvement in median OS (from 6.8 month to 21.3 month, respectively). The CTC count prior to and following initiation of treatment was the strongest prognostic factor, superior to prostate-specific antigen (PSA) and many established prognostic variables.

In the next paragraphs, we will address the main open question about the clinical management of mPCa, with the intent to underscore how the extended use of CTC detection and characterization can offer further benefit to these patients.

5.2 Can We Use the Enumeration of CTCs for Planning PCa Prevention Strategies?

Increasing age, ethnic origin, and heredity have been associated with higher risk of developing clinical PCa. However, if the frequency of incidentally- and autopsy-detected cancers is roughly the same in different parts of the world [10], the incidence of clinical PCa differs widely between different geographical areas. Notably, if Japanese men move from Japan to Hawaii, their risk of PCa increases; if they move to California, their risk increases even more, approaching that of American men [11].

These findings indicate that exogenous factors affect the risk of progression from latent to clinical PCa, including alimentary and sexual behavior, alcohol consumption, exposure to ultraviolet radiation, chronic inflammation [12, 13], and occupational exposure [13]. On this basis, PCa may be an ideal candidate for exogenous preventive measures that might include dietary and pharmacological prevention, particularly if we considered the high prevalence and long latency of this endocrine-dependent malignancy.

However, the availability of serum markers and the identification of prostatic intraepithelial lesions are mandatory to plan efficacious prevention. Indeed, if hereditary factors are important in determining the risk of developing clinical PCa, exogenous factors play a role in the risk of progression. Unfortunately, due to the lack of a reliable marker for identifying these patients, there is, as yet, insufficient evidence to recommend lifestyle changes (such as a reduced intake of animal fat and an increased intake of fruit, cereals and vegetables) in order to decrease this last risk [14].

Unlike early breast cancer, in which prognostic and predictive impact of tumor cells in peripheral blood or bone marrow was largely provided [15–17], the role of CTCs in localized PCa is far from clear. Whereas some authors were unable to find a significantly higher number of CTCs in the setting of localized PCa [18], more recently close to 50 % of CTC-positive patients have been reported in men candidates to undergo radical prostatectomy because of positive biopsy for cancer [19]. If we can use CTC count to plan any prevention strategy at least in these patients remains an open question that deserves ad hoc designed studies.

5.3 Can We Use the Enumeration of CTCs for Choosing the Treatment of mPCa?

Discriminating among widely advanced disease versus locally advanced disease (clinical stage T3) drives the treatment choice of PCa. Generally, after a radical prostatectomy, the PSA level should be less than 0.2 ng/mL, and after radiation therapy the level should be less than 0.5 ng/mL [20]. The most common presentation of advanced PCa is a patient with a rising PSA level in whom initial local therapy has failed; this condition is defined as "biochemical failure," and it determines a change of treatment.

Historically, systemic therapy for metastatic and advanced prostate cancer has included androgen suppression. In metastatic disease, this palliative therapy has yielded a median progression-free survival (PFS) of 18–20 months and an overall survival (OS) of 24–36 months. However, virtually all patients develop hormone-refractory disease.

Despite the steady decline in the incidence of newly diagnosed mPCa and microscopic lymph node metastasis, from 20 % in the 1970s to 3.4 % in the 1990s, the risk of extra-prostatic disease in patients with clinically localized disease remains high, at 30–60 %, despite initial treatment with intent to cure. In some cases of hormone-refractory prostate cancer, the prostate cancer may continue to exhibit hormone dependence; however, so far we cannot predict whether these patients may benefit from androgen withdrawal versus continued hormone therapy.

Indeed, despite the great effort employed, often rewarded by a net improving of clinical results, we still live in an imperfect world, so the main clinical and research unanswered question in CRPC has been to define and standardize *progression as an objective end point*, in order to optimize duration of any systemic therapy [21]

The definition of a rising PSA level is not consistent in the literature, but many agree that the occurrence of two consecutive PSA level elevations can be considered biochemical failure. Other important prognostic indicators include the PSA velocity, time to PSA nadir, time to PSA recurrence, and pattern of PSA recurrence. Denham et al. reported that the PSA doubling time and the time to biochemical failure could provide useful surrogate endpoints for prostate cancer-specific mortality, potentially meaning that the follow-up period in clinical trials can be significantly reduced. However, further studies are still needed [22].

Speaking about other clinical-pathological criteria (and putative surrogate endpoints), pretreatment Gleason score, clinical stage, PSA level, and percentage of positive core biopsy results have been found to be reliable predictors of failure following local therapy. Unfortunately, no means of identifying recurrences limited to the pelvis is reliable. Although a Gleason grade of 7 or less is associated with a better prognosis than a grade of 8 or more, if the PSA level rise occurs after 2 years following local treatment, the associated survival likelihood is greater than if the rise occurs before 2 years.

In a study, based on an evaluation of data from the Radiation Therapy and Oncology Group 92–02 randomized trial, Ray et al. determined that distant metastasis and general failure of clinical treatment at 3 years might be candidates as surrogate endpoints for prostate cancer-specific survival at 10 years, potentially shortening the duration of clinical trials for prostate cancer. According to investigators' conclusions, these endpoints still need to be validated in other datasets [23].

On this basis, we should not be surprised if the decision algorithm for initiation of treatment for biochemical failure is controversial. Certain factors to consider include the type of local therapy previously instituted (if any), the patient's life expectancy, the intention and likelihood of cure, the risk for increased morbidity, and the patient's quality of life. So far, no guidelines have been set for treating patients with advanced PCa in whom local therapy has failed.

The enumeration of CTCs in the peripheral blood of mPCa patients might contribute to address this issue, and several clinical studies reported results concerning the potential of this parameter as surrogate marker of overall survival (OS) in mPCa (reviewed by de Bono et al. [24]).

For example, Goldkorn and colleagues [25] published the result of SWOG S0421 that addressed the prognostic and predictive value of CTC enumeration prospectively, in a large phase III cohort treated homogenously with docetaxel—the standard first-line chemotherapy for mCRPC. The authors could validate baseline CTC counts as prognosticator and demonstrated that rising CTCs at 3 weeks heralded significantly worse OS, potentially serving as an early metric to help redirect and optimize therapy in this clinical setting. The prognostic value of CTCs was also reported in metastatic hormone-sensitive PCa by SWOG S0925 [26], despite that the little number of evaluable patients ($n=39$) included in the study requires to be confirmed in larger studies.

A comparison of individual prognostic value of CTCs and objective response criteria has been also prospectively conducted in mCRPC treated by first-line docetaxel [27]. The authors included morphological RECIST and clinical criteria, as well as PSA decline, for evaluating patients' survival. This small pilot study ($n=33$) offers the rationale to larger validation studies, and the authors concluded that CTC counts appear to be an earlier and more sensitive predictor for survival and treatment response than current objective response approaches. In other words, CTCs might provide complementary information for individualized treatment strategies.

Notably, the use of CTCs as an earlier surrogate marker of OS might contribute to reduce the time and the cost of clinical studies focused to identify men likely to respond to new available therapies. Indeed, CTC enumeration was included as an outcome measure into the abiraterone acetate phase III registration trial (COU-AA-301) in patients with mCRPC previously treated with docetaxel [28].

Similarly, CTC count was embedded as a biomarker endpoint into the AFFIRM trial that conducted to the approval of enzalutamide for post-chemotherapy CRPC, based on the OS benefit. In this trial, the higher rate of conversion from unfavorable to favorable CTC count and the lower conversion from favorable to unfavorable CTC count for enzalutamide relative to placebo were consistent with the observed OS benefit [29].

5.4 CTC Detection Methods: Looking to Consensus Criteria

The main reason of the CTC success as potential surrogate endpoint comes from afar and depends on a strong biological evidence, sustained by the robustness of detection methods.

In 1869, for the first time, CTCs were observed in the blood of a man with metastatic cancer by Thomas Ashworth, who postulated that "cells identical with those of the cancer itself being seen in the blood may tend to throw some light upon the mode of origin of multiple tumors existing in the same person." A thorough comparison of the morphology of the circulating cells to tumor cells from different lesions led Ashworth to conclude that "One thing is certain, that if they [CTC] came from an existing cancer structure, they must have passed through the greater part of the circulatory system to have arrived at the internal saphena vein of the sound leg" [30].

In 1874 De Morgan postulated that cells derived from a primary tumor could escape and travel through environ tissue and invade new areas, using lymphatic or blood vessels [31].

Twenty years after Ashworth, Stephan Paget, a surgeon in the UK, proposed the "seed and soil" theory, the theory that suggests that a tumor cell – the seed – either sleeps or thrives within the unique environment of each organ [32].

The first systematic study using smears blood from cancer patients, in 1934, demonstrated the presence of CTC in 43 % of cases [33].

Only in 2003 the soil theory was verified, an analysis of CTCs that is a "seed" in the blood has been considered to be a very important field in clinical prediction. In 2004, a clinical study was reported showing the importance of CTC as a prognostic factor. Strong evidence for CTCs as prognostic markers has been documented for breast cancer [34], but CTC detection is also connected to metastatic relapse and progression in other tumor entities, including prostate, lung, and colorectal cancer.

The process of metastatic spread from the primary tumor site into distal organs is still not well understood. Recent studies suggest an early spread of tumor cells to lymph nodes or bone marrow (BM) referred as "disseminated tumor cells" (DTCs) or as "circulating tumor cells" (CTCs) when present in the peripheral blood (PB) [17, 35].

The rate of tumor cells that are released by cancer is not known, but different studies estimate that millions of cells are dispersed into the body. The evidence demonstrated that only few tumor cells are able to overcome the lack of cell matrix interaction and escape the immunosurveillance, thus, to survive in the bloodstream and reach a distant organ and eventually grow into a metastasis.

Only in 2007, for the first time, the American Society of Clinical Oncology (ASCO) cited CTC and DTC in recommendations on tumor markers. Recently, the American Joint Committee on Cancer has proposed a new category, M0(i+), for TNM staging in breast cancer (BC). This category is defined as "no clinical or radiographic evidence of distant metastases, but deposits of molecularly or microscopically detected tumor cells (no larger than 0.2 mm) in blood, bone marrow, or other non-regional nodal tissue in a patient without symptoms or signs of metastases."

More recently, Bidard and colleagues demonstrated the clinical validity of the CTC assay, as performed by the CellSearch platform, reaching the level I of evidence by the pooled analysis of individual data obtained from close to two thousand European metastatic BC [36].

CTCs are very rare cells as only one CTC is contained in about 1×10^8 or 1×10^9 of blood cells in cancer patients' blood, thus their detection and characterization requires highly sensitive and specific methods. To date, the only method FDA approved is the CellSearch system. This platform takes advantage of the fact that carcinomas derive from epithelial cells that are not normally found in the bloodstream. From 7.5 ml of blood, CTCs are immune-magnetically enriched with a specific antibody for epithelial cell adhesion molecule (EpCAM) coupled with ferrofluid. In a second step, the enriched cells were stained with a nucleic acid dye, DAPI, and a monoclonal antibody directed against cytokeratins (CK) 8, 18, and 19; in order to exclude contaminating leukocytes, an antibody that identifies CD45 is included. An automated microscope collects the images of any fluorescent event and proposes a photo gallery to a trained operator for the manual scoring of CTCs (see Fig. 5.1).

Currently there are many methods in order to isolate and detect CTCs, follow you find an overview of strategies used to capture CTCs and specific examples from every kind (see Table 5.1).

Methods that use immunoaffinity purification strategy have proven to be an efficient way to capture CTCs and for this is the most widely used. They typically use anti-EpCAM antibodies but also other antibodies that recognized tumor-associated antigen, acting as capturing elements for CTCs from human whole blood. The main example is the CellSearch platform, but there are also CTC-chip, an array of 78,000 microspots coated with anti-EpCAM antibodies, Adna Test and Mag-Sweeper Isoflux that use a cocktail of antibodies specific to kind of cancer, and the GILUPI CellCollector® that is the first in vivo CTC isolation product worldwide which is CE

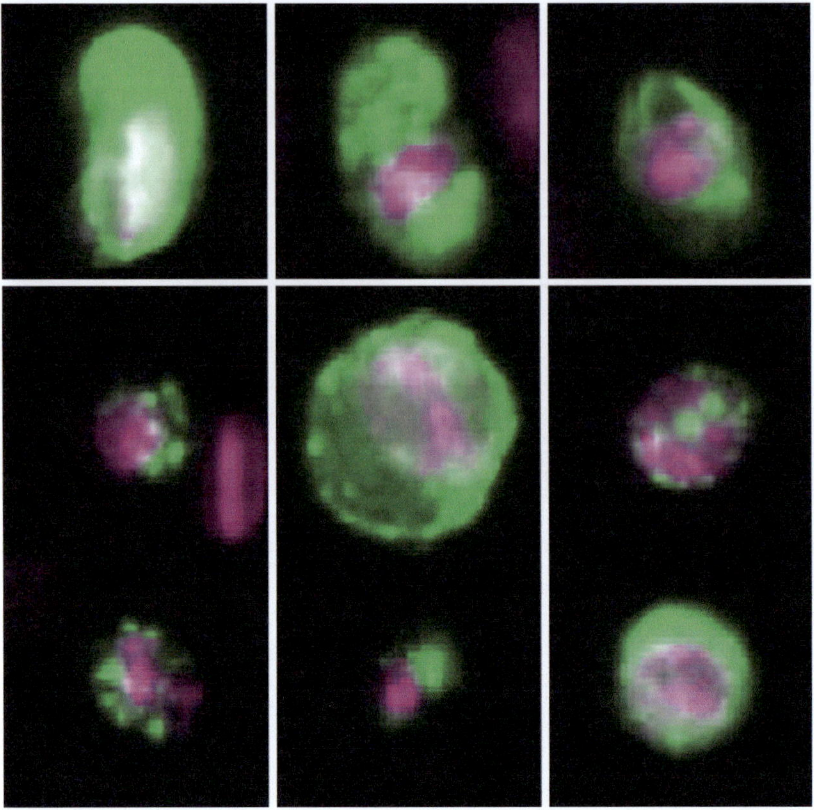

Fig. 5.1 In this picture, it is possible to see CTCs with different morphology detected with CellSearch platform. CTCs are immune-magnetically enriched with a specific antibody for epithelial cell adhesion molecule (EpCAM) coupled with ferrofluid. In a second step, the enriched cells were stained with a nucleic acid dye, DAPI (in *purple*), and a monoclonal antibody directed against cytokeratins (CK) 8, 18, and 19 (in *green*)

Table 5.1 Methods for CTC detection

Assay	Enrichment	Detection	Key features
CellSearch®	EpCAM mAb coupled ferrofluid	Immunofluorescence: CTC is positive for CKs 8, 18, and 19 and nucleus positive for DAPI negative for CD45	Semiautomated system with FDA approval for metastatic breast, colon, and prostate cancer. CTC can be enumerated and visualized
Adna Test	Antibody cocktail (MUC1, EpCAM) coupled microbeads	Molecular biology: RT-PCR positive for at least one of the following markers: MUC1, Her2, EpCAM	This system does not quantify the tumor cell load; false-positive results are due to unspecific amplification
MACS	EpCAM mAb coupled beads	Microscope visualization: morphology, high surface area to volume	Possibility to positive/negative enrichment
MagSweeper	EpCAM mAb coupled ferrofluid	Microscope visualization: morphology	High purity can process WB, 9 ml/h throughput
Ariol system	CK antibodies and EpCAM antibodies coupled to microbeads	Positive markers: CKs	Possibility to detect of EpCAM+and EpCAM-

Table 5.1 (continued)

Assay	Enrichment	Detection	Key features
CTC-Chip	Microsoft array: EpCAM coupled microspots	Immunofluorescence: CTC is positive for CKs 8, 18, and 19 and nucleus positive for DAPI negative for CD45	Microspots are optimized for cell-antibody contact, 1–2 ml/h, high detection rate even in M0 patients
Ephesia	Self-assembly of magnetic beads in columns	Immunofluorescence or immunocytochemistry: CTC is positive for CKs 8, 18, and 19 and nucleus positive for DAPI negative for CD45	Flexibility with capture antibody
Isoflux	EpCAM-coated magnetic beads combined with microfluidic processing	Immunocytochemistry for cytokeratin, CD45, and Hoechst	Automated, continuous flow
CTC iChip®	Magnetic bead capture combined with microfluidic inertial focusing	Immunocytochemistry or RT-PCR	Positive/negative enrichment, remove nucleated cells from whole blood by size-based deflection by using a specially designed array of posts performed in CTC-iChip1, inertial focusing to line up cells to prepare for precise magnetic separation and magnetophoresis for sensitive separation of bead-labeled WBCs and unlabeled CTCs
GILUPI cell collector	Functionalized EpCAM-coated medical wire	Immunocytochemistry for EpCAM, cytokeratin, and DAPI	In vivo collection
Ficoll-Paque®	Density	Immunocytochemistry	Inexpensive, easy to use
OncoQuick	Density/size	Immunocytochemistry/RT-PCR	Density gradient centrifugation with OncoQuick results in higher relative tumor cell enrichment than Ficoll density gradient centrifugation
ISET®	Filtration based on cell size	Immunocytochemistry/FISH	Epithelial and mesenchymal tumor cells can be isolated
ScreenCell®	Filtration based on cell size	Immunocytochemistry/FISH	Epithelial and mesenchymal tumor cells can be isolated
VyCAP	Filtration based on cell size	Filtration based on cell size	Epithelial and mesenchymal tumor cells can be isolated

(continued)

Table 5.1 (continued)

Assay	Enrichment	Detection	Key features
Dean flow fractionation	Size-based selection using centrifugal force	Immunocytochemistry for cytokeratin, EpCAM, CD45, and Hoechst	Non-epithelial cells can be isolated
Dielectrophoretic field-flow fractionation	Membrane capacitance	Immunocytochemistry	CTCs selected are viable
DEPArray™	Enables movement of cells within chip by electric field changes	Fluorescence imaging	Requires pre-enrichment step/isolation of purified single cells for downstream analysis
ApoStream®	Dielectrophoretic technology in a microfluidic flow chamber	Fluorescence imaging	Isolation of purified single cells for downstream analysis
EPISPOT assay	CD45 depletion and short-term culture in plates coated in antibody against MUC-1, PSA, or cytokeratin-19	Immunofluorescence secondary antibodies to MUC-1, PSA, or cytokeratin-19	Detection of only viable CTCs
Vita-Assay™ or Collagen Adhesion Matrix (CAM) technology	Density gradient centrifugation and cells applied to CAM for short-term culture	Immunocytochemistry for cell-surface markers	Detection of only viable CTCs with the invasive phenotype

approved. This device resembles a venous blood withdrawal. The GILUPI CellCollector® is placed directly into the bloodstream of a patient via an indwelling catheter (size 20 G, pink), remains in the arm vein for 30 min, and thus enables the capture of a large number of CTCs in vivo [37].

It is also known that tumor cells are a heterogeneous population, and EpCAM is not constantly expressed on them. Furthermore, it has been noted that circulating tumor microemboli (CTM) or CTCs with epithelial mesenchymal transition (EMT) which are attracting attention these years show no or weak expression of EpCAM, and therefore they are not detectable by the method above. For this reason, methods to isolate CTCs based on their *physical properties, including density, size, deformability, and electrical properties have been developed.*

Some groups use **density gradient centrifugation methods** for separating CTCs in mononuclear fraction based on cell density as centrifugation with Ficoll-Paque solution or OncoQuick (combine a porous filter for size-based separation in conjunction with gradient centrifugation). The isolation is in general followed by an RT-PCR specific for CK. The most promising method is leukapheresis in which white blood cells are separated from a sample of blood. In this way, a large volume of patient's blood could be analyzed for CTCs; the result is an improvement in the number of CTCs isolated and in sensitivity for downstream analysis and characterization.

Microfiltration and microfluidics are also employed: with microfiltration CTCs are retained on the basis of size, assuming that CTCs are larger than leukocytes. The two main techniques are ISET [38] that uses a polycarbonate filter with 8 μm diameter circular pores for CTC enrichment and ScreenCell that uses circular track-etched filters; the pores' range is 7.5–6.5 μm. This methods' advantage is that CTCs can be isolated as living cells without fixation. Nowadays, inexpensive and convenient devices are available, but they are disadvantageous in that the blood samples have to be isolated in a short time after drawing. Recently De Wit and colleagues [39] were able to isolate CTCs onto a silicon membrane with 5 μm diameter circular pores. Using microfluidic tool to retain CTCs, the size and deformability of these cells can be explored.

The dielectrophoresis (DEP) exploits the electrical properties of CTCs, to discriminate them from leukocytes by applying a nonuniform electric field. Gupta and colleagues developed ApoStream instrument for file flow fractionation [40], and Manaresi and colleague [41] developed DEPArray, based on a microfluidic cartridge that contains an array of individually controllable electrodes, each with embedded sensors. This circuitry enables the creation of dielectrophoretic (DEP) cages around cells. After imaging, individual cells of interest are gently moved to specific locations on the cartridge, e.g. for cell-cell interaction studies or into the holding chamber for isolation and recovery.

Functional assay CTCs could also be enriched by an approach that utilizes the functional aspect of CTCs as invasiveness and secretion of specifics protein. So far, only two technologies use this strategy, namely, EPISPOT and VitaAssay™. By the first, membrane immune-captures specific proteins secreted near of the cells. The second method takes advantage of the propensity of cells to invade into collagenous matrices.

Notably, the numbers of CTCs reported vary widely between different platforms; for this reason, there is a need of a uniform, clear, and concordant definition of criteria for defining an event as a CTCs. About CellSearch platform, many studies have been performed, and all this show a high level of concordance also if the classification is operator dependent [42–44].

However, the same level of evidence has not been yet obtained for other different platforms; the studies are few, and the great majority of them are lacking of automation in the classification of CTCs.

Hopefully, this step will be overcome in a few years through the results of the CANCER-ID (IMI-JU-11-2013, EoL no. 115749-1, "Cancer treatment and monitoring through identification of circulating tumor cells and tumour related nucleic acids in blood"), an EU-founded project that, among other, is working to an open source computer program to identify CTCs from image obtained by different platforms. Indeed, the main purpose of the consortium, which so far collected 37 partners among academic and industry world, is to construct a consensus about the minimum criteria necessary and sufficient to define an event as a CTC (http://www.cancer-id.eu/).

5.5 Molecular Characterization of CTCs in mPCa

CTCs represent a source of tumor specimen useful for molecular studies without the invasiveness of a tumor biopsy; at the same time, by collecting sequential blood samples, CTC study allows longitudinal analyses in order to assess the effect or lack of effect of treatments.

Especially in prostate cancer (PCa), and into the age of target therapy, molecular characterization of CTCs should bring advances in the current lack of biomarkers specific for individualized treatment. Characterization of CRPC disease in clinical studies is challenging, for its heterogeneity and because often metastases are exclusive to the bone, a site which is difficult to reach.

A wide assortment of protein- and genome-based assay can be performed on CTCs. The most common ones are immunohistochemistry, immunofluorescence, gene-copy-number analysis using comparative genomic hybridization (aCGH), genomic sequencing analysis, epigenetic studies, and finally next-generation sequencing (NGS).

The common approach of immunophenotyping of CTCs is the complemented assay of enumeration; the only drawback is that the number of antibodies necessary to identify CTCs limits the number of characterizations. By using CellSearch system, it is possible to introduce an additional antibody conjugated to a fluorochrome in order to evaluate the CTC expression of specific antigens. Many studies in CRPC focus on the expression of androgen receptor (AR) by using an antibody directed against AR, and the presence of genomic AR amplification is then confirmed by FISH analysis [45].

This approach is aimed at monitoring the response to the AR targeting agents, like enzalutamide and abiraterone. In fact, prostate cancer could develop resistance to androgen receptor therapy by way of amplification, mutation, or spliced variant of AR or autocrine androgen synthesis [46–49].

M. Crespo [45] analyzed 94 samples from 48 patients affected by metastatic CRCP using CellSearch platform with an additional antibody specific for AR. In this study, the authors compared patients grouped by the absence of prior exposure vs. resistance to abiraterone or enzalutamide. A large intra- and inter-patient heterogeneity of AR expression in CTCs was observed. Crespo and colleagues did not observe a difference in nuclear AR expression in CTCs in CRCP, suggesting that there are no changes in nuclear AR expression following development of resistance to novel endocrine agents in CRCP. However, we observed that the antibody chosen by the authors did not distinguish AR full length from AR-V7 or other spliced isoforms of this protein.

Speaking about the expression of AR and AR-V7 variant, Miyamoto uses the CTC-iChip, a microfliudic device, in order to sequence RNA of 77 single CTCs from 13 PCa patients, of whom 11 were CRCP [50]. This study provided several important observations, firstly that about one-sixth of CTCs co-expressed more than one AR splice variant (AR-V7). This finding does not agree with the common opinion that several variants are co-expressed in tumor tissue and/or CTCs and that they may be competing with full-length AR (AR-FL) for dimerization, which is required for transcriptional activity. They also observed the presence of other AR variants, like AR-V1, AR-V3, and AR-V4 in 5 out of 11 patients and AR-V7 and AR-V12 in 8 out of 11 patients. These results revealed a more complex and heterogeneous pattern regarding AR spliced-variant expression in the CTC compartment that was not revealed in primary tumors. Interestingly, the researchers also observed an inverse relationship between glucocorticoid receptor (GR) and non-canonical Wnt signaling in enzalutamide-progressing patients; both these pathways can be activated in drug resistance in PCa, and the finding suggests the presence in a part of CTC population of an AR-independent drug resistance pathway. In the small group observed by Miyamoto, he did not find a substantial enrichment in AR-V7 expression in patients treated with enzalutamide compared with the cohort enzalutamide naïve.

This is in contrast with the Antonarakis and colleagues study that demonstrated that the resistance to treatment with enzalutamide and abiraterone was associated with expression of AR-V7 in CTCs. Notably, Antonorakis and colleagues studied the outcomes of 31 CRCP patients according to the presence of AR-V7 RNA, as detected by AlereTM CTC Adna Test. These authors concluded by proposing the presence of AR-V7 as a predictive biomarker for lack of clinical benefit of this target drug [51].

Genomic changes showed by CGH array and limited sequencing have been reported on CTCs isolated by using CellSearch platform. Analysis in pared tumors, metastasis, and CTCs suggests that most mutations detected in CTCs were present at a low level in the primary tumors [52].

By using different methods to count and isolate CTC (HD-CTC), Dago and colleagues characterized 41 CTCs collected at four clinical time points. They were able to demonstrate the emergence of distinct CTC subpopulations with specific molecular alterations that were associated to the clinical course of disease and the treatment with targeted ADT [53].

A study carried out with Epic CTC platform, a system without enrichment that spots nucleated cells onto glass microscope slides, revealed that CTCs and WBC are characterized by distinct PTEN and CEP10 genotypes, and CTCs showed an increased ploidy and a heterogeneous status of PTEN. By using FISH analysis, the authors [54] demonstrated a good correlation between PTEN in CTCs and in fresh tumor tissue. Notably, PTEN loss in CTCs (as well as in tumor biopsy) was associated with a worse prognosis.

Recently, a study also revealed that in metastatic neuroendocrine prostate cancer, the CTCs were heterogenic for CK and AR expressions; the expression of AR was much lower, and the presence of AR was localized into the cytoplasm, contrary to CRPC that show AR in the nucleus. This characteristic in addition to morphology has a diagnostic potential in distinguishing NEPC from CRPC [55].

Finally yet importantly, if we will be able to address the full molecular characterization of CTCs, we will probably realize the right concept of "liquid biopsy," i.e., a minimally invasive procedure to investigate the malignancies throughout the disease course.

Conclusions

The great majority of the studies that we have briefly discussed here underscore the limits deriving from the need to enlarge the cohorts of patients studied and to receive an external validation as further independent confirmation. However, all of them indicate that CTC evaluation could provide information about disease heterogeneity, its clonal evolution, metastatic dissemination, and development of resistance to therapeutics in individual patient, throughout the continuum of the care. The study of this particular compartment of malignancy offers firstly the opportunity to design the patient treatment onto the biology of his/her disease.

References

1. Hayes DF (2015) Biomarker validation and testing. Mol Oncol 9(5):960–966
2. Zhang T, Armstrong AJ (2016) Clinical utility of circulating tumor cells in advanced prostate cancer. Curr Oncol Rep 18(1):3
3. De Angelis R, Sant M, Coleman MP, Francisci S, Baili P, Pierannunzio D, Trama A, Visser O, Brenner H, Ardanaz E et al (2014) Cancer survival in Europe 1999-2007 by country and age: results of EUROCARE – 5-a population-based study. Lancet Oncol 15(1):23–34
4. Bill-Axelson A, Holmberg L, Garmo H, Rider JR, Taari K, Busch C, Nordling S, Haggman M, Andersson SO, Spangberg A et al (2014) Radical prostatectomy or watchful waiting in early prostate cancer. N Engl J Med 370(10):932–942
5. Luengo-Fernandez R, Leal J, Gray A, Sullivan R (2013) Economic burden of cancer across the European Union: a population-based cost analysis. Lancet Oncol 14(12):1165–1174
6. Allard WJ, Matera J, Miller MC, Repollet M, Connelly MC, Rao C, Tibbe AG, Uhr JW, Terstappen LW (2004) Tumor cells circulate in the peripheral blood of all major carcinomas but not in healthy subjects or patients with nonmalignant diseases. Clin Cancer Res 10(20):6897–6904
7. Moreno JG, O'Hara SM, Gross S, Doyle G, Fritsche H, Gomella LG, Terstappen LW (2001) Changes in circulating carcinoma cells in patients with metastatic prostate cancer correlate with disease status. Urology 58(3):386–392
8. Danila DC, Heller G, Gignac GA, Gonzalez-Espinoza R, Anand A, Tanaka E, Lilja H, Schwartz L, Larson S, Fleisher M et al (2007) Circulating tumor cell number and prognosis in progressive castration-resistant prostate cancer. Clin Cancer Res 13(23):7053–7058
9. de Bono JS, Scher HI, Montgomery RB, Parker C, Miller MC, Tissing H, Doyle GV, Terstappen LW, Pienta KJ, Raghavan D (2008) Circulating tumor cells predict survival benefit from treatment in metastatic castration-resistant prostate cancer. Clin Cancer Res 14(19):6302–6309
10. Lawrentschuk N, Haider MA, Daljeet N, Evans A, Toi A, Finelli A, Trachtenberg J, Zlotta A, Fleshner N (2010) 'Prostatic evasive anterior tumours': the role of magnetic resonance imaging. BJU Int 105(9): 1231–1236
11. Breslow N, Chan CW, Dhom G, Drury RA, Franks LM, Gellei B, Lee YS, Lundberg S, Sparke B, Sternby NH et al (1977) Latent carcinoma of prostate at autopsy in seven areas. The International Agency for Research on Cancer, Lyons, France. Int J Cancer 20(5):680–688
12. Nelson WG, De Marzo AM, Isaacs WB (2003) Prostate cancer. N Engl J Med 349(4):366–381
13. Leitzmann MF, Rohrmann S (2012) Risk factors for the onset of prostatic cancer: age, location, and behavioral correlates. Clin Epidemiol 4:1–11
14. Richman EL, Kenfield SA, Stampfer MJ, Giovannucci EL, Chan JM (2011) Egg, red meat, and poultry intake and risk of lethal prostate cancer in the prostate-specific antigen-era: incidence and survival. Cancer Prev Res (Phila) 4(12):2110–2121
15. Lucci A, Hall CS, Lodhi AK, Bhattacharyya A, Anderson AE, Xiao L, Bedrosian I, Kuerer HM, Krishnamurthy S (2012) Circulating tumour cells in non-metastatic breast cancer: a prospective study. Lancet Oncol 13(7):688–695
16. Rack B, Schindlbeck C, Juckstock J, Andergassen U, Hepp P, Zwingers T, Friedl TW, Lorenz R, Tesch H, Fasching PA et al (2014) Circulating tumor cells predict survival in early average-to-high risk breast cancer patients. J Natl Cancer Inst 106(5)
17. Braun S, Vogl FD, Naume B, Janni W, Osborne MP, Coombes RC, Schlimok G, Diel IJ, Gerber B, Gebauer

G et al (2005) A pooled analysis of bone marrow micrometastasis in breast cancer. N Engl J Med 353(8):793–802
18. Davis JW, Nakanishi H, Kumar VS, Bhadkamkar VA, McCormack R, Fritsche HA, Handy B, Gornet T, Babaian RJ (2008) Circulating tumor cells in peripheral blood samples from patients with increased serum prostate specific antigen: initial results in early prostate cancer. J Urol 179(6):2187–2191; discussion 2191
19. Rossi E et al (2015) AACR Annu Meet poster #379
20. Amling CL, Bergstralh EJ, Blute ML, Slezak JM, Zincke H (2001) Defining prostate specific antigen progression after radical prostatectomy: what is the most appropriate cut point? J Urol 165(4):1146–1151
21. Armstrong AJ, Eisenberger MA, Halabi S, Oudard S, Nanus DM, Petrylak DP, Sartor AO, Scher HI (2012) Biomarkers in the management and treatment of men with metastatic castration-resistant prostate cancer. Eur Urol 61(3):549–559
22. Denham JW, Steigler A, Wilcox C, Lamb DS, Joseph D, Atkinson C, Matthews J, Tai KH, Spry NA, Christie D et al (2008) Time to biochemical failure and prostate-specific antigen doubling time as surrogates for prostate cancer-specific mortality: evidence from the TROG 96.01 randomised controlled trial. Lancet Oncol 9(11):1058–1068
23. Ray ME, Bae K, Hussain MH, Hanks GE, Shipley WU, Sandler HM (2009) Potential surrogate endpoints for prostate cancer survival: analysis of a phase III randomized trial. J Natl Cancer Inst 101(4):228–236
24. Mehra N, Zafeiriou Z, Lorente D, Terstappen LW, de Bono JS (2015) CCR 20th anniversary commentary: circulating tumor cells in prostate cancer. Clin Cancer Res 21(22):4992–4995
25. Goldkorn A, Ely B, Quinn DI, Tangen CM, Fink LM, Xu T, Twardowski P, Van Veldhuizen PJ, Agarwal N, Carducci MA et al (2014) Circulating tumor cell counts are prognostic of overall survival in SWOG S0421: a phase III trial of docetaxel with or without atrasentan for metastatic castration-resistant prostate cancer. J Clin Oncol 32(11):1136–1142
26. Yu EY, Li H, Higano CS, Agarwal N, Pal SK, Alva A, Heath EI, Lam ET, Gupta S, Lilly MB et al (2015) SWOG S0925: a randomized phase II study of androgen deprivation combined with cixutumumab versus androgen deprivation alone in patients with new metastatic hormone-sensitive prostate cancer. J Clin Oncol 33(14):1601–1608
27. Thalgott M, Heck MM, Eiber M, Souvatzoglou M, Hatzichristodoulou G, Kehl V, Krause BJ, Rack B, Retz M, Gschwend JE et al (2015) Circulating tumor cells versus objective response assessment predicting survival in metastatic castration-resistant prostate cancer patients treated with docetaxel chemotherapy. J Cancer Res Clin Oncol 141(8):1457–1464
28. Scher HI, Heller G, Molina A, Attard G, Danila DC, Jia X, Peng W, Sandhu SK, Olmos D, Riisnaes R et al (2015) Circulating tumor cell biomarker panel as an individual-level surrogate for survival in metastatic castration-resistant prostate cancer. J Clin Oncol 33(12):1348–1355
29. Fleisher M et al (2015) J Clin Oncol 33(suppl; abstr 5035)
30. Ashworth TR (1869) A case of cancer in which cells similar to those in the tumours were seen in the blood after death. Aust Med J 14:146
31. De Morgan C (1874) Observations on cancer: its pathology, and its relations to the organism and to other morbid growths. Lancet 103(2636):325–329
32. Paget S (1889) The distribution of secondary growths in cancer of the breast. 1989. Cancer Metastasis Rev 8(2):98–101
33. Pool EH, Dunlop GR (1934) Cancer cells in the blood stream. Am J Cancer 21:99–102
34. Cristofanilli M, Budd GT, Ellis MJ, Stopeck A, Matera J, Miller MC, Reuben JM, Doyle GV, Allard WJ, Terstappen LW et al (2004) Circulating tumor cells, disease progression, and survival in metastatic breast cancer. N Engl J Med 351(8):781–791
35. Braun S, Cevatli BS, Assemi C, Janni W, Kentenich CR, Schindlbeck C, Rjosk D, Hepp F (2001) Comparative analysis of micrometastasis to the bone marrow and lymph nodes of node-negative breast cancer patients receiving no adjuvant therapy. J Clin Oncol 19(5):1468–1475
36. Bidard FC, Peeters DJ, Fehm T, Nole F, Gisbert-Criado R, Mavroudis D, Grisanti S, Generali D, Garcia-Saenz JA, Stebbing J et al (2014) Clinical validity of circulating tumour cells in patients with metastatic breast cancer: a pooled analysis of individual patient data. Lancet Oncol 15(4):406–414
37. Saucedo-Zeni N, Mewes S, Niestroj R, Gasiorowski L, Murawa D, Nowaczyk P, Tomasi T, Weber E, Dworacki G, Morgenthaler NG et al (2012) A novel method for the in vivo isolation of circulating tumor cells from peripheral blood of cancer patients using a functionalized and structured medical wire. Int J Oncol 41(4):1241–1250
38. Vona G, Sabile A, Louha M, Sitruk V, Romana S, Schutze K, Capron F, Franco D, Pazzagli M, Vekemans M et al (2000) Isolation by size of epithelial tumor cells: a new method for the immunomorphological and molecular characterization of circulating tumor cells. Am J Pathol 156(1):57–63
39. de Wit S, van Dalum G, Lenferink AT, Tibbe AG, Hiltermann TJ, Groen HJ, van Rijn CJ, Terstappen LW (2015) The detection of EpCAM(+) and EpCAM(-) circulating tumor cells. Sci Rep 5:12270
40. Gupta V, Jafferji I, Garza M, Melnikova VO, Hasegawa DK, Pethig R, Davis DW (2012) ApoStream(™), a new dielectrophoretic device for antibody independent isolation and recovery of viable cancer cells from blood. Biomicrofluidics 6(2):24133
41. Bolognesi C, Forcato C, Buson G, Fontana F, Mangano C, Doffini A, Sero V, Lanzellotto R, Signorini G, Calanca A et al (2016) Digital sorting of pure cell populations enables unambiguous genetic analysis of heterogeneous formalin-fixed paraffin-

embedded tumors by next generation sequencing. Sci Rep 6:20944

42. Riethdorf S, Fritsche H, Muller V, Rau T, Schindlbeck C, Rack B, Janni W, Coith C, Beck K, Janicke F et al (2007) Detection of circulating tumor cells in peripheral blood of patients with metastatic breast cancer: a validation study of the Cell Search system. Clin Cancer Res 13(3):920–928
43. Kraan J, Sleijfer S, Strijbos MH, Ignatiadis M, Peeters D, Pierga JY, Farace F, Riethdorf S, Fehm T, Zorzino L et al (2011) External quality assurance of circulating tumor cell enumeration using the Cell Search((R)) system: a feasibility study. Cytometry B Clin Cytom 80(2):112–118
44. Cummings J, Morris K, Zhou C, Sloane R, Lancashire M, Morris D, Bramley S, Krebs M, Khoja L, Dive C (2013) Method validation of circulating tumour cell enumeration at low cell counts. BMC Cancer 13:415
45. Crespo M, van Dalum G, Ferraldeschi R, Zafeiriou Z, Sideris S, Lorente D, Bianchini D, Rodrigues DN, Riisnaes R, Miranda S et al (2015) Androgen receptor expression in circulating tumour cells from castration-resistant prostate cancer patients treated with novel endocrine agents. Br J Cancer 112(7):1166–1174
46. Koivisto P, Kononen J, Palmberg C, Tammela T, Hyytinen E, Isola J, Trapman J, Cleutjens K, Noordzij A, Visakorpi T et al (1997) Androgen receptor gene amplification: a possible molecular mechanism for androgen deprivation therapy failure in prostate cancer. Cancer Res 57(2):314–319
47. Stanbrough M, Bubley GJ, Ross K, Golub TR, Rubin MA, Penning TM, Febbo PG, Balk SP (2006) Increased expression of genes converting adrenal androgens to testosterone in androgen-independent prostate cancer. Cancer Res 66(5):2815–2825
48. Dehm SM, Schmidt LJ, Heemers HV, Vessella RL, Tindall DJ (2008) Splicing of a novel androgen receptor exon generates a constitutively active androgen receptor that mediates prostate cancer therapy resistance. Cancer Res 68(13):5469–5477
49. Taylor BS, Schultz N, Hieronymus H, Gopalan A, Xiao Y, Carver BS, Arora VK, Kaushik P, Cerami E, Reva B et al (2010) Integrative genomic profiling of human prostate cancer. Cancer Cell 18(1):11–22
50. Miyamoto DT, Lee RJ, Stott SL, Ting DT, Wittner BS, Ulman M, Smas ME, Lord JB, Brannigan BW, Trautwein J et al (2012) Androgen receptor signaling in circulating tumor cells as a marker of hormonally responsive prostate cancer. Cancer Discov 2(11):995–1003
51. Antonarakis ES, Lu C, Wang H, Luber B, Nakazawa M, Roeser JC, Chen Y, Mohammad TA, Fedor HL, Lotan TL et al (2014) AR-V7 and resistance to enzalutamide and abiraterone in prostate cancer. N Engl J Med 371(11):1028–1038
52. Heitzer E, Auer M, Gasch C, Pichler M, Ulz P, Hoffmann EM, Lax S, Waldispuehl-Geigl J, Mauermann O, Lackner C et al (2013) Complex tumor genomes inferred from single circulating tumor cells by array-CGH and next-generation sequencing. Cancer Res 73(10):2965–2975
53. Dago AE, Stepansky A, Carlsson A, Luttgen M, Kendall J, Baslan T, Kolatkar A, Wigler M, Bethel K, Gross ME et al (2014) Rapid phenotypic and genomic change in response to therapeutic pressure in prostate cancer inferred by high content analysis of single circulating tumor cells. PLoS One 9(8):e101777
54. Punnoose EA, Ferraldeschi R, Szafer-Glusman E, Tucker EK, Mohan S, Flohr P, Riisnaes R, Miranda S, Figueiredo I, Rodrigues DN et al (2015) PTEN loss in circulating tumour cells correlates with PTEN loss in fresh tumour tissue from castration-resistant prostate cancer patients. Br J Cancer 113(8): 1225–1233
55. Beltran H, Jendrisak A, Landers M, Mosquera JM, Kossai M, Louw J, Krupa R, Graf RP, Schreiber NA, Nanus DM et al (2016) The initial detection and partial characterization of circulating tumor cells in neuroendocrine prostate cancer. Clin Cancer Res 22(6): 1510–1519

6 Nuclear Medicine Modalities to Image Bone Metastases with Bone-Targeting Agents: Conventional Scintigraphy and Positron-Emission Tomography

Werner Langsteger, Alireza Rezaee, and Mohsen Beheshti

6.1 Introduction

Prostate cancer is the second most diagnosed malignancy and the sixth cause of cancer-related death across the globe [1, 2]. There are some known risk factors for this cancer, including advanced age, lifestyle, race, using tobacco products, geographic area of living, positive history in immediate relatives, and distinct genetic mutations [1–10].

More early-stage prostate cancers with resultant less metastatic disease were diagnosed in the recent decades by using prostatic-specific antigen (PSA) as a screening examination worldwide. This also expectedly caused less cancer death. Nowadays, the clinicians use pathologic Gleason score, the PSA level, and patients' clinical stage for risk stratification before treatment. They widely use PSA in patients' follow-up after therapy [1, 11–14].

W. Langsteger • A. Rezaee • M. Beheshti, MD, FEBNM, FASNC (✉)
Department of Nuclear Medicine and Endocrinology, PET – CT Center LINZ, St Vincent's Hospital, Seilerstaette 4 A-4020, Linz, Austria
e-mail: mohsen.beheshti@bhs.at

The imaging-guided tissue biopsy is routinely used for diagnosis confirmation. Locally advanced malignancy is seen in about 20 % of prostate cancer patients, and up to 35 % of cases present with metastatic disease [15].

Prostate cancer can potentially invade the surrounding pelvic structures or distantly metastasize to the bone and lymph nodes, using either lymphatics or the bloodstream [16, 17]. Axial skeleton with high content of active bone marrow is the main destination for cancerous cells [18].

Prostate cancer could be fatal particularly in aggressive type if the malignancy extensively spread to the bone and distant soft tissue. However, most of the time, it is a slow-growing cancer, and given increased prevalence in advanced age, these patients often die from causes not related to prostate cancer. From those who die of prostate cancer, 80–90 % has already developed osseous metastases [1, 17, 19].

In order to choose the best treatment earlier and reduce morbidity in future, it is crucial to diagnose the skeletal metastases as soon as possible [20]. The first-line treatment for such patients is composed of androgen depravation with routine evaluation of serum testosterone and PSA levels [14]. If it fails, the next step will be the application of chemotherapy or radionuclide treatment [21].

F. Bertoldo et al. (eds.), *Bone Metastases from Prostate Cancer*,
DOI 10.1007/978-3-319-42327-2_6

6.2 Conventional Radionuclide Imaging

6.2.1 ^{99m}Tc-Bisphosphonate Planar Scintigraphy

Different radiotracers have been tried to evaluate bone metastases from prostate cancer; however, Tc-99 m-bisphosphonates such as Tc-99 m-methylene diphosphonate (^{99m}Tc-MDP) and Tc-99 m 3,3-diphosphono-1,2-propanedicarboxylic acid (^{99m}Tc-DPD) are the most common tracers which are widely used for this purpose [22–26].

Although it is not clearly recognized how ^{99m}Tc-MDP is accumulated in pathologic bone lesions, however, it is assumed that ^{99m}Tc-MDP will be chemically adsorbed onto, and into, the crystalline structure of hydroxyapatite on osseous surface. The uptake is in close relation with osteoblastic function and blood flow. Considering blastic nature of bone metastases from prostate cancer, those lesions will be clearly detectable on whole-body bone scintigraphy [27].

The reason that conventional ^{99m}Tc-MDP whole-body bone scintigraphy is wildly used to image bone metastases is because it is not only greatly sensitive and affordable but also easily reachable even in small nuclear medicine centers [28]. The planar whole-body scintigraphy is recommended for detection of skeletal lesions by major guidelines for prostate cancer [29]. However, large retrospective analysis demonstrated that bone metastases occurs in <1 % of patients with a serum PSA level of less than 20 ng/ml (negative predictive value of approximately 100 %) [30]. In order to limit futile diagnostic imaging and procedures, the guidelines such as American Urological Association (AUA) and European Association of Urology (EAU) recommend whole-body bone scintigraphy for cancers with Gleason score of >7 or patients with serum PSA level >20 ng/ml [29, 31]. It is also suggested by the National Institute for Clinical Excellence (NICE) of the United Kingdom for the assessment of bone metastases in intermediate and high-risk prostate cancer patients with a PSA level of greater than 10 ng/ml and Gleason score of greater than 6 [32].

Nevertheless, urologists prefer to evaluate their metastatic prostate cancer patients who complain of skeletal pain with bone scintigraphy. But they believe it is not needed if the patient is asymptomatic or the level of serum PSA is below 10 ng/ml [33]. Also, 70 % of them who participated in a survey considered the whole-body bone scintigraphy as their follow-up method for the patients with rising PSA levels after surgery or radiation therapy [34]. Hence, ^{99m}Tc-MDP bone scan is applied to evaluate treatment response in patients with bone metastases from prostate cancer [35, 36]. However, the nuclear physicians need to differentiate between disease progression and "flare phenomenon," the former with development of new metastatic lesions but the latter with increased intensity of previously seen metastases from prostate or breast cancer within the first week after hormonal therapy which may even persist by 6 months [37, 38].

Although the lesions which cannot trigger a reactive process or grow extremely slowly may cause a false-negative result on whole-body bone scintigraphy, this modality is still more sensitive when compared with plain x-ray imaging and may be able to demonstrate functional findings related to bone metastases several months earlier than anatomical changes detected by plain radiography do [17, 39–42].

Despite a desirable sensitivity, the major limitation of ^{99m}Tc-MDP bone scintigraphy is its relatively low-specificity and false-positive results due to radiotracer accumulation in traumatic, degenerative, and infectious as well as postsurgical changes [43].

6.2.2 Bone Scan Index

Similar to many other nuclear medicine images, the whole-body bone scintigraphy is usually qualitatively and visually interpreted. In order to evaluate the metastatic disease from prostate cancer quantitatively on ^{99m}Tc-MDP scintigraphy, Imbriaco and colleagues invented a method in the late 1990s, renowned as bone scan index (BSI) [44], in which the percentage of total skeletal mass involved with metastases is reported [44, 45].

It is strongly correlated with changes of serum PSA level, thus, used as a parameter for metastases progression and evaluation of response to treatment as well as a prognostic factor [18, 44, 46, 47]. Reza and colleagues demonstrated significantly different survival among patients with BSI of 0, ≤1 and >1 in baseline and follow-up whole-body bone scans [48]. Of the cons of this manual method is its time-consuming nature and dependency on interpreter for an appropriate report. To solve the problem and use the method in daily clinical practice, an automated method was developed which is faster and much more reproducible [49–51].

Another prognostic aspect of ^{99m}Tc-MDP whole-body bone scan is revealed by Rigaud and colleagues in a retrospective study. The prostate cancer patient with axial skeletal metastases demonstrated more favorable survival, compared with patients who had metastases within appendicular skeleton ($p=0.048$). By reviewing the total of 86 patients, the median survival was determined as 53 % versus 29 % in patients with axial and appendicular metastases, respectively [14].

6.2.3 ^{99m}Tc-Bisphosphonate SPECT and SPECT/CT

For complex skeleton such as the spine, hip, pelvis, and knee as well as small carpal and tarsal bones, it may be difficult to precisely detect or localize the bony lesions, using planar bone scintigraphy. The calculated range of sensitivity and specificity for detection of bone metastases by conventional planar bone scintigraphy is 70–95 % and 60–75 %, respectively [17, 29].

To mitigate this shortcoming of reduced specificity, a supplemental modality such as single-photon emission-computed tomography (SPECT) can be applied [52]. SPECT provides useful information when analyzing the lesions in the spine as the prominent site for ^{99m}Tc-MDP-positive degenerative lesions. SPECT enhances the sensitivity, specificity, negative predictive value (NPV), positive predictive value (PPV), and accuracy of ^{99m}Tc-MDP bone scan up to 92 %, 91 %, 94 %, 82 %, and 90 %, respectively [53]. It is more specific and sensitive than planar bone scintigraphy particularly for detection of lumbosacral lesions [54].

Although correlation of planar and SPECT bone scintigraphy with other imaging modalities such as magnetic resonance imaging (MRI), computed tomography (CT), or even plain radiography will improve the accuracy, however, it will be in the expense of more imaging performance and delayed in patient management [55]. Indeed, the hybrid SPECT/CT equipments mitigate this limitation by combining two techniques in a single performance and extracting both functional and anatomic data. It is also capable of better localization of abnormal ^{99m}Tc-MDP uptakes and determining the osseous metastatic lesions more accurately. This is particularly required for some skeletal regions such as the spine and thorax, in which a combination of SPECT and CT or MRI is necessary for a correct diagnosis (Fig. 6.1).

Another application of hybrid SPECT/CT imaging is in the assessment of ^{99m}Tc-MDP-positive benign bone abnormalities such as spondylopathy, spondylarthrosis, and osteochondrosis. Interesting results revealed by Gnanasegaran and colleagues showed a better diagnostic confidence in differentiating benign from malignant skeletal lesions for interpreters when they used SPECT/CT images compared with SPECT images alone or side-by-side CT correlation [56]. A total of 57 patients with bone metastases from prostate cancer which were interpreted as indeterminate on SPECT images had been enrolled in a study, performed by Römer and colleagues. Among those equivocal lesions which approximately 64 % of them were localized in the spine, more than 90 % were clarified by additional hybrid SPECT/CT modality [57]. Helyar and colleagues retrospectively evaluated 50 skeletal lesions from prostate cancer and found 61 % versus 8 % of equivocal lesions on planar/SPECT and SPECT/CT, respectively. They concluded that in comparison with SPECT or planar bone scintigraphy, SPECT/CT is more accurate with better diagnostic confidence in assessment of osseous metastases from prostate cancer [58]. These data were confirmed in another study by Ndlovu and colleagues. They recruited 42 patients who had a total of 189 bone metastatic

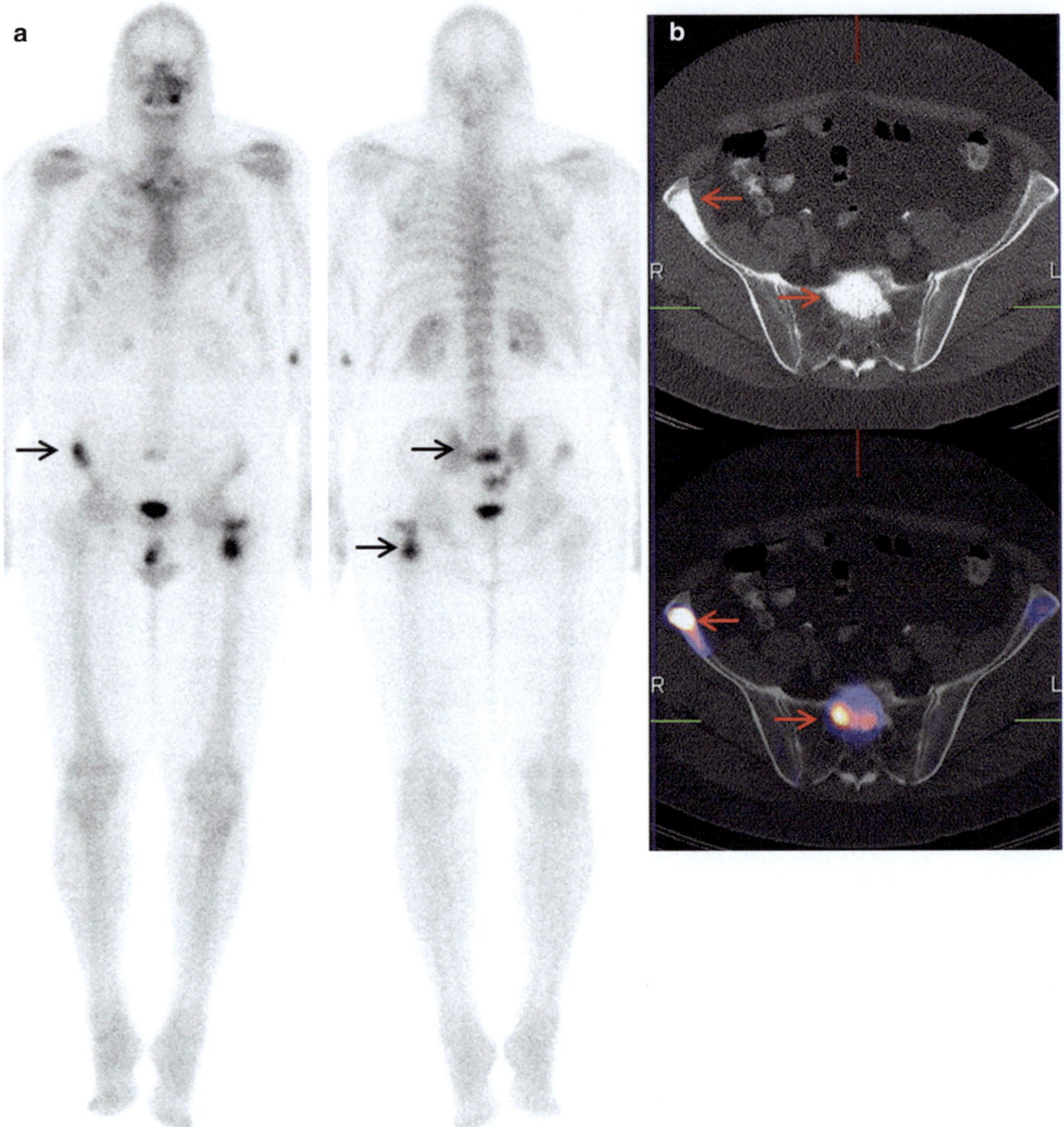

Fig. 6.1 Prostate cancer patient with increased PSA level after radical prostatectomy. (**a**) ^{99m}Tc-MDP planar whole-body bone scan in anterior (*left*) and posterior (*right*) views shows multiple increasing tracer uptakes (*arrows*) suggestive of bone metastases. (**b**) SPECT/CT from pelvis skeleton (CT upper, fusion lower) is able to better determine the suspicious lesions on whole-body scan (*arrows*)

lesions. When compared with SPECT imaging alone, the SPECT/CT significantly reduced the number of indeterminate lesions (31 % vs 9 %, $p<0.0001$). It also outperformed SPECT alone with an overall accuracy of 92 % versus 67 % ($p<0.0001$) on a lesion-wise basis [59]. In another study, Sharma and colleagues realized that from 49 indeterminate lesions on planar imaging, 48 (96 %) were clarified with SPECT/CT method ($p<0.001$) which shows a superiority for latter in correctly differentiate osseous metastases from prostate cancer. They also revealed that the management was changed in 61 % of patients based on SPECT/CT data compared with planar whole-body bone scintigraphy [60]. In a most recent study, Palmedo and colleagues discovered significantly better ($p<0.01$) specificity (94 % vs 78 %) and positive predictive value (88 % vs 59 %) in the detection of osseous metastases for SPECT/CT scan compared with ^{99m}Tc-MDP bone scintigraphy and SPECT alone. The sensitivity calculated as 97 % versus 93 % and NPV as 97 % versus 95 %. There was an approximately 30 % downstaging for enrolled patients based on SPECT/CT data [61]. The abovementioned findings are supported in a review article by Ghosh who emphasized that SPECT/CT imaging provides higher accuracy and better diagnostic confidence in metastases localization and characterization of solitary or indeterminate skeletal lesions [62]. Indeed, the fact was confirmed by other investigators as well [17, 61, 63–67].

6.3 ^{18}F-NaF PET/CT

Conventional whole-body scintigraphy is relatively inexpensive method of imaging and has some other advantages such as desirable sensitivity and widespread availability that makes it the first choice in diagnosing skeletal metastases from different cancers, including the lung, breast, and prostate. However, due to reduced spatial resolution, most notably within the spine, pelvic bones, and calvarium, the application of a high-resolution imaging technique such as hybrid positron-emission tomography/computed tomography (PET/CT) is warranted. More accurate than ^{99m}Tc-MDP planar bone scintigraphy or SPECT, the ^{18}F-sodium fluoride (^{18}F-NaF) PET/CT had been used to assess skeletal metastatic disease (Figs. 6.2 and 6.3) [68].

As a positron-emitting radiopharmaceutical, the ^{18}F-NaF had been firstly utilized to image osseous structures more than four decades ago. However, the application was limited due to its high energy of 511 keV which was not optimal for gamma cameras and short half-life of only 110 min. By the introduction of ^{99m}Tc-bisphosphonates with desirable peak photon energy, the latter replaced completely for bone imaging. Then, the application of new modality had extended dramatically when its accuracy improved by development of SPECT and SPECT/CT scans later [69]. Nonetheless, the use of PET scanners which are perfectly capable of detecting photons with 511 keV energy is markedly increased in the last decade, which, in turn, introduced ^{18}F agents again for research as well as in clinical studies.

The skeletal uptake of ^{18}F-NaF and ^{99m}Tc-MDP is in almost the same way. The agents chemisorb to hydroxyapatite, with the production of fluoroapatite and a hydroxyl group [OH^{-}]:

$$Ca_5\left(PO_4\right)_3 OH + F^- \rightarrow Ca_5\left(PO_4\right)_3 F + OH^-$$

This way, the radiotracers attach to the areas of new formation and mainly represent osteoblastic activity [27, 70].

^{18}F-NaF has a first-pass clearance of approximately 100 %[71]. The bone structures take up to the half of the dose and another 30 % diffuse within the red blood cells. The remaining amount will be excreting by the kidneys within 6 h of injection [72]. Accordingly, the patients that undergo ^{18}F-NaF PET/CT should be perfectly hydrated by drinking more than half a liter of water before and after imaging and more frequently empty the bladder to hasten radiotracer excretion from the body and diminish radiation exposure to urinary bladder as the target organ [72, 73].

The recommended adult dose of ^{18}F-NaF is 40–100 μCi/kg (1.5–3.7 MBq/kg) or a maximum of 10 mCi (370 MBq) for oncologic PET/CT imaging [73]. It is usually 20–25 mCi (740–925 MBq) for ^{99m}Tc-MDP [28]. The effective radiation dose is 0.021 mrem and 0.089 mrem per mCi of ^{99m}Tc-MDP and ^{18}F-NaF, respectively. However, due to less injected dose and shorter half-life of ^{18}F-NaF (110 min vs 6 h), the total actual radiation absorbed dose is quite similar [72–74].

The indications for ^{18}F-NaF PET/CT are resembling to ^{99m}Tc-MDP whole-body bone scan and include the assessment of primary and secondary bone malignancies, evaluation of equivocal findings of other imaging or lab modalities, as well as determination of response to therapy [17].

In a study by Langsteger and colleagues on 22 patients with prostate cancer who underwent

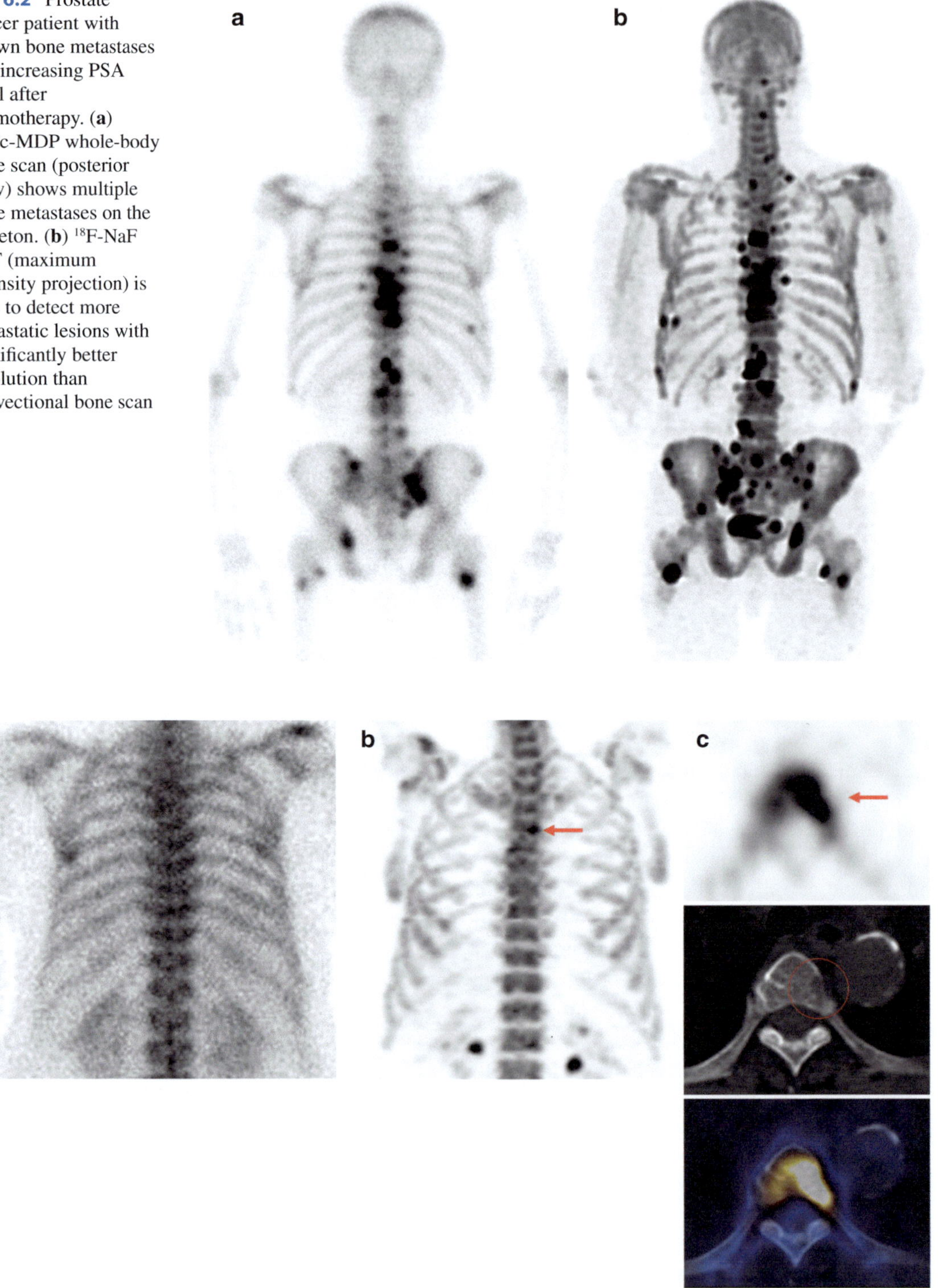

Fig. 6.2 Prostate cancer patient with known bone metastases and increasing PSA level after chemotherapy. (**a**) ^{99m}Tc-MDP whole-body bone scan (posterior view) shows multiple bone metastases on the skeleton. (**b**) ^{18}F-NaF PET (maximum intensity projection) is able to detect more metastatic lesions with significantly better resolution than convectional bone scan

Fig. 6.3 Staging from a high-risk cancer patient. (**a**) ^{99m}Tc-MDP planar bone scan (posterior view) is unremarkable. (**b**) ^{18}F-NaF PET (maximum intensity projection) shows suspicious increased tracer uptake on a thoracic spine. (**c**) ^{18}F-NaF PET/CT (transaxial images): intensive ^{18}F-NaF uptake on a thoracic spine (*upper*, *arrow*) with corresponding cortical destruction on CT (*Mid*), fusion image (*lower*) confirms the findings on PET and CT

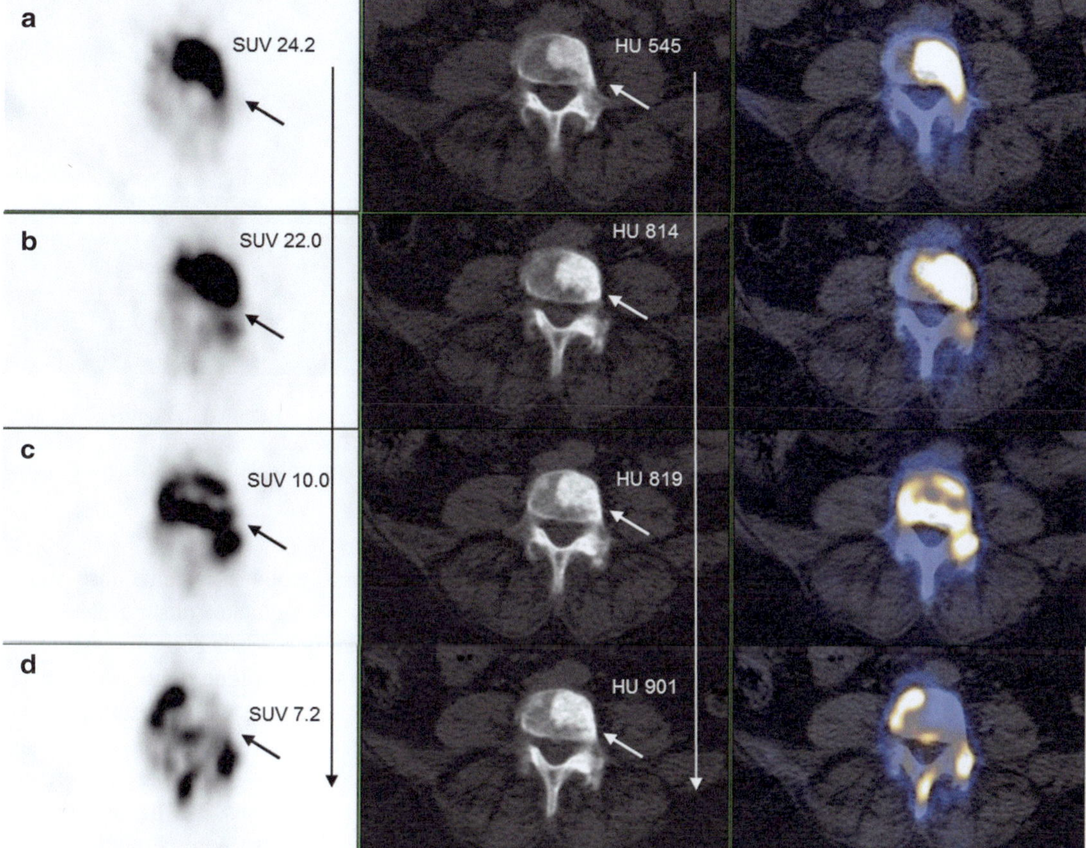

Fig. 6.4 ^{18}F-NaF PET/CT (transaxial views); treatment monitoring of a prostate cancer patient with bone metastases before and after therapy. (**a**) PET image (*left*) shows a markedly increased 18 F-NaF uptake (*left upper row, arrow*) corresponding with a sclerotic lesion (*mid upper row, arrow*) on fourth lumbar spine on CT; fusion PET/CT (*right*). (**b–d**) Follow-up ^{18}F-NaF PET/CT shows decreasing pattern of ^{18}F-NaF uptake on PET (*left, arrows*); however with increasing in Hounsfield unit (*HU*) of the sclerotic lesion (*mid, arrows*); clearly shows higher impact of functional (PET) over anatomical (CT) imaging for therapy monitoring

^{18}F-NaF PET/CT, the modality was calculated to be 91 % sensitive, 83 % specific, and 88 % accurate in evaluation of osseous metastases [75].

Considering high sensitivity of ^{18}F-NaF PET to detect osseous lesions, however, interpreting all focal uptakes as metastasis causes an increased number of false-positive reports and reduced specificity of the modality. In fact, an integrated hybrid PET/CT system guides the interpreters to differentiate benign from malignant lesions. This is specifically an important issue in the spinal lesions in most often old prostate cancer patients who are bearing extensive degenerative changes. Therefore, any abnormal focal uptake which is not correlated to joint surface or end plate should be considered as suspicious [76]. Similar to PET/CT scans with other radiopharmaceuticals, a shortcoming of ^{18}F-NaF PET/CT is the inability of tiny lesions to provoke a blastic reaction with resultant tracer uptake, particularly within the spine [77, 78].

Similar to conventional whole-body bone scintigraphy, the interpreters should be aware of "flare phenomenon" when reviewing ^{18}F-NaF PET/CT images for skeletal metastases from prostate cancer [79].

^{18}F-NaF PET/CT scan has the potential for monitoring response to treatment in patients with osseous metastatic disease (Fig. 6.4). Hillner and colleagues released data based on the American National Oncologic PET Registry (NOPR) which demonstrated the impact of ^{18}F-NaF PET/CT on

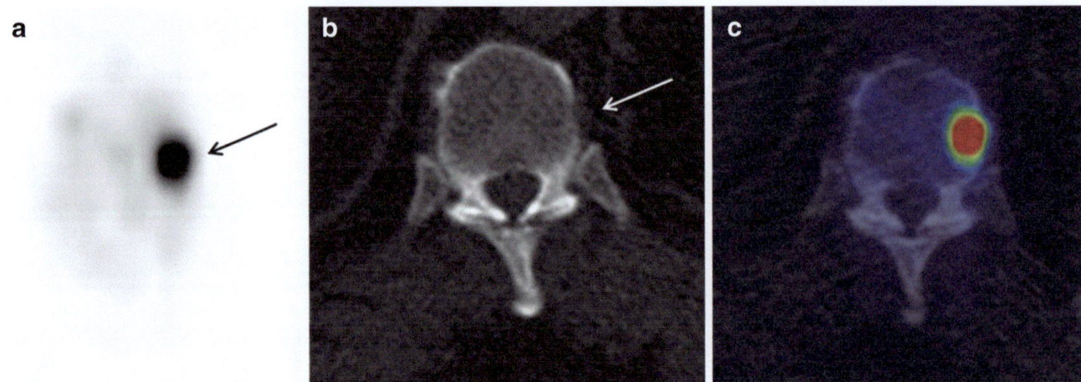

Fig. 6.5 ^{18}F-NaF PET/CT in staging of a prostate cancer patient. (**a**) ^{18}F-NaF PET image (transaxial) shows a focal increased 18 F-NaF uptake (*arrow*) in a thoracic spine. (**b**) CT (transaxial) is unremarkable regarding bone metastases. (**c**) Fusion PET/CT image (transaxial) confirms the findings of PET and CT which are suggestive of early bone metastases without any morphological changes detected by ^{18}F-NaF PET

management of these patients. The total of 2217 patients with 2839 imaging studies (68 % prostate, 17 % breast, 6 % lung, 8 % other cancers) was evaluated. ^{18}F-NaF PET/CT caused alteration in 40 % of the treatments, and the impact was particularly high in patients with evidence of progressive skeletal metastatic disease [80].

As a fact, the sooner recognition of bone metastases in prostate cancer patients, the better planning for successful therapy as well as evaluation of prognosis (Fig. 6.5). Recently, Apolo and colleagues introduced ^{18}F-NaF PET/CT as a tool with prognostic values. They reviewed 60 patients with bone metastases from prostate cancer and discovered a significant correlation between overall survival and changes of SUV on 6-month follow-up images ($p=0.018$) as well as the number of metastases on primary examination ($p=0.017$) [81]. However, regarding few investigations, more studies are still needed to establish the prognostic role for ^{18}F-NaF PET/CT in patients with prostate cancer and skeletal metastases.

6.4 Conventional Bone Scintigraphy Versus ^{18}F-NaF PET/CT

There are pros and cons for ^{18}F-NaF PET/CT, compared with conventional ^{99m}Tc-MDP whole-body bone scintigraphy. The former has less binding to plasma proteins which cause much more availability with quicker plasma clearance; higher uptake rate by osseous cells and target-to-background ratio with resultant double concentration in metastatic lesions, as well as better imaging quality with better spatial resolution (4–5 versus 10–15 mm); earlier imaging after radiotracer administration (0.5–1 versus 2–3 h); and greater sensitivity [74, 82–84]. Also, some studies reported that ^{18}F-NaF PET/CT is able to image both blastic and lytic skeletal metastatic lesions (Fig. 6.6) [85].

Despite the aforementioned advantages, PET/CT scanners are less available than gamma cameras, and the study is more expensive. On the other hand, the insurance reimbursement is more organized for conventional nuclear medicine imaging compared with ^{18}F-NaF PET/CT. While the ^{99m}Tc is produced readily by generator, the production of ^{18}F needs a cyclotron which makes an extra cost. Overall, the PET/CT cost-effectiveness needs to be further investigated in the future studies [17].

Generally, the sensitivity and specificity to detect bone metastases from prostate cancer are higher for ^{18}F-NaF PET/CT than whole-body bone scintigraphy. Even-Sapir and colleagues reviewed 23 patients and calculated a patient-based sensitivity of 100 % and 70 % and specificity of 100 % and 57 % for ^{18}F-NaF PET/CT and planar whole-body bone scintigraphy, respectively. This superiority approved on a lesion-based analysis as well. They

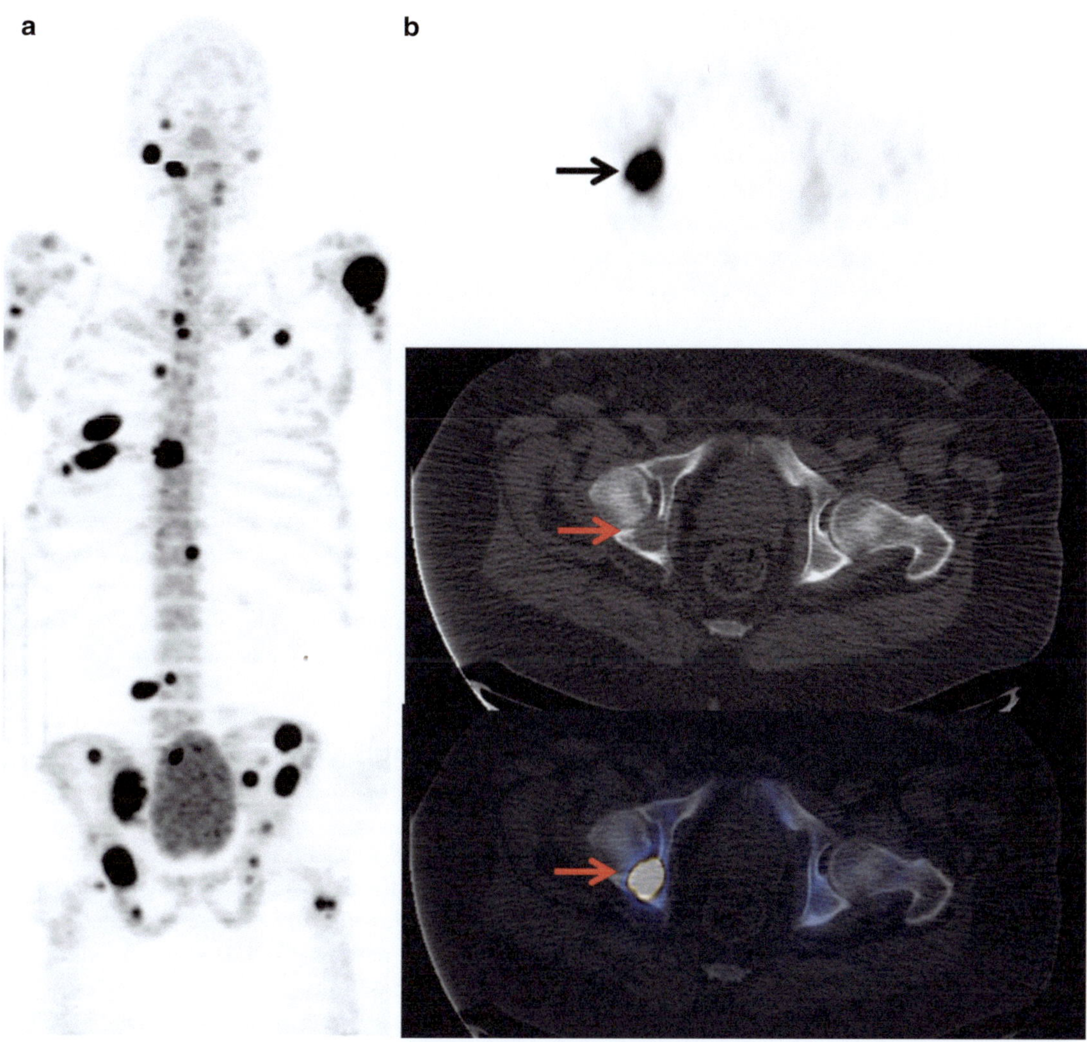

Fig. 6.6 ^{18}F-NaF PET/CT in primary staging of a prostate cancer patient with highly increased PSA level. (**a**) ^{18}F-NaF PET (maximum intensity projection) shows multiple metastatic lesions in the skeleton. (**b**) ^{18}F-NaF PET/CT (transaxial images): intensive ^{18}F-NaF uptake on the right acetabulum (*upper*, *arrow*) with corresponding osteolytic lesion on CT (*Mid*, *arrow*). Fusion image (*lower*, *arrow*) shows that ^{18}F-NaF PET/CT is also able to detect osteolytic bone metastases

also realized that compared with SPECT imaging, PET/CT shows significantly better sensitivity and specificity ($p<0.05$) [17]. Also, Evangelista and colleagues revealed in their review an article that the ^{18}F-NaF PET/CT has the best median sensitivity (with a range of 81–100 %) among the nuclear medicine modalities in evaluation of bone metastases from prostate cancer [83].

Bombardieri and colleagues revealed that ^{18}F-NaF PET/CT is more sensitive and superior to whole-body bone scan in evaluation of osseous metastases from prostate cancer, most likely due to fast uptake of radiotracer by bone lesions and quick excretion by urinary system, leading to higher target-to-background ratio. Also, some other investigators had almost similar conclusion [17, 67, 75, 86–89].

Furthermore, the ^{18}F-NaF PET/CT depicts more number of lesions and earlier in the course of disease when compared with conventional bone scintigraphy [81].

The superiority of ^{18}F-NaF PET/CT over conventional bone scan in sensitivity, NPV, and accuracy was the conclusion of a study by Poulsen and colleagues, in which they evaluated 50 patients with 526 metastatic bone lesions from prostate cancer. With a sensitivity of 93 %, however, the specificity was reported as low as 54 %, most likely due to false-positive lesions from inflammatory or degenerative process among the enrolled old-age patients. The sensitivity, specificity, accuracy, and positive and negative predictive values were reported as 93 % vs 51 %, 54 % vs 82 %, 81 % vs 61 %, 82 % vs 86 %, and 78 % vs 43 % for ^{18}F-NaF PET/CT versus ^{99m}Tc-MDP whole-body scintigraphy, respectively [70].

^{18}F-NaF PET/CT is more accurate for evaluation of response to treatment among patients with prostate cancer osseous metastatic disease [90].

Jadvar and colleagues investigated 37 patients with history of localized prostate cancer, followed by a definitive therapy such as radiation or radical prostatectomy, who presented with evidence of PSA biochemical recurrence but negative conventional studies. They demonstrated that the ^{18}F-NaF PET/CT is capable of detecting occult skeletal metastatic lesion in lower serum PSA levels than conventional imaging [91].

When compared with conventional whole-body bone scan, semiquantitative evaluation of skeletal lesions with calculation of standardized uptake value (SUV) is a unique advantage of ^{18}F-NaF PET/CT. This is actually important in the spine as the most frequent site of both ^{18}F-NaF-positive degenerative changes and metastases from prostate cancer [92]. Muzahir and colleagues performed a pilot investigation in which the results showed a significantly lower SUV_{max} for degenerative (<12) versus metastases from castrate-resistant prostate cancer (>50) in the spine ($p<0.001$). They enrolled 17 patients with history of castrate-resistant prostate cancer and 65 metastatic as well as 56 degenerative ^{18}F-NaF-positive lesions, differentiated according to low-dose CT scan. The range of SUV_{max} was calculated as 11–188 (mean of 160) for metastatic versus 3–50 (mean of 6.2) for degenerative lesions. The authors concluded that semiquantitative measurements can play a complementary role for qualitative analysis in order to better differentiate osseous metastatic from degenerative lesions [93].

A retrospective study by our group examined the value of semiquantitative analysis (SUV) in differentiation of benign versus malignant bone lesions on ^{18}F-NaF PET/CT. We found that a differentiation between benign and malignant lesions is not possible in SUV levels less than 45. However, all malignant lesions interestingly showed an SUV of over 45 [94]. Nevertheless, further research studies are strongly needed to define the real value of SUV in this differentiation.

In summary, this is our belief that based on increasing number of established PET/CT scanners and decreasing price for PET radiotracers, as well as better accuracy in detecting metastatic lesions, ^{18}F-NaF PET/CT will supplant conventional ^{99m}Tc-MDP whole-body bone scintigraphy in the near future for evaluation of skeletal metastatic disease from prostate cancer [78].

6.5 Single Combined ^{18}F-FDG/^{18}F-NaF PET/CT

Although ^{18}F-FDG PET/CT is not competent to routinely evaluate prostate cancer. Unremarkable glucose metabolism by prostate cancer tumor cells and excretion of radioactive urine into the bladder at proximity of prostate gland are two major reasons which make ^{18}F-FDG PET/CT a noncompetent method for routine prostate cancer assessment [95, 96]. However, since high-grade prostate cancers (with Gleason score$\geq$8) could be FDG avid, the FDG avidity is assumed to be an independent prognostic factor in this group of patients [46], mostly due to largely reduced glucose metabolism by tumor; however, it can play a supplemental role for ^{18}F-NaF PET/CT to detect extra-skeletal metastatic involvement.

Nonetheless, it could be a supplement for ^{18}F-NaF PET/CT in the evaluation of bone metastases in patients with prostate cancer [97] as well as assessment of soft tissue and lymph node involvement [98, 99]. Merging the two modalities in a single examination is more soothed for patients and also more affordable for insurance companies due to reduced cost. This way, involvements beyond the osseous structures can be more accurately evaluated [100, 101]. Moreover, ^{18}F-FDG avidity of prostate tumor is considered as an independent prognostic factor and represents a high-grade malignancy.

Recently, the combination ^{18}F-NaF with other specific PET tracers (e.g., ^{18}F-choline) in a single PET/CT (i.e., dual tracer PET/CT) is introduced as a promising imaging technique in the evaluation of prostate cancer patients which allows more accurate assessment of both skeletal and soft tissue malignancies [100, 101].

References

1. Center MM, Jemal A, Lortet-Tieulent J et al (2012) International variation in prostate cancer incidence and mortality rates. Eur Urol 61:1079–1092
2. Ferlay J, Shin HR, Bray F, Forman D, Mathers C, Parkin DM (2010) Estimates of worldwide burden of cancer in 2008: GLOBOCAN 2008. Int J Cancer 127:2893–2917
3. Castro E, Goh C, Olmos D et al (2013) Germline BRCA mutations are associated with higher risk of nodal involvement, distant metastasis, and poor survival outcomes in prostate cancer. J Clin Oncol 31:1748–1757
4. Goh CL, Eeles RA (2014) Germline genetic variants associated with prostate cancer and potential relevance to clinical practice. Recent Results Cancer Res 202:9–26
5. Hemminki K, Ankerst DP, Sundquist J, Mousavi SM (2013) Prostate cancer incidence and survival in immigrants to Sweden. World J Urol 31:1483–1488
6. Huncharek M, Haddock KS, Reid R, Kupelnick B (2010) Smoking as a risk factor for prostate cancer: a meta-analysis of 24 prospective cohort studies. Am J Public Health 100:693–701
7. Karlsson R, Aly M, Clements M et al (2014) A population-based assessment of germline HOXB13 G84E mutation and prostate cancer risk. Eur Urol 65:169–176
8. Kicinski M, Vangronsveld J, Nawrot TS (2011) An epidemiological reappraisal of the familial aggregation of prostate cancer: a meta-analysis. PLoS One 6, e27130
9. Merrill RM, Sloan A (2012) Risk-adjusted incidence rates for prostate cancer in the United States. Prostate 72:181–185
10. Zu K, Giovannucci E (2009) Smoking and aggressive prostate cancer: a review of the epidemiologic evidence. Cancer Causes Control 20:1799–1810
11. Bastian PJ, Boorjian SA, Bossi A et al (2012) High-risk prostate cancer: from definition to contemporary management. Eur Urol 61:1096–1106
12. Espey DK, Wu XC, Swan J et al (2007) Annual report to the nation on the status of cancer, 1975–2004, featuring cancer in American Indians and Alaska Natives. Cancer 110:2119–2152
13. Farwell WR, Linder JA, Jha AK (2007) Trends in prostate-specific antigen testing from 1995 through 2004. Arch Intern Med 167:2497–2502
14. Rigaud J, Tiguert R, Le Normand L et al (2002) Prognostic value of bone scan in patients with metastatic prostate cancer treated initially with androgen deprivation therapy. J Urol 168:1423–1426
15. Fowler JE Jr, Sanders J, Bigler SA, Rigdon J, Kilambi NK, Land SA (2000) Percent free prostate specific antigen and cancer detection in black and white men with total prostate specific antigen 2.5 to 9.9 ng./ml. J Urol 163:1467–1470
16. Bubendorf L, Schopfer A, Wagner U et al (2000) Metastatic patterns of prostate cancer: an autopsy study of 1,589 patients. Hum Pathol 31:578–583
17. Even-Sapir E, Metser U, Mishani E, Lievshitz G, Lerman H, Leibovitch I (2006) The detection of bone metastases in patients with high-risk prostate cancer: 99mTc-MDP Planar bone scintigraphy, single- and multi-field-of-view SPECT, 18F-fluoride PET, and 18F-fluoride PET/CT. J Nucl Med 47:287–297
18. Dennis ER, Jia X, Mezheritskiy IS et al (2012) Bone scan index: a quantitative treatment response biomarker for castration-resistant metastatic prostate cancer. J Clin Oncol 30:519–524
19. Norgaard M, Jensen AO, Jacobsen JB, Cetin K, Fryzek JP, Sorensen HT (2010) Skeletal related events, bone metastasis and survival of prostate cancer: a population based cohort study in Denmark (1999 to 2007). J Urol 184:162–167
20. Coleman RE (2006) Clinical features of metastatic bone disease and risk of skeletal morbidity. Clin Cancer Res 12:6243s–6249s
21. Thoreson GR, Gayed BA, Chung PH, Raj GV (2014) Emerging therapies in castration resistant prostate cancer. Can J Urol 21:98–105
22. Fogelman I (1982) Diphosphonate bone scanning agents – current concepts. Eur J Nucl Med 7:506–509
23. Lam AS, Kettle AG, O'Doherty MJ, Coakley AJ, Barrington SF, Blower PJ (1997) Pentavalent 99Tcm-DMSA imaging in patients with bone metastases. Nucl Med Commun 18:907–914
24. Lin J, Leung WT, Ho SK et al (1995) Quantitative evaluation of thallium-201 uptake in predicting chemotherapeutic response of osteosarcoma. Eur J Nucl Med 22:553–555
25. Salvatore M, Carratu L, Porta E (1976) Thallium-201 as a positive indicator for lung neoplasms: preliminary experiments. Radiology 121:487–488
26. Weiner RE (1996) The mechanism of 67Ga localization in malignant disease. Nucl Med Biol 23:745–751
27. Fogelman I, Bessent RG, Cohen HN, Hart DM, Lindsay R (1980) Skeletal uptake of diphosphonate. Method for prediction of post-menopausal osteoporosis. Lancet 2:667–670

28. Love C, Din AS, Tomas MB, Kalapparambath TP, Palestro CJ (2003) Radionuclide bone imaging: an illustrative review. Radiographics 23:341–358
29. Bombardieri E, Setti L, Kirienko M, Antunovic L, Guglielmo P, Ciocia G (2015) Which metabolic imaging, besides bone scan with 99mTc-phosphonates, for detecting and evaluating bone metastases in prostatic cancer patients? An open discussion. Q J Nucl Med Mol Imaging 59:381–399
30. Briganti A, Passoni N, Ferrari M et al (2010) When to perform bone scan in patients with newly diagnosed prostate cancer: external validation of the currently available guidelines and proposal of a novel risk stratification tool. Eur Urol 57:551–558
31. Scher HI, Sawyers CL (2005) Biology of progressive, castration-resistant prostate cancer: directed therapies targeting the androgen-receptor signaling axis. J Clin Oncol 23:8253–8261
32. National Institute for Clinical Excellence. Improving outcomes in urological cancers. 2002. London, UK. www.nice.org.uk. ISBN: 1-84257-210-5
33. Minoves M (2003) Bone and joint sports injuries: the role of bone scintigraphy. Nucl Med Commun 24:3–10
34. de Jong IJ, Pruim J, Elsinga PH, Vaalburg W, Mensink HJ (2003) Preoperative staging of pelvic lymph nodes in prostate cancer by 11C-choline PET. J Nucl Med 44:331–335
35. Krasnow AZ, Hellman RS, Timins ME, Collier BD, Anderson T, Isitman AT (1997) Diagnostic bone scanning in oncology. Semin Nucl Med 27:107–141
36. Rosenthal DI (1997) Radiologic diagnosis of bone metastases. Cancer 80:1595–1607
37. Cook GJ, Fogelman I (2001) The role of nuclear medicine in monitoring treatment in skeletal malignancy. Semin Nucl Med 31:206–211
38. Koizumi M, Matsumoto S, Takahashi S, Yamashita T, Ogata E (1999) Bone metabolic markers in the evaluation of bone scan flare phenomenon in bone metastases of breast cancer. Clin Nucl Med 24:15–20
39. Horiuchi-Suzuki K, Konno A, Ueda M et al (2004) Skeletal affinity of Tc(V)-DMS is bone cell mediated and pH dependent. Eur J Nucl Med Mol Imaging 31:388–398
40. Jacobson A, Fogelman I, Rosenthall L (1996) Skeletal nuclear medicine: bone scanning in metastatic disease. Mosby, St Louis, pp 87–123
41. O'Mara RE (1976) Skeletal scanning in neoplastic disease. Cancer 37:480–486
42. Roland J, van den Weyngaert D, Krug B, Brans B, Scalliet P, Vandevivere J (1995) Metastases seen on SPECT imaging despite a normal planar bone scan. Clin Nucl Med 20:1052–1054
43. Oesterling JE, Martin SK, Bergstralh EJ, Lowe FC (1993) The use of prostate-specific antigen in staging patients with newly diagnosed prostate cancer. JAMA 269:57–60
44. Imbriaco M, Larson SM, Yeung HW et al (1998) A new parameter for measuring metastatic bone involvement by prostate cancer: the Bone Scan Index. Clin Cancer Res 4:1765–1772
45. Ellis RE (1961) The distribution of active bone marrow in the adult. Phys Med Biol 5:255–258
46. Meirelles GS, Schoder H, Ravizzini GC et al (2010) Prognostic value of baseline [18F] fluorodeoxyglucose positron emission tomography and 99mTc-MDP bone scan in progressing metastatic prostate cancer. Clin Cancer Res 16:6093–6099
47. Sabbatini P, Larson SM, Kremer A et al (1999) Prognostic significance of extent of disease in bone in patients with androgen-independent prostate cancer. J Clin Oncol 17:948–957
48. Reza M, Bjartell A, Ohlsson M et al (2014) Bone Scan Index as a prognostic imaging biomarker during androgen deprivation therapy. EJNMMI Res 4:58
49. Kaboteh R, Damber JE, Gjertsson P et al (2013) Bone Scan Index: a prognostic imaging biomarker for high-risk prostate cancer patients receiving primary hormonal therapy. EJNMMI Res 3:9
50. Sadik M, Suurkula M, Hoglund P, Jarund A, Edenbrandt L (2009) Improved classifications of planar whole-body bone scans using a computer-assisted diagnosis system: a multicenter, multiple-reader, multiple-case study. J Nucl Med 50:368–375
51. Ulmert D, Kaboteh R, Fox JJ et al (2012) A novel automated platform for quantifying the extent of skeletal tumour involvement in prostate cancer patients using the Bone Scan Index. Eur Urol 62:78–84
52. Sarikaya I, Sarikaya A, Holder LE (2001) The role of single photon emission computed tomography in bone imaging. Semin Nucl Med 31:3–16
53. Savelli G, Maffioli L, Maccauro M, De Deckere E, Bombardieri E (2001) Bone scintigraphy and the added value of SPECT (single photon emission tomography) in detecting skeletal lesions. Q J Nucl Med 45:27–37
54. Sedonja I, Budihna NV (1999) The benefit of SPECT when added to planar scintigraphy in patients with bone metastases in the spine. Clin Nucl Med 24:407–413
55. Savelli G, Chiti A, Grasselli G, Maccauro M, Rodari M, Bombardieri E (2000) The role of bone SPET study in diagnosis of single vertebral metastases. Anticancer Res 20:1115–1120
56. Gnanasegaran G, Barwick T, Adamson K, Mohan H, Sharp D, Fogelman I (2009) Multislice SPECT/CT in benign and malignant bone disease: when the ordinary turns into the extraordinary. Semin Nucl Med 39:431–442
57. Romer W, Nomayr A, Uder M, Bautz W, Kuwert T (2006) SPECT-guided CT for evaluating foci of increased bone metabolism classified as indeterminate on SPECT in cancer patients. J Nucl Med 47:1102–1106
58. Helyar V, Mohan HK, Barwick T et al (2010) The added value of multislice SPECT/CT in patients with equivocal bony metastasis from carcinoma of the prostate. Eur J Nucl Med Mol Imaging 37:706–713

59. Ndlovu X, George R, Ellmann A, Warwick J (2010) Should SPECT-CT replace SPECT for the evaluation of equivocal bone scan lesions in patients with underlying malignancies? Nucl Med Commun 31:659–665
60. Sharma P, Dhull VS, Reddy RM et al (2013) Hybrid SPECT-CT for characterizing isolated vertebral lesions observed by bone scintigraphy: comparison with planar scintigraphy, SPECT, and CT. Diagn Interv Radiol 19:33–40
61. Palmedo H, Marx C, Ebert A et al (2014) Whole-body SPECT/CT for bone scintigraphy: diagnostic value and effect on patient management in oncological patients. Eur J Nucl Med Mol Imaging 41:59–67
62. Ghosh P (2014) The role of SPECT/CT in skeletal malignancies. Semin Musculoskelet Radiol 18:175–193
63. Ben-Haim S, Israel O (2009) Breast cancer: role of SPECT and PET in imaging bone metastases. Semin Nucl Med 39:408–415
64. Horger M, Eschmann SM, Pfannenberg C et al (2004) Evaluation of combined transmission and emission tomography for classification of skeletal lesions. AJR Am J Roentgenol 183:655–661
65. Shen G, Deng H, Hu S, Jia Z (2014) Comparison of choline-PET/CT, MRI, SPECT, and bone scintigraphy in the diagnosis of bone metastases in patients with prostate cancer: a meta-analysis. Skeletal Radiol 43:1503–1513
66. Utsunomiya D, Shiraishi S, Imuta M et al (2006) Added value of SPECT/CT fusion in assessing suspected bone metastasis: comparison with scintigraphy alone and nonfused scintigraphy and CT. Radiology 238:264–271
67. Withofs N, Grayet B, Tancredi T et al (2011) ^{18}F-fluoride PET/CT for assessing bone involvement in prostate and breast cancers. Nucl Med Commun 32:168–176
68. Schirrmeister H, Guhlmann A, Elsner K et al (1999) Sensitivity in detecting osseous lesions depends on anatomic localization: planar bone scintigraphy versus 18F PET. J Nucl Med 40:1623–1629
69. Beheshti M, Langsteger W, Fogelman I (2009) Prostate cancer: role of SPECT and PET in imaging bone metastases. Semin Nucl Med 39:396–407
70. Poulsen MH, Petersen H, Hoilund-Carlsen PF et al (2014) Spine metastases in prostate cancer: comparison of technetium-99m-MDP whole-body bone scintigraphy, [(18) F]choline positron emission tomography(PET)/computed tomography (CT) and [(18) F]NaF PET/CT. BJU Int 114:818–823
71. Wootton R, Dore C (1986) The single-passage extraction of 18F in rabbit bone. Clin Phys Physiol Meas 7:333–343
72. Grant FD, Fahey FH, Packard AB, Davis RT, Alavi A, Treves ST (2008) Skeletal PET with 18F-fluoride: applying new technology to an old tracer. J Nucl Med 49:68–78
73. Beheshti M, Mottaghy FM, Payche F et al (2015) ^{18}F-NaF PET/CT: EANM procedure guidelines for bone imaging. Eur J Nucl Med Mol Imaging 42:1767–1777
74. Segall G, Delbeke D, Stabin MG et al (2010) SNM practice guideline for sodium 18F-fluoride PET/CT bone scans 1.0. J Nucl Med 51:1813–1820
75. Langsteger W, Balogova S, Huchet V et al (2011) Fluorocholine (18F) and sodium fluoride (18F) PET/CT in the detection of prostate cancer: prospective comparison of diagnostic performance determined by masked reading. Q J Nucl Med Mol Imaging 55:448–457
76. Schirrmeister H (2007) Detection of bone metastases in breast cancer by positron emission tomography. Radiol Clin North Am 45:669–676, vi
77. Cook GJ, Fogelman I (1999) Skeletal metastases from breast cancer: imaging with nuclear medicine. Semin Nucl Med 29:69–79
78. Langsteger W, Heinisch M, Fogelman I (2006) The role of fluorodeoxyglucose, 18F-dihydroxyphenylalanine, 18F-choline, and 18F-fluoride in bone imaging with emphasis on prostate and breast. Semin Nucl Med 36:73–92
79. Wade AA, Scott JA, Kuter I, Fischman AJ (2006) Flare response in 18F-fluoride ion PET bone scanning. AJR Am J Roentgenol 186:1783–1786
80. Hillner BE, Siegel BA, Hanna L, Duan F, Quinn B, Shields AF (2015) 18F-fluoride PET used for treatment monitoring of systemic cancer therapy: results from the National Oncologic PET Registry. J Nucl Med 56:222–228
81. Apolo AB, Lindenberg L, Shih JH et al (2016) Prospective study evaluating Na18F-positron emission tomography/computed tomography (NaF-PET/CT) in predicting clinical outcomes and survival in advanced prostate cancer. J Nucl Med 57:886–892
82. Blau M, Ganatra R, Bender MA (1972) 18 F-fluoride for bone imaging. Semin Nucl Med 2:31–37
83. Evangelista L, Bertoldo F, Boccardo F et al (2016) Diagnostic imaging to detect and evaluate response to therapy in bone metastases from prostate cancer: current modalities and new horizons. Eur J Nucl Med Mol Imaging 43:1546–1562
84. Park-Holohan SJ, Blake GM, Fogelman I (2001) Quantitative studies of bone using (18)F-fluoride and (99m)Tc-methylene diphosphonate: evaluation of renal and whole-blood kinetics. Nucl Med Commun 22:1037–1044
85. Araz M, Aras G, Kucuk ON (2015) The role of 18F-NaF PET/CT in metastatic bone disease. J Bone Oncol 4:92–97
86. Beheshti M, Vali R, Waldenberger P et al (2008) Detection of bone metastases in patients with prostate cancer by 18F fluorocholine and 18F fluoride PET-CT: a comparative study. Eur J Nucl Med Mol Imaging 35:1766–1774
87. Damle NA, Bal C, Bandopadhyaya GP et al (2013) The role of 18F-fluoride PET-CT in the detection of bone metastases in patients with breast, lung and prostate carcinoma: a comparison with FDG PET/CT and 99mTc-MDP bone scan. Jpn J Radiol 31:262–269

88. Iagaru A, Mittra E, Dick DW, Gambhir SS (2012) Prospective evaluation of (99m)Tc MDP scintigraphy, (18)F NaF PET/CT, and (18)F FDG PET/CT for detection of skeletal metastases. Mol Imaging Biol 14:252–259
89. Minamimoto R, Loening A, Jamali M et al (2015) Prospective comparison of 99mTc-MDP scintigraphy, combined 18F-NaF and 18F-FDG PET/CT, and whole-body MRI in patients with breast and prostate cancer. J Nucl Med 56:1862–1868
90. Zukotynski KA, Kim CK, Gerbaudo VH et al (2015) ^{18}F-FDG-PET/CT and ^{18}F-NaF-PET/CT in men with castrate-resistant prostate cancer. Am J Nucl Med Mol Imaging 5:72–82
91. Jadvar H, Desai B, Ji L et al (2012) Prospective evaluation of 18F-NaF and 18F-FDG PET/CT in detection of occult metastatic disease in biochemical recurrence of prostate cancer. Clin Nucl Med 37:637–643
92. Rosen RS, Fayad L, Wahl RL (2006) Increased 18F-FDG uptake in degenerative disease of the spine: characterization with 18F-FDG PET/CT. J Nucl Med 47:1274–1280
93. Muzahir S, Jeraj R, Liu G et al (2015) Differentiation of metastatic vs degenerative joint disease using semi-quantitative analysis with (18)F-NaF PET/CT in castrate resistant prostate cancer patients. Am J Nucl Med Mol Imaging 5:162–168
94. Vali R, Beheshti M, Waldenberger P et al (2008) Assessment of malignant and benign bone lesions by static F-18 Fluoride PET-CT: Additional value of SUV! J Nucl Med 49(Supplement 1):150P
95. Beauregard JM, Blouin AC, Fradet V et al (2015) FDG-PET/CT for pre-operative staging and prognostic stratification of patients with high-grade prostate cancer at biopsy. Cancer Imaging 15:2
96. Liu IJ, Zafar MB, Lai YH, Segall GM, Terris MK (2001) Fluorodeoxyglucose positron emission tomography studies in diagnosis and staging of clinically organ-confined prostate cancer. Urology 57:108–111
97. Iagaru A, Mittra E, Mosci C et al (2013) Combined 18F-fluoride and 18F-FDG PET/CT scanning for evaluation of malignancy: results of an international multicenter trial. J Nucl Med 54:176–183
98. Jadvar H, Pinski JK, Conti PS (2003) FDG PET in suspected recurrent and metastatic prostate cancer. Oncol Rep 10:1485–1488
99. Shiiba M, Ishihara K, Kimura G et al (2012) Evaluation of primary prostate cancer using 11C-methionine-PET/CT and 18F-FDG-PET/CT. Ann Nucl Med 26:138–145
100. Iagaru A, Mittra E, Yaghoubi SS et al (2009) Novel strategy for a cocktail 18F-fluoride and 18F-FDG PET/CT scan for evaluation of malignancy: results of the pilot-phase study. J Nucl Med 50:501–505
101. Lin FI, Rao JE, Mittra ES et al (2012) Prospective comparison of combined 18F-FDG and 18F-NaF PET/CT vs. 18F-FDG PET/CT imaging for detection of malignancy. Eur J Nucl Med Mol Imaging 39:262–270

Detection of Bone Metastases and Evaluation of Therapy Response in Prostate Cancer Patients by Radiolabelled Choline PET/CT

7

Elena Incerti, Paola Mapelli, and Maria Picchio

Index Acronyms

11C-CHO	11C-choline
18F-CHO	18F-choline
ADT	Androgen deprivation therapy
BS	Bone scintigraphy
CRPC	Castration-resistant prostate cancer
CT	Computed tomography
18F-FDG	Fluorodeoxyglucose
MRI	Magnetic resonance imaging
PET	Positron emission tomography
PSA	Prostate-specific antigen
RECIST	Response Evaluation Criteria in Solid Tumours
RT	Radiation therapy
SBRT	Stereotactic body RT
SUV	Standardised uptake value

E. Incerti, MSc • P. Mapelli, MD • M. Picchio, MD (✉)
Unit of Nuclear Medicine, IRCCS San Raffaele Scientific Institute, IRCCS San Raffaele Scientific Institute, Via Olgettina 60, 20132 Milan, Italy
e-mail: incerti.elena@hsr.it; mapelli.paola@hsr.it; picchio.maria@hsr.it

7.1 Rationale for Choline PET in Prostate Cancer

Choline positron emission tomography/computed tomography (PET/CT) has been largely investigated in prostate cancer patients, particularly in restaging phase. Choline is a critical molecule in phospholipid metabolism, transmembrane signalling and lipid transport and metabolism [1]. Intracellular choline is phosphorylated to phosphoryl choline by the enzyme choline kinase. Phosphoryl choline is then trapped within the cell. Prior investigations have demonstrated increased phosphoryl choline as well as increased choline kinase activity in prostate cancer cells relative to normal prostatic tissue [2] Fig. 7.1.

Choline radiopharmaceuticals can be labelled by both 11C (11C-CHO) and 18F (18F-CHO). The most striking difference between the two tracers is the urinary elimination that is high for 18F-CHO, being an important disadvantage for imaging prostate region. Conversely, 18F-CHO imaging has the advantage of a longer half-life (approximately 110 min versus 20 min of 11C-CHO) allowing transportation from one single cyclotron centre to several PET centres [3, 4]. 18F-CHO provides more flexibility concerning imaging protocols and availability and presents a very similar behaviour to 11C-CHO in prostate cancer

F. Bertoldo et al. (eds.), *Bone Metastases from Prostate Cancer*,
DOI 10.1007/978-3-319-42327-2_7

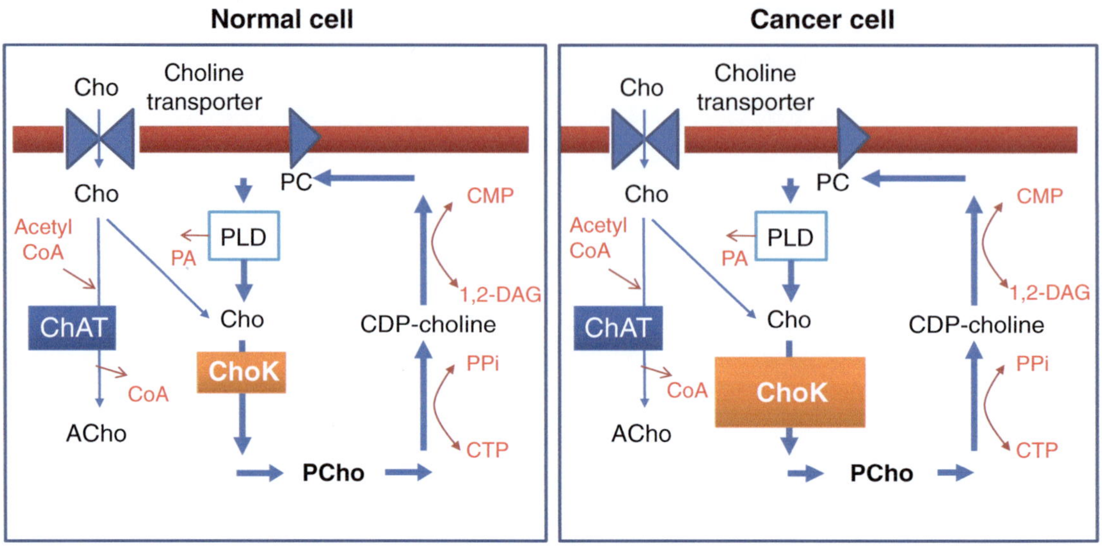

Fig. 7.1 Pathway of choline metabolism in normal and cancer cell (*Cho* choline, *ChAT* choline acetyltransferase, *ACho* acetylcholine, *ChoK* choline kinase, *CMP* cytidylate, *DAG* diacylglycerol, *PCho* phosphocholine, *CDP* diphosphocholine, *PPi* Inorganic pyrophosphate, *PC* phosphocholine, *PA* phosphatic acid, *PLD* phospholipase D)

patients. Both 11C- and 18F-CHO PET/CT are actually an established imaging modality in the evaluation of patients with prostate cancer [5, 6].

7.2 Diagnostic Accuracy of Radiolabelled Choline in Skeletal Metastases

Although most studies of choline in prostate cancer evaluated localised or lymph node disease [7, 8], their results provided additional evidence to support the use of choline also for the detection of early osseous metastatic disease in newly diagnosed and recurrent prostate cancer patients [9]. In a retrospective analysis, 11C-CHO PET/CT was valuable in the assessment of metastatic bone disease in terms of detection, localisation and characterisation [10]. It remains unclear whether 11C-CHO PET/CT is more sensitive than conventional BS, but it has higher specificity, with fewer indeterminate lesions [6, 11, 12]. 11C-CHO PET/CT may detect multiple bone metastases in patients showing a single metastases on bone scan and may be positive for bone metastases in up to 15 % of patients with biochemical failure after radical prostatectomy and negative bone scan [13]. The specificity of 11C-CHO PET/CT is also higher than bone scan with less false-positive and indeterminate findings [14, 15]. An important advantage of CHO PET/CT is the opportunity to discover the presence of medullary bone involvement, before that the cortical part is taken. Fig. 7.2 is reported in example of a patient with bone medullary involvement at 18F-CHO PET/CT that was later confirmed by MRI.

Beheshti et al. have investigated whether 18F-CHO PET/CT is of value for the detection of bone metastases and found that 18F-CHO PET/CT showed a sensitivity, specificity and accuracy of 79 %, 97 % and 84 % [16]. Onyeuku et al. observed similar radiographic results to Beheshti et al. when compared to conventional methods in two of the four patients with positive findings on imaging [17]. In a recent study by Kjolhede et al., 90 high-risk prostate cancer patients presenting a negative or inconclusive bone scan underwent 18F-CHO PET/CT [18]. Authors concluded that choline PET/CT imaging could detect metastases in high-risk prostate cancer patients with negative or inconclusive bone scan, with a change in the planned treatment (from curative to palliative) in 20 % of them. Poulsen et al. [19] evaluated the value of 18F-CHO PET/CT in the initial staging of 210 patients. Even if the goal of the study was to assess the value of PET/CT in lymph

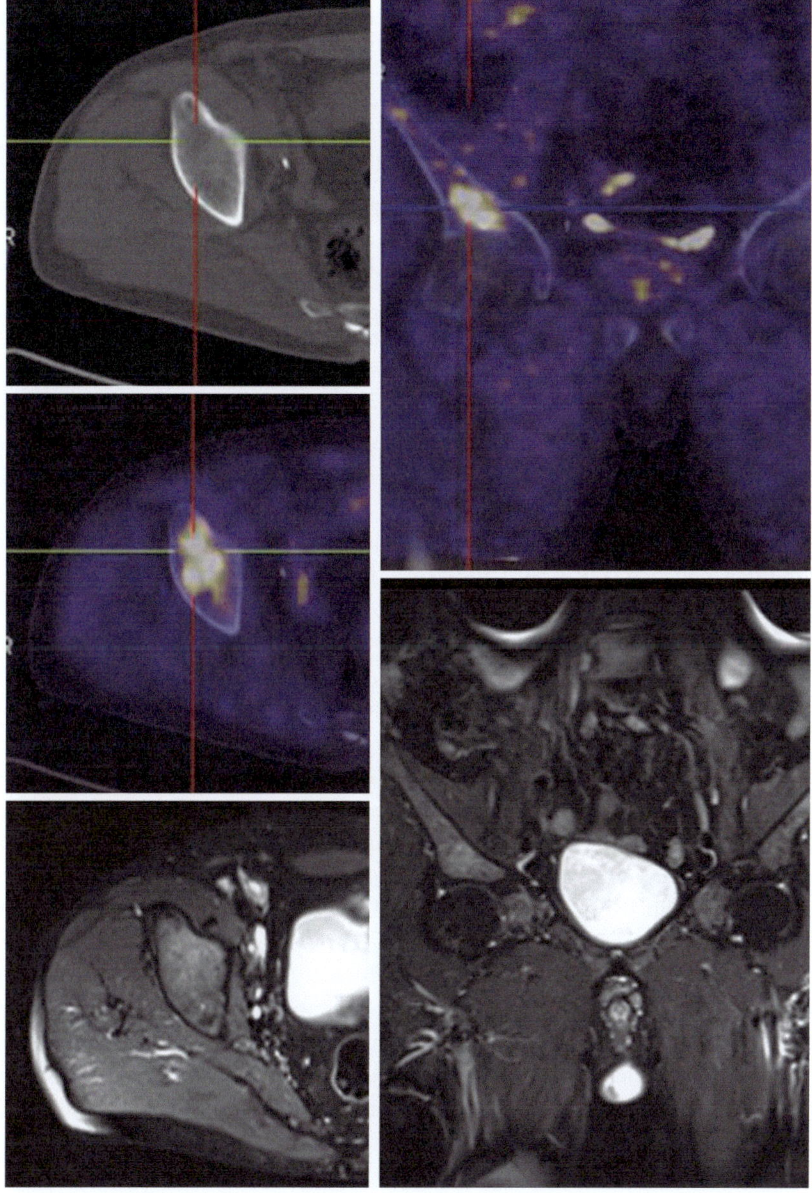

Fig. 7.2 A 78-year-old man underwent 18F-CHO PET/CT for a biochemical recurrence of prostate cancer. A significant uptake of CHO was shown in the right ischium (*up*; *left* and *right*), without any morphological changes at co-registrated CT images (*up*, *left*). An MRI scan confirmed the presence of medullary involvement in the same site (*down*, *left* and *right*) (Courtesy Dr. Laura Evangelista, Nuclear Medicine and Molecular Imaging Unit, Veneto Institute of Oncology IOV – IRCCS, Padua, Italy)

node staging, authors underlined that a high focal bone uptake, consistent with bone metastases, was seen in 18 patients, 12 of which presented histologically proven benign lymph nodes. However, 18F-CHO presented limitations in detecting densely sclerotic malignant lesions [14]. In particular, in restaging prostate cancer, both 11C- and 18F-CHO PET/CT have been demonstrated to be superior to 18F-FDG PET/CT in detecting recurrences, including bone metastatic lesions (Figs. 7.3, 7.4 and 7.5) [20].

Picchio et al. showed that 11C-CHO PET/CT exhibits a lower sensitivity but a higher specificity than those of bone scan in the detection of bone metastases in prostate cancer patients with biochemical progression. Equivocal findings occurred in 1 of 78 (1 %) cases in 11C-CHO PET/CT and in 21 of 78 (27 %) cases in bone scan. Depending on their attribution as either positive or negative, the ranges of sensitivity, specificity, positive predictive value, negative predictive value and accuracy for 11C-CHO

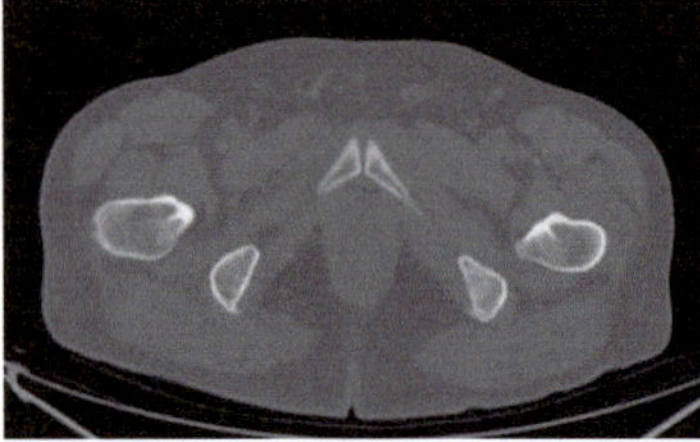
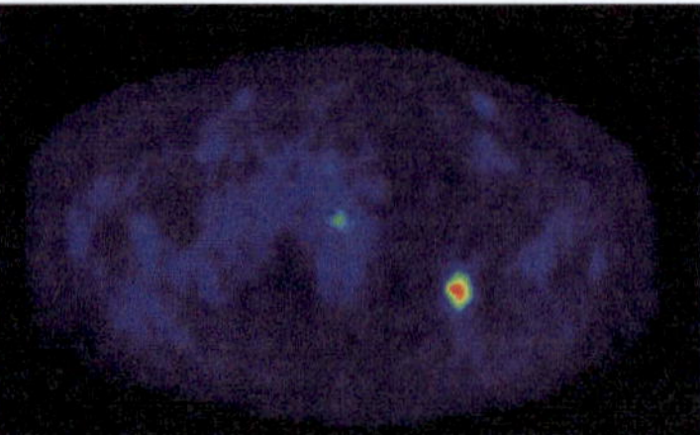
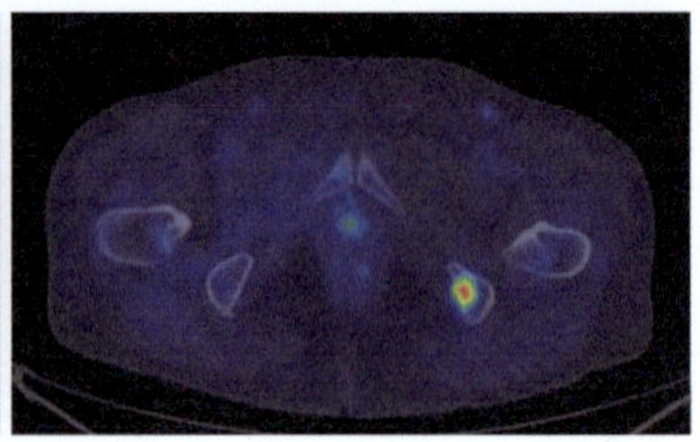

Fig. 7.3 A 61-year-old man treated with radical prostatectomy for prostate cancer (GS 7 (4+3), pT2cR1N0), who performed 11C-CHO PET/CT for biochemical recurrence (PSA: 14.62 ng/mL). 11C-CHO PET/CT showed a pathological uptake in the left ischial tuberosity as documented on CT (**a**), PET (**b**) and PET/CT-fused (**c**) transaxial images. After androgen deprivation therapy (PSA: 0.07 ng/mL), helical tomotherapy (HTT) was performed on the positive 11C-CHO PET/CT lesion. One year after HTT, patient showed a complete response with a PSA value of 0.03 ng/mL

PET/CT were 89–89 %, 98–100 %, 96–100 %, 94–96 % and 95–96 %, respectively. For bone scan they were 100–70 %, 75–100 %, 68–100 %, 100–86 % and 83–90 %, respectively. Concordant findings between 11C-CHO PET/CT and bone scan occurred in 55 of 78 (71 %) cases [6]. Fig. 7.6 is reported with discordant images between 18F-CHO PET/CT and bone scan.

Another PET tracer, 18F-fluoride, traditionally used in the evaluation of bone metastases, showed a better sensitivity compared with traditional bone scan. However, 18F-fluoride PET/CT scans suffer from the same lack of specificity of bone scan. Poulsen et al. [21] studied detection of spine metastases with 18F-fluoride, 18F-CHO and bone scan and found that 18F-fluoride is superior in sensitivity to 18F-CHO (93 vs 85 %). However, 18F-CHO is superior to 18F-fluoride in specificity (81 vs 91 %). Both tracers were better than bone scan in hormone-naïve patients. Thus, 18F-fluoride PET is most useful in high-risk patients to confidently detect or eliminate bone disease and potentially monitor the effects of therapy on bone metastases. In another review by Wondergem et al. [5], data on the performances of 11C- or 18F-CHO and 18F-fluoride PET/CT in bone metastases detection has been reported. On a lesion basis, authors reported sensitivity and specificity rates of 84 % and 98 % for 11C-CHO and 18F-CHO and 89 % and 91 % for 18 F-fluoride, respectively. On a patient basis, the reported sensitivity and specificity rates were 85 % and 96 % for 11C-CHO and 18F-CHO and 87 % and 80 % for 18F-fluoride, respectively. No significant differences were found between the sensitivity and specificity of 11C-CHO or 18F-CHO and 18F-fluoride reporting a general high sensitivity for PET/CT [14, 22–24]. In addition, Ceci et al. also evaluated the semi-quantitative data of 11C-CHO in 304 bone lesions (184 osteoblastic, 99 osteolytic and 21 bone marrow lesions) of 140 patients during biochemical recurrence. They could demonstrate differences in PSA kinetics and SUVmax between osteolytic (higher values) and osteoblastic (lower values) lesions. 11C-CHO PET/CT may identify patients that could benefit from early targeted therapies, depending on the type of bone lesions expressed [25]. The reported method could also help in delineating the extension and severity of skeletal involvement and classifying lesions as predominantly osteoblastic, lytic or mixed type, with crucial impact on treatment plan. In the management of prostate cancer patients, radiotherapy (RT) and diagnostic imaging have always enjoyed a close relationship: advances in diagnostic imaging and RT techniques have in fact resulted in a significant improvement of planning delineation [26, 27]. In general, PET may improve the target definition with a decrease in inter-observer variations, also in bone lesions, being potentially considered as a valuable tool in guiding tailored treatment on bone metastatic lesions [28–32]. Beheshti et al. comparing 18F-CHO and 18F-fluoride in 38 patients with biopsy-proven prostate cancer documented a sensitivity, specificity and accuracy in the detection of bone metastases of 81 %, 93 % and 86 % for 18F-fluoride and 74 % ($p=0.12$), 99 % ($p=0.01$) and 85 % for 18F-CHO, respectively. In addition, 18F-CHO could lead to a change in the management in two out of 38 patients due to the early detection of bone marrow metastases [14].

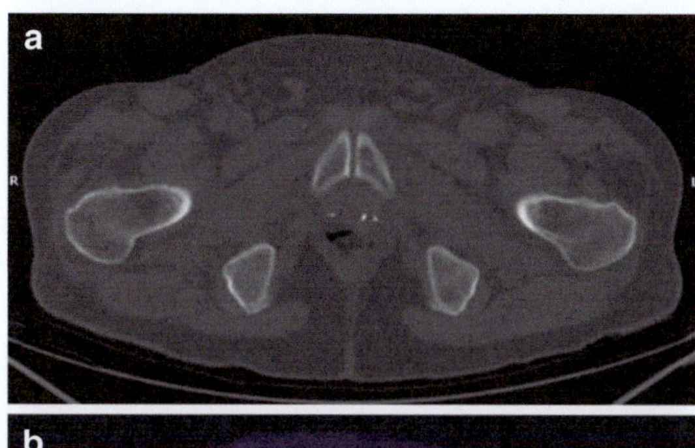

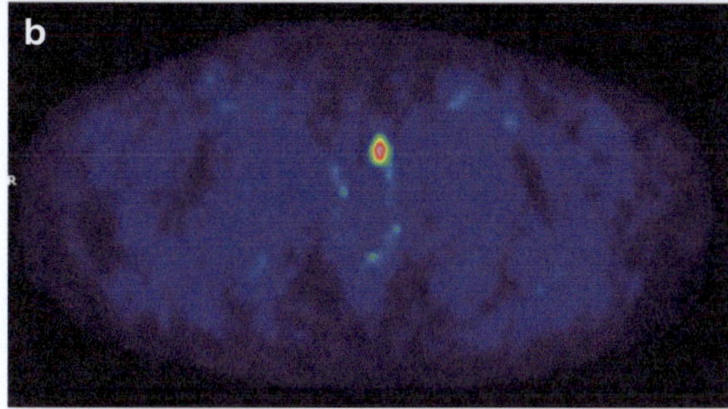

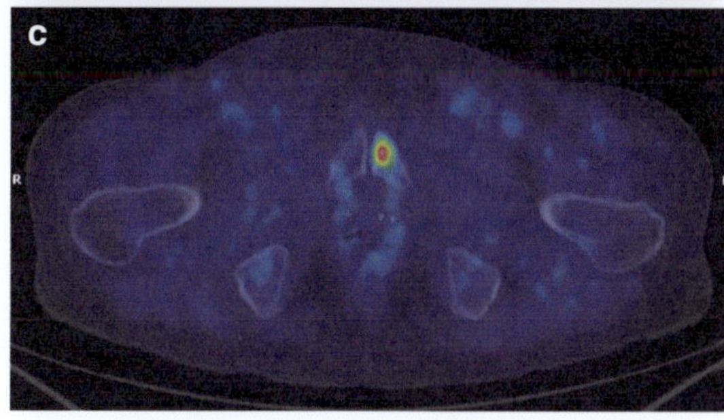

Fig. 7.4 A 75-year-old man treated with radical prostatectomy for prostate cancer (GS 7 (3+4), pT2cN0), who performed 11C-CHO PET/CT for biochemical recurrence (PSA: 4.00 ng/mL). 11C-CHO PET/CT showed a pathological uptake in the left groyne as documented on CT (**a**), PET (**b**) and fused PET/CT (**c**) transaxial images. After androgen deprivation therapy (PSA: 0.60 ng/mL), helical tomotherapy (HTT) was performed on the positive 11C-CHO PET/CT lesion. Nine months after HTT, patient showed a complete response with an undetectable PSA serum value

7.3 Response to Treatment with Radiolabelled Choline Agents

Oligometastatic subjects are a group of prostate cancer patients with a limited number of metastases (≤3 lesion). The number of metastases may reflect the biological aggressiveness of the tumour and may determine the possibility of curative potential interventions such as surgery or high-dose targeted RT [33]. However, there are very few data on the irradiation of oligometastases in recurrent disease, and they are mainly exclusively focused to lymph node lesions [34–36]. Interestingly, the extent of osseous metastatic disease is an independent prognostic factor in evaluating newly diagnosed advanced prostate cancer [37, 38]. A recent study showed that skeletal complications result in significant decreases in quality-of-life scores [39]. Therefore, therapies preventing skeletal complications could translate into improvements in quality of life and prolong physical activity. Besides analgesics, different treatment options are available for further palliation in case of symptomatic local and systemic progression. They include drug treatment, surgery, chemotherapy, hormonal therapy, RT and radionuclide treatment. It has been reported that androgen deprivation therapy (ADT) is strongly associated with bone metabolism modifications in prostate cancer, significantly decreasing bone mineral density [40]. In addition to conventional treatments, in patients with bone oligometastatic disease, a tailored approach on bone lesions by using either high-dose targeted RT or surgery could be proposed when an accurate imaging is available. Choline PET/CT can be a valuable imaging technique to monitor the disease in prostate cancer patients, as reported in a study in 40 patients with 64 bone metastases referred to after image-guided single fraction robotic stereotactic radiosurgery. The advantage of PET/CT in the evaluation of bone metastases is that this method combines the detection and the morphologic assessment of bone lesions with information concerning the metabolic activity of the metastases and can help to triage patients with metastatic prostate cancer and also in the evaluation of therapy response [41]. The potential influence of anti-androgenic treatment in patients who undergone 11C-CHO PET/CT study is still controversial. A significant reduction of 11C-CHO uptake following treatment with the nonsteroidal androgenic antagonist bicalutamide has been reported during the staging phase of prostate cancer patients [42]. In particular, in a series of 14 hormone-sensitive patients with recurrent prostate cancer, it was

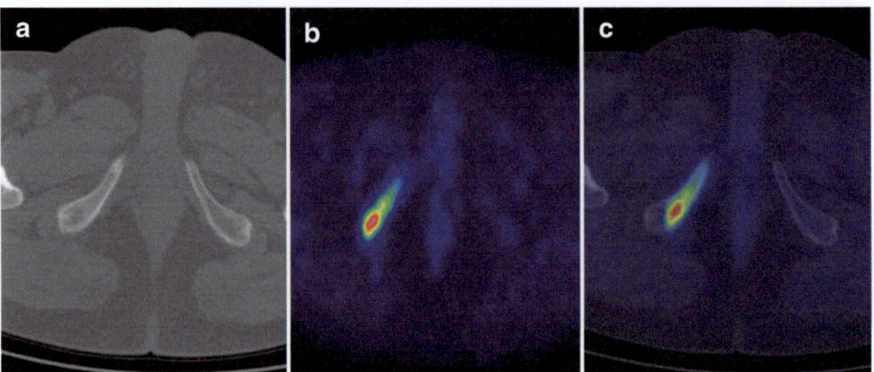

Fig. 7.5 A 57-year-old man treated with radical prostatectomy for prostate cancer (GS 7 (4+3), pT3aN0), who performed 11C-CHO PET/CT for biochemical recurrence (PSA: 15.14 ng/mL). 11C-CHO PET/CT showed a pathological uptake in the right ischio-pubic branch as documented on CT (**a**), PET (**b**) and fused PET/CT (**c**) transaxial images. After androgen deprivation therapy (PSA: 0.63 ng/mL), helical tomotherapy (HTT) was performed on the positive 11C-CHO PET/CT lesion. Two years after HTT, patient showed a complete response with a PSA value of 0.03 ng/mL

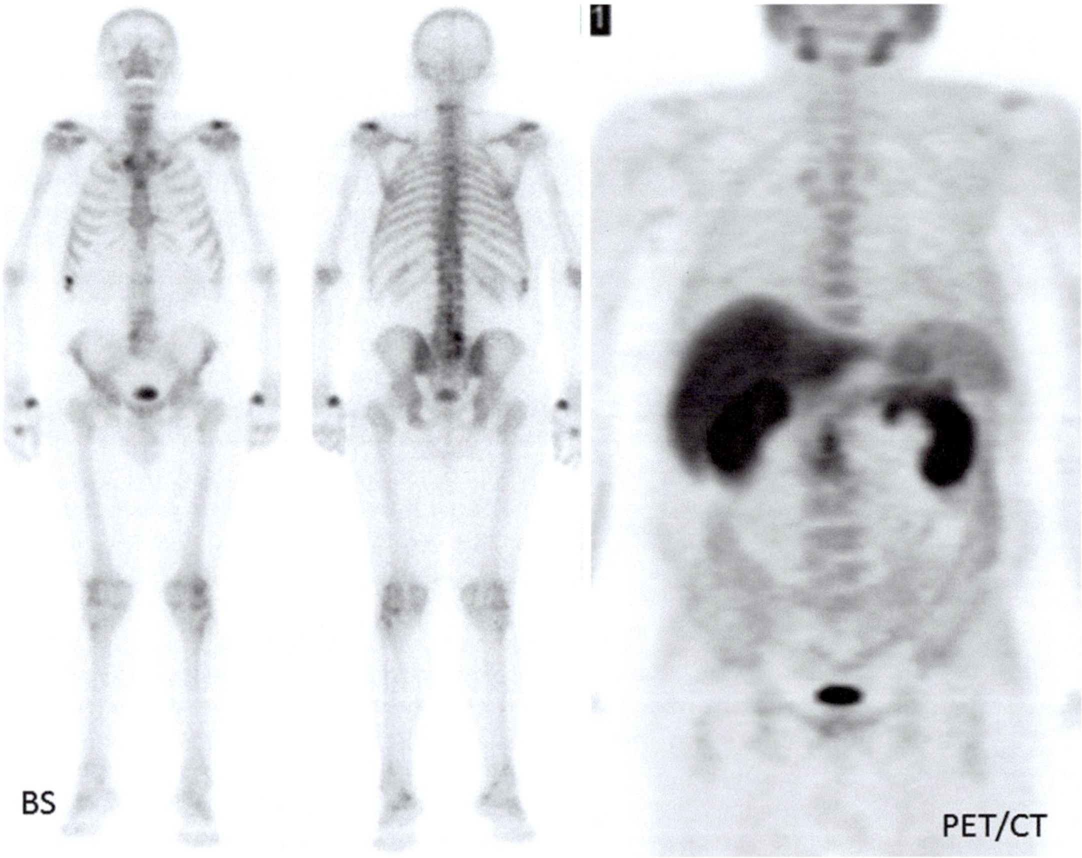

Fig. 7.6 A 65-year-old man with a suspicion for bone recurrence at bone scan was sent to 18F-CHO PET/CT. PSA level at the time of bone scan was 2.3 ng/mL. Bone scan resulted falsely negative, while PET/CT was truly negative (Courtesy Dr. Laura Evangelista, Nuclear Medicine and Molecular Imaging Unit, Veneto Institute of Oncology IOV – IRCCS, Padua, Italy)

stated that ADT influences the uptake of 11C-CHO PET/CT [43]. Berkovic et al. [44] investigated whether repeated stereotactic body RT (SBRT) of oligometastatic disease is able to defer the initiation of ADT in patients with low-volume metastases. They enrolled 24 recurrent prostate cancer patients with biochemical recurrence after radical therapy and 1–3 synchronous metastases (bone and/or lymph nodes) assessed by 18F-CHO PET/CT.

Patients were treated with repeated SBRT, and the ADT-free survival defined as the time interval between the first day of SBRT and the initiation of ADT was the primary end point. Authors concluded that repeated salvage SBRT is feasible, well tolerated and defers palliative ADT with a median of 38 months in patients with limited bone or lymph node prostate cancer metastases. SBRT is indicated in patients with oligometastatic or traditionally resistant disease, who often present with minimal or no associated symptoms [45, 46]. Assessing response to treatment is therefore difficult and must rely on evaluation by changes in the tumour itself and any related symptoms. The objective of the study by Costelloe et al. [47] was to compare the assessment of the RECIST 1.1 [48] and the University of Texas MD Anderson Cancer Center criteria [49] in evaluating tumour response for bone metastases. Tumour response measures in clinical trials are in continued evolution as molecular imaging techniques gain increasing acceptance in clinical oncology. However, the replacement of morphometric measures with molecular markers as measures of disease progression should proceed cautiously through the validation of these techniques by existing criteria and clinical outcome. Comparisons with RECIST appear feasible for evaluations of 18F-CHO PET/CT as a therapeutic response marker [50]. The clinical relevance of prostatic and skeletal lesions detected by 18F-CHO PET/CT is under investigation, not being taken into account by conventional RECIST. Figures 7.7 and 7.8 illustrate examples of monitoring the response to therapy by using serial 18F-CHO PET/CT scans.

Although the pain response is the most important end point for patients with metastatic bone disease receiving palliative care, the use of imaging response criteria may allow an objective evaluation of the therapeutic outcome, being also possible to be quantified by monitoring changes of several imaging parameters. Three sets (CT, MRI and PET) of criteria for assessing the therapeutic response of bone metastases are known. These techniques are able to detect the early infiltration of the bone marrow by cancer and to quantify this infiltration using morphologic images, quantitative parameters and functional approaches. Choline PET modality can potentially become an early response biomarker in prostate cancer metastases [51]. Long-term event/progression/survival follow-up in osteolytic cancers could justifiably consider the use of bone scan. However, for early response assessment, particularly when evaluating new drugs in clinical trials, or if radical changes in therapy are considered, MRI and PET are recommended [52].

Consequently, changes in imaging parameters have been advocated as important markers of disease response and progression. De Giorgi et al. used 18F-CHO PET/CT for outcome prediction and tumour monitoring in castration-resistant prostate cancer (CRPC) [53]. The correlation between the prognostic value of PSA and 18F-CHO PET/CT response to therapy suggests that PSA levels are linked to a tumour metabolic activity. Furthermore, in multivariate analysis, 18F-CHO PET/CT (progression vs non-progression) was superior to PSA with respect to progression-free survival and overall survival prediction, supporting the hypothesis of an essential role of 18F-CHO PET/CT to improve therapy management. PSA decline ≥50 % concurred with the 18F-CHO PET/CT response/non-response in 71 % of patients and with the 18F-CHO PET/CT progression/non-progression in 22 out of 26 (81 %) of patients. PET/CT progression/non-progression proved capable of predicting outcome in patients with other tumours, including bone metastases [54]. Clinical studies have demonstrated that PET can

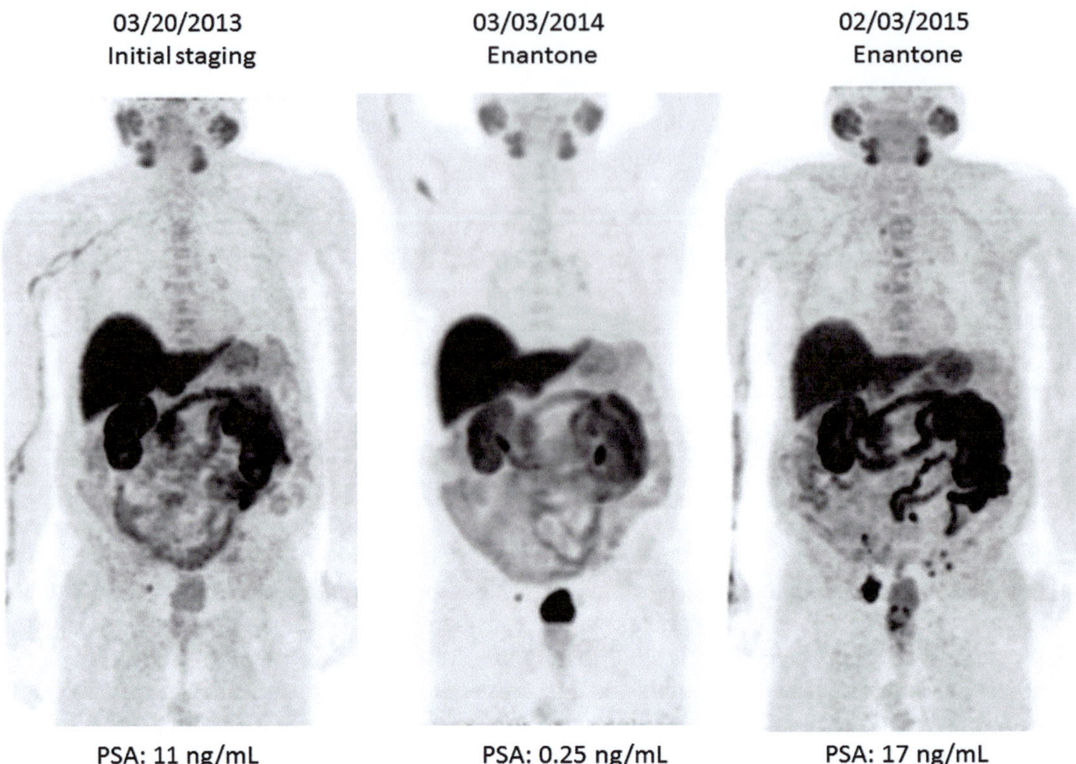

Fig. 7.7 Serial 18F-CHO PET/CT in patients undergoing with Enantone for a biochemical recurrence of prostate cancer. A significant uptake of 18F-CHO was found in the first scan (*left*) in a right obturator lymph node. After the administration of Enantone, a significant reduction in PSA was reported, although the uptake in the lymph node was stable (*middle*). After one from the last 18F-CHO PET/CT scan, a significant increase of PSA was compatible with an extensive metabolic progression of disease, either in the obturator lymph node or in others (Courtesy Dr. Laura Evangelista, Nuclear Medicine and Molecular Imaging Unit, Veneto Institute of Oncology IOV – IRCCS, Padua, Italy)

predict response to chemotherapy and targeted therapy in several tumours [55, 56]. The early identification of therapeutic response supports the clinician in the decision-making.

Quantification is necessary for characterising metabolic response. A newly proposed system for measuring functional response with 18F-FDG PET/CT, PET Response Criteria in Solid Tumours (PERCIST), might also be applied to radiolabelled choline PET as biomarker for response evaluation in prostate cancer [57, 58]. In a prospective study, Kwee et al. [59] found that 18F-CHO PET/CT parameters based on metabolically active tumour volume and total lesion activity of 18F-CHO are associated to overall survival. In another study of Oprea-Lager et al., different PET parameters were used, and 18F-CHO was reported as a potential biomarker for response evaluation in prostate cancer. In patients with metastatic prostate cancer, repeatability of SUV, normalised to the area under the curve, was comparable to that of standard SUV and indicated that repeatability coefficient of 18F-CHO PET/CT uptake differences of 30 % or more are likely to represent treatment effects [60].

Being well known, the limitations of BS for treatment monitoring, such as the misinterpretation of the “flare” reaction due to the persistence of uptake at the sites of bone metastases responding to treatment, PET and MRI, could be of help in assisting clinical data interpretation as reported by the Prostate Cancer Working Group 2 (PCWG2) who stated that bone scan is to be recommended to monitor the extent and the response of bone metastases, due to its wide availability and low cost, but they recognise that standards for using MRI and PET to assess bone metastases are to be investigated [61].

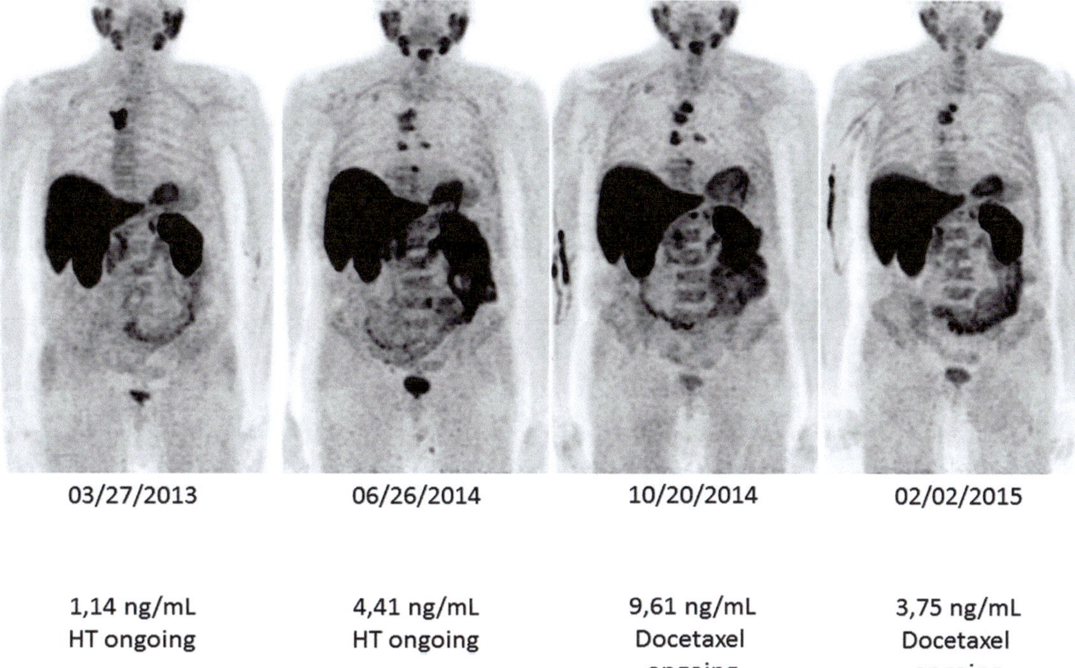

Fig. 7.8 Serial 18F-CHO PET/CT scans in a patient with metastatic prostate cancer. The patient was initially treated with hormonal therapy (HT) and later with chemotherapy for the development of a castrate-resistant condition (Courtesy Dr. Laura Evangelista, Nuclear Medicine and Molecular Imaging Unit, Veneto Institute of Oncology IOV – IRCCS, Padua, Italy)

More recently, McCarthy et al. [62] assessed 18F-CHO PET in comparison with standard imaging (BS and CT) for evaluating the extension of CRPC in 26 patients. Concordance rate between lesions shown on 18F-CHO and on either bone scan or CT was 81 %. In discordant results, analysis of follow-up data determined that 18F-CHO was correct in 79 % of these cases. A careful interpretation of 18F-CHO PET/CT made it possible to avoid the confusion between diffuse bone marrow infiltration by cancer and bone marrow activation in response to colony growth factors, generally administered for correcting bone marrow toxicity of chemotherapy implying cytotoxic agents. A pilot study conducted by Balogova et al. [51] confirm that 18F-CHO PET/CT may detect prostate cancer lesions at the CRPC stage. In addition, 18F-CHO PET/CT may represent an adding value with respect to MRI and PSA assay in monitoring various types of treatment regimen in CRPC.

Conclusions

Data from literature support the use of choline PET/CT in PCa patients with bone metastatic disease as a valuable tool to detect bone lesions, to guide tailored treatment and to monitor different therapeutical approaches.

References

1. Podo F (1999) Tumour phospholipid metabolism. NMR Biomed 12(7):413–439
2. Janardhan S, Srivani P, Sastry GN (2006) Choline kinase: an important target for cancer. Curr Med Chem 13(10):1169–1186
3. Hara T, Kosaka N, Kishi H (1998) PET imaging of prostate cancer using carbon-11-choline. J Nucl Med Off Publ Soc Nucl Med 39(6):990–995
4. Torizuka T et al (2003) Imaging of gynecologic tumors: comparison of (11)C-choline PET with (18) F-FDG PET. J Nucl Med Off Publ Soc Nucl Med 44(7):1051–1056

5. Wondergem M et al (2013) A literature review of 18F-fluoride PET/CT and 18F-choline or 11C-choline PET/CT for detection of bone metastases in patients with prostate cancer. Nucl Med Commun 34(10):935–945
6. Picchio M et al (2012) [11C]Choline PET/CT detection of bone metastases in patients with PSA progression after primary treatment for prostate cancer: comparison with bone scintigraphy. Eur J Nucl Med Mol Imaging 39(1):13–26
7. Messiou C, Cook G, deSouza NM (2009) Imaging metastatic bone disease from carcinoma of the prostate. Br J Cancer 101:1225–1232
8. Evangelista L et al (2013) Utility of choline positron emission tomography/computed tomography for lymph node involvement identification in intermediate- to high-risk prostate cancer: a systematic literature review and meta-analysis. Eur Urol 63(6):1040–1048
9. De Bari B et al (2014) Choline-PET in prostate cancer management: the point of view of the radiation oncologist. Crit Rev Oncol Hematol 91(3):234–247
10. Tuncel M et al (2008) [(11)C]Choline positron emission tomography/computed tomography for staging and restaging of patients with advanced prostate cancer. Nucl Med Biol 35(6):689–695
11. Langsteger W et al (2012) Imaging of bone metastases in prostate cancer: an update. Q J Nucl Med Mol Imaging Off Publ Ital Assoc Nucl Med 56(5):447–458
12. von Eyben FE, Kairemo K (2014) Meta-analysis of (11)C-choline and (18)F-choline PET/CT for management of patients with prostate cancer. Nucl Med Commun 35(3):221–230
13. Fuccio C et al (2012) Role of 11C-choline PET/CT in the re-staging of prostate cancer patients with biochemical relapse and negative results at bone scintigraphy. Eur J Radiol 81(8):e893–e896
14. Beheshti M et al (2008) Detection of bone metastases in patients with prostate cancer by 18F fluorocholine and 18F fluoride PET-CT: a comparative study. Eur J Nucl Med Mol Imaging 35(10):1766–1774
15. Beer AJ et al (2011) Radionuclide and hybrid imaging of recurrent prostate cancer. Lancet Oncol 12(2):181–191
16. Beheshti M et al (2010) The use of F-18 choline PET in the assessment of bone metastases in prostate cancer: correlation with morphological changes on CT. Mol Imaging Biol MIB Off Publ Acad Mol Imaging 12(1):98–107
17. Ayala-Peacock DN et al (2013) A pilot 11C-choline PET/CT imaging study investigating the ability to detect occult metastatic osseous disease in newly diagnosed high-risk prostate adenocarcinoma. Pract Radiat Oncol 3(2 Suppl 1):S27
18. Kjolhede H et al (2012) Combined 18F-fluorocholine and 18F-fluoride positron emission tomography/computed tomography imaging for staging of high-risk prostate cancer. BJU Int 110(10):1501–1506
19. Poulsen MH et al (2012) [18F]fluoromethylcholine (FCH) positron emission tomography/computed tomography (PET/CT) for lymph node staging of prostate cancer: a prospective study of 210 patients. BJU Int 110(11):1666–1671
20. Fuccio C et al (2010) Role of 11C-choline PET/CT in the restaging of prostate cancer patients showing a single lesion on bone scintigraphy. Ann Nucl Med 24(6):485–492
21. Poulsen MH et al (2014) Spine metastases in prostate cancer: comparison of technetium-99m-MDP whole-body bone scintigraphy, [(18) F]choline positron emission tomography(PET)/computed tomography (CT) and [(18) F]NaF PET/CT. BJU Int 114(6):818–823
22. Even-Sapir E et al (2006) The detection of bone metastases in patients with high-risk prostate cancer: 99mTc-MDP Planar bone scintigraphy, single- and multi-field-of-view SPECT, 18F-fluoride PET, and 18F-fluoride PET/CT. J Nucl Med Off Publ Soc Nucl Med 47(2):287–297
23. Brogsitter C, Zophel K, Kotzerke J (2013) ^{18}F-Choline, (11)C-choline and (11)C-acetate PET/CT: comparative analysis for imaging prostate cancer patients. Eur J Nucl Med Mol Imaging 40(Suppl 1):18–27
24. Fanti S et al (2011) Re: Nicolas Mottet, Joaquim Bellmunt, Michel Bolla, et al. EAU guidelines on prostate cancer. Part II: treatment of advanced, relapsing, and castration-resistant prostate cancer. Eur Urol 2011;59:572–83. Eur Urol 60(5):e37–e38; author reply e39–41
25. Ceci F et al (2015) 11C-choline PET/CT identifies osteoblastic and osteolytic lesions in patients with metastatic prostate cancer. Clin Nucl Med 40(5):e265–e270
26. Zhu A, Lee D, Shim H (2011) Metabolic positron emission tomography imaging in cancer detection and therapy response. Semin Oncol 38(1):55–69
27. Pinkawa M, Eble MJ, Mottaghy FM (2011) PET and PET/CT in radiation treatment planning for prostate cancer. Expert Rev Anticancer Ther 11(7): 1033–1039
28. Das SK, Ten Haken RK (2011) Functional and molecular image guidance in radiotherapy treatment planning optimization. Semin Radiat Oncol 21(2):111–118
29. Shi X et al (2014) PET/CT imaging-guided dose painting in radiation therapy. Cancer Lett 355(2):169–175
30. Kunkler IH et al (2014) Review of current best practice and priorities for research in radiation oncology for elderly patients with cancer: the International Society of Geriatric Oncology (SIOG) task force. Ann Oncol Off J Eur Soc Med Oncol/ESMO 25(11):2134–2146
31. Husarik DB et al (2008) Evaluation of [(18)F]-choline PET/CT for staging and restaging of prostate cancer. Eur J Nucl Med Mol Imaging 35(2):253–263
32. Soyka JD et al (2012) Clinical impact of 18F-choline PET/CT in patients with recurrent prostate cancer. Eur J Nucl Med Mol Imaging 39(6):936–943
33. Schick U et al (2013) Androgen deprivation and high-dose radiotherapy for oligometastatic prostate cancer

patients with less than five regional and/or distant metastases. Acta Oncol 52(8):1622–1628
34. Decaestecker K et al (2014) Surveillance or metastasis-directed Therapy for OligoMetastatic Prostate cancer recurrence (STOMP): study protocol for a randomized phase II trial. BMC Cancer 14:671
35. Ost P et al (2015) Metastasis-directed therapy of regional and distant recurrences after curative treatment of prostate cancer: a systematic review of the literature. Eur Urol 67(5):852–863
36. Gandaglia G et al (2014) Impact of the site of metastases on survival in patients with metastatic prostate cancer. Eur Urol 68(2):325–334
37. Rigaud J et al (2002) Prognostic value of bone scan in patients with metastatic prostate cancer treated initially with androgen deprivation therapy. J Urol 168(4 Pt 1):1423–1426
38. Sabbatini P et al (1999) Prognostic significance of extent of disease in bone in patients with androgen-independent prostate cancer. J Clin Oncol Off J Am Soc Clin Oncol 17(3):948–957
39. Weinfurt KP et al (2004) The impact of skeletal-related events on preferences and health-related quality of life of patients with metastatic prostate cancer. J Urol 171(4):42
40. Serpa Neto A et al (2010) A systematic review and meta-analysis of bone metabolism in prostate adenocarcinoma. BMC Urol 10:9
41. Muacevic A et al (2013) Safety and feasibility of image-guided robotic radiosurgery for patients with limited bone metastases of prostate cancer. Urol Oncol 31(4):455–460
42. Giovacchini G et al (2008) [(11)C]choline uptake with PET/CT for the initial diagnosis of prostate cancer: relation to PSA levels, tumour stage and anti-androgenic therapy. Eur J Nucl Med Mol Imaging 35(6):1065–1073
43. Fuccio C et al (2011) Androgen deprivation therapy influences the uptake of 11C-choline in patients with recurrent prostate cancer: the preliminary results of a sequential PET/CT study. Eur J Nucl Med Mol Imaging 38(11):1985–1989
44. Berkovic P et al (2013) Salvage stereotactic body radiotherapy for patients with limited prostate cancer metastases: deferring androgen deprivation therapy. Clin Genitourin Cancer 11(1):27–32
45. Ahmed KA et al (2012) Stereotactic body radiation therapy in the treatment of oligometastatic prostate cancer. Front oOncol 2:215
46. Milano MT et al (2012) Oligometastases treated with stereotactic body radiotherapy: long-term follow-up of prospective study. Int J Radiat Oncol Biol Phys 83(3):878–886
47. Costelloe CM et al (2010) Cancer response criteria and bone metastases: RECIST 1.1, MDA and PERCIST. J Cancer 1:80–92
48. Eisenhauer EA et al (2009) New response evaluation criteria in solid tumours: revised RECIST guideline (version 1.1). Eur J Cancer 45(2):228–247
49. Hamaoka T et al (2004) Bone imaging in metastatic breast cancer. J Clin Oncol Off J Am Soc Clin Oncol 22(14):2942–2953
50. Kwee SA et al (2009) (18)F-Choline PET/CT imaging of RECIST measurable lesions in hormone refractory prostate cancer. Ann Nucl Med 23(6):541–548
51. Balogova S et al (2014) Whole-body 18F-fluorocholine (FCH) PET/CT and MRI of the spine for monitoring patients with castration-resistant prostate cancer metastatic to bone: a pilot study. Clin Nucl Med 39(11):951–959
52. Lecouvet FE et al (2014) Monitoring the response of bone metastases to treatment with Magnetic Resonance Imaging and nuclear medicine techniques: a review and position statement by the European Organisation for Research and Treatment of Cancer imaging group. Eur J Cancer 50(15):2519–2531
53. De Giorgi U et al (2014) Early outcome prediction on 18F-fluorocholine PET/CT in metastatic castration-resistant prostate cancer patients treated with abiraterone. Oncotarg et 5(23):12448–12458
54. De Giorgi U et al (2010) 18F-FDG PET/CT findings and circulating tumor cell counts in the monitoring of systemic therapies for bone metastases from breast cancer. J Nucl Med Off Publ Soc Nucl Med 51(8):1213–1218
55. Ell PJ (2006) The contribution of PET/CT to improved patient management. Br J Radiol 79(937):32–36
56. Juweid ME, Cheson BD (2006) Positron-emission tomography and assessment of cancer therapy. N Engl J Med 354(5):496–507
57. Wahl RL et al (2009) From RECIST to PERCIST: Evolving Considerations for PET response criteria in solid tumors. J Nucl Med Off Publ Soc Nucl Med 50(Suppl 1):122S–150S
58. Morisson C, Jeraj R, Liu G (2013) Imaging of castration-resistant prostrate cancer: development of imaging response biomarkers. Curr Opin Urol 23(3):230–236
59. Kwee SA et al (2014) Prognosis related to metastatic burden measured by (1)(8)F-fluorocholine PET/CT in castration-resistant prostate cancer. J Nucl Med Off Publ Soc Nucl Med 55(6):905–910
60. Oprea-Lager DE et al (2015) Repeatability of quantitative 18F-fluoromethylcholine PET/CT studies in prostate cancer. J Nucl Med Off Publ Soc Nucl Med 57(5):721–727
61. Scher HI et al (2008) Design and end points of clinical trials for patients with progressive prostate cancer and castrate levels of testosterone: recommendations of the Prostate Cancer Clinical Trials Working Group. J Clin Oncol Off J Am Soc Clin Oncol 26(7):1148–1159
62. McCarthy M et al (2011) (1)(8)F-Fluoromethylcholine (FCH) PET imaging in patients with castration-resistant prostate cancer: prospective comparison with standard imaging. Eur J Nucl Med Mol Imaging 38(1):14–22

Imaging of Glycolysis with 18F-FDG PET

8

Hossein Jadvar and Laura Evangelista

8.1 Physiopathology and FDG PET in Prostate Cancer

18F-Fluorodeoxyglucose (FDG) is an analogue of glucose and is the most common PET radiotracer for oncological applications. Its wide use in clinical practice is primarily due to the Warburg effect, which leads to higher glucose consumption in the malignant cells in comparison to normal tissue. The malignancy-induced hypermetabolism is generally based upon overexpression of cellular membrane glucose transporters (mainly glucose transporter 1, GLUT-1) and enhanced hexokinase enzymatic activity in tumors [1, 2].

Some studies have demonstrated that GLUT-1 is overexpressed in poorly differentiated prostate cancer cell lines [3] and that the level of FDG uptake may be affected by the androgens [4, 5]. This latter characteristic may be due to the modulatory effects of androgens on GLUT-1 and hexokinase expression [3]. Kukuk et al. [6] reported a statistically significant decrease in FDG uptake by androgen-sensitive xenograft tumor model after surgical castration. The effects of androgen of prostate cancer cells can be demonstrated by a significant reduction in proliferation index (Ki67) after the administration of androgen ablation. GLUT-1 gene expression is also significantly higher in prostate cancer than in benign prostatic hyperplasia tissue, and it is correlated with Gleason score [7]. In Fig. 8.1, the biological processes related to the hyperexpression of GLUT-1 are shown. It has been shown that the expressions of GLUT-1 and prostate-specific antigen (PSA) are induced by the activation of HIF-1 and androgen receptor, respectively [8–10].

H. Jadvar, MD, PhD, MPH, MBA (✉)
Division of Nuclear Medicine, Department of Radiology, Keck School of Medicine of USC, University of Southern California,
2250 Alcazar Street, CSC 102, Los Angeles, CA 90033, USA
e-mail: jadvar@med.usc.edu

L. Evangelista
Nuclear Medicine and Molecular Imaging Unit, Veneto Institute of Oncology IOV – IRCCS, Padua, Italy

8.2 Comparative Diagnostic Accuracy among Imaging Modalities

Early studies in mid-1990s showed discrepancy between bone scintigraphy and FDG PET with bone scans showing more lesions than FDG PET [11, 12]. However, the clinical setting was mixed, and more studies in specific clinical settings were needed to decipher the unique utility of FDG PET. One prospective investigation compared FDG PET and conventional bone scan in 16 patients with prostate cancer [13]. Overall bone

F. Bertoldo et al. (eds.), *Bone Metastases from Prostate Cancer*,
DOI 10.1007/978-3-319-42327-2_8

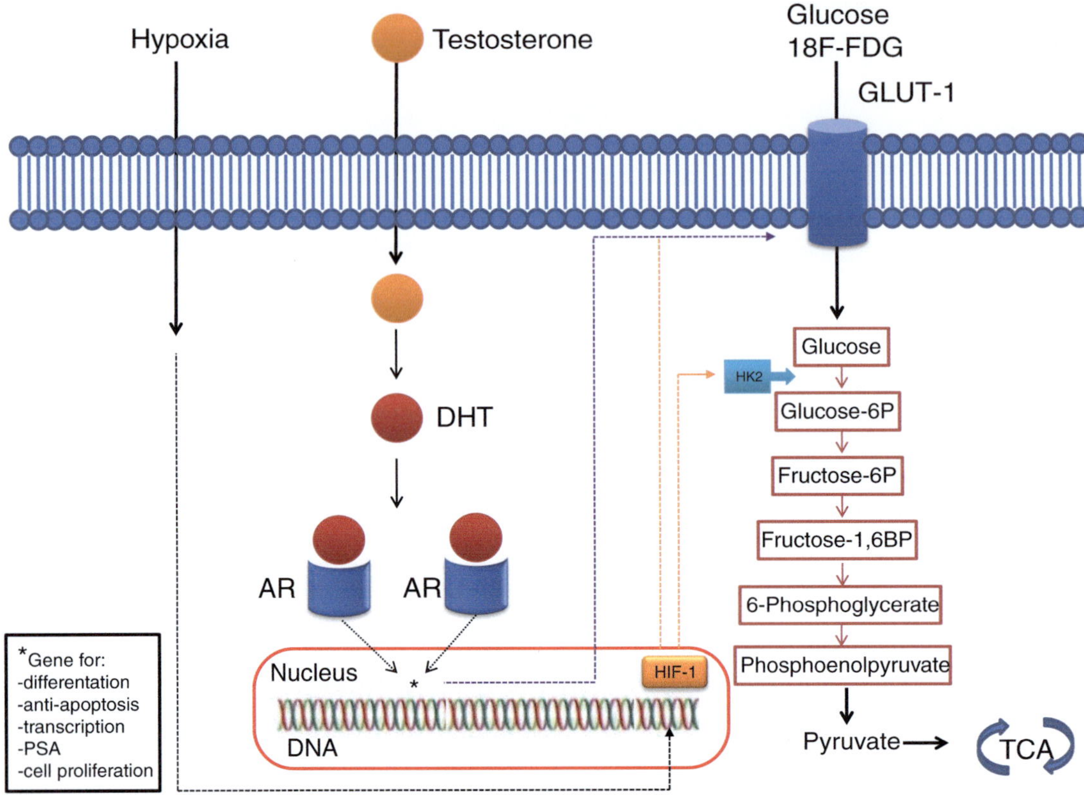

Fig. 8.1 Physiopathological processes correlate with the entrance of FDG in the prostatic cancer cell. *DHT* dihydrotestosterone, *AR* androgen receptors, *TCA* tricarboxylic acid cycle

scan detected more suspicious metastatic bony lesions than FDG PET; however, PET also revealed some marrow-only disease sites and many metastatic soft tissue lesions. The apparent false-negative FDG PET findings at some bony sites may have in fact been true negative with regard to favorable response to treatment with metabolically inactive disease, while bone scan may have displayed false-positive flare or healing reaction at these sites. The authors concluded that bone scan and FDG PET could be complementary in the management of patients with metastatic prostate cancer (Fig. 8.2).

In a prospective study of patients with breast, lung, and prostate cancer, FDG PET-CT was compared with 18F-NaF PET-CT and standard 99mTc-methylene diphosphonate (99mTc-MDP) bone scan at the time of initial staging or restaging [14]. Sensitivity and negative predictive value of 18F-NaF PET-CT was 100 % for all 3 cancers. In prostate cancer, the sensitivity, specificity, negative predictive value, and positive predictive value were 72 %, 65 %, 100 %, and 100 %, respectively. Conventional bone scan displayed superior sensitivity and negative predictive value compared to FDG PET-CT but had lower specificity and positive predictive value. Langsteger et al. contended in a review article that 18F-NaF PET provides a more sensitive "conventional" bone scan and also that FDG PET in early disease (marrow only involvement) is more advantageous than 18F-NaF PET [15]. It is interesting to note that FDG PET-CT may also display extensive hypermetabolic osseous metastatic disease similar to "superscan" described previously for bone scintigraphy [16]. The use of combined 18F-NaF and FDG has been advocated by some investigators who contend that such co-injected radiotracer PET study can provide synergistic diagnostic information with reduced overall cost

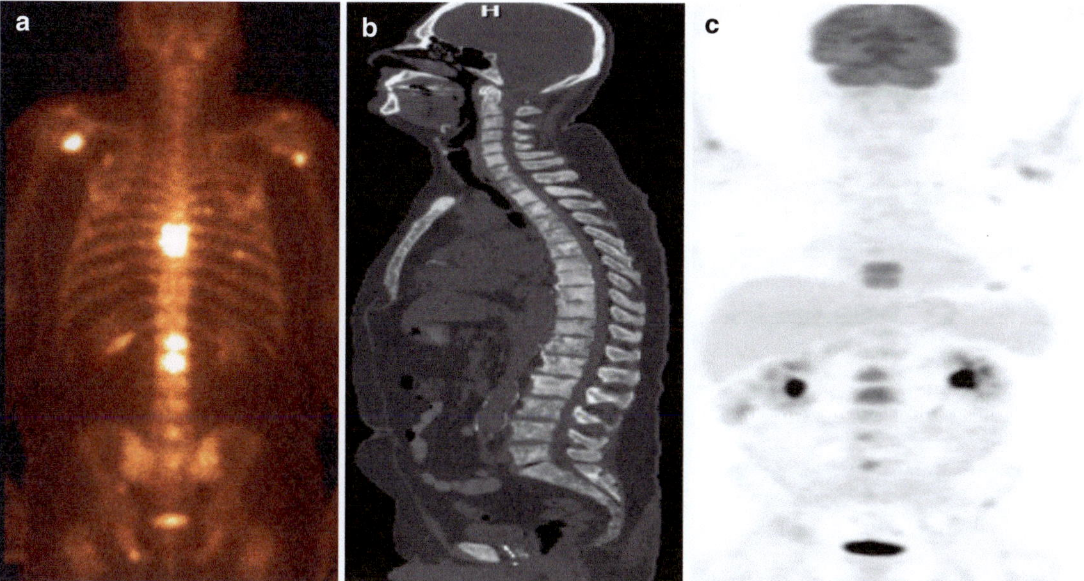

Fig. 8.2 Metastatic castrate-resistant prostate cancer (PSA 168.6 ng/mL). 99mTc-MDP bone scan (**a**) shows multiple randomly distributed osseous lesions while sagittal CT scan at bone window level (**b**) shows many more sclerotic lesions and FDG PET maximal intensity projection image (**c**) demonstrating fewer metabolically active lesions than bone scan

and patient radiation exposure from the CT component and enhanced patient convenience [17, 18]. Mianamimoto et al. from Stanford University, Stanford, CA, prospectively evaluated the use of combined 18F-NaF and FDG in 15 men with prostate cancer and 15 women with breast cancer [19]. For detection of skeletal lesions, combined PET scintigraphy showed significantly higher sensitivity compared to whole-body magnetic resonance imaging (MRI) alone (96.2 % vs. 81.4 %, $p<0.001$) and 99mTc-MDP bone scan alone (96.2 % vs. 64.6 %, $p<0.001$). For extra-skeletal lesions, there was no statistically difference between PET scintigraphy and whole-body MRI. In one retrospective study of 91 men with PSA relapse following prostatectomy and validation of PET findings by biopsy or clinical and imaging follow-up, mean serum PSA levels were higher in the FDG PET-positive patients than in the FDG PET-negative patients (9.5 ± 2.2 ng/mL vs. 2.1 ± 3.3 ng/mL) with an overall PET detection rate of 31 % [20]. However, the reported detection rate was likely overestimated since some patients had disease already evident on conventional imaging; as such the unique diagnostic contribution of FDG PET in this clinical setting was unclear. Nevertheless, PET-CT with FDG in patients with prostate cancer has a prognostic meaning, being able to assess the aggressiveness of the lesions and therefore the long-term survival ([7]; Fig. 8.3).

Jadvar et al. reported on a prospective investigation of FDG PET-CT and 18F-NaF PET-CT in detection of occult metastases in 37 men with biochemical recurrence (range, 0.5–40.2 ng/mL) and negative standard imaging studies [21]. The occult metastasis detection rate for FDG PET-CT was only 8.1 %, which was much lower than that reported previously and likely represented the unique diagnostic information provided by FDG PET-CT in this clinical setting (Fig. 8.4).

8.3 Treatment Response Evaluation and Outcome Prediction

It has become evident that conventional imaging methods are inadequate for the assessment of changes in bone metastases in response to

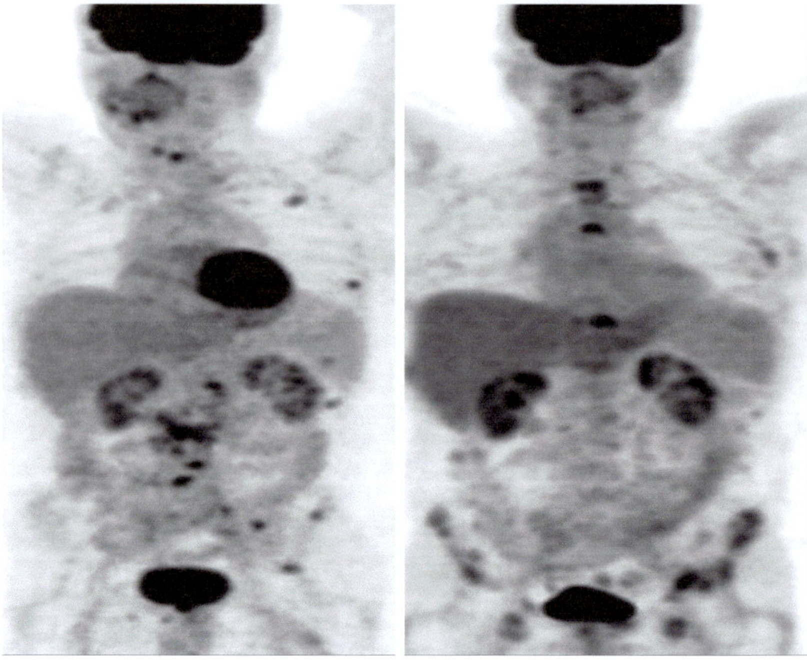

Fig. 8.3 Prognostic utility of FDG PET-CT in metastatic prostate cancer. Maximum intensity projection PET images show clinical states of castrate-sensitive predominantly lymph node disease at baseline (*left*) developing into castrate-resistant predominantly bone metastatic disease after 12 months (*right*). The patient died at 28.5 months after the baseline scan (This research was originally published in Jadvar [7]. Figure 3)

various treatments. Challenges include flare phenomenon, insensitivity to capture degrees of biological response, and the need to interpret imaging changes in the context of other clinical and nonimaging data. The situation is even more problematic since bone lesions are considered nonmeasurable targets in the commonly used structure-based response criteria (e.g., RECIST 1.0 and RECIST 1.1). New international consensus response criteria specific for bone metastases using the newer imaging modalities (PET, multiparametric MR imaging) will need to be developed and then adopted to improve treatment response assessment of bony lesions [22]. Preclinical studies have shown the feasibility of assessing response to therapy quantitatively. Zhang et al. performed FDG microPET scans before, during, and after treatment with bortezomib (a proteasome inhibitor) in immunodeficient mice harboring prostate tumor cell line CWR22 xenografts [23]. Decline in tumor FDG uptake was advantageous over tumor volume reduction in measuring response to therapy. In the clinical arena, Zukotynski and colleagues performed FDG PET-CT, 18F-NaF PET-CT, and standard 99mTc-MDP bone scan in 9 men with castrate-resistant prostate cancer before and after 8 weeks of therapy with abiraterone and cabozantinib [24]. The authors found that 18F-NaF-avid disease was not predictive of treatment response. However, FDG PET-CT was noted to have the potential to stratify men into three groups (widespread vs. oligometastatic FDG-avid vs. non-FDG avid metastases) that could tailor appropriate therapy. Simoncic and colleagues compared dynamic 18F-NaF and FDG PET-CT for assessment of response to zibotentan in men with bone metastases from prostate cancer [25]. All patients initially received a diagnostic CT and bone scan, followed by 18F-NaF and FDG PET-CT and MR imaging at baseline (before therapy), and then again after 4 weeks of therapy (peak therapy effect). Zibotentan was then held for 2 weeks (therapy break with maximum drug washout) followed by the final 18F-NaF and FDG PET-CT and MR imaging scans. It was assumed that a change in imaging metrics from baseline scan to week 4 scan would be most suggestive of a true therapy effect if the scan at week 6 (i.e., after 2 weeks of drug break) showed a change back toward baseline scan. Conversely, a change from baseline scan to week 4 scan that still persisted at week 6 (after drug break), might have represented a change that was probably not due to treatment

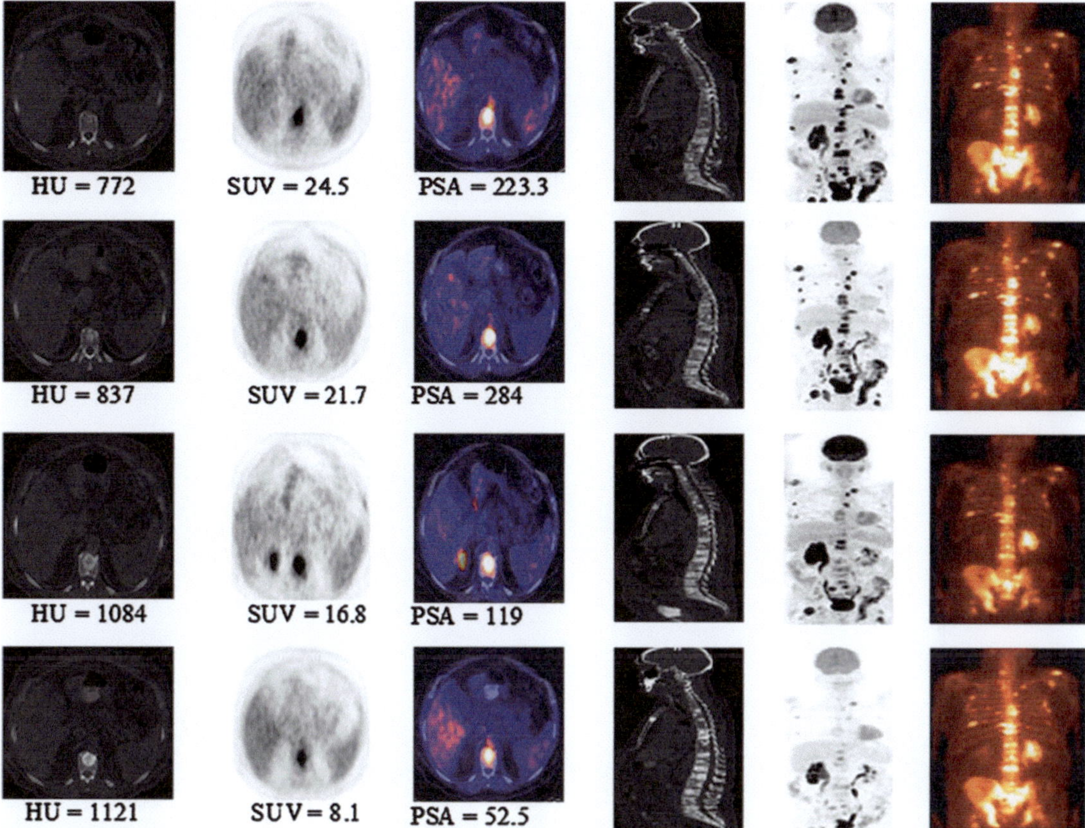

Fig. 8.4 Serial 18F-FDG PET-CT and bone scans of 63-year-old man with castrate-resistant metastatic prostate cancer with original primary cancer Gleason score of 9. Rows from top to bottom are scans at baseline (before chemotherapy) and at 4, 8, and 12 months after initiation of chemotherapy. Columns from the left to right are axial CT scans (bone window level), 18F-FDG PET scan, fused PET-CT scans, mid sagittal CT scan (bone window level), PET maximum intensity projection images, and 99mTc-methylene diphosphonate bone scans. Concordant decline in overall metabolic activity of metastatic lesions and PSA level is seen with treatment. Sclerosis of osseous lesions increases as corresponding metabolic activity declines with treatment (This research was originally published in *JNM*. Jadvar [34]. Fig. 8.2 © by the Society of Nuclear Medicine and Molecular Imaging, Inc.)

effect (or possibly reflected drug resistant colonies). The 2-week drug washout was based on the half-life of zibotentan, with complete drug washout at the time of week 6 scan. Late (week 6) 18F-NaF and FDG uptake responses were correlated, but earlier uptake responses (4 week scan) were unrelated suggesting that 18F-NaF and FDG uptakes in the setting of response assessment may be spatially dislocated and that both radiotracers may provide complementary information. A recent investigation showed that FDG PET could be useful in assessing treatment with the mTOR inhibitor, everolimus, in combination with docetaxel [26]. Yu et al. compared 11C-acetate and FDG in assessing treatment response to androgen deprivation therapy in 8 patients with >3 prostate cancer metastases on bone scintigraphy [27]. The authors' overall conclusion was that acetate PET is complementary to FDG PET in bone metastases detection, probably reflecting the underlying complex tumor biology. Morris et al. from Memorial Sloan Kettering Cancer Center in New York, NY, performed a lesion-by-lesion analysis of FDG PET in progressive metastatic prostate cancer in 17 patients with 134 osseous lesions [28]. Ninety-five lesions (71 %) were evident on both FDG PET and bone scans, 31 lesions (23 %) were only seen on bone

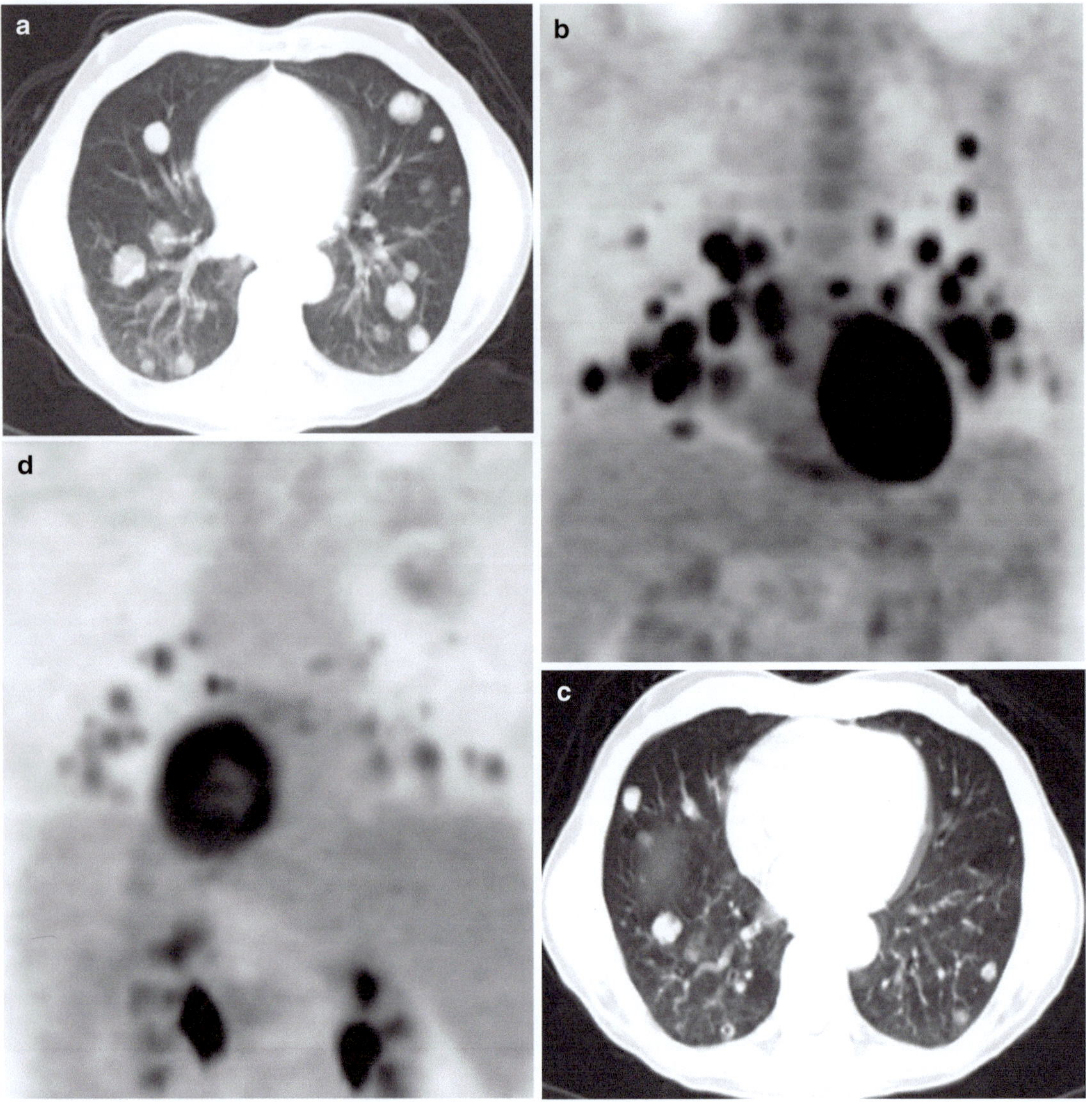

Fig. 8.5 Treatment response to docetaxel in a patient with metastatic castrate-resistant prostate cancer. Pretreatment (PSA 0.09 ng/mL) chest CT at lung window level (**a**), and FDG PET maximal intensity projection image (**b**) show multiple bilateral hypermetabolic pulmonary nodules. Post-treatment (PSA 0.04 ng/mL) chest CT (**c**) and FDG PET maximal intensity projection image (**d**) show decline in number, size, and metabolic activity of the metastatic pulmonary nodules compatible with favorable response to docetaxel chemotherapy

scan, and 8 lesions (6 %) were seen only on FDG PET. All metabolically active lesions on FDG PET were noted to be active on the follow-up bone scans (suggesting true positive findings on PET). The authors concluded that FDG PET could discriminate metabolically active bony lesions from scintigraphically quiescent lesions in men with progressive metastatic prostate cancer. Along the same line of rationale, the same group of investigators showed that FDG PET could be used as an outcome measure in patients with metastatic castrate-resistant prostate cancer undergoing treatment with antimicrotubule chemotherapy [29] (Fig. 8.5).

The authors found that a >33 % increase in the average of the maximum standardized uptake value (SUVmax) of metastatic lesions or appearance of new lesions could optimally dichotomize patients as progressors or nonprogressors. Meirelles and colleagues compared the prognostic value of bone scan and FDG PET in a prospective imaging trial of 43 men with metastatic castrate-resistant prostate cancer [30]. Overall survival correlated inversely with SUVmax of the osseous lesions with a median survival of 14.4 months for SUVmax >6.10 vs. 32.8 months with SUVmax ≤ 6.10 ($p = 0.002$). Although a defined calculated bone scan index was also prognostic (overall survival 14.7 months vs. 28.2 months if BSI >1.27 vs. <1.27; $p = 0.004$), in the multivariate analysis, only SUVmax was an independent factor in predicting survival. Vargas et al. reported on a retrospective study of 38 patients with metastatic castration-resistant prostate cancer who underwent CT, FDG PET, and 16β-fluoro-5-dihydrotestosterone (18F-FDHT) [31]. The number of lesions on CT, FDG, and FDHT PET were significantly associated with overall survival. Interestingly while higher FDHT uptake was associated with significantly shorter overall survival, such association was not seen with FDG uptake intensity. In another prospective clinical imaging trial of 87 men with metastatic castrate-resistant prostate cancer, Jadvar et al. showed in a multivariate analysis, controlling for confounding factors (age, serum PSA level, serum alkaline phosphatase level, the use of pain medication, prior chemotherapy, and Gleason score at initial diagnosis) that the sum of the SUVmax of up to 25 metabolically active lesions (lymph nodes, bone, and soft tissue metastases) was statistically significant with a hazard ratio of 1.01 (95 % confidence interval [CI]: 1.001–1.020; $p = 0.053$) in predicting overall survival [32]. The moving hazards of death (interpreted as chance of death per person per month) showed a marked increase in chance of death for sum of SUVmax greater than 20. These latter two studies together suggest that the number of lesions and the intensity of FDG uptake in lesions might be independent prognostic variables for overall survival in patients with metastatic castrate resistant prostate cancer [33]. This prognostic information can be helpful for management decisions and comparative evaluation of current and emerging new therapies in this clinical space.

Conclusions

Accurate detection, localization, and determination of pre-therapy extent and therapy-induced changes of bone metastases in patients with prostate cancer are of pivotal importance in clinical management decisions and in outcome prediction. Conventional imaging is inadequate in achieving these goals. PET with various targeted radiotracers may be helpful to fill this void. In this chapter, we focused on the potential role of FDG, which is the most commonly available PET radiotracer in the world. Evidence suggests that FDG PET (whether combined with CT or MRI) can be useful in determination of the extent of metabolically active disease and potentially in treatment response evaluation and in prognostication.

Acknowledgment Supported in part by the United States of America National Institutes of Health grants R01-CA111613, R21-CA142426, R21-EB017568, and P30-CA014089

Financial Disclosure No conflict of interest.

References

1. Macheda ML, Rogers S, Bets JD (2005) Molecular and cellular regulation of glucose transport (GLUT) proteins in cancer. J Cell Physiol 202:654–662
2. Smith TA (2000) Mammalian hexokinases and their abnormal expression in cancer. Br J Biomed Sci 57:170–178
3. Effert P, Beniers AJ, Tamimi Y et al (2004) Expression of glucose transporter 1 (GLUT-1) in cell lines and clinical specimen from human prostate adenocarcinoma. Anticancer Res 24:3057–3063
4. Clavo AC, Brown RS, Wahl RL (1995) Fluorodeoxyglucose uptake in human cancer cell lines is increased by hypoxia. J Nucl Med 36:1625–1632
5. Moon JS, Jin WJ, Kwak JH, Kim HJ, Yun MJ, Kim JW et al (2011) Androgen stimulates glycolysis for de novo lipid synthesis by increasing activities of hexokinase 2 and 6-phosphofructo-2-kinase/fructose-2,

6-biphosphatase 2 in prostate cancer cells. Biochem J 433:225–233
6. Kukuk D, Reischl G, Raguin O, Wiehr S, Judenhofer MS, Calaminus C et al (2011) Assessment of PET tracer uptake in hormone-independent and hormone-dependent xenograft prostate cancer mouse models. J Nucl Med 52:1654–1663
7. Jadvar H (2013) Imaging evaluation of prostate cancer with 18F-fluorodeoxyglucose PET/CT: utility and limitations. Eur J Nucl Med Mol Imaging 40:S5–S10
8. Gelmann EP (2002) Molecular biology of the androgen receptor. J Clin Oncol 20(13):3001–3015
9. Balk SP, Ko YJ, Burbley GJ (2003) Biology of prostate-specific antigen. J Clin Oncol 21(2):383–391
10. Schofield CJ, Ratcliffe PJ (2004) Oxygen sensing by HIF hydroxylases. Nat Rev Mol Cell Biol 5(5):343–354
11. Shreve PD, Grossman HB, Gross MD, Wahl RL (1996) Metastatic prostate cancer: initial findings of PET with 2-deoxyglucose-2-[F-18]fluoro-D-glucose. Radiology 199:751–756
12. Yeh SD, Imbriaco M, Larson SM et al (1996) Detection of bony metastases of androgen-independent prostate cancer by PET FDG. Nucl Med Biol 23:693–697
13. Tiwari BP, Jangra S, Nair N et al (2010) Complimentary role of FDG PET imaging and skeletal scintigraphy in the evaluation of patients with prostate carcinoma. Indian J Cancer 47:385–390
14. Damle NA, Bal C, Bandopadhyaya GP et al (2013) The role of 18F-fluoride PET-CT in the detection of bone metastases in patients with breast, lung, and prostate carcinoma: a comparison with FDG PET/CT and 99mTc-MDP bone scan. Jpn J Radiol 31:262–269
15. Langsteger W, Heinisch M, Fogelman I (2006) The role of fluorodeoxyglucose, 18F-dishydroxyphenylalanine, 18F-choline, and 18F-fluoride in bone imaging with emphasis on prostate and breast. Semin Nucl Med 36:73–92
16. Bailly M, Besse H, Kerdraon R et al (2014) 18F-FDG PET/CT superscan in prostate cancer. Clin Nucl Med 39:912–914
17. Iagaru A, Mittra E, Yaghoubi SS et al (2009) Novel strategy for a cocktail 18F-fluoride and 18F-FDG PET/CT scan for evaluation of malignancy: results of the pilot-phase study. J Nucl Med 50:501–505
18. Lin FI, Rao JE, Mittra ES et al (2012) Prospective comparison of combined 18F-FDG and 18F-NaF PET/CT vs. 18F-FDG PET/CT imaging for detection of malignancy. Eur J Nucl Med Mol Imaging 39:262–270
19. Minamimoto R, Loening A, Jamali M et al (2015) Prospective comparison of 99mTc-MDP scintigraphy, combined 18F-NaF and 18F-FDG PET/CT, and whole-body MRI in patients with breast and prostate cancer. J Nucl Med 56:1862–1868
20. Schoder H, Hermann K, Gonen M et al (2005) 2-[18F] fluoro-2-deoxyglucose positron emission tomography for the detection of disease in patients with prostate-specific antigen relapse after radical prostatectomy. Clin Cancer Res 11:4761–4769
21. Jadvar H, Desai B, Ji L et al (2012) Prospective evaluation of 18F-NaF and 18F-FDG PET/CT in detection of occult metastatic disease in biochemical recurrence of prostate cancer. Clin Nucl Med 37:637–643
22. Vassiliou V, Andreopoulos D, Frangos S et al (2011) Bone metastases: assessment of therapeutic response through radiological and nuclear medicine imaging modalities. Clin Oncol (R Coll Radiol) 23:632–645
23. Zhang Y, Saylor M, Wen S et al (2006) Longitudinally quantitative 2-deoxy-2-[18F]fluoro-D-glucose micro positron emission tomography imaging for efficacy of new anticancer drugs: a case study with bortezomib in prostate cancer murine model. Mol Imaging Biol 8:300–308
24. Zukotynski KA, Kim CK, Gerbaudo VH et al (2014) (18F)F-FDG-PET/CT and (18F)F-NaF-PET/CT in men with castrate-resistant prostate cancer. Am J Nucl Med Mol Imaging 5:72–82
25. Simoncic U, Perlman S, Liu G et al (2015) Comparison of NaF and FDG PET/CT for assessment of treatment response in castrate-resistant prostate cancers with osseous metastases. Clin Genitourin Cancer 13:e7–e17
26. Courtney KD, Manola JB, Elfiky AA et al (2015) A phase I study of everolimus and docetaxel in patients with castration-resistant prostate cancer. Clin Genitourin Cancer 13:113–123
27. Yu EY, Muzi M, Hackenbracht JA et al (2011) C11-acetate and F-18 FDG PET for men with prostate cancer bone metastases: relative findings and response to therapy. Clin Nucl Med 36:192–198
28. Morris MJ, Akhurst T, Osman I et al (2002) Fluoridated deoxyglucose positron emission tomography imaging in progressive metastatic prostate cancer. Urology 59:913–918
29. Morris MJ, Akhurst T, Larson SM et al (2005) Fluorodeoxyglucose positron emission tomography as an outcome measure for castrate metastatic prostate cancer treated with antimicrotubule chemotherapy. Clin Cancer Res 11:3210–3216
30. Meirelles GS, Schoder H, Ravizzini GC et al (2010) Prognostic value of baseline [18F]fluorodeoxyglucose positron emission tomography and 99mTc-MDP bone scan in progressing metastatic prostate cancer. Clin Cancer Res 16:6093–6096
31. Vargas HA, Wassberg C, Fox JJ et al (2014) Bone metastases in castration-resistant prostate cancer: associations between morphologic CT patterns, glycolytic activity, and androgen receptor expression on PET and overall survival. Radiology 271:220–229
32. Jadvar H, Desai B, Ji L et al (2013) Baseline 18F-FDG PET/CT parameters as imaging biomarkers of overall survival in castrate-resistant metastatic prostate cancer. J Nucl Med 54:1195–1201
33. Jadvar H, Groshen SG, Quinn DI (2015) Association of overall survival with glycolytic activity of castrate-resistant prostate cancer metastases. Radiology 274:624–625
34. Jadvar H (2011) Prostate cancer: PET with 18F-FDG, 18F-or 11C-Acetate, and 18F- or 11C-choline. J Nucl Med 52(1):81–89

New Radiopharmaceutical Markers for Metabolism and Receptor

9

Francesco Ceci, Joshua James Morigi, Lucia Zanoni, and Stefano Fanti

9.1 Introduction

Recently new radiopharmaceuticals have been proposed for investigating prostate cancer patients, including metabolic radiotracer such as anti1-amino-3-18F-fluorocyclobutane-1-carboxylic acid (^{18}F-FACBC) or probe targeting the prostate-specific membrane antigen (PSMA). These radiotracers showed in literature better performance in the detection of prostate cancer recurrence as compared to choline PET/CT imaging [1, 2].

18F-FACBC is a synthetic L-leucine analogue that has excellent in vitro uptake in the DU145 prostate cancer cell line [3]. Its uptake is likely mediated via the sodium-independent L large-neutral amino acid transport system which is composed of some transporters overexpressed in several types of cancer and linked to angiogenesis, proliferation and metastatic potential [4].

F. Ceci, MD • J.J. Morigi, MD • L. Zanoni, MD
Service of Nuclear Medicine, S.Orsola-Malpighi University Hospital, University of Bologna, Bologna, Italy
e-mail: francesco.ceci83@gmail.com; joshuamorigi@me.com; lucia.zanoni84@gmail.com

S. Fanti, MD, PhD (✉)
Service of Nuclear Medicine, PAD.30, S.Orsola-Malpighi University Hospital, University of Bologna, Via Massarenti, 9, Bologna 40138, Italy
e-mail: stefano.fanti@aosp.bo.it

PSMA-based PET imaging agents fall into three categories: (1) antibodies, (2) aptamers and (3) PSMA inhibitors of low molecular weight. J591 is a deimmunised monoclonal antibody that is specific for the extracellular domain of PSMA and has been radiolabelled with 89Zr and 64Cu for preclinical PET imaging in mice. Compared with these latter radiolabelled agents, the Glu-NH-CO-NH-Lys-(Ahx)-(68Ga[HBED-CC]) (68Ga-PSMA) derivative showed reduced unspecific binding and considerable higher specific internalisation in PCa cells, resulting in improved in vivo properties.

In the management of metastatic prostate cancer, the incidence of bone metastasis is a frequent event, occurring in 65–75% of men with advanced disease [5], with a median survival of approximately 2–3 years after the bone metastases diagnosis, depending on hormone responsiveness of the disease [6, 7]. Choline PET/CT provided good performance for detecting bone metastases in prostate cancer, both in case of osteoblastic and osteolytic lesions [8]. Considering the promising performance of ^{18}F-FACBC and ^{68}Ga-PSMA for investigating prostate cancer patients with BCR, it should be of interest to understand the accuracy of these new imaging procedures in the assessment of bone metastases. Therefore, the aim of this chapter is to investigate the role of new PET/CT radiopharmaceuticals for the evaluation of the bone involvement in prostate cancer patients.

F. Bertoldo et al. (eds.), *Bone Metastases from Prostate Cancer*,
DOI 10.1007/978-3-319-42327-2_9

9.2 Role of ^{18}F-FACBC PET/CT for Detecting Bone Metastases in Prostate Cancer

In recent years, an investigational amino acidic PET compound, anti1-amino-3-18F-fluoro-cyclobutane-1-carboxylic acid (^{18}F-FACBC), a synthetic L-leucine analogue, was developed and tested in prostate cancer patients with biochemical recurrence after radical treatment. Its uptake is mainly mediated via the sodium-independent "L" large-neutral amino acid transport system (particularly, LAT1/4F2hc); secondly, the sodium-dependent alanine-serine-cysteine (ASC) system (particularly, ASCT1), the sodium-independent ASC system (asc-1/4F2hc) and the sodium-independent T system (TAT1) are involved [9]. In literature, few promising studies confirming the good performance of these new radiopharmaceuticals, when compared to ^{11}C-choline PET/CT, are already present. However, there are no studies up to now that aimed to specifically explore skeletal involvement.

Few studies evaluated ^{18}F-FACBC biodistribution and radiation dosimetry in healthy volunteers. The four organs with the highest initial uptake were the liver, red bone marrow (11.1 %; range 4.8–20.4 %), lung and pancreas. Bone marrow demonstrated moderate and frequently heterogeneous or patchy ^{18}F-FACBC uptake, which decreased over time and was related with locations of red marrow, thus representing a complex background for the evaluation of metastases. Skeletal muscle also had mild uptake initially, which increased with time and over that of marrow at approximately 30–60 min after radiotracer injection [10–13].

Considering bone marrow, in a study by Emory et al., despite significant difference in average SUVmean at 4 min ($p=0.04$) was observed, the average absolute mean difference was minimal (0.3), mean percent difference was 10.7 % (±6.5), and there was a very high inter-class correlation coefficient ICC (0.8) [14]. Results of a prospective clinical trial comparing ^{18}F-FACBC PET/CT and ProstaScint for recurrent prostate carcinoma were presented by the group from Emory University headed by Schuster et al. [15]. Abnormal moderate focal ^{18}F-FACBC uptake greater than marrow that deviated from the expected biodistribution and persisted from early to delayed images was interpreted as positive. For bone involvement, histological proof or a characteristic appearance on no fewer than two other imaging studies (MR, CT and/or bone scan) was accepted. Of 93 ^{18}F-FACBC scans, 77 (82.8 %) were positive, including 49 (63.6 %) in the prostate/bed only, 24 (31.2 %) in the prostate/bed and extraprostatically and 4 (5.2 %) extraprostatically only. In the 70 of 93 patients with a definitive consensus on extraprostatic disease, ^{18}F-FACBC demonstrated 55 % sensitivity, 96.7 % specificity, 72.9 % accuracy, 95.7 % PPV and 61.7 % NPV, significantly superior than the conventional competitor. In Fig. 9.1, an example of a patient with a bone metastasis at FACBC PET/CT is illustrated.

Recently, Nanni et al. compared the accuracy of ^{18}F-FACBC and ^{11}C-choline PET/CT in 89 pts, consecutively and prospectively enrolled, with BCR after RP, ^{11}C-choline and ^{18}F-FACBC PET/CT performed within 1 week and off ADT at the time of the scans. PET positivity criterion was the presence of abnormal focal areas of uptake, more intense than background, and a semiquantitative SUV ratio (SUVmax in the lesion/SUVmean in surrounding background) ≥ 1.5 was used to aid the visual analysis. Different from the Emory group, they considered as background not the marrow but the healthy tissues surrounding the focal pathological uptake, wherever it was. Considering only the bone region analysis, overall seven patients resulted positive with at least one of the two tracers. Four patients were equally positive (TP) at the two tracers (lesion appearances in corresponding low-dose CT images were no evidence of bone remodelling in 2 pts, degenerative-like in one patient, multiple small osteosclerotic in one patient). Two patients were positive at choline (1FP, 1TP) but negative at FACBC (1TN, 1FN) in osteosclerotic lesions (Fig. 9.2).

One patient was negative at choline (FN) but positive at FACBC (TP) in a lesion that could be misinterpreted for its degenerative-like aspect. Standard of reference was clinical evaluation and

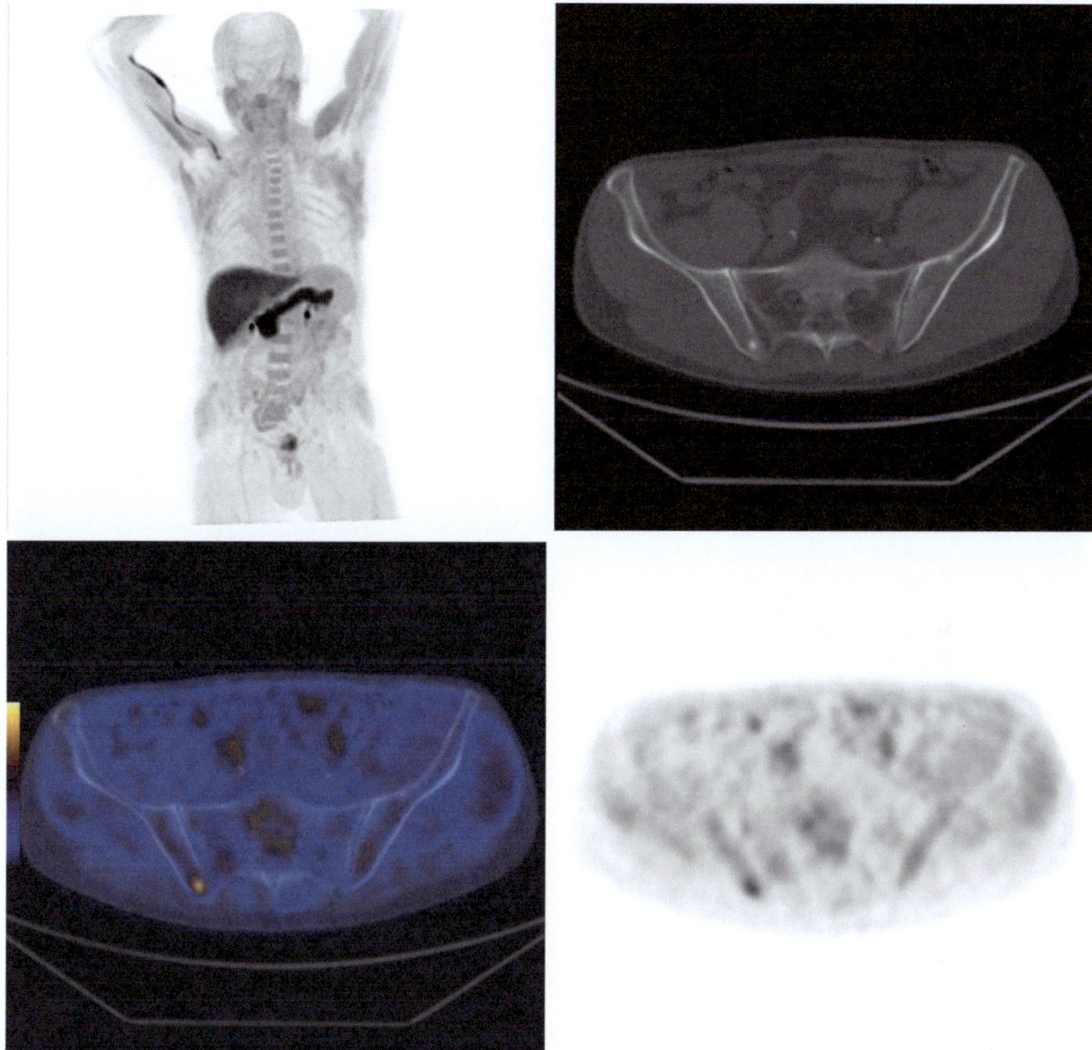

Fig. 9.1 18F-FACBC positive bone metastases in high-risk prostate cancer at staging evaluation. A 71-year-old patient diagnosed with high-risk prostate cancer (PSA 6.8 ng/ml; cT2; GS 4+4) underwent the standard staging flow chart and was scheduled for radical surgery. He was enrolled in a prospective study for staging lymph nodes with 18F-FACBC PET/CT. The experimental compound showed increased focal uptake in a single osteosclerotic lesion in the right iliac bone in keeping with bone metastasis. The detection of distant secondary lesions leads to an exclusion from surgery procedure and a change in treatment management . Project granted by "Programma di ricerca Regione-Università 2013, Regione Emilia Romagna, Area 1- Bando Giovani ricercatori Alessandro Liberati"

imaging in all cases (i.e. bone scan, MRI, follow-up 11C-choline PET/CT). Among the 82 patients who presented a concordant negative test with both compounds, at least four turned out FN at clinical evaluation and imaging (two CT images, one follow-up 11C-choline PET/CT, one bone scan + MRI both depicting a lesion in the tibia outside the PET field of view). At least 32 pts turned out disease-free for bone involvement (TN); reference standard was PSA drop after target treatment on prostate bed or lymph nodes (i.e. RT prostate bed and/or ln; lymphadenectomy) or imaging (negative for bone metastases but positive for local relapse or nodal involvement or other site dissemination) in most cases and a clinical evaluation in two cases. The remaining 46 were actually inde-

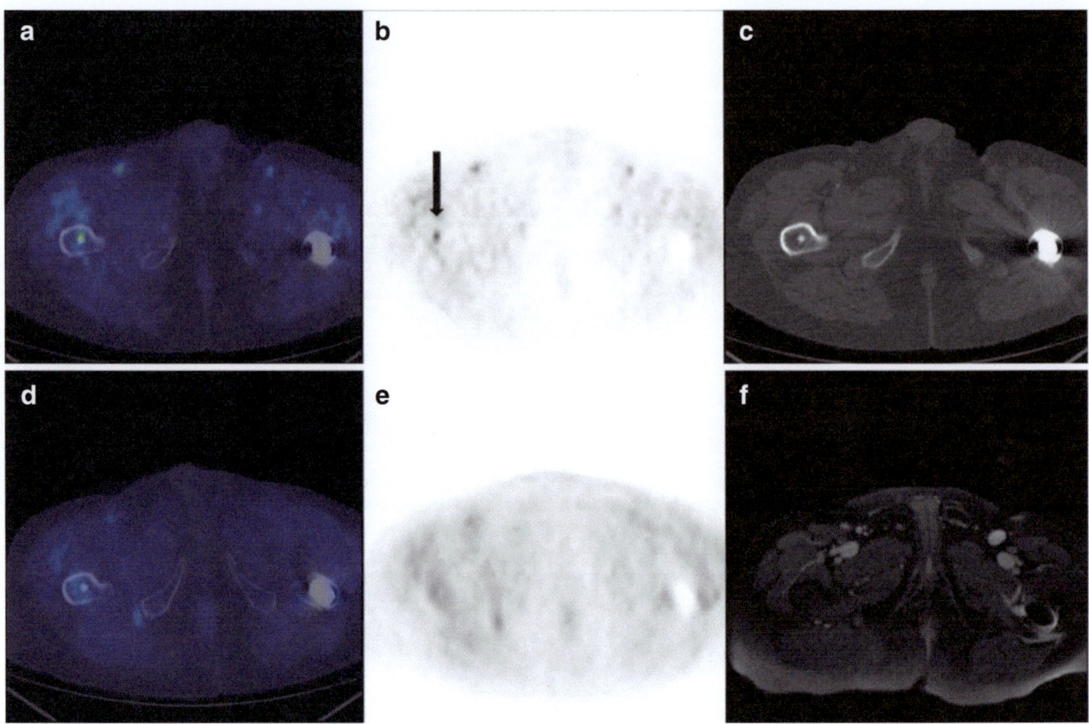

Fig. 9.2 False-positive 11C-choline and true-negative 18F-FACBC benign bone island, confirmed by MRI. A 74-year-old-patient radically treated for prostate cancer presenting with biochemical recurrence (PSA 1.57 ng/ml, PSA doubling time (dt) 16.4 months, PSA velocity 0.7 ng/ml/year). 11C-choline PET/CT showed focal increased uptake in the right femur (**a** axial fused choline PET/CT; **b** axial choline PET; see *black arrow*), corresponding with a subcentimetric osteosclerotic lesion in low-dose CT images (**c**). The bone finding resulted non-avid with 18F-FACBC, performed within 1 week (**d** axial fused FACBC PET/CT; **e** axial FACBC PET). A dedicated MRI (**f** axial T2 fatsat) and the subsequent clinical follow-up excluded bone relapse defining the lesion as benign bone island . Project granted by "Programma di ricerca Regione-Università 2010–2012, Regione Emilia Romagna, Bando Giovani Ricercatori"

terminate TN or FN because of insufficient evidences at follow-up data [1, 16, 17].

Kairemo et al. in a cohort of 26 patients concluded that ^{18}F-FACBC may play a role for restaging prostate cancer, especially in patients with a fast PSAdt. In particular, 26 (44.8 %) metabolically active lesions were reported in the skeleton [18]. Data about staging primary prostate cancer come from a Japanese multicenter phase IIb clinical trial with NMK36, trans-1-amino-318F-FACBC, by Suzuki et al. In their population (radical prostatectomy cohort, 42 patients; hormone therapy cohort, 24 patients), the concordance rate and k coefficient for diagnosis of bone metastasis by NMK36-PET/CT and combined conventional exams (bone scan and whole-body contrast-enhanced CT) were 83.3 % and 0.557, respectively. These results showed moderate concordance, and seven subjects were positive only with NMK36-PET/CT suggesting that the experimental compound might visualise early stage of bone metastases [19].

Few limitations should be considered when approaching ^{18}F-FACBC in this limited topic: the low intrinsic spatial resolution makes PET not suitable for the detection of bone micrometastases; the majority of population investigated so far are often small, clinically heterogeneous and with a limited number of positive findings; the reference standard is mainly based on a longitudinal follow-up because bone biopsy is rarely feasible; treatment decisions are often undertaken without a matching imaging or reliable biopsy, which makes it difficult to determine if and where exactly the metastases were present; and of the absence of validation for most of negative PET scans (TN or FN actually remains indeterminate) [17].

9.3 Role of ^{68}GA-PSMA PET/CT for Detecting of Bone Metastases in Prostate Cancer

A new molecular probe targeting PSMA has been recently developed [20]. PSMA is a membrane-bound enzyme with significantly elevated expression in prostate cancer cells in comparison to benign prostatic tissue [21]. The localisation of the catalytic site of PSMA in the extracellular domain allowed for the development of small specific inhibitors that are internalised after ligand binding [21]. Preliminary studies demonstrated that ^{68}Ga-PSMA (Glu-NH-CO-NH-Lys-(Ahx)-[68Ga(HBED-CC)]), an extracellular PSMA inhibitor for PET/CT imaging, is characterised by a significantly higher accuracy in the detection of early recurrence as compared to ^{18}F-choline PET/CT [2, 22]. These investigations also reported a higher tumour-to-background ratio for ^{68}Ga-PSMA PET/CT for the detection of suspected prostate cancer metastases when compared to ^{18}F-choline PET/CT [22] and very promising performances also at very low PSA levels [2, 23]. In Fig. 9.3, an example of a patient with bone metastasis at 68Ga-PSMA and 11C-choline PET/CT is reported.

Despite these promising results, the results obtained by ^{68}Ga-PSMA PET/CT in recurrent prostate cancer have not been extensively validated with either histology (namely, biopsy of the suspicious metastatic site) or with lesion-directed imaging provided with high specificity [24]. More specifically literature lacks studies specifically aimed to evaluate the accuracy of PSMA PET/CT for investigating bone metastatic disease. In the largest patient series published so far, however [25], Afshar-Oromieh and colleagues evaluated the role of ^{68}Ga-PSMA PET/CT in a cohort of 319 recurrent prostate cancer patients. Despite inhomogeneous characteristics in the population (mean PSA 161 ng/mL; median PSA 4.59 ng/mL; 28 patients not treated with radical therapies), authors assessed an overall positivity rate of 82.8 %. A total of 901 lesions were assessed by ^{68}Ga-PSMA PET/CT and considered suspicious for malignancy, with a mean per-lesion SUVmax of 13.4 (±14.6). According to the published data, on a per-lesion analysis, bone lesions were observed in the 39.8 % of cases (359 out of 901 lesions observed) with a mean per-lesion SUVmax value of 14.3 (±14.0). This data suggests the good value of this new imaging procedure for evaluating a possible skeletal involvement in recurrent prostate cancer patients. In particular, in this large cohort of patients, a high tumour-to-background ratio (TBR) for ^{68}Ga-PSMA PET/CT allowing a proper visualisation of the suspected lesions was confirmed. Eiber et al. [26] later confirmed these results. In a cohort of 248 recurrent patients, the authors observed an overall positivity rate of 89.5 % for ^{68}Ga-PSMA PET/CT. On a per-patient analysis, bone lesions were documented in the 35.9 % of patients (89 out of 248 patients). In particular, in the data reported by authors, in the 10.1 % of these 89 patients, the bone metastases were exclusively identified with PSMA focal uptake in the bone marrow, without any morphological alterations in CT. Thus, according to these results, in this patient series, with median PSA of 1.99 ng/mL, in the 3.7 % of the overall population, bone marrow metastases were suspected. Recently, Ceci et al. [23] investigated the role of ^{68}Ga-PSMA PET/CT for restaging prostate cancer patients and evaluated which clinical and pathological features were associated with PET/CT positivity rate. In their patient series (mean/median PSA 3.5/1.7 ng/mL), positive bone lesions were observed in the 17.1 % of the overall population (12 out of 70). On a per-lesion analysis, bone lesions were observed in the 14.5 % of the 152 positive lesions analysed with a mean/median SUVmax of 16.1/10.9 (range 4.2–33.7). It is interesting to report that according to data not published in this article (reported as courtesy of the authors), in the 12 patients with positive bone lesions, the mean/median PSA values observed were relatively low (mean/median PSA 4.3/1.3 ng/mL). Furthermore, these patients showed fast PSA kinetics (mean PSA doubling time 3.5 months). This data is in accordance with the statistical analysis presented by the authors, in which PSAdt was a significant predictor of the detection of distant lesions, including bone metastases ($p=0.011$).

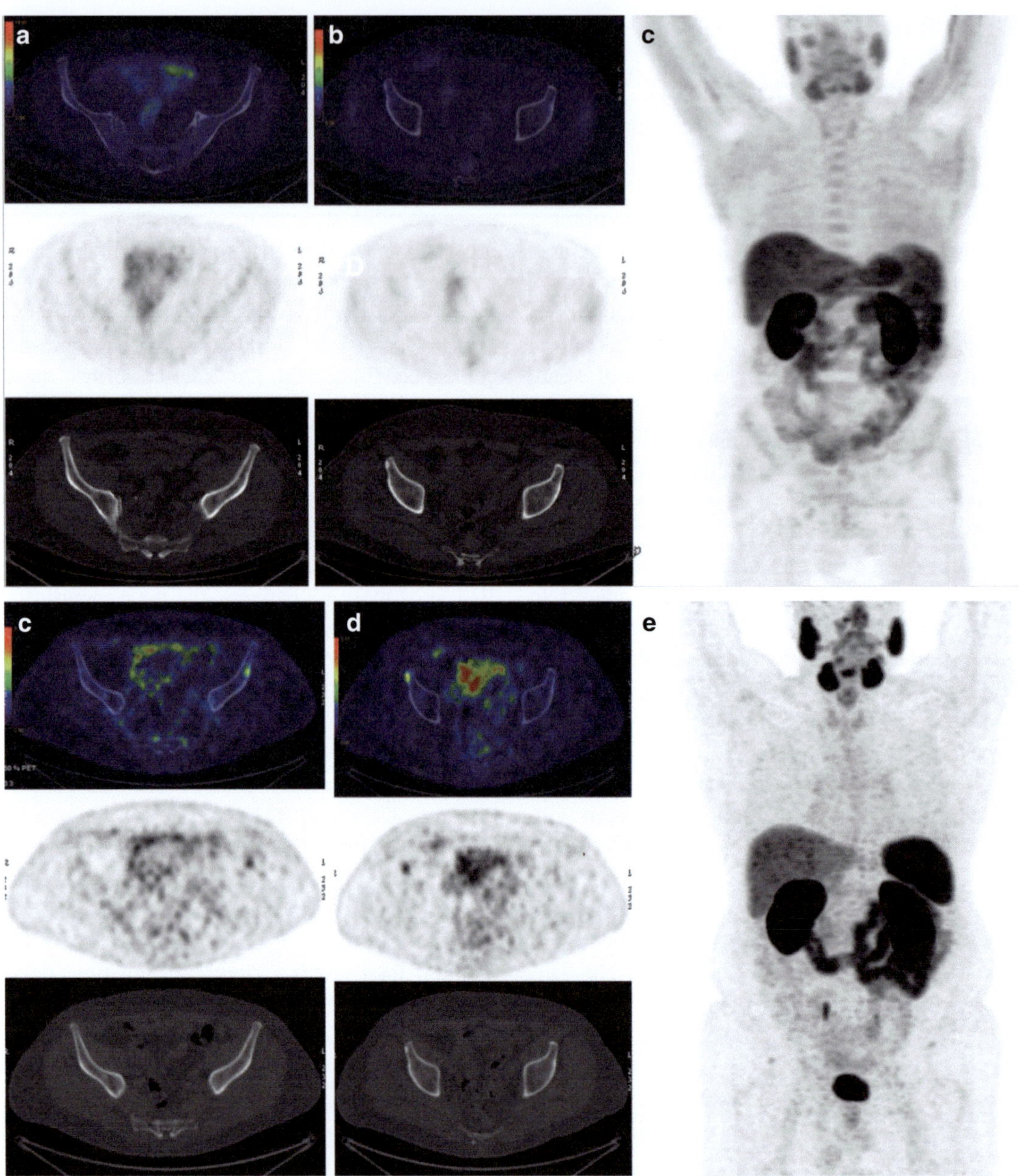

Fig. 9.3 F.P. is a 68-year-old patient treated with RP for PCa, GS 4+3, T2cN0(0/22)MxR0 in 20/7/2012. No adjuvant therapies have been performed after RP. In February 2015, the patient was addressed to salvage radiotherapy on the prostatic bed for biochemical relapse. PSA nadir after salvage therapy was 0.01 ng/mL. On June 2015, patient experienced a biochemical failure with PSA=0.24 ng/mL and was referred in March 2016 to choline PET/CT which resulted negative (**a**–**c**) (PSA=0.73 ng/mL). As a consequence, the patient was investigated with 68Ga-PSMA PET/CT that showed the presence of two bone osteoblastic lesions. According to 68Ga-PSMA PET/CT results, the patient was addressed to androgen deprivation therapy

A prospective comparative study between ^{18}F-fluoromethylcholine (CHO) and ^{68}Ga-PSMA PET/CT (PSMA) was performed on 38 patients in early 2015. The study specifically addressed patients in the low and very low PSA area, also remarking possible changes in clinical

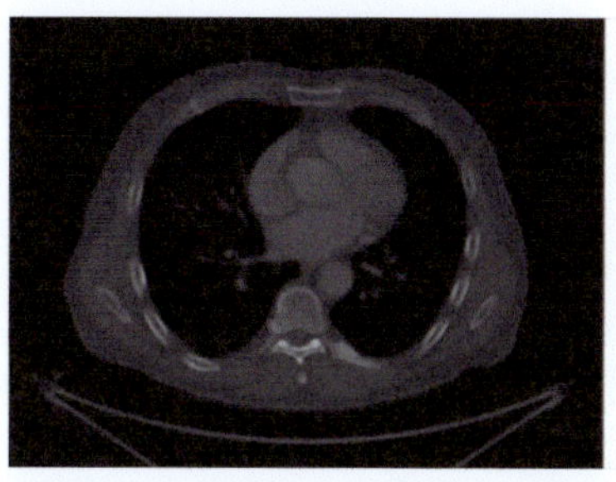
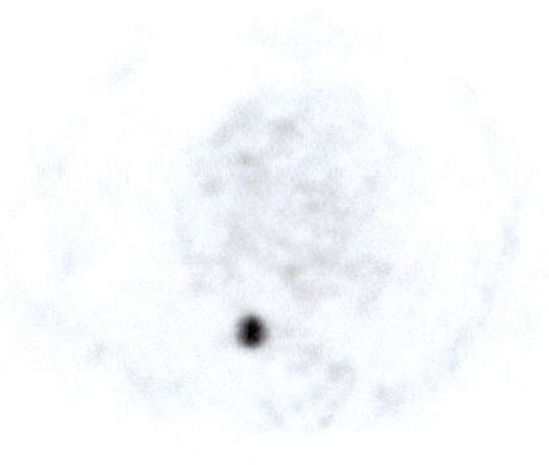
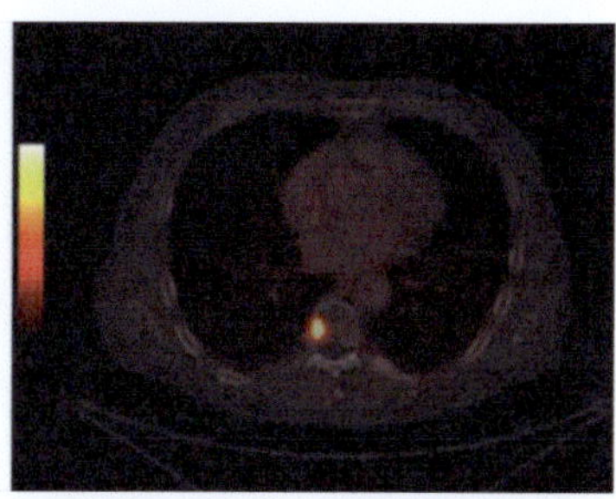

Fig. 9.4 A 72-year-old patient with prostate cancer GS 4+3, pT2cN0(0/15)Mx, initial PSA=7.9 ng/ml treated with RP without adjuvant RT. PSA nadir<0.01 ng/mL. BCR occurred 22 months after RP. The patient, with PSA of 0.83 ng/mL, PSAdt of 5.5 months and PSAvel of 0.88 ng/mL/year, was referred to 68Ga-PSMA PET/CT that showed a single bone lesion involving the VIII dorsal vertebra (SUVmax=6.1). Patient was referred to metastases-directed EBRT on the bone lesion with a PSA response (PSA=0.4 ng/mL) after the treatment (Courtesy from Dr. Llanos Geraldo and Prof. Irene Virgolini (Department of Nuclear Medicine, Medizinische Universität Innsbruck, Austria))

management of these patients. The study confirmed a major detection rate for PSMA over CHO regardless of the PSA level. Within this patient cohort, a total of 16 bone lesions were identified by PSMA (Fig. 9.4) (CHO identified 9 lesions; *this data was not published in this article and is reported as courtesy of the authors*).

The mean value of PSA for these patients was 1.91 ng/ml. Regardless of the limited number of patients presenting with bone metastases (7/38, 18 %), in patients with rising PSA being evaluated for curative intent therapy with low PSA levels, ^{68}Ga-PSMA-HBED-CC PET/CT demonstrated a significantly higher detection rate (DR) for recurrent disease than CHO and impacted on management in a high proportion of subjects imaged. Management impact is a topic of main interest when addressing the issue of bone involvement in prostate cancer as it will change the therapeutic approach, for example, shifting from salvage RT to systemic treatment [2].

A recently published paper by Mottaghy and colleagues on 151 patients specifically inquired the extent of disease in recurrent prostate cancer determined by ^{68}Ga-PSMA PET/CT in relation to PSA levels, PSA doubling time (PSAdt) and Gleason score (GS). In this study, the presence of bone lesions was demonstrated in 4/27 patients (15 %) with PSA<1ng/ml, 3/19 patients (16 %) with PSA between 1 and 2 and 43/109 patients (39 %) with PSA>2. When focusing on PSA kinetics, even more interesting data emerges, as fast PSA-kinetics (PSAdt shorter than 6 months) bone lesions are identified in 32/60 patients (53 %), with a PSAdt between 6 and 12 months: 9/27 patients (33 %) and 0/21 patients with a PSAdt >12 months. With regard to GS, values of less than 8 were associated with a 30 % DR of bone disease, while values from 8 to 10 were associated with a 32 % DR [27]. This finding confirms other data suggesting that PSMA overexpression is not directly related to Gleason score and that fast PSA kinetics are more likely to relate to a positive PSMA scan (Fig. 9.5).

There is however a lack of strong prospective studies involving large patient populations, and none of them specifically address bone metastases detection or response to therapy. Also, it is important to be aware of other potential causes of increased PSMA uptake within the bone district: there are two case reports indicating how Paget's disease might show intense PSMA uptake 17. The author theorises a mechanism of stimulation by secreted angiogenic as the probable cause of this false-positive uptake.

There are also a number of alternatives to gallium PSMA that are being proposed, most of them being PSMA-based fluorinated compounds. Advantages of ^{18}F over ^{68}Ga are mostly due to a higher feasibility of these compounds and possibly to higher quality standards of fluorinated isotopes N [28]. Among them, ^{18}F-DCFBC (N-[N-{(S)-1,3-dicarboxpropyl]carbamoyl} 4-18F-fluorobenzyl-L-cysteine] or DCFBC) and ^{18}F-DCFPyLis

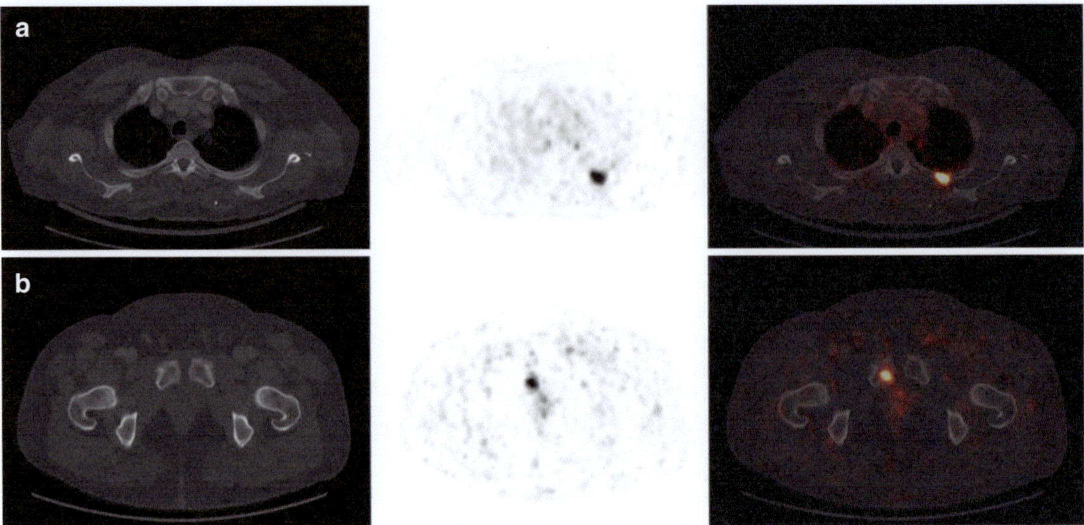

Fig. 9.5 A 59-year-old patient with prostate cancer GS 4+5, pT3bN1(2/15)MxR1, initial PSA=18.9 ng/ml treated with RP with adjuvant RT. PSA nadir <0.02 ng/mL. BCR occurred 10 months after treatments. The patient presented a PSA of 1.1 ng/mL, PSAdt of 4.9 months and PSAvel of 1.5 ng/mL/year and was addressed to S-RT on prostate bed and iliac lymph node chains. The patient was referred to 68Ga-PSMA PET/CT, to restage the disease before S-RT. PET/CT showed prostate bed and pelvic lymph node relapse together with bone metastases (**a**, **b**). According to PET/CT results, the patient treatment strategy was changed from S-RT to palliative ADT (Courtesy from Dr. Llanos Geraldo and Prof. Irene Virgolini (Department of Nuclear Medicine, Medizinische Universität Innsbruck, Austria))

(2-[3-{1-carboxy-5-[(6-[18F]fluoro-pyridine-3-carbonyl)-amino]-pentil}-ureido]-pentanedioic acid or DCFPyLis) are of particular interest. DCFBC and DCFPyLis both present favourable dosimetry and biodistribution [29, 30], and preliminary data published on only small patient populations suggest a superiority of both over conventional imaging in terms of detection of bone lesions in prostate cancer patients [31, 32].

Bombesin-based radiotracers and antagonists of gastrin-releasing peptide (GRP) receptor are also of interest [33, 34], and a recently hybrid PSMA-GRP PET tracer developed and first tested on murine samples [35] suggests that this field is ever evolving towards new and hopefully more accurate diagnostic tools.

Conclusions

In accordance with the most used guidelines of urology such as EAU and NCCN guidelines, conventional bone imaging should be limited to patients with high PSA values during BCR, since these patients are more likely to present with distant metastases. However, considering the limited value of PSA as a specific biomarker, more useful prognostic factors that might help in predicting disease aggressiveness and possibly drive better treatment decisions are needed. New data emerging from PET/CT imaging, both considering choline and new radiopharmaceuticals (PSMA and FACBC), suggests that bone imaging with PET/CT should be considered for restaging PCa patients in case of BCR, regardless of the PSA values. In fact, even in patients presenting low PSA levels at the time of imaging, and particularly in patients with fast PSA kinetics, the demonstration of bone involvement will prevent these patients from futile aggressive local treatment, like S-RT on prostate bed. In this context, the assessment of bone invasion with PET/CT could have a considerable impact on patient clinical decision-making process, addressing these patients to more tailored therapy schemes. PET/CT, with the abovementioned promising PSMA or FACBC, may help to better define the setting of a specific bone-dominant vs. non-bone-dominant disease in order to select further imaging options and treatment strategies specifically directed on bone metastases.

Acknowledgement The authors would like to thank Dr. Llanos Geraldo and Prof. Irene Virgolini (Department of Nuclear Medicine, Medizinische Universität Innsbruck, Austria) for providing the 68Ga-PSMA PET/CT cases reported in Figs. 9.4 and 9.5.

References

1. Nanni C, Schiavina R, Boschi S et al (2013) Comparison of 18F-FACBC and 11C-choline PET/CT in patients with radically treated prostate cancer and biochemical relapse: preliminary results. Eur J Nucl Med Mol Imaging 40(Suppl 1):S11–S17. doi:10.1007/s00259-013-2373-3
2. Morigi JJ, Stricker PD, van Leeuwen PJ et al (2015) Prospective comparison of 18F-fluoromethylcholine versus 68Ga-PSMA PET/CT in prostate cancer patients who have rising PSA after curative treatment and are being considered for targeted therapy. J Nucl Med 56(8):1185–1190. doi:10.2967/jnumed.115.160382
3. Oka S, Hattori R, Kurosaki F et al (2007) A preliminary study of anti-1-amino-3-18F-fluorocyclobutyl-1-carboxylic acid for the detection of prostate cancer. J Nucl Med 48:46–55
4. Sörensen J, Owenius R, Lax M, Johansson S (2013) Regional distribution and kinetics of [18F]fluciclovine (anti-[18F]FACBC), a tracer of amino acid transport, in subjects with primary prostate cancer. Eur J Nucl Med Mol Imaging 40:394–402
5. Coleman RE (2001) Metastatic bone disease: clinical features, pathophysiology and treatment strategies. Cancer Treat Rev 27(3):165–176. doi:10.1053/ctrv.2000.0210
6. Bogdanos J, Karamanolakis D, Tenta R et al (2003) Endocrine/paracrine/autocrine survival factor activity of bone microenvironment participates in the development of androgen ablation and chemotherapy refractoriness of prostate cancer metastasis in skeleton. Endocr Relat Cancer 10(2):279–289, http://www.ncbi.nlm.nih.gov/pubmed/12790789. Accessed 9 Mar 2016
7. Coleman RE (1997) Skeletal complications of malignancy. Cancer 80(8 Suppl):1588–1594, http://www.ncbi.nlm.nih.gov/pubmed/9362426. Accessed 25 Jan 2016
8. Ceci F, Castellucci P, Graziani T et al (2015) 11C-choline PET/CT identifies osteoblastic and osteolytic lesions in patients with metastatic prostate cancer. Clin Nucl Med 40(5):e265–e270. doi:10.1097/RLU.0000000000000783
9. Okudaira H, Shikano N, Nishii R et al (2011) Putative transport mechanism and intracellular fate of trans-1-amino-3-18F-fluorocyclobutanecarboxylic acid in human prostate cancer. J Nucl Med 52(5):822–829. doi:10.2967/jnumed.110.086074
10. Nye JA, Schuster DM, Yu W, Camp VM, Goodman MM, Votaw JR (2007) Biodistribution and radiation dosimetry of the synthetic nonmetabolized amino acid analogue anti-18F-FACBC in humans. J Nucl Med 48(6):1017–1020. doi:10.2967/jnumed.107.040097
11. Asano Y, Inoue Y, Ikeda Y et al (2011) Phase I clinical study of NMK36: a new PET tracer with the synthetic amino acid analogue anti-[18F]FACBC. Ann Nucl Med 25(6):414–418. doi:10.1007/s12149-011-0477-z
12. McParland BJ, Wall A, Johansson S, Sørensen J (2013) The clinical safety, biodistribution and internal radiation dosimetry of [18F]fluciclovine in healthy adult volunteers. Eur J Nucl Med Mol Imaging 40(8):1256–1264. doi:10.1007/s00259-013-2403-1
13. Schuster DM, Nanni C, Fanti S et al (2014) Anti-1-amino-3-18F-fluorocyclobutane-1-carboxylic acid: physiologic uptake patterns, incidental findings, and variants that may simulate disease. J Nucl Med 55(12):1986–1992. doi:10.2967/jnumed.114.143628
14. Odewole OA, Oyenuga OA, Tade F et al (2015) Reproducibility and reliability of anti-3-[18F]FACBC uptake measurements in background structures and malignant lesions on follow-up PET-CT in prostate carcinoma: an exploratory analysis. Mol Imaging Biol 17(2):277–283. doi:10.1007/s11307-014-0797-1
15. Schuster DM, Nieh PT, Jani AB et al (2014) Anti-3-[(18)F]FACBC positron emission tomography-computerized tomography and (111)In-capromab pendetide single photon emission computerized tomography-computerized tomography for recurrent prostate carcinoma: results of a prospective clinical trial. J Urol 191(5):1446–1453. doi:10.1016/j.juro.2013.10.065
16. Brunocilla E, Schiavina R, Nanni C et al (2014) First case of 18F-FACBC PET/CT-guided salvage radiotherapy for local relapse after radical prostatectomy with negative 11C-Choline PET/CT and multiparametric MRI: new imaging techniques may improve patient selection. Arch Ital di Urol Androl organo Uff [di] Soc Ital di Ecogr Urol e Nefrol/Assoc Ric Urol 86(3):239–240. doi:10.4081/aiua.2014.3.239
17. Nanni C, Zanoni L, Pultrone C et al (2016) (18) F-FACBC (anti1-amino-3-(18)F-fluorocyclobutane-1-carboxylic acid) versus (11)C-choline PET/CT in prostate cancer relapse: results of a prospective trial. Eur J Nucl Med Mol Imaging 43(9):1601–1610. doi:10.1007/s00259-016-3329-1. Epub 2016 Mar 10. PubMed PMID: 26960562.
18. Kairemo K, Rasulova N, Partanen K, Joensuu T (2014) Preliminary clinical experience of trans-1-Amino-3-(18)F-fluorocyclobutanecarboxylic Acid (anti-(18)F-FACBC) PET/CT imaging in prostate cancer patients. Biomed Res Int 2014:305182. doi:10.1155/2014/305182
19. Suzuki H, Inoue Y, Fujimoto H et al (2016) Diagnostic performance and safety of NMK36 (trans-1-amino-3-

[18F]fluorocyclobutanecarboxylic acid)-PET/CT in primary prostate cancer: multicenter Phase IIb clinical trial. Jpn J Clin Oncol 46(2):152–162. doi:10.1093/jjco/hyv181

20. Sweat SD, Pacelli A, Murphy GP, Bostwick DG (1998) Prostate-specific membrane antigen expression is greatest in prostate adenocarcinoma and lymph node metastases. Urology 52(4):637–640, http://www.ncbi.nlm.nih.gov/pubmed/9763084. Accessed 9 Mar 2016
21. Silver DA, Pellicer I, Fair WR, Heston WD, Cordon-Cardo C (1997) Prostate-specific membrane antigen expression in normal and malignant human tissues. Clin Cancer Res 3(1):81–85, http://www.ncbi.nlm.nih.gov/pubmed/9815541. Accessed 9 Mar 2016
22. Afshar-Oromieh A, Zechmann CM, Malcher A et al (2013) Comparison of PET imaging with a 68Ga-labelled PSMA ligand and 18F-choline-based PET/CT for the diagnosis of recurrent prostate cancer. Eur J Nucl Med Mol Imaging 41(1):11–20. doi:10.1007/s00259-013-2525-5
23. Ceci F, Uprimny C, Nilica B et al (2015) (68) Ga-PSMA PET/CT for restaging recurrent prostate cancer: which factors are associated with PET/CT detection rate? Eur J Nucl Med Mol Imaging. doi:10.1007/s00259-015-3078-6
24. Sterzing F, Kratochwil C, Fiedler H et al (2016) (68) Ga-PSMA-11 PET/CT: a new technique with high potential for the radiotherapeutic management of prostate cancer patients. Eur J Nucl Med Mol Imaging 43(1):34–41. doi:10.1007/s00259-015-3188-1
25. Afshar-Oromieh A, Avtzi E, Giesel FL et al (2015) The diagnostic value of PET/CT imaging with the (68)Ga-labelled PSMA ligand HBED-CC in the diagnosis of recurrent prostate cancer. Eur J Nucl Med Mol Imaging 42(2):197–209. doi:10.1007/s00259-014-2949-6
26. Eiber M, Maurer T, Souvatzoglou M et al (2015) Evaluation of hybrid 68Ga-PSMA-ligand PET/CT in 248 patients with biochemical recurrence after radical prostatectomy. J Nucl Med. doi:10.2967/jnumed.115.154153
27. Verburg FA, Pfister D, Heidenreich A et al (2016) Extent of disease in recurrent prostate cancer determined by [(68)Ga]PSMA-HBED-CC PET/CT in relation to PSA levels, PSA doubling time and Gleason score. Eur J Nucl Med Mol Imaging 43(3):397–403. doi: 10.1007/s00259-015-3240-1. Epub 2015 Nov 12. PubMed PMID: 26563121.
28. Evangelista L, Briganti A, Fanti S et al (2016) New clinical indications for 18F/11C-choline, new tracers for positron emission tomography and a promising hybrid device for prostate cancer staging: a systematic review of the literature. Eur Urol. doi:10.1016/j.eururo.2016.01.029
29. Cho SY, Gage KL, Mease RC et al (2012) Biodistribution, tumor detection, and radiation dosimetry of 18F-DCFBC, a low-molecular-weight inhibitor of prostate-specific membrane antigen, in patients with metastatic prostate cancer. J Nucl Med 53(12):1883–1891. doi:10.2967/jnumed.112.104661
30. Chen Y, Pullambhatla M, Foss CA et al (2011) 2-(3-{1-Carboxy-5-[(6-[18F]fluoro-pyridine-3-carbonyl)-amino]-pentyl}-ureido)-pentanedioic acid, [18F]DCFPyL, a PSMA-based PET imaging agent for prostate cancer. Clin Cancer Res 17(24):7645–7653. doi:10.1158/1078-0432.CCR-11-1357
31. Rowe SP, Mana-Ay M, Javadi MS et al (2016) PSMA-based detection of prostate cancer bone lesions with (18)F-DCFPyL PET/CT: a sensitive alternative to (99m)Tc-MDP bone scan and Na(18)F PET/CT? Clin Genitourin Cancer 14(1):e115–e118. doi:10.1016/j.clgc.2015.09.011
32. Rowe SP, Macura KJ, Ciarallo A et al (2016) Comparison of prostate-specific membrane antigen-based 18F-DCFBC PET/CT to conventional imaging modalities for detection of hormone-naïve and castration-resistant metastatic prostate cancer. J Nucl Med 57(1):46–53. doi:10.2967/jnumed.115.163782
33. Wieser G, Mansi R, Grosu AL et al (2014) Positron emission tomography (PET) imaging of prostate cancer with a gastrin releasing peptide receptor antagonist – from mice to men. Theranostics 4(4):412–419. doi:10.7150/thno.7324
34. Sah B-R, Burger IA, Schibli R et al (2015) Dosimetry and first clinical evaluation of the new 18F-radiolabeled bombesin analogue BAY 864367 in patients with prostate cancer. J Nucl Med 56(3):372–378. doi:10.2967/jnumed.114.147116
35. Liolios CC, Schaefer M, Haberkorn U, Eder M, Kopka K (2016) Novel bispecific PSMA/GRPr targeting radioligands with optimized pharmacokinetics for improved PET imaging of prostate cancer. Bioconjug Chem. doi:10.1021/acs.bioconjchem.5b00687

10 Bone Metastases from Prostate Cancer: Hormonal Therapy

Elisa Zanardi, Carlo Cattrini, and Francesco Boccardo

10.1 Introduction

Skeletal metastases occur in more than 80 % of prostate cancer patients diagnosed with metastatic disease [1]. The majority of these patients initially benefit from hormone therapies, namely, androgen deprivation therapies (ADT); however, virtually all of them develop castration-resistant prostate cancer (CRPC), a condition which is defined by losing response to ADT [2, 3]. In most cases, bone metastases are already present at this stage of disease. However, in other cases that also harbor CRPC according to the criteria most widely employed, bone metastases develop later in the course of the disease. In a paper by Smith et al., 33 % of patients who had no metastases at CRPC diagnosis developed one or more bone localizations within 2 years of CRPC diagnosis [4]. The median survival of patients affected by CRPC is highly variable. In a recent review by Kirby et al. [1], a pooled sample-weighted survival estimate was 14 months. Survival expectation in these patients is the result of tumor bulk and disease spread to other sites beyond the skeleton. The survival of patients affected by visceral metastasis is in fact usually poorer than that of patients affected only by skeletal metastases. However, the number of metastatic sites and site of involvement is closely correlated with life expectancy. Life expectancy is also unfavorably affected by skeletal-related events, like bone fractures or spinal cord compression, which can complicate the course of disease. If untreated, about half of advanced prostate cancer patients with bone metastases will experience at least one skeletal event over a 2-year period [5]. Beyond shortening patients' life expectancy, these events are usually associated with pain and other troublesome symptoms, which can seriously affect patient quality of life and can represent a cause of temporary or permanent disability. Costs are also increased in patients with bone metastases in relation to the management of these adverse events and disability. Bone-related parameters are not the only factors able to predict for patient survival, though they play a major role in this regard. In a recent analysis reported by Fizazi et al., including nearly 2,000 patients enrolled in an international multicenter study, 15 potential prognostic variables were investigated, 12 of which were included into multiparametric models [6].

E. Zanardi • C. Cattrini • F. Boccardo (✉)
Academic Unit of Medical Oncology, IRCCS AOU San Martino – IST, San Martino University Hospital and National Cancer Research Institute, Genoa 16132, Italy

Department of Internal Medicine, School of Medicine, University of Genoa, Genoa 16132, Italy
e-mail: fboccardo@unige.it

F. Bertoldo et al. (eds.), *Bone Metastases from Prostate Cancer*,
DOI 10.1007/978-3-319-42327-2_10

Seven bone-related variables were associated with longer survival: lower alkaline phosphatase and bone-specific alkaline phosphatase serum levels, lower corrected urinary N-telopeptide concentration, mild or no pain, no previous skeletal-related events, longer time from initial diagnosis to first bone metastasis, and longer time from first bone metastasis to randomization. The morphologic pattern on CT scan, glycolytic activity, and androgen receptor (AR) expression on PET also appear to be associated with overall survival (OS) [7]. More recently, other researchers have investigated whether novel molecular approaches might provide additional prognostic variables in patients affected by bone metastases. Indeed, it has been shown that bone metastases of CRPC patients express higher levels of AR splice variants, like AR-V7 or AR567e, than those of hormone-naïve patients [8]. The overexpression of AR variants is usually correlated with a poorer prognosis and resistance to endocrine therapies [9]. Moreover, induced capacity of converting adrenal-gland-derived steroids into more potent androgens was also demonstrated in a subgroup of bone metastases [10]. However, these molecular changes appear to correlate more with the probability to respond to second-line endocrine manipulations than with the probability of survival [10]. These premises highlight the complexity of the issues to be addressed in patients affected by bone metastases, starting from the mechanisms involved in the development of this manifestation of disease as the logical premise to implement adequate treatment strategies. Concerning bone metastases pathogenesis (see Chap. 1 to have more information about this topic), the central role of the bone niches must be underlined [11]. In fact, the specific molecular changes which drive the activation of osteoclasts and osteoblasts are essential to the attachment and proliferation of cancer stem cells. The extracellular matrix and some of its main components, like periostin, play a crucial role in tumor cell proliferation at the niche level. These components are involved in promoting neo-angiogenesis or activating alternative signaling pathways which advantage the growth of phenotypically aggressive tumor clones, able to drive tumor spreading to other bone sites or to other organs [12, 13]. These novel theories open the door to the concept of "precision medicine" and to the implementation of new strategies based on the combination of systemic and local treatment modalities, beyond the old purpose of improving disease palliation. Waiting for the results based on the new emerging paradigms, a multidisciplinary approach is often required in everyday clinical practice to correctly approach patients affected by bone metastases. In fact, local treatments are usually aimed at bone stabilization, and symptomatic treatments are usually aimed at pain control; however, these strategies must be integrated with systemic treatments more specifically aimed at disease control, at preventing the consequences of bone involvement, and at minimizing the side effects of oncologic treatments on bone health. Both can in fact contribute to the development of serious adverse events, like bone fractures or spinal cord compression. Among systemic treatments, hormone therapies still represent the mainstay to manage bone metastases both in hormone-naïve and in castration-resistant patients, due to the central role played by androgen receptor (AR) in sustaining disease progression in both situations. Endocrine manipulations can target both the seed, i.e., cancer cells which generate the metastasis, and the soil, i.e., the mechanisms operating at the level of the bone niches which interfere with bone resorption, which, in turn, is responsible for the majority of the adverse events occurring at this stage of disease. This evidence, though often underestimated, provides further support to the use of endocrine manipulations and to consider the concurrent administration of other bone-targeting therapies, like bisphosphonates or denosumab. In fact, it has been shown that androgens modulate Runx2 activity in prostate cancer cells, promoting EMT and metastatic potential, but also stimulate Wnt signaling in osteoblasts, causing Runx2 overexpression, osteoblast differentiation, and enhanced secretion of RANKL, which in turn promotes osteoclast differentiation [14, 15]. Mature osteoclasts initiate bone resorption with the release of TGF-beta, which can further stimulate prostate cancer growth. Therefore, the interference with androgen synthesis or function through appropriate pharmacological manipulations interrupts this vicious circle, arresting both prostate cancer proliferation and bone resorption [16]. These data have been obtained in preclinical models. However, they are supported by the fact that both tumor control and the reduction in the adverse events more strictly related to bone resorption have been observed in the clinical trials testing the novel generation endocrine therapies which will be described in the next paragraphs.

10.2 Hormonal Therapy: Options

Prostate tissue, whether benign or malignant, is heavily dependent on AR signaling for growth and proliferation. Therefore, the inhibition of this pathway by hormonal therapy has historically been the mainstay of treatment for prostate cancer, namely, of patients with bone metastases. Gonads are the main source of androgens, with adrenal biosynthesis providing only 5–10% of total male sex hormones. Testosterone is converted to 5-α-dihydrotestosterone (DHT), a compound which is about ten times more powerful than testosterone, within the prostate cells and at the stromal level [17]. The first important results in prostate cancer treatment were obtained with ADT. ADT, formerly achieved through orchiectomy or major surgical procedures, like adrenalectomy, is now achieved through different pharmacological approaches. The use of steroidal and nonsteroidal compounds able to bind the AR with a higher affinity than that of the natural ligand and, as a consequence, to inhibit AR transcription also proved to effectively inhibit prostate cancer proliferation (Table 10.1).

10.2.1 Inhibitors of Gonadal Androgen Synthesis

As already mentioned, the surgical ablation of the gonads is the most effective and cheap way to obtain androgen deprivation and doesn't expose the patient to any risk of paradoxical flare of the disease [18]. Medical castration is achieved by interfering with the release of gonadotropins at the pituitary level, and this treatment is considered an acceptable alternative to surgical castration, which is better tolerated by patients from a psychological point of view due to its putative reversibility [18–20]. Medical androgen deprivation has been accomplished through estrogens (diethylstilbestrol), luteinizing hormone-releasing hormone (LH-RH) agonists, and LH-RH antagonists. However, severe thromboembolic and cardiac side effects have limited the use of estrogenic therapy over time [20].

LH-RH (also known as gonadotropin-releasing hormone or GnRH) is secreted in the hypothalamic area of the brain in a pulsatile fashion, with pulses occurring every 60–90 min. The binding of LH-RH to specific plasma membrane receptors on pituitary gonadotrope cells is the step necessary to activate the synthesis and release of LH and FSH. Once LH enters the general circulation, it acts on the Leydig cells in the testes to control testosterone synthesis [21]. LH-RH agonists (buserelin, goserelin, leuprolide, and triptorelin) override this pulsatile control of the pituitary by providing continuous stimulation, which eventually leads to the down-regulation of pituitary LH-RH receptors, the consequent reduction in LH and FSH release, and, therefore, the consequent suppression of testosterone levels [22] (Fig. 10.2). The chronic administration of LH-RH agonists achieves a deep and long-standing serum testosterone fall [19]; however, at the beginning of treatment, the physiological spiking of LH levels with consequent testosterone surge can determinate a transient disease flare, sometimes causing patients clinical worsening due to pain increase, spinal cord compression, or urethral obstruction [23, 24]. For this reason, the concurrent administration of an anti-androgen at the beginning of treatment with LH-RH agonists is usually recommended, especially in patients with bone metastases who have a higher risk of clinical complications from the flare caused by the early surge of testosterone [25, 26]. LH-RH antagonists (abarelix, degarelix) bind directly to LH-RH receptor at the pituitary cell level competing with native LH-RH, thus inducing an immediate suppression of LH, FSH, and testosterone circulating levels. Therefore, they are not associated with the initial surge of testosterone observed after agonist administration, and for this reason they don't require the concurrent administration of an antiandrogen [27]. Two randomized trials evaluated the efficacy of the LH-RH antagonist abarelix depot in suppressing testosterone levels compared to leuprolide or leuprolide plus an antiandrogen. Abarelix not only achieved a comparable suppression of testosterone levels in the range of castrated levels but also achieved a more prompt reduction in the serum levels of this hormone without any flare effect [27, 28]. However, in 2009, this drug was withdrawn by the US FDA because of the occurrence of severe systemic allergic reactions subsequent to its administration. Allergic reactions are very uncommon with degarelix, a second-generation LH-RH antagonist. Therefore, this compound was approved by the US FDA and EMA for the treatment of prostate cancer as an alternative to LH-RH agonists [28]. The approval was granted based on the results of a phase III study which demonstrated the non-inferiority of degarelix compared with leuprolide in maintaining castration levels of testosterone (i.e., ≤0.5 ng/ml) for 1 year of treatment (primary endpoint of the study) in patients candidates to ADT [29].

Adverse events generally related to ADT include flushes, weight increase, impotence, loss of libido, fatigue, decreased muscle mass, osteoporosis, anemia, metabolic syndrome, and cardiovascular disorders [30–32]. Recent evidences also suggest the possible association between ADT and the appearance of cognitive disorders [33, 34]. A recent meta-analysis of five randomized trials comparing antagonists to agonists provides initial evidence about the putative superiority of antagonists on OS as well as on the lower incidence of ischemic cardiovascular events, particularly in patients with pre-existing cardiovascular disorders [35]. Noteworthy, the different incidence of cardiovascular events among patients allocated to degarelix was more evident during the first 6 months of treatment [30]. It is still unclear why the "protective effect" of LH-RH antagonists comes out especially in the first months of treatment. It was assumed that it might be mediated by the effect of treatment on the early detachment of arterial plaques, which, in turn, is probably mediated by the different behavior of FSH during treatment with agonists or antagonists or by immunologic mechanisms involving IL-2 [36, 37]. The previously mentioned meta-analysis also showed a reduced incidence of joint, musculoskeletal, and urinary tract adverse events in favor of LH-RH antagonists [35]. Noteworthy, LH-RH antagonists do not appear to be cross-resistant with LH-RH agonists, as shown in the retrospective study by Crawford et al., who demonstrated that patients initially progressed during treatment with an LH-RH agonist could be rescued after switching them to degarelix [23]. More recently, the results achieved with TAK 385, an oral LH-RH antagonist, confirmed the ability of this compound in achieving a prompt and durable suppression of testosterone levels, almost comparable to that induced by LH-RH agonist, with the advantage of being devoid of the local effects at the injection site that occur in about 40 % of the patients treated with degarelix [38]. Large prospective trials, specifically designed to compare the toxicity profile and survival outcomes of LH-RH agonists and antagonists, are still missing, and up to now the preference for antagonists is supported in selected patients, namely, those with cardiovascular comorbidities or at higher risk of tumor flare.

10.2.2 Inhibitors of Adrenal Androgen Synthesis

Abiraterone acetate was developed to interfere with residual androgen synthesis in castrated patients in a more selective and safer manner compared to the older adrenal steroidogenesis inhibitors, such as ketoconazole [39, 40]. In fact, this novel steroidal antiandrogen selectively inhibits the cytochrome P450 17α-hydroxylase/17,20-lyase (CYP17) activities. CYP17 is located in the endoplasmic reticulum of the testes and of the adrenals [41] and catalyzes two sequential reactions leading to the conversion of pregnenolone and progesterone into their 17α-hydroxy-derivatives and, subsequently, to dehydroepiandrosterone (DHEA) and androstenedione (ASD) [40]. ASD and DHEA are converted to testosterone through 17-beta-hydroxy-steroid dehydrogenase activity; testosterone is, in turn, converted to dihydrotestosterone (DHT), the biologically active compound, by 5α reductase. The inhibition of CYP17 thus decreases circulating levels of DHEA, ASD, testosterone, and DHT (Fig. 10.2). However, the blockade of abovementioned enzymatic pathways leads to the suppression of the negative adrenocorticotropic feedback, which, in turn, results in an exceeding production of precursor steroids with high mineralocorticoid activity. This effect is responsible for the most frequent adverse events observed during abiraterone treatment, namely, hypokalemia, hypertension, and fluid overload. The concomitant use of low-dose glucocorticoids, which block the adrenocorticotropic feedback, is therefore required to decrease the frequency and severity of these events [42, 43]. Initial phase I dose escalation studies with abiraterone showed a strict relationship between the degree of testosterone suppression and the percentage of objective tumor responses [44, 45]. Indeed, a significant inhibition in testosterone levels was demonstrated in both castrate and non-castrate patients; however, a reactive LH rise was observed in non-castrate males, suggesting the opportunity of maintaining gonadal suppression during treatment with abiraterone [45]. Li et al. have recently demonstrated that abiraterone is converted to a more active metabolite, the delta-4-abiraterone (D4A). Beyond blocking the enzymatic pathways required to DHT synthesis through an increased affinity for CYP17, this metabolite directly competes for AR transcription, through a mechanism similar to enzalutamide. These findings provide an additional explanation for abiraterone's activity in prostate cancer [46]. Moreover, interfering with abiraterone pharmacodynamics by adding an inhibitor of 5-alpha-reductase, which induces an increase in D4A levels, might increase treatment efficacy and overcome the resistance to this drug [46]. The use of dexamethasone in place of prednisone might also overcome the resistance to abiraterone, due to the higher affinity of dexamethasone for the glucocorticoid receptors which might be also involved in abiraterone resistance [47, 48]. Orteronel (TAK-700) is another inhibitor of adrenal androgen synthesis. Differently from abiraterone, this is a nonsteroidal, reversible inhibitor of CYP17. Results of a phase II trial preliminarily showed that orteronel (with or without prednisone) greatly decreased the plasma concentrations of testosterone, DHEA-S, and prostate-specific antigen (PSA) in patients with metastatic CRPC (mCRPC) [49]. However, two subsequent phase III trials in patients previously treated with docetaxel or chemo-naïve (ELM-PC 5 and ELM-PC 4 trials) failed to confirm the ability of orteronel to impact on patients' survival (as it was the case for abiraterone; see next paragraphs); therefore, this drug did not obtain the US FDA approval [50, 51].

10.2.3 First-Generation Antiandrogens

Differently from therapies which act by interfering with the hypothalamic–pituitary–gonadal axis, antiandrogens compete directly with circulating androgens for binding sites on their receptors within the prostate cells, thus promoting apoptosis and inhibiting prostate cancer growth [52, 53] (Fig. 10.1). These effects can be achieved either by steroidal compounds like cyproterone acetate or by nonsteroidal moieties (bicalutamide, flutamide, nilutamide) [54]. Differently from nonsteroidal antiandrogens, cyproterone acetate also blocks gonadotropin release at the pituitary level (depending on the dose employed) causing a decrease in testosterone plasma levels too, leading to a sort of maximal androgen blockade [55, 56]. However, cardiovascular adverse events have been observed in more than 20 % of patients treated with this progestin [37]. These relevant side effects, which also include liver toxicity and fulminant hepatitis, have progressively narrowed the indications to the use of cyproterone acetate in prostate cancer [57, 58]. In contrast to cyproterone acetate, which causes loss of libido and sexual impotence, nonsteroidal antiandrogens have been shown to preserve sexual function if used as monotherapy. These drugs are also associated with a better physical capacity and quality of life; moreover, the treatment with these compounds has favorable effects on hemoglobin levels and bone mineral density

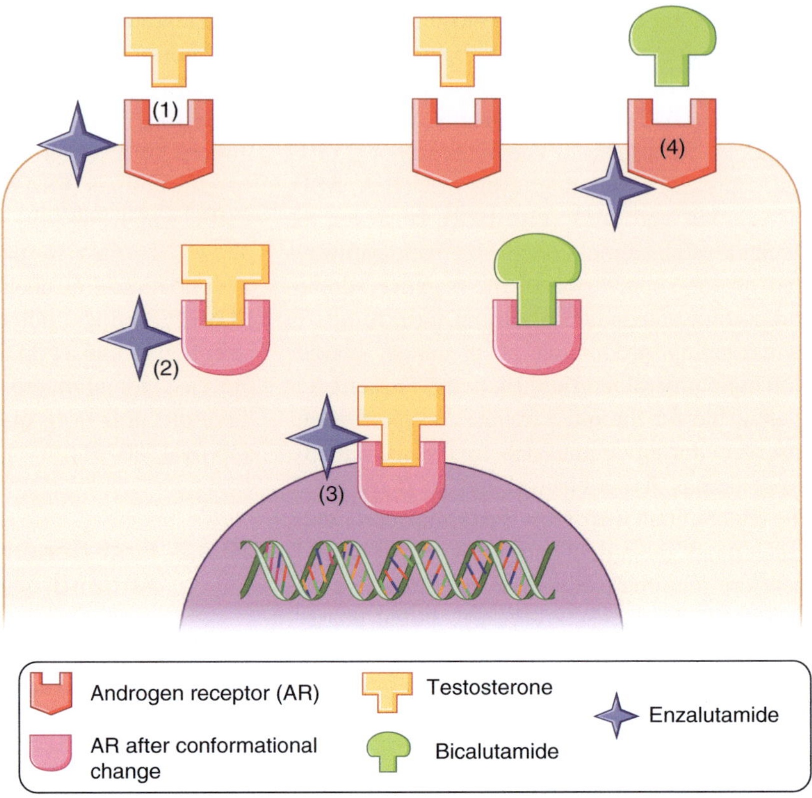

Fig. 10.1 Mechanisms of action of bicalutamide and enzalutamide. Bicalutamide competes directly with circulating androgens for binding sites on their receptors within the prostate cells. Enzalutamide inhibits prostate cancer cells acting at different levels: (1) It inhibits AR–testosterone binding with higher affinity than bicalutamide. (2) Receptor inhibition blocks the activational change induced by AR–testosterone binding. (3) It inhibits AR–testosterone nuclear translocation and DNA transcription. (4) Enzalutamide lacks partial AR agonist activity that occurs with bicalutamide resistance (From: Hoffman-Censits and Kelly [103])

[52, 59–61]. However, mild- to moderate-grade gynecomastia and mastalgia occur virtually in all patients, due to the increase in circulating estrogen levels which is the consequence of antiandrogen monotherapy [62]. This mechanism explains the efficacy of tamoxifen in preventing or in managing gynecomastia and breast pain in these patients [63]. Abnormal liver function tests have been observed with all nonsteroidal therapies [52]. Serious hepatotoxicity was rarely observed with bicalutamide and nilutamide, but a few cases of fulminant liver failure have been described with flutamide [62, 64]. Nilutamide has been associated with a higher incidence of adverse effects than the other nonsteroidal antiandrogens, including some peculiar toxicities like interstitial pneumonitis, delayed adaptation to darkness, and alcohol intolerance [62, 65]. Although no direct comparisons are available, bicalutamide appears to be the first-generation antiandrogen with the most favorable safety and tolerability profile [52]. As it will be discussed in the next paragraphs, these compounds have been developed to be used in combination with ADT, to prevent tumor flare or to improve treatment efficacy in the frame of a total androgen-blockade strategy [66]. However, they have been proven to be also effective as monotherapy, but only in selected groups of nonmetastatic patients. There is no indication that they might replace ADT in patients with metastatic disease, namely, those with bone metastases.

10.2.4 Second-Generation Antiandrogens

First-generation antiandrogens, such as bicalutamide or flutamide, have modest efficacy in the setting of AR overexpression or of specific mutations in the AR ligand-binding domain [67]. New antiandrogens, like enzalutamide, were developed to overcome these limits. Enzalutamide has fourfold greater binding affinity for AR than bicalutamide; it reduces the efficiency of AR nuclear translocation and impairs both DNA binding to androgen response elements and recruitment of co-activators [54, 68, 69] (Figs. 10.1 and 10.2). Enzalutamide is also active against prostate cancer cell lines bearing the

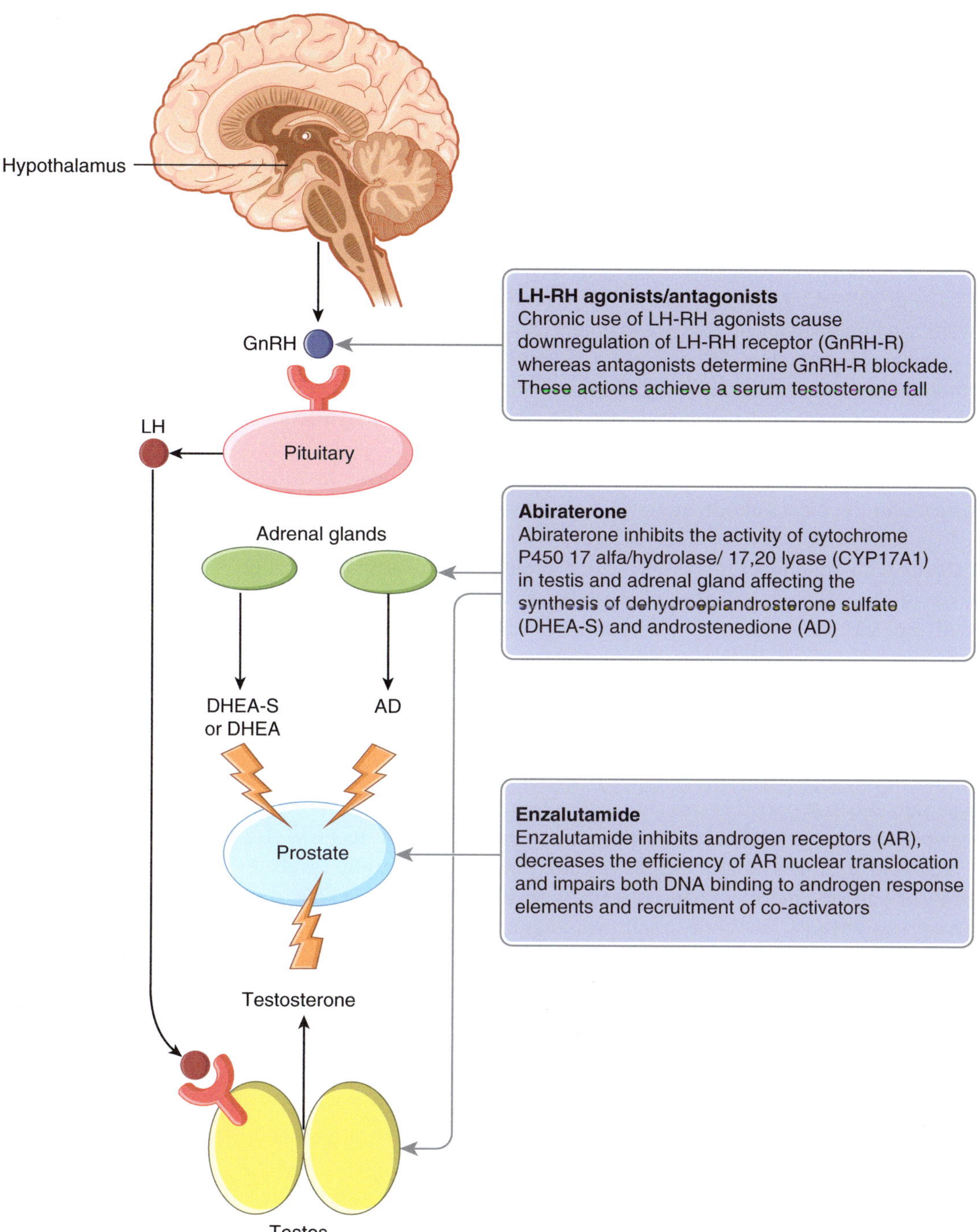

Fig. 10.2 Mechanisms of action of LH-RH agonists/antagonists, enzalutamide, and abiraterone. Chronic use of LH-RH agonists leads to downregulation of the LH-RH receptor (GnRH-R), whereas antagonists provide immediate GnRH-R blockade, achieving a deep and long-standing serum testosterone fall (**a**). Abiraterone selectively inhibits the cytochrome P450 17α-hydroxylase/17,20-lyase (CYP17A1) activities, located in the endoplasmic reticulum of testes and adrenals (**b**). Enzalutamide inhibits androgen receptor (AR) with high affinity, reduces the efficiency of AR nuclear translocation, and impairs both DNA binding to androgen response elements and recruitment of co-activators. *DHEA* dehydroepiandrosterone, *GnRH* gonadotropin-releasing hormone, *LH* luteinizing hormone, *DHEA-S* dehydroepiandrosterone sulfate, *AD* androstenedione, II (From: Watson et al. [104])

W741C AR point mutation that is known to confer resistance to bicalutamide. The superiority of enzalutamide over bicalutamide was recently demonstrated by two randomized controlled trials: the TERRAIN trial, which compared these two drugs in combinations with ADT in mCRPC [70], and the STRIVE trial, which compared enzalutamide versus bicalutamide in nonmetastatic or metastatic CRPC [71]. In the TERRAIN trial, a double-blind phase II study, 375 patients were randomly assigned to enzalutamide (184 patients) or bicalutamide (191 patients). Castrated levels of testosterone were maintained in both arms. Patients in the enzalutamide group had significantly improved median progression-free survival (PFS) duration (15.7 months) compared to patients in the bicalutamide group (5.8 months; HR: 0.44; $p<0.0001$). In the STRIVE trial, patients with bone metastases represented about 55 % of the whole population on study. In this trial too, castrated levels of testosterone were required. Again enzalutamide was associated with a significant improvement in all study endpoints, including median time to PSA progression (HR: 0.19, $p<0.001$) and PFS (median PFS duration: 16.5 vs. 5.5 months HR: 0.24, $p<0.001$). The side effects reported in this study were comparable between groups; in fact, grade ≥3 adverse events and treatment-related deaths occurred in 36 % of patients and in 3 % of patients in each group, respectively. This study confirmed fatigue and hypertension being the most common clinically relevant adverse events. Seizures were not reported in this study but were previously observed in pivotal trials. Seizures are dose dependent and are thought to be related to the inhibition of gamma-aminobutyric acid (GABA) receptors in the brain [72]. Although the incidence of seizures in pivotal trials was small, it should be taken into account that patients eligible to these studies were required to have a low seizure risk at the time of enrolment (no prior seizures, no brain metastases, no recent stroke, no concomitant medications known to lower the seizure threshold), suggesting that the true incidence of seizures in an unselected patient population might be higher. Therefore, the administration of enzalutamide must be carefully evaluated in patients with a medical history of seizures or predisposing conditions.

ARN-509 (ARN) is another potent and selective AR antagonist, which, similarly to enzalutamide, inhibits AR nuclear translocation and DNA binding without significant AR agonist properties [73]. The efficacy of this compound is now being tested in randomized trials [74].

10.3 Hormonal Therapy: Indications

10.3.1 Hormone-Naïve Patients

As already mentioned, ADT represents the common treatment suggested to manage hormone-naïve patients with bone metastases. The results achievable with either surgical or pharmacological castration (LH-RH agonists or antagonists) are comparable. More than two-thirds of patients benefit from ADT, with both symptoms and disease improvement, though it is still difficult to measure tumor response at bone level (see Chap. 16). However, the benefit is commonly limited to 12–24 months. After ADT failure, defined by tumor progression according to PCWG 2 criteria in the presence of castration levels of testosterone (possibly ≤0.20 ng/ml) [75], it is usually suggested to add an antiandrogen to ADT in patients initially managed with ADT alone or to switch from an antiandrogen to another one in patients initially managed through maximal androgen blockade (MAB); discontinuing the antiandrogen in patients initially receiving combined treatment is another alternative. In fact, about 20–30 % of patients managed in this latter way may experience symptom control and/or PSA decrease ("withdrawal response"), though response is usually short lived. Attempts have been made in order to increase response rate and duration in hormone-naïve patients by combining ADT with chemotherapy in selected patients (see Chap. 10) or by combining ADT with antiandrogen therapy (MAB). This approach is based on the evidence that pharmacological or surgical castration is able to reduce more than 95 %

Table 10.1 Hormonal therapies in prostate cancer: mechanisms of action and side effects

Therapy	Mechanism of action	Side effects
LH-RH agonists (buserelin, goserelin, leuprolide, and triptorelin)	Downregulation of LH-RH receptor	Flushes, weight increase, impotence, loss of libido, fatigue, decreased muscle mass, osteoporosis, anemia, metabolic syndrome, cardiovascular disorders, cognitive disorders, and "testosterone flare"
LH-RH antagonists (degarelix)	Competitive occupancy of LH-RH receptor	The same side effects of agonists with a putative lower incidence of cardiovascular, joint, musculoskeletal, and urinary tract events; no "testosterone flare"
Nonsteroidal antiandrogens (bicalutamide, flutamide, and nilutamide)	Competitive occupancy of AR	Anemia, liver toxicities, gynecomastia, mastalgia, and gastrointestinal disorders
Steroidal antiandrogens (cyproterone acetate)	Competitive occupancy of AR and gonadotropin release blockade	Cardiovascular events, gynecomastia, mastalgia, loss of libido, and sexual impotence
Abiraterone acetate	Inhibition of residual and adrenal androgen synthesis	Hypokalemia, hypertension, and fluid overload
Orteronel	Reversible inhibition of residual and adrenal androgen synthesis	Nausea, vomiting, fatigue, hypokalemia, and hypertension
Enzalutamide	Competitive occupancy of AR with high affinity, inhibition of AR nuclear translocation, and interaction with DNA	Cephalea, fatigue, hypertension, flushes, and seizures

LH-RH luteinizing hormone-releasing hormone, *AR* androgen receptor

of the daily testosterone production; however, residual androgen synthesis is retained by adrenal glands and the tumor itself [76], and relevant androgen levels can be found in prostatectomy samples of patients subjected to chemical or surgical castration [77]. Numerous studies have addressed the problem of the potential superiority of MAB compared to monotherapy with LH-RH agonists, with contradictory results [78–86] (there are no studies comparing MAB vs. LH-RH antagonists). The Prostate Cancer Trialists' Collaborative Group examined the results of 27 randomized trials comparing MAB versus medical or surgical castration [66]. Although MAB implies increased cost and toxicities, this meta-analysis showed a small but significant advantage favoring this approach, when the trials with cyproterone acetate were excluded. These trends have been confirmed by a couple of subsequent meta-analyses and by a recent Cochrane overview [84, 87]. In view of these data, MAB has become a common treatment option for patients with metastatic disease in many countries [25].

As already mentioned, the use of enzalutamide in combination with a LH-RH agonist might prove to be superior to MAB with first-generation antiandrogens, like flutamide or bicalutamide, similarly to what has been observed in mCRPC in the TERRAIN and STRIVE trials [70]. Other approaches tending to "maximize" androgen deprivation are based on the use of pharmacological castration combined with drugs able to interfere with adrenal or tumor androgen synthesis like abiraterone acetate [88, 89]. However, results from these trials are not available yet.

Combination of ADT with bone-targeting treatments has been also proposed as a putative way to increase the therapeutic efficacy of hormonal therapy. This combination failed to improve patients' survival as well as to decrease the incidence of skeletal adverse events. The CALGB 90202 study analyzed the efficacy of zoledronic acid in delaying the development of skeletal-related events (SREs) in hormone-naïve patients; no differences were observed between patients treated with the combo compared to patients assigned to ADT alone. In fact, time to first SRE was 31.9 months in the ADT/zoledronic acid arm versus 29.8 months in the ADT/placebo arm (HR 0.97; 95 % CI, 0–1.17; $p=0.39$) [90]. Accordingly, the recent data of the British trial STAMPEDE confirmed that the addition of zoledronic acid to ADT, in the presence or in the absence of docetaxel, was neither able to improve patients' survival nor to reduce the incidence of SREs [91]. In view of previous findings, it could be concluded that treatment with bisphosphonates or RANKL inhibitors should not be considered for the management of hormone-naïve patients.

As it has been shown in the previous paragraphs, ADT is not devoid of clinically relevant side effects; for this reason, it has been long debated whether this treatment could be delayed in asymptomatic or low tumor burden patients. The UK Medical Research Council randomized 934 patients with locally advanced or asymptomatic prostate cancer either to immediate ADT or to the same treatment deferred until disease indication. The immediate treatment conferred significant benefits either regarding OS ($p=0.02$) or prostate cancer-specific survival ($p=0.001$) [92]. The incidence and severity of adverse events like metastatic pain, spinal cord compression, and urethral obstruction favored also men in the immediate treatment arm. Meta-analysis data confirmed the superiority of immediate treatment but indicated a significant increase in adverse events. Moreover, available data were considered insufficient to support firm conclusions, especially in patients with metastatic disease. Therefore, while early ADT is strongly recommended in patients with high-risk locally advanced disease treated with radiation therapy [93, 94], the advantages in patients with metastatic disease are probably less defined in respect to OS. Immediate treatment of patients with bone metastases, even in the absence of symptoms, is however supported by the fact that, independently of the effect on expected survival, ADT can benefit these patients through preventing bone pain and complications.

The intermittent administration of ADT was also suggested in order to minimize the consequences of ADT. The rationale for testing intermittent androgen deprivation (IAD) was provided by preclinical data demonstrating that IAD could prolong time to castration resistance by threefold compared to continuous androgen deprivation therapy (CAD) [95]. A number of trials testing CAD versus IAD reached inconclusive and contradictory results, and a recent meta-analysis indicated non-inferiority in respect to OS with IAD versus CAD [96]. However, a subgroup analysis of individual trials suggested that IAD could be inferior to CAD in patients with metastatic disease, and CAD should remain the standard for these patients. Moreover, IAD could imply a higher risk of cardiovascular events, since the risk of developing such events during ADT appears to be higher during the first 6 months, but it declines afterward [30]. Restarting ADT more times could thus hamper, rather than limit, the risk of cardiovascular events in patients receiving IAD compared to patients treated continuously.

10.3.2 CRPC Patients

The treatment options available for this stage of disease have increased significantly within the last few years: some options, namely, chemotherapy or radio-metabolic treatments, have been considered in detail in other chapters (Chaps. 9 and 14). Here we will analyze the results achieved with abiraterone acetate and enzalutamide, the two hormonal therapies that have profoundly changed the management of mCRPC.

Abiraterone acetate has been approved for the treatment of mCRPC after the results of the COU-AA-301 study. This was a phase III randomized trial, in which patients already undergoing chemotherapy with taxanes were randomized to receive abiraterone acetate 1,000 mg/daily ($N=797$) or placebo ($N=398$), in both cases in combination with prednisone, 5 mg orally, twice a day [97]. The great majority of patients in both arms had bone metastases. The median OS, which represented the primary study endpoint, was 14.8 months in the abiraterone plus prednisone group compared to 10.9 months in the placebo plus prednisone group (HR 0.64; 95 % CI, 0.54–0.77; P <0.0001), the survival benefit being evident virtually in all patient subgroups. Time to radiographic progression (5.6 months vs. 3.6 months), PSA response rate (29 % vs. 6 %), and pain control rate (44 % vs. 27 %) also favored abiraterone in a statistically significant way (all p values <0.0001) [97]. This trial demonstrated that abiraterone was highly effective in bone metastases treatment. In fact, the exploratory analysis of data from the COU-AA-301 trial showed that in patients with clinically significant pain at baseline, abiraterone acetate and prednisone resulted in a significantly greater pain palliation rate (157 of 349 [45 %] patients vs. 47 of 163 [28.8 %]; p=0.0005) and a faster time to pain palliation (median time to palliation 5.6 months [95 % CI 3.7–9.2] vs. 13.7 months [5.4-not estimable]; p=0.0018) compared to prednisone and placebo. Palliation of pain interference (134 of 223 [60.1 %] vs. 38 of 100 [38 %], p=0.0002), median time to palliation of pain interference (1.0 months [95 % CI 0.9–1.9] vs. 3.7 months [2.7-not estimable], p=0.0004), and median duration of palliation of pain intensity (4.2 months [95 % CI 3.0–4.9] vs. 2.1 months [1.4–3.7]; p=0·005) were also significantly longer with abiraterone acetate and prednisone than with prednisone and placebo. Finally, median time to occurrence of the first SRE was also significantly longer with abiraterone acetate and prednisone than with prednisone and placebo (25.0 months [95 % CI 25.0-not estimable] vs. 20.3 months [16.9-not estimable]; p=0.0001).

The results achieved by abiraterone acetate plus prednisone on bone metastases provided the rationale for testing the efficacy of the combo abiraterone acetate and radium 223 dichloride (Ra-223), an alpha-emitting radioisotope approved as monotherapy for the treatment of mCRPC with symptomatic bone metastases. This trial is still ongoing and no results are available so far [95].

The more recent COU-AA-302 study evaluated the efficacy of abiraterone acetate in chemo-naïve patients. In this phase III study, patients with asymptomatic or oligosymptomatic metastatic disease, without visceral metastases, were randomly allocated to abiraterone acetate plus prednisone or to a placebo plus prednisone [42]. Again abiraterone plus prednisone showed superiority over prednisone and placebo in respect of opiate use in cancer-related pain, in PSA progression, as well as in radiological progression (radiological PFS: 16.5 months vs. 8.3 months; HR: 0.53; 95 % CI, 0.45–0.62; P < 0.001) and OS (34.7 months vs. 30.3 months; HR 0.81 [95 % CI, 0.70–0.93]; p=0.003), both being the primary study endpoints [98, 99]. Again the benefit induced by abiraterone acetate plus prednisone was evident in all subgroups and, relative to OS, was higher in patients with bone metastases only.

Analogously to abiraterone acetate, enzalutamide was first tested in patients failing front-line treatment with docetaxel. The AFFIRM trial compared enzalutamide, 160 mg/daily, versus a placebo in 1199 patients, virtually all of whom had bone metastases [72]. OS duration was the primary endpoint of this study. The superiority of enzalutamide was shown in respect to either OS, the primary study endpoint (median OS duration: 18.4 months vs. 13.6 months; HR: 0.63; 95 % CI: 0.52–0.75; p < 0.0001), or the secondary study endpoints, including time to radiographic progression (8.3 months vs. 2.9 months; HR: 0.40, p<0.0001), PSA progression (8.3 months vs. 3.0 months; HR: 0.25; p<0.001), PSA response rate (54 % vs. 2 %, p<0.0001), and improvement in quality of life (43 % vs. 18 %, p<0.0001). Noteworthy, also in the case of enzalutamide, treatment did significantly prolong the time to the first skeletal event (16.7 months vs. 13.3 months, HR 0.69, p<0.0001).

Enzalutamide was then evaluated in chemo-naïve patients through a large phase III study (the PREVAIL trial), which enrolled 1.717 patients, most of whom were affected by bone metastases, though they were asymptomatic or mildly symptomatic. As in the previous trial, the patients were randomized to receive either enzalutamide or a placebo [100]. The results of this study showed a significant benefit of enzalutamide relative to all endpoints, including the risk of death and the risk of radiographic progression, representing the two co-primary endpoints of the study. The trial was closed early after the interim analysis, programmed after the first 540 deaths, which showed a 12-month radiographic PFS of 65 % in the patients treated with enzalutamide compared to a PFS of 14 % in patients treated with the placebo (HR: 0.19, $p < 0.001$). This preliminary analysis also showed a significant survival benefit favoring patients in the enzalutamide group (72 % alive at 12 months compared to 63 % in the placebo group; HR: 0.71, $p < 0.001$). The results favored enzalutamide also relative to the secondary study endpoints, namely, the time to first SRE (HR 0.72), time to PSA progression (HR 0.17), and PSA response (78 % vs. 3 %) ($p < 0.001$ for all comparisons). On the basis of these results, the indication for enzalutamide use was extended to chemo-naïve patients.

Abiraterone and enzalutamide are currently used in the management of mCRPC in both patients previously treated with docetaxel and in chemo-naïve patients. At present, there are no robust evidences about sequencing abiraterone, enzalutamide, and docetaxel, which represent the three major options to manage mCRPC. Currently available treatment algorithms are based on the presence and severity of symptoms, patient comorbidities, performance status, and tumor spreading to distant sites other than bones (i.e., soft tissues, viscera) [101]. Recently, Antonarakis et al. evaluated the androgen receptor isoform encoded by splice variant 7 (AR-V7) as a possible factor of resistance to abiraterone and enzalutamide. AR-V7 lacks the ligand-binding domain, which is the target of enzalutamide and abiraterone, and remains constitutively active as a transcription factor [9]. These investigators have prospectively evaluated AR-V7 in circulating tumor cells of patients receiving either enzalutamide or abiraterone. A total of 31 enzalutamide-treated patients and 31 abiraterone-treated patients were enrolled, of whom 39 % and 19 %, respectively, had detectable AR-V7 in circulating tumor cells. Among men receiving enzalutamide, AR-V7-positive patients had lower PSA response rates than AR-V7-negative patients (0 % vs. 53 %, $P=0.004$) and shorter PSA PFS (median: 1.4 months vs. 6.0 months; $P<0.001$), clinical or radiographic PFS (median: 2.1 months vs. 6.1 months; $P<0.001$), and OS (median: 5.5 months vs. not reached; $P=0.002$). Similarly, among men receiving abiraterone, AR-V7-positive patients had lower PSA response rates than AR-V7 negative patients (0 % vs. 68 %, $P=0.004$) and shorter PSA PFS (median: 1.3 months vs. not reached; $P<0.001$), clinical or radiographic PFS (median, 2.3 months vs. not reached; $P<0.001$), and OS (median, 10.6 months vs. not reached, $P=0.006$).

Conclusions

Hormonal therapy still represents a cornerstone in the management of prostate cancer, and ADT represents the first step in the inhibition of AR pathway. The identification of molecular targets and mutations of AR pathway could allow to identify patients less responsive to hormonal therapy as well as candidates to novel approaches based on the combination of multiple hormonal manipulations, hormone therapy plus chemotherapy, or therapies targeting specific gene alterations. ADT is the treatment of choice to manage hormone-naïve patients with bone metastases, independently of tumor burden and presence or absence of symptoms. New-generation hormonal therapies have profoundly changed the management of CRPC patients, who are commonly affected by bone metastases. Trial findings demonstrate that both abiraterone and enzalutamide are highly effective in bone metastases treatment and in preventing the complications related to this specific type of tumor spreading. As already mentioned in the introductory remarks, a multidisciplinary approach is required in everyday clinical practice to correctly approach the health of patients affected by bone metastases. Local and symptomatic treatments are, in fact, often required to achieve "optimal" disease control and to prevent or minimize the consequences of bone involvement and the effects of oncologic treatments on bone health. Bone clinics could represent the best response to patients' needs in this frame, being able to guarantee appropriate multidisciplinary evaluation and monitoring [102].

References

1. Kirby M, Hirst C, Crawford ED (2011) Characterising the castration-resistant prostate cancer population: a systematic review. Int J Clin Pract 65(11):1180–92
2. Karantanos T, Corn PG, Thompson TC (2013) Prostate cancer progression after androgen deprivation therapy: mechanisms of castrate resistance and novel therapeutic approaches. Oncogene 32(49):5501–11
3. Mitsiades N (2013) A road map to comprehensive androgen receptor axis targeting for castration-resistant prostate cancer. Cancer Res 73(15):4599–605
4. Smith MR et al (2005) Natural history of rising serum prostate-specific antigen in men with castrate nonmetastatic prostate cancer. J Clin Oncol 23(13):2918–25
5. Saad F et al (2004) Long-term efficacy of zoledronic acid for the prevention of skeletal complications in patients with metastatic hormone-refractory prostate cancer. J Natl Cancer Inst 96(11):879–82
6. Fizazi K et al (2015) Bone-related parameters are the main prognostic factors for overall survival in Men with bone metastases from castration-resistant prostate cancer. Eur Urol 68(1):42–50
7. Vargas HA et al (2014) Bone metastases in castration-resistant prostate cancer: associations between morphologic CT patterns, glycolytic activity, and androgen receptor expression on PET and overall survival. Radiology 271(1):220–9
8. Hornberg E et al (2011) Expression of androgen receptor splice variants in prostate cancer bone metastases is associated with castration-resistance and short survival. PLoS One 6(4), e19059
9. Antonarakis ES et al (2014) AR-V7 and resistance to enzalutamide and abiraterone in prostate cancer. N Engl J Med 371(11):1028–38
10. Jernberg E et al (2013) Characterization of prostate cancer bone metastases according to expression levels of steroidogenic enzymes and androgen receptor splice variants. PLoS One 8(11), e77407
11. Ren G, Esposito M, Kang Y (2015) Bone metastasis and the metastatic niche. J Mol Med (Berl) 93(11):1203–12
12. Nuzzo PV et al (2014) Periostin: a novel prognostic and therapeutic target for genitourinary cancer? Clin Genitourin Cancer 12(5):301–11
13. Nuzzo PV et al (2012) Prognostic value of stromal and epithelial periostin expression in human prostate cancer: correlation with clinical pathological features and the risk of biochemical relapse or death. BMC Cancer 12:625
14. Baniwal SK et al (2009) Repression of Runx2 by androgen receptor (AR) in osteoblasts and prostate cancer cells: AR binds Runx2 and abrogates its recruitment to DNA. Mol Endocrinol 23(8):1203–14
15. Liu XH et al (2007) Androgen-induced Wnt signaling in preosteoblasts promotes the growth of MDA-PCa-2b human prostate cancer cells. Cancer Res 67(12):5747–53
16. Yang W, Levine AC (2011) Androgens and prostate cancer bone metastases: effects on both the seed and the soil. Endocrinol Metab Clin North Am 40(3):643–53, x
17. Berman DM, Rodriguez R, Veltri RW (2012) Development, molecular biology and physiology of the prostate. In: Wein AJ et al (eds) Campbell-Walsh urology. 10th edn. Elsevier, Philadelphia, pp 2533–2569
18. Seidenfeld J et al (2000) Single-therapy androgen suppression in men with advanced prostate cancer: a systematic review and meta-analysis. Ann Intern Med 132(7):566–77
19. Lepor H, Shore ND (2012) LHRH agonists for the treatment of prostate cancer: 2012. Rev Urol 14(1–2):1–12
20. Lam JS et al (2006) Secondary hormonal therapy for advanced prostate cancer. J Urol 175(1):27–34
21. Lincoln D (1997) Gonadotropin-releasing hormone (GnRH): basic physiology. In: DeGroot LJ et al. (eds) Endrocrinology. W.B. Saunders, Co., Philadelphia, pp 142–151
22. Cook T, Sheridan WP (2000) Development of GnRH antagonists for prostate cancer: new approaches to treatment. Oncologist 5(2):162–8
23. Crawford ED et al (2011) A phase III extension trial with a 1-arm crossover from leuprolide to degarelix: comparison of gonadotropin-releasing hormone agonist and antagonist effect on prostate cancer. J Urol 186(3):889–97
24. Bubley GJ (2001) Is the flare phenomenon clinically significant? Urology 58(2 Suppl 1):5–9
25. Heidenreich A et al (2014) EAU guidelines on prostate cancer. Part II: treatment of advanced, relapsing, and castration-resistant prostate cancer. Eur Urol 65(2):467–79
26. Labrie F et al (1987) Flutamide eliminates the risk of disease flare in prostatic cancer patients treated with a luteinizing hormone-releasing hormone agonist. J Urol 138(4):804–6
27. Trachtenberg J et al (2002) A phase 3, multicenter, open label, randomized study of abarelix versus leuprolide plus daily antiandrogen in men with prostate cancer. J Urol 167(4):1670–4
28. McLeod D et al (2001) A phase 3, multicenter, open-label, randomized study of abarelix versus leuprolide acetate in men with prostate cancer. Urology 58(5):756–61
29. Klotz L et al (2008) The efficacy and safety of degarelix: a 12-month, comparative, randomized, open-label, parallel-group phase III study in patients with prostate cancer. BJU Int 102(11):1531–8
30. O'Farrell S et al (2015) Risk and timing of cardiovascular disease after androgen-deprivation therapy in men with prostate cancer. J Clin Oncol 33(11):1243–51
31. Nguyen PL et al (2011) Association of androgen deprivation therapy with cardiovascular death in patients with prostate cancer: a meta-analysis of randomized trials. Jama 306(21):2359–66

32. Moinpour CM et al (1998) Quality of life in advanced prostate cancer: results of a randomized therapeutic trial. J Natl Cancer Inst 90(20):1537–44
33. Gardiner RA et al (2015) Patients who receive androgen deprivation therapy risk adverse cognitive changes. J Clin Oncol 33(36):4314–5
34. Gonzalez BD et al (2015) Course and predictors of cognitive function in patients with prostate cancer receiving androgen-deprivation therapy: a controlled comparison. J Clin Oncol 33(18):2021–7
35. Klotz L et al (2014) Disease control outcomes from analysis of pooled individual patient data from five comparative randomised clinical trials of degarelix versus luteinising hormone-releasing hormone agonists. Eur Urol 66(6):1101–8
36. Chen HF et al (1999) Human peripheral blood mononuclear cells express gonadotropin-releasing hormone (GnRH), GnRH receptor, and interleukin-2 receptor gamma-chain messenger ribonucleic acids that are regulated by GnRH in vitro. J Clin Endocrinol Metab 84(2):743–50
37. Tanriverdi F et al (2005) GnRH-I and GnRH-II have differential modulatory effects on human peripheral blood mononuclear cell proliferation and interleukin-2 receptor gamma-chain mRNA expression in healthy males. Clin Exp Immunol 142(1):103–10
38. Shore N et al (2015) TAK-385, an oral GnRH antagonist: efficacy and safety results from a randomized phase 2 trial in prostate cancer patients (pts). Eur J Cancer 51 Supp. 3:S474
39. Small EJ et al (2004) Antiandrogen withdrawal alone or in combination with ketoconazole in androgen-independent prostate cancer patients: a phase III trial (CALGB 9583). J Clin Oncol 22(6): 1025–33
40. Attard G, Belldegrun AS, de Bono JS (2005) Selective blockade of androgenic steroid synthesis by novel lyase inhibitors as a therapeutic strategy for treating metastatic prostate cancer. BJU Int 96(9):1241–6
41. Rehman Y, Rosenberg JE (2012) Abiraterone acetate: oral androgen biosynthesis inhibitor for treatment of castration-resistant prostate cancer. Drug Des Devel Ther 6:13–8
42. Ryan CJ et al (2013) Abiraterone in metastatic prostate cancer without previous chemotherapy. N Engl J Med 368(2):138–48
43. Attard G et al (2012) Clinical and biochemical consequences of CYP17A1 inhibition with abiraterone given with and without exogenous glucocorticoids in castrate men with advanced prostate cancer. J Clin Endocrinol Metab 97(2):507–16
44. Attard G et al (2009) Selective inhibition of CYP17 with abiraterone acetate is highly active in the treatment of castration-resistant prostate cancer. J Clin Oncol 27(23):3742–8
45. O'Donnell A et al (2004) Hormonal impact of the 17alpha-hydroxylase/C(17,20)-lyase inhibitor abiraterone acetate (CB7630) in patients with prostate cancer. Br J Cancer 90(12):2317–25
46. Li Z et al (2015) Conversion of abiraterone to D4A drives anti-tumour activity in prostate cancer. Nature 523(7560):347–51
47. Lorente D et al (2014) Tumour responses following a steroid switch from prednisone to dexamethasone in castration-resistant prostate cancer patients progressing on abiraterone. Br J Cancer 111(12): 2248–53
48. Romero-Laorden N et al (2016) Prospective evaluation of the response to prednisone-dexamethasone switch in castration-resistant prostate cancer patients treated with abiraterone pre- and post-docetaxel. J Clin Oncol 34(Suppl 2S; abstr 327)
49. Petrylak DP et al (2015) Phase 1/2 study of orteronel (TAK-700), an investigational 17,20-lyase inhibitor, with docetaxel-prednisone in metastatic castration-resistant prostate cancer. Invest New Drugs 33(2): 397–408
50. Saad F et al (2015) Orteronel plus prednisone in patients with chemotherapy-naive metastatic castration-resistant prostate cancer (ELM-PC 4): a double-blind, multicentre, phase 3, randomised, placebo-controlled trial. Lancet Oncol 16(3): 338–48
51. Fizazi K et al (2015) Phase III, randomized, double-blind, multicenter trial comparing orteronel (TAK-700) plus prednisone with placebo plus prednisone in patients with metastatic castration-resistant prostate cancer that has progressed during or after docetaxel-based therapy: ELM-PC 5. J Clin Oncol 33(7):723–31
52. Gillatt D (2006) Antiandrogen treatments in locally advanced prostate cancer: are they all the same? J Cancer Res Clin Oncol 132(Suppl 1):S17–26
53. Helsen C et al (2012) Structural basis for nuclear hormone receptor DNA binding. Mol Cell Endocrinol 348(2):411–7
54. Gioeli DG (2010) The promise of novel androgen receptor antagonists. Cell Cycle 9(3):440–1
55. Isurugi K et al (1980) Endocrine effects of cyproterone acetate in patients with prostatic cancer. J Urol 123(2):180–3
56. Anderson J (2003) The role of antiandrogen monotherapy in the treatment of prostate cancer. BJU Int 91(5):455–61
57. Migliari R et al (1999) Antiandrogens: a summary review of pharmacodynamic properties and tolerability in prostate cancer therapy. Arch Ital Urol Androl 71(5):293–302
58. Ricci F et al (2014) Safety of antiandrogen therapy for treating prostate cancer. Expert Opin Drug Saf 13(11):1483–99
59. Iversen P et al (2000) Bicalutamide monotherapy compared with castration in patients with nonmetastatic locally advanced prostate cancer: 6.3 years of followup. J Urol 164(5):1579–82
60. Boccardo F et al (1999) Bicalutamide monotherapy versus flutamide plus goserelin in prostate cancer patients: results of an Italian Prostate Cancer Project study. J Clin Oncol 17(7):2027–38

61. Sieber PR et al (2004) Bicalutamide 150 mg maintains bone mineral density during monotherapy for localized or locally advanced prostate cancer. J Urol 171(6 Pt 1):2272–6, quiz 2435
62. McLeod D, Fourcade RO (2004) Tolerability of Nonsteroidal Antiandrogens in the treatment of Advanced Prostate Cancer. McLeod DG Oncologist 1997;2(1):18–27
63. Boccardo F et al (2005) Evaluation of tamoxifen and anastrozole in the prevention of gynecomastia and breast pain induced by bicalutamide monotherapy of prostate cancer. J Clin Oncol 23(4):808–15
64. Famularo G et al (2003) Flutamide-associated acute liver failure. Ann Ital Med Int 18(4):250–3
65. Dole EJ, Holdsworth MT (1997) Nilutamide: an antiandrogen for the treatment of prostate cancer. Ann Pharmacother 31(1):65–75
66. Maximum androgen blockade in advanced prostate cancer: an overview of the randomised trials. Prostate Cancer Trialists' Collaborative Group (2000) Lancet 355(9214):1491–1498
67. Kelly WK, Scher HI (1993) Prostate specific antigen decline after antiandrogen withdrawal: the flutamide withdrawal syndrome. J Urol 149(3):607–9
68. Bambury RM, Scher HI (2015) Enzalutamide: development from bench to bedside. Urol Oncol 33(6):280–8
69. Tran C et al (2009) Development of a second-generation antiandrogen for treatment of advanced prostate cancer. Science 324(5928):787–90
70. Shore ND et al (2016) Efficacy and safety of enzalutamide versus bicalutamide for patients with metastatic prostate cancer (TERRAIN): a randomised, double-blind, phase 2 study. Lancet Oncol 17(2): 153–63
71. Penson DF et al (2016) Enzalutamide versus Bicalutamide in Castration-Resistant Prostate Cancer: The STRIVE Trial. J Clin Oncol August 20, 2016, 34(24).
72. Scher HI et al (2012) Increased survival with enzalutamide in prostate cancer after chemotherapy. N Engl J Med 367(13):1187–97
73. Clegg NJ et al (2012) ARN-509: a novel antiandrogen for prostate cancer treatment. Cancer Res 72(6):1494–503
74. Raymond Smith M et al (2013) ARN-509 in men with high-risk nonmetastatic castration-resistant prostate cancer (CRPC). J Clin Oncol 31(Suppl 6; abstr 7)
75. Saad F et al (2015) The 2015 CUA-CUOG Guidelines for the management of castration-resistant prostate cancer (CRPC). Can Urol Assoc J 9(3–4):90–6
76. Montgomery RB et al (2008) Maintenance of intratumoral androgens in metastatic prostate cancer: a mechanism for castration-resistant tumor growth. Cancer Res 68(11):4447–54
77. Mostaghel EA et al (2007) Intraprostatic androgens and androgen-regulated gene expression persist after testosterone suppression: therapeutic implications for castration-resistant prostate cancer. Cancer Res 67(10):5033–41
78. Tyrrell CJ et al (1993) Multicenter randomized trial comparing Zoladex with Zoladex plus flutamide in the treatment of advanced prostate cancer. Survival update. International Prostate Cancer Study Group. Cancer 72(12 Suppl):3878–9
79. Denis LJ et al (1998) Maximal androgen blockade: final analysis of EORTC phase III trial 30853. EORTC Genito-Urinary Tract Cancer Cooperative Group and the EORTC Data Center. Eur Urol 33(2):144–51
80. Eisenberger MA et al (1998) Bilateral orchiectomy with or without flutamide for metastatic prostate cancer. N Engl J Med 339(15):1036–42
81. Boccardo F et al (1993) Goserelin acetate with or without flutamide in the treatment of patients with locally advanced or metastatic prostate cancer. The Italian Prostatic Cancer Project (PONCAP) Study Group. Eur J Cancer 29a(8):1088–93
82. Janknegt RA et al (1993) Orchiectomy and nilutamide or placebo as treatment of metastatic prostatic cancer in a multinational double-blind randomized trial. J Urol 149(1):77–82; discussion 83
83. Crawford ED et al (1989) A controlled trial of leuprolide with and without flutamide in prostatic carcinoma. N Engl J Med 321(7):419–24
84. Schmitt B et al (2000) Maximal androgen blockade for advanced prostate cancer. Cochrane Database Syst Rev (2):CD001526
85. Schmitt B et al (2001) Combined androgen blockade with nonsteroidal antiandrogens for advanced prostate cancer: a systematic review. Urology 57(4):727–32
86. Moul JW (2009) Twenty years of controversy surrounding combined androgen blockade for advanced prostate cancer. Cancer 115(15):3376–8
87. Samson DJ et al (2002) Systematic review and meta-analysis of monotherapy compared with combined androgen blockade for patients with advanced prostate carcinoma. Cancer 95(2):361–76
88. Efstathiou E et al (2014) Enzalutamide (ENZA) in combination with abiraterone acetate (AA) in bone metastatic castration resistant prostate cancer (mCRPC). J Clin Oncol 32:5s(Suppl; abstr 5000)
89. NCT01949337 Clinical Trial.gov. Enzalutamide with or without abiraterone and prednisone in treating patients with castration-resistant metastatic prostate cancer
90. Smith MR et al (2014) Randomized controlled trial of early zoledronic acid in men with castration-sensitive prostate cancer and bone metastases: results of CALGB 90202 (alliance). J Clin Oncol 32(11):1143–50
91. James ND et al (2016) Addition of docetaxel, zoledronic acid, or both to first-line long-term hormone therapy in prostate cancer (STAMPEDE): survival results from an adaptive, multiarm, multistage, platform randomised controlled trial. 387(10024):1163–77.

92. Immediate versus deferred treatment for advanced prostatic cancer: initial results of the Medical Research Council Trial. The Medical Research Council Prostate Cancer Working Party Investigators Group (1997) Br J Urol 79(2):235–246
93. Bolla M et al (2002) Long-term results with immediate androgen suppression and external irradiation in patients with locally advanced prostate cancer (an EORTC study): a phase III randomised trial. Lancet 360(9327):103–6
94. Bolla M et al (2009) Duration of androgen suppression in the treatment of prostate cancer. N Engl J Med 360(24):2516–27
95. Akakura K et al (1993) Effects of intermittent androgen suppression on androgen-dependent tumors. Apoptosis and serum prostate-specific antigen. Cancer 71(9):2782–90
96. Magnan S et al (2015) Intermittent vs continuous androgen deprivation therapy for prostate cancer: a systematic review and meta-analysis. JAMA Oncol 1(9):1261–9
97. de Bono JS et al (2011) Abiraterone and increased survival in metastatic prostate cancer. N Engl J Med 364(21):1995–2005
98. Morris MJ et al (2015) Radiographic progression-free survival as a response biomarker in metastatic castration-resistant prostate cancer: COU-AA-302 results. J Clin Oncol 33(12):1356–63
99. Ryan CJ et al (2015) Abiraterone acetate plus prednisone versus placebo plus prednisone in chemotherapy-naive men with metastatic castration-resistant prostate cancer (COU-AA-302): final overall survival analysis of a randomised, double-blind, placebo-controlled phase 3 study. Lancet Oncol 16(2):152–60
100. Beer TM et al (2014) Enzalutamide in metastatic prostate cancer before chemotherapy. N Engl J Med 371(5):424–33
101. Maines F et al (2015) Sequencing new agents after docetaxel in patients with metastatic castration-resistant prostate cancer. Crit Rev Oncol Hematol 96(3):498–506
102. Goh P et al (2007) New multidisciplinary prostate bone metastases clinic: first of its kind in Canada. Curr Oncol 14(1):9–12
103. Hoffman-Censits J, Kelly WK (2013) Enzalutamide: a novel antiandrogen for patients with castrate-resistant prostate cancer. Clin Cancer Res 19(6):1335–9
104. Watson PA, Arora VK, Sawyers CL (2015) Emerging mechanisms of resistance to androgen receptor inhibitors in prostate cancer. Nat Rev Cancer 15(12):701–11

Chemotherapy

11

Giovanni Luca Ceresoli, Maria Bonomi, and Maria Grazia Sauta

11.1 Introduction

Nearly all patients with metastatic prostate cancer (PC) become resistant to the initial approach with androgen deprivation therapy (ADT), developing the state known as metastatic castration-resistant prostate cancer (mCRPC) [1]. Up to 30 % of patients can respond to additional hormonal manipulations but responses are usually short lasting [2]. In this setting, chemotherapy has represented for a long time the only available treatment, although its role in providing palliation was in the past controversial [3]. In an early trial published in 1996, treatment with mitoxantrone and prednisone provided palliation in a significantly higher percentage of patients with symptomatic mCRPC, as compared with prednisone alone [4]. Most responding patients had an improvement in quality-of-life (QoL) scales and a decrease in serum prostate-specific antigen (PSA) level; however, no difference in overall survival (OS) between the two treatment arms was found. In 2004, two landmark phase III trials reported a survival advantage and an improvement in QoL over mitoxantrone with the use of docetaxel chemotherapy in men with mCRPC [5, 6]. For nearly a decade, chemotherapy with docetaxel has been the only established standard of care for men with mCRPC. In recent years, treatment of mCRPC has changed dramatically due to the improvement in the understanding of CRPC biology, which has revealed that during the progression to the castrate status, PC cells remain dependent on androgens and on the androgen receptor (AR) signaling pathway [7]. Multiple novel agents that have demonstrated to improve OS, symptom control, and QoL in mCRPC have been approved, including sipuleucel-T, cabazitaxel, abiraterone acetate, enzalutamide, and radium-223 [8–12]. Since docetaxel became the first approved therapy in mCRPC, two registration-driven therapeutic spaces have evolved in this scenario, defined as pre-docetaxel (or chemotherapy-naïve) and post-docetaxel settings [13]. However, this division does not take into account the disease biology. As for many other cancers, it has become clear that PC is a highly heterogeneous disease, characterized by the presence of AR-dependent and AR-independent cellular clones in the same patient [14].

Although several treatments are available for mCRPC, the development of resistance and some degree of cross-resistance between abiraterone

G.L. Ceresoli (✉) • M. Bonomi • M.G. Sauta
Department of Medical Oncology, Cliniche Humanitas Gavazzeni, Bergamo, Italy
e-mail: giovanni_luca.ceresoli@gavazzeni.it

F. Bertoldo et al. (eds.), *Bone Metastases from Prostate Cancer*,
DOI 10.1007/978-3-319-42327-2_11

and enzalutamide limits the efficacy of these drugs; there is therefore still a high medical need for new treatment options. CRPC molecular profiling studies have shown that up to 30% of patients harbor DNA repair defects [15]. Some of these alterations have been associated with the antitumor activity of the poly-ADP-ribose polymerase (PARP) inhibitor olaparib in patients with mCRPC [16]. Interestingly, the same biomarkers have been correlated with sensitivity to platinum agents in preclinical studies, renewing the interest in the use of these compounds in molecularly selected patients [17].

Therefore, chemotherapy with docetaxel, cabazitaxel, and possibly platinum agents in selected patients remains an important therapeutic option for patients with mCRPC [18, 19]. In particular, the therapeutic effect of chemotherapy (mainly with docetaxel and cabazitaxel) on bone metastases, which are very frequent in this setting, is well known. It has been reported in terms of pain control or incidence of skeletal-related events (SREs), usually defined as a composite end point, including pathological bone fractures, spinal cord compression, and the need for radiation therapy on symptomatic areas [20].

11.2 Early Experience with Chemotherapy in Metastatic CRPC

Palliative chemotherapy has represented for a long time the only available treatment in mCRPC, although its role in this patient setting was in the past controversial, due to the lack of OS gain with any agent. Methodological limitations, mainly in study design and response assessment, hampered the comparison of different trials [3, 21]. Most agents were tested in the phase II setting. Moreover, PC metastasizes primarily to the bone, and changes in bony disease were often not measurable radiographically. PSA was not evaluated in these early studies. Cyclophosphamide, 5-fluorouracil, streptozotocin, and estramustine phosphate, either alone or in combination, were the most widely used agents [22]. In particular, oral cyclophosphamide was extensively studied in several single-agent and combination studies, with some evidence of both PSA and objective response [23]. Estramustine phosphate is a nitrogen mustard–estradiol conjugate that has both hormonal and nonhormonal effects [24]. Upon uptake into cells, the two parts of the compound split. Its metabolic products include estrone and estradiol, which exert antigonadotropic properties leading to decrease in serum testosterone. The cytotoxic metabolite causes microtubule depolymerization through a direct tubulin interaction. Single-agent estramustine demonstrated only modest activity. Based on a strong in vitro synergy with several other chemotherapeutic agents, a number of combination trials were conducted [25]. The most successful was the phase III Southwest Oncology Group (SWOG) 9916 study that demonstrated a survival advantage with the combination of estramustine and docetaxel compared to mitoxantrone [6].

11.2.1 Mitoxantrone

Mitoxantrone is a synthetic anthracenedione originally developed to improve the therapeutic profile of the anthracyclines. Early single-arm studies suggested some palliative benefit with its association with steroids for patients with metastatic PC progressing on androgen deprivation therapy [26, 27]. Mitoxantrone was subsequently investigated in patients with symptomatic mCRPC using end points of palliation in a Canadian randomized phase III trial [4]. Overall, 161 men with mCRPC and bone pain were randomized to receive mitoxantrone plus prednisone versus prednisone alone. Nonresponding patients on prednisone could cross to mitoxantrone/prednisone. The primary end point was a palliative response, defined as a 2-point decrease in pain assessed using a 6-point pain scale (or complete loss of pain if initially 1+). Palliative response was observed in 23 of 80 patients (29%) who received mitoxantrone plus prednisone and in 10 of 81 patients (12%) who received prednisone alone ($p = .01$).

However, no significant difference in PSA response rates and in OS was observed between the two treatment groups. QoL analysis showed a significant improvement in the mitoxantrone-treated patient group ($p=.009$) [28]. The Canadian mitoxantrone trial was not powered to detect a difference in OS between patients receiving mitoxantrone versus those that did not. A larger trial was therefore conducted by the Cancer and Leukemia Group B (CALGB) [29]. Two hundred forty-two patients with mCRPC were randomized to receive either mitoxantrone and hydrocortisone or hydrocortisone alone. Patients were monitored for OS, time to disease progression (TTP), time to treatment failure (TTF), response, and QoL parameters. Although PSA responses were more common with mitoxantrone (38% vs 22%, $p=0.008$), and there was a significant delay in TTF and TTP in favor of mitoxantrone arm, there was no difference in OS (12.3 versus 12.6 months for mitoxantrone and hydrocortisone alone arms, respectively). QoL was not improved globally, with an improvement just for a few pain items in mitoxantrone arm.

Due to the effectiveness of taxanes, after the approval of docetaxel and cabazitaxel, mitoxantrone has been no longer used very commonly. In the post-docetaxel setting, it was inferior to cabazitaxel in the TROPIC trial [9]. Also in this setting, mitoxantrone offered no demonstrated survival benefit. In a retrospective analysis comparing control arm data from two large randomized clinical studies (the TROPIC [9] and the SUN 1120 [30] trials), no significant OS benefit was observed for mitoxantrone plus prednisone versus prednisone alone among patients with mCRPC pretreated with docetaxel therapy [31]. Of note, pain response rate of mitoxantrone in a more heavily pretreated population such as that enrolled in TROPIC trial was 7.7% only [9], far less than the 29% of palliation reported in the original first-line trial [4]. However, mitoxantrone remains a possible option in docetaxel-pretreated patients with symptomatic skeletal metastases who may not tolerate cabazitaxel due to poor bone marrow function or poor performance status [22].

11.3 Taxanes

11.3.1 General Mechanism of Action

Microtubules are dynamic proteins composed of polymerized tubulin, which is a heterodimer of alpha- and beta-tubulin subunits. They are involved in different cellular functions including mitosis, cellular architecture and transport, cell signaling, and gene expression [32]. The main mechanism of action of taxanes is a dysfunction of the mitotic spindle, which causes a mitotic block and eventually activates the apoptotic cascade [33]. Interestingly, microtubules are implicated in AR signaling, particularly in AR nuclear localization and AR-mediated transcription [34, 35]. In a small study evaluating the effect of taxanes on AR localization in circulating tumor cells of PC patients, 12/17 patients (70.6%) with response or stable disease had cytoplasmic AR localization, while 13/18 (72%) of progressors had nuclear AR localization [36]. This complex mechanism of action could at least partially explain why taxanes, which function as microtubule inhibitors, are the most effective chemotherapeutic agents in PC.

11.3.2 Docetaxel

Docetaxel is a semisynthetic taxane that in several early phase II trials had proved active with either a weekly or every-3-week schedule at a dose of 30 and 75 mg/m^2, respectively [37–39]. Based on these encouraging data, docetaxel was moved to phase III testing and was approved in the mCRPC setting on the basis of two landmark phase III trials: the TAX 327 study and the SWOG 9916 study [5, 6].

In the TAX 327 trial, 1006 men with mCRPC received 10 mg of prednisone daily and were randomly assigned to receive 12 mg/m^2 of mitoxantrone every 3 weeks, 75 mg/m^2 of docetaxel every 3 weeks, or 30 mg/m^2 of docetaxel weekly for five of every 6 weeks. The primary end point was OS. Secondary end points were pain, PSA levels, and QoL. The median OS for patients treated with docetaxel every 3 weeks was 18.9 months, compared to 16.5 months for patients in the control mitoxantrone arm (HR 0.76, 95% CI 0.62–0.94, $p=0.009$). Patients given weekly docetaxel had a median OS of 17.4 months (HR 0.91, 95% CI 0.75–1.11; $p=0.36$). PSA decrease of at least 50% occurred in 32%, 45%, and 48% of men in the mitoxantrone, every-3-week docetaxel, and weekly docetaxel, respectively ($p<0.001$ for both comparisons with mitoxantrone). Among these three groups, 22%, 35%($p=0.01$), and 31% ($p=0.08$) of patients had predefined reductions in pain, and 13%, 22% ($p=0.009$), and 23% ($p=0.005$) had improvements in the QoL. Adverse events were more common in the groups that received docetaxel. However, most adverse events associated with docetaxel were of low grades. An updated survival analysis confirmed the OS benefit with docetaxel given every 3 weeks [40]. More patients survived 3 years when treated with docetaxel either every 3 weeks or weekly (18.6% and 16.6%, respectively, as compared to 13.5% with mitoxantrone); however, the survival benefit with weekly docetaxel was not statistically significant; moreover, men treated with weekly docetaxel were more likely to experience early deterioration of QoL. Therefore, there is general consensus that weekly docetaxel schedule should not be adopted, with the possible exception of patients with poor performance status who are at high risk of hematological toxicity (mainly febrile neutropenia). The TAX 327 trial included patients with and without symptoms. The OS benefit was consistent through all the patient subgroups. In general, the chances of prolonging survival with docetaxel seemed similar among patients with higher and lower disease burden, as indicated by level of serum PSA, the presence or absence of pain, and the QoL or performance score [40]. Visceral disease, pain, poorer performance status, and higher values of baseline PSA were negative prognostic factors across all the study arms.

The SWOG 9916 was a phase III randomized study, in which 770 patients with mCRPC were randomized to receive 280 mg of estramustine three times daily on days 1 through 5, 60 mg/m^2 of docetaxel on day 2, and 60 mg of dexamethasone in three divided doses before docetaxel or 12 mg/m^2 of mitoxantrone on day 1 plus 5 mg of prednisone twice daily [6]. Both treatments were given in 21-day cycles. The primary end point was OS; secondary end points were PFS, objective response rate, and PSA response. In an intention-to-treat analysis, the median OS was longer in the group given docetaxel and estramustine (17.5 months vs 15.6 months, HR 0.80, 95% CI 0.67–0.97, $p=0.02$). PFS (6.3 versus 3.2 months, $p<0.001$) and PSA response rate were significantly superior in the docetaxel arm, while no significant difference was observed in objective response rate between the two arms. Pain relief was similar in both groups. Grade 3–4 febrile neutropenia, nausea and vomiting, and cardiovascular events were more common in the docetaxel arm. HR and median OS in the docetaxel arm were similar to those reported in the TAX 327 study; however, the SWOG 9916 trial failed to meet its primary aim of detecting a 33% improvement in median OS with estramustine and docetaxel. Of note, the median OS of 15.6 months among men treated with mitoxantrone and prednisone was longer than that reported in the original Canadian trial [4], probably due to different eligibility criteria, in particular as regards the inclusion of symptomatic patients only in that study.

It is difficult to compare these two landmark trials. However, the addition of estramustine seems to add no benefit, while increasing toxicity. A randomized phase II trial conducted on 150 patients evaluating docetaxel/prednisone either with or without estramustine found no statistically significant difference in PSA response rates between the two arms, while grade 3–4 toxicities were increased with the addition of estramustine to docetaxel (45% versus 21%, $p=0.005$). Of special concern is the reported association of estramustine with venous thromboembolic events [41].

11.3.3 Docetaxel-Based Combinations

A number of novel agents have been investigated in combination with docetaxel/prednisone, in the attempt to improve response rates and survival outcomes. However, no combination proved superior to the reference regimen. Despite a preclinical rationale, the combinations of docetaxel with anti-angiogenic agents, including bevacizumab [42] and aflibercept [43], have been consistently disappointing. Similarly, no efficacy improvement was found with the addition of bone-targeting agents such as atrasentan [44], dasatinib [45], and ZD4054 [46]. Another phase III trial evaluated docetaxel with or without custirsen (previously called OGX-011), an antisense oligonucleotide inhibitor of the production of clusterin. Clusterin is a chaperone protein associated with treatment resistance and upregulated by apoptotic stressors such as chemotherapy. The SYNERGY trial evaluated docetaxel ± custirsen as first-line therapy in men with mCRPC ($N=1022$). Median OS was 23.4 months vs. 22.2 m for custirsen and control arms, respectively (HR 0.93; $p=0.42$). When the study population was retrospectively split in two prognostic categories according to a trial-specific nomogram, patient with poor prognosis appeared to benefit from the addition of custirsen [47].

Reasons for the failure of these combination regimens are probably the marginal activity of the added compound on mCRPC and also the dose reduction of docetaxel due to the overlapping toxicities.

11.3.4 Docetaxel Rechallenge

Several treatment options are currently available for men with mCRPC, including second-line chemotherapy with cabazitaxel, hormonal therapy with abiraterone and enzalutamide, and radiopharmaceuticals such as radium-223. A great benefit is expected by their combined and sequential use [48]. However, until a few years ago, chemotherapy with docetaxel was the only established standard of care in this setting. Selected patients with a prior response to docetaxel could therefore be candidate for re-treatment with the same drug, although the risk of cumulative toxicity could potentially outweigh the treatment benefit. This strategy has been never assessed in a randomized trial [49]. However, some retrospective studies and a few small prospective series have explored this therapeutic modality. Di Lorenzo et al. [50] reported a PSA response in 25 % of patients, with a medium PFS of 5 months and a median OS of 13 months. Peripheral neurotoxicity was the most relevant adverse event. Oudard et al. evaluated in a retrospective study 270 mCRPC patients with prior response to docetaxel; 223 of them were rechallenged with docetaxel. The treatment was associated with PSA response and symptom relief; however, no improvement in OS was reported in comparison to 47 patients not receiving docetaxel rechallenge [51]. Finally, Caffo et al. assessed in 46 patients factors predicting the efficacy of docetaxel rechallenge [52]. Response to previous treatment with docetaxel and time from previous chemotherapy were predictive of response to rechallenge in multivariate analysis. Sensory neuropathy and nail toxicity were the main cumulative adverse events.

In the modern multidrug scenario, data about the use of docetaxel rechallenge in patients pretreated with novel hormonotherapy and/or cabazitaxel are so far lacking. However, due to the increasing use of early docetaxel in castration-sensitive PC, the number of patients re-treated with docetaxel is probably going to increase steadily. Emerging data on the presence of splice variants of AR (namely, AR-V7) in circulating tumor cells as a potential predictive factor of resistance to abiraterone and enzalutamide [53], and of response to chemotherapy [54, 55], will hopefully contribute to identify the optimal candidates to this therapeutic option.

11.3.5 Cabazitaxel

Cabazitaxel is a novel taxane that showed activity against docetaxel-resistant PC in cell lines in vitro and in vivo animal models [33, 56]. Like other taxanes, cabazitaxel exerts its antitumor cytotoxic activity through the mitotic arrest at the metaphase to anaphase transition, leading to cell death by apoptosis. Cabazitaxel demonstrated a lower binding affinity as compared to docetaxel for multidrug resistance (MDR) proteins, considered a major mechanism of resistance [57]. Another attractive property of cabazitaxel is its enhanced solubility in water-based solutions compared with other taxanes, enabling better blood–brain barrier penetration and higher central nervous system concentrations with systemic administration in mouse models [58]. Two phase I studies evaluated the safety and pharmacokinetic properties of cabazitaxel across various solid tumor types [59, 60]. In the first study [59], cabazitaxel was generally well tolerated up to 25 mg/m^2, grade 4 neutropenia was commonly observed at this dose, and the investigators concluded that a dose of 20 mg/m^2 every 3 weeks was appropriate for further clinical testing. Of three patients who achieved partial responses to treatment, two had mCRPC, including one who had previously been treated with docetaxel. Another phase I study concluded that the hematologic dose-limiting toxicity was seen at 30 mg/m^2 [60]. Two separate phase II studies were conducted in women with metastatic breast cancer, showing efficacy and safety of cabazitaxel despite prior progression on taxane therapy [61, 62]. Based on these results, and without first conducting phase II studies in PC, cabazitaxel was evaluated in a phase III study (the TROPIC trial) in men with docetaxel-resistant mCRPC [9]. To ensure docetaxel resistance, a cumulative dose of docetaxel greater than 225 mg/m^2 was required. The TROPIC trial evaluated cabazitaxel in association with prednisone compared with mitoxantrone and prednisone in 775 mCRPC patients with disease progression during (29 %) or after (71 %) docetaxel-based chemotherapy. The primary end point was OS. Secondary end points included PFS, safety, and pain control. At the cutoff for the final analysis, median OS was 15.1 months in the cabazitaxel group and 12.7 months in the mitoxantrone group, with an HR of 0.70 (95 % CI 0.59–0.83, $p<0.0001$). Median PFS was 2.8 months in the cabazitaxel group and 1.4 months in the mitoxantrone group (HR 0.74, 0.64–0.86, $p<0.0001$). PSA and tumor response rates, as well as pain control, were also significantly higher in the cabazitaxel group. An updated analysis of the TROPIC trial with longer follow-up confirmed a sustained OS benefit for treatment with cabazitaxel, which was predictive of survival over 2 years [63]. The most common grade 3 or higher adverse event with cabazitaxel was neutropenia, observed in 82 % of cabazitaxel patients versus 58 % of mitoxantrone; febrile neutropenia was registered in 8 % of patients in the cabazitaxel group and in 1 % in the mitoxantrone group. Grade 3–4 anemia (11 %) and thrombocytopenia (4 %) were far less common. Frequent nonhematologic toxicities were gastrointestinal disturbances such as diarrhea, nausea/vomiting, and constipation. Importantly in a population of patients pretreated with docetaxel, a severe peripheral neuropathy was observed in less than 1 % of cases. Fatal adverse reactions with cabazitaxel were reported in five patients due to infections and in four due to renal failure [9, 63].

The high degree of neutropenia reported in the TROPIC trial has raised some concern about the use of the drug, particularly in unfit and elderly patients. Several retrospective reports of patient series treated in a "real-world" setting have therefore analyzed the issue of cabazitaxel toxicity [64–68]. The results of these studies suggest that cabazitaxel has a manageable safety profile in everyday clinical practice. In the largest series, including 746 men with mCRPC, multivariate analysis showed that age ≥75 years, treatment cycle 1, and neutrophil count <4000/mm^3 before cabazitaxel administration were associated with increased risk of developing grade ≥3 neutropenia and/or neutropenic complications. Prophylactic use of G-CSF significantly reduced this risk by 30 % [64]. Another study investigated in 112 patients with mCRPC, from 12 UK institutions, the impact of cabazitaxel on QoL [68]. This study provided the evidence, even though by a non-randomized analysis, that cabazitaxel improved QoL, particularly with regard to pain scores.

A prognostic model of OS in the post-docetaxel, second-line chemotherapy, mCRPC setting was developed and validated [69]. This model incorporates novel prognostic factors and can be used to provide predicted probabilities for individual patients. The nine prognostic variables in the final model were Eastern Cooperative Oncology Group performance status, time since last docetaxel use, measurable disease, presence of visceral disease, pain, duration of hormonal use, hemoglobin, PSA, and alkaline phosphatase. Based on these variables, a prognostic nomogram for patients treated with cabazitaxel was proposed.

Even after the regulatory approval of cabazitaxel in the treatment of docetaxel-refractory mCRPC, many issues remain open with regard to its optimal use. In order to optimize the toxicity profile, the 25 mg/m^2 dose used in the TROPIC trial has been compared in a randomized trial with a 20 mg/m^2 dose [70]. Overall, 1200 patients were randomized. The median OS did not differ significantly between the two arms, and the HR boundaries were within the non-inferiority margins assumptions, therefore meeting the study's non-inferiority end point. Cabazitaxel at the dose of 20 mg/m^2 showed an improved overall safety profile. In addition, alternative (weekly) schedules of administration are being evaluated. Due to its pharmacological properties, cabazitaxel was supposed to be more potent than docetaxel. Therefore, a superiority phase III study has randomized patients with mCRPC to receive either docetaxel 75 mg/m^2 (D75), cabazitaxel 25 mg/m^2 (C25), or cabazitaxel 20 mg/m^2 (C20) as first-line cytotoxic therapy (FIRSTANA trial) [71]. The primary end point was OS. Key secondary end points were safety, PFS, tumor response (RECIST 1.1), PSA response, PSA PFS, pain response, pain PFS, time to SREs, and health-related QoL. Overall, 1168 patients were randomized. The median number of treatment cycles was nine for all dose groups. In the ITT analysis, median OS was 24.5 months for C20, 25.2 months for C25, and 24.3 months for D75. HR for C20 vs. D75 was 1.009 (95% CI 0.85–1.197, $p=0.9967$) and for C25 vs. D75 was 0.97 (95% CI 0.819–1.16, $p=0.7574$), indicating that C20 and C25 were not superior to D75 in terms of OS. PFS did not differ between the three arms. Among secondary end points, only tumor responses were significantly superior for C25. The remaining secondary end points did not significantly differ across treatment groups. Febrile neutropenia, diarrhea, and hematuria were more frequent in C25; peripheral neuropathy, peripheral edema, alopecia, and nail disorders were more frequent in D75. Adverse events were less frequent in C20 for most categories. In conclusion, the final results of the study showed that docetaxel remains the standard first-line chemotherapy in patients with mCRPC [71].

11.4 Platinum Agents

Platinum compounds have been studied in several clinical trials in patients with advanced PC, both as single agents and in combination regimens [17]. Most of these studies were small phase II single-arm trials, with heterogeneous patient populations and response criteria. Platinum-based chemotherapy was evaluated mainly in mCRPC, with only a few small trials reported in the castration-sensitive setting. Overall, antitumor activity was in the range of 10–40 % for radiological response and 20–70 % for PSA decline. Response rates were generally higher with combination therapies, such as carboplatin/taxanes [72, 73] or oxaliplatin/gemcitabine [74], at the expense of higher toxicity, mainly hematological. However, no regimen showed a significant OS benefit, and no treatment has received regulatory approval. Only satraplatin, a novel oral platinum compound, was investigated in a large phase III trial [75]. Satraplatin, like the other platinum compounds, exerts its activity through the formation of covalent platinum–DNA adducts and cross-links, resulting in DNA damage; however, its resistance mechanisms are partially distinct from those of other platinum compounds [76]. Interestingly, satraplatin showed preclinical activity in PC cell lines resistant to taxanes [76, 77]. The SPARC (Satraplatin and Prednisone Against Refractory Cancer) study was a multinational, double-blind, randomized, placebo-controlled trial that assessed the efficacy and tolerability of satraplatin in patients with mCRPC progressing after one prior chemotherapy regimen [75]. Nine hundred fifty patients were randomly assigned (2:1) to receive oral satraplatin 80 mg/m^2 on days 1–5 of a 35-day cycle and prednisone 5 mg twice daily or placebo and prednisone 5 mg twice daily. Primary end points were PFS and OS. The secondary end points comprised QoL and time to pain progression. Satraplatin was generally well tolerated, with an increased rate of myelosuppression and gastrointestinal adverse effects. The results of the study showed a statistically significant, but clinically irrelevant, benefit of satraplatin in PFS, with a median PFS of 11.1 weeks versus 9.7 weeks, and an HR of 0.67 for satraplatin versus placebo (95 % CI 0.57–0.77, $p<0.001$). This effect was maintained irrespective of prior docetaxel treatment. There was also a benefit in terms of PSA response, time to pain progression, and QoL. However, no significant difference in OS was reported between the two arms. Median OS was 61.3 weeks for satraplatin and 61.4 weeks for placebo (HR 0.98; 95 % CI, 0.84–1.15, $p=0.8$). In docetaxel-pretreated patients, median OS was 66.1 v 62.9 weeks in satraplatin and placebo arms, respectively (HR_0.91; 95 % CI, 0.72–1.14). Unfortunately, no correlative and translational studies were performed to assess potential predictive markers, and further development of satraplatin was stopped.

Recently, several studies of next-generation sequencing have shed new light on the mutational landscape of PC. Characterization of the PC transcriptome and genome has identified chromosomal rearrangements and copy number gains/losses that drive PC development and progression to lethal mCRPC [15, 78, 79]. As in other tumor types, current efforts are aimed toward bringing sequencing discoveries into the clinic in the form of biomarkers and biomarker-driven clinical trials [15, 80, 81]. All sequencing studies of advanced PC have found a high incidence (in the range of 20–30 %) of genomic alterations involving key genes important for DNA repair, such as BRCA2 and ATM (ataxia telangiectasia-mutated gene). These mutations have been associated with sensitivity to platinum compounds and poly-(ADP)-ribose polymerase (PARP) inhibitors in preclinical models [82–85]. Olaparib, an oral PARP inhibitor with activity in germ line BRCA1 and BRCA2 – associated breast and ovarian cancers – has been recently evaluated in a spectrum of different BRCA1/2-associated cancers, including PC with progression on hormonal and one systemic therapy [86]. Responses to olaparib were observed across different tumor types; of eight PC patients, four had a partial response and two were classified as having stable disease. Mateo et al. conducted a phase II trial of olaparib, given orally at a dose of 400 mg twice a day, in 50 mCRPC patients [16]. All had received prior treatment with docetaxel, 49 (98 %) had received abiraterone or enzalutamide, and 29 (58 %) had received cabazitaxel. Overall, 16 of 49 evaluable patients (33 %) had a response (defined as objective response, PSA decrease ≥50 %, or reduction in the circulating tumor-cell count). Next-generation sequencing identified mutations in DNA repair genes, including BRCA1/2, ATM, Fanconi's anemia genes, and CHEK2 in 16 cases (33 % of the whole study population). Of these 16 patients, 14 (88 %) had a response to olaparib, including all 7 patients with BRCA2 loss and 4 of 5 with ATM aberrations. Anemia (in 20 %) and fatigue (in 12 % of patients) were the most common grade 3 or 4 adverse events. Although it is currently unclear whether the biomarkers associated with response to olaparib in mCRPC are also associated with response to platinum-based chemotherapy, the interest in platinum compounds in mCRPC has been revived, and trials are currently ongoing in molecularly selected patients. The optimal compound, dosing regimen, and potential combination partners are yet to be identified. A phase II pilot trial of carboplatin in patients with evidence of pTEN loss and/or DNA repair defects is currently enrolling (NCT02311764); another phase II trial with carboplatin in combination with docetaxel is ongoing in mCRPC patients carrying BRCA1/2 mutations (NCT02598895) [87].

In patients with histologically proven small-cell PC, platinum-containing chemotherapy is considered the standard of care, despite the lack of prospective trials. In fact, the available evidence is based on case reports and small clinical series, none of which including exclusively patients with small-cell PC [88, 89]. Recent studies have provided insights into neuroendocrine PC as an aggressive evolution of mCRPC [14, 90, 91]; however, this diagnosis is rarely achieved in clinical practice, due to the challenges in carrying out fresh tumor biopsies in advanced PC.

In conclusion, there is new interest in trials exploring platinum compounds in selected patients with mCRPC. Possible challenges of their use in this setting are toxicities and patient selection. Treatment with cisplatin and oxaliplatin is often limited by impaired renal function and preexisting taxane-induced neuropathy. Carboplatin is generally better tolerated, but hematological toxicity can limit its use. Moreover, further studies of biomarker validation with an extensive use of tumor sampling in mCRPC patients are needed to identify optimal candidates to platinum therapy.

11.5 Effect of Chemotherapy on Bone Metastases (Summary)

The incidence of bone metastases (BM) in patients with mCRPC who are treated with chemotherapy is very high [92]. For each agent, the therapeutic effect on skeletal disease has been assessed in terms of pain control and incidence of SREs [20].

11.5.1 Mitoxantrone

As previously discussed in this chapter, the primary end point of the Canadian randomized trial of mitoxantrone plus prednisone versus prednisone alone was a palliative response, defined as a decrease in pain [4]. Despite the lack of improvement in OS, pain control was more frequent (29 %) in patients who received mitoxantrone plus prednisone as compared to the group receiving prednisone alone (12 %) (p=.01). QoL was also improved in the mitoxantrone-treated patient group (p=.009) [28]. SREs were not reported. Similar results were observed in the confirmation trial reported by XX et al. [29].

11.5.2 Docetaxel

Both the TAX 327 and the SWOG 9916 trials had OS as primary end point, while the effect on pain related to BM was among the secondary end points [5, 6]. Pain response was higher in patients receiving docetaxel in the TAX 327 study. However, although baseline pain was recorded in a high percentage of patients, an OS benefit with docetaxel was observed also in asymptomatic patients [93, 94]. In the SWOG 9916 study, pain relief was similar in the two arms, despite an OS improvement in men treated with docetaxel/estramustine. In both these randomized trials, no specific SREs description was available.

Interestingly, in the STAMPEDE trial (discussed in another chapter of this book) conducted in castration-sensitive PC patients, the addition of docetaxel to ADT not only improved OS but also significantly increased the time to first SRE [95]. This end point was not indagated in the other randomized trials of docetaxel plus ADT in that setting [96, 97].

11.5.3 Cabazitaxel

In the randomized phase III TROPIC trial, cabazitaxel plus prednisone was associated with a significant prolongation of OS as compared to mitoxantrone plus prednisone in patients with mCRPC after docetaxel failure [9]. More than 80 % of patients had bone metastases, and about 45 % had baseline pain. Pain response and time to pain progression were included among the secondary end points of the study. However, pain improvement with cabazitaxel/prednisone was similar to that achieved in the mitoxantrone arm [63]. No specific description of SREs was reported in the TROPIC study. An expanded access study conducted in the UK investigated the impact of cabazitaxel on QoL in 112 patients with mCRPC [68]. This study provided a nonrandomized evidence that cabazitaxel improved QoL, particularly with regard to pain scores.

11.5.4 Platinum Agents

As reported previously, satraplatin/prednisone was compared to placebo/prednisone in patients with mCRPC progressing after one prior chemotherapy regimen. Primary end points of the trial were PFS and OS. The secondary end points included time to pain progression. Although no significant difference in OS was reported between the two arms, patients treated with satraplatin had a benefit in terms of time to pain progression and quality of life [75].

Conclusions

Important advances have been achieved in the knowledge of biology and in the treatment of mCRPC, which remains however an incurable disease, with a heterogeneous behavior. Several treatments consisting of hormonal, chemotherapeutic, immunotherapeutic agents, radiopharmaceuticals, and bone-targeted therapies are available; most of them have been shown to improve QoL and survival. Chemotherapy with docetaxel and cabazitaxel remains an important therapeutic option for patients with mCRPC, with potential clinical effect on bone metastases. The optimal sequencing and combination of treatments still need to be defined. Studies of circulating biomarkers have introduced the concept of treatment selection, which in the near future will hopefully drive an individualized treatment choice and sequence [98]. Until these assays are validated in prospective clinical trials, physicians should continue to use the approved treatments in a patient-specific sequence according to good clinical judgment.

References

1. Attard G, Parker C, Eeles RA et al (2016) Prostate cancer. Lancet 387:70–82
2. Ryan CJ, Small EJ (2003) Role of secondary hormonal therapy in the management of recurrent prostate cancer. Urology 62(Suppl 1):87–94
3. Tannock IF (1985) Is there evidence that chemotherapy is of benefit to patients with carcinoma of the prostate? J Clin Oncol 3:1013–1021
4. Tannock IF, Osoba D, Stockler MR et al (1996) Chemotherapy with mitoxantrone plus prednisone or prednisone alone for symptomatic hormone-resistant prostate cancer: a Canadian randomized trial with palliative endpoints. J Clin Oncol 14:1756–1764
5. Tannock IF, de Wit R, Berry WR et al (2004) Docetaxel plus prednisone or mitoxantrone plus prednisone for advanced prostate cancer. N Engl J Med 351:1502–1512
6. Petrylak DP, Tangen CM, Hussain MHA et al (2004) Docetaxel and estramustine compared with mitoxantrone and prednisone for advanced refractory prostate cancer. N Engl J Med 351:1513–1520
7. Mostaghel EA, Page ST, Lin DW et al (2007) Intraprostatic androgens and androgen-regulated gene expression persist after testosterone suppression: therapeutic implications for castration-resistant prostate cancer. Cancer Res 67:5033–5041
8. Kantoff PW, Higano CS, Shore ND et al (2010) Sipuleucel-T immunotherapy for castration-resistant prostate cancer. N Engl J Med 363:411–422
9. de Bono JS, Oudard S, Ozguroglu M et al (2010) Prednisone plus cabazitaxel or mitoxantrone for metastatic castration-resistant prostate cancer progressing after docetaxel treatment: a randomised open-label trial. Lancet 376:1147–1154
10. de Bono JS, Logothetis CJ, Molina A et al (2011) Abiraterone and increased survival in metastatic prostate cancer. N Engl J Med 364:1995–2005
11. Scher HI, Fizazi K, Saad F et al (2012) Increased survival with enzalutamide in prostate cancer after chemotherapy. N Engl J Med 367:1187–1197
12. Parker C, Nilsson S, Heinrich D et al (2013) Alpha emitter radium-223 and survival in metastatic prostate cancer. N Engl J Med 369:213–223
13. Gillessen S, Omlin A, Attard G et al (2016) Management of patients with advanced prostate cancer: recommendations of the St Gallen Advanced Prostate Cancer Consensus Conference (APCCC) 2015. Ann Oncol 26(8):1589–1604
14. Gundem G, Van Loo P, Kremeyer B et al (2015) The evolutionary history of lethal metastatic prostate cancer. Nature 520:353–357
15. Beltran H, Yelensky R, Frampton GM et al (2013) Targeted next-generation sequencing of advanced prostate cancer identifies potential therapeutic targets and disease heterogeneity. Eur Urol 63:920–926
16. Mateo J, Carreira S, Sandhu S et al (2015) DNA-repair defects and olaparib in metastatic prostate cancer. N Engl J Med 373:1697–1708
17. Hager S, Ackermann CJ, Joerger M et al (2016) Anti-tumour activity of platinum compounds in advanced prostate cancer—a systematic literature review. Ann Oncol 27:975–984

18. Petrylak DP (2014) Practical guide to the use of chemotherapy in castration resistant prostate cancer. Can J Urol 21(Suppl 1):77–83
19. Hurwitz M (2015) Chemotherapy in prostate cancer. Curr Oncol Rep 17:44–53
20. Vignani F, Bertaglia V, Buttigliero C et al (2016) Skeletal metastases and impact of anticancer and bone-targeted agents in patients with castration-resistant prostate cancer. Cancer Treat Rev 44:61–73
21. Eisenberger MA, Simon R, O'Dwyer PJ et al (1985) A reevaluation of nonhormonal cytotoxic chemotherapy in the treatment of prostatic carcinoma. J Clin Oncol 3:827–841
22. Schweizer T, Antonarakis ES (2014) Chemotherapy and its evolving role in the management of advanced prostate cancer. Asian J Androl 16:334–340
23. Glode LM, Barqawi A, Crighton F et al (2003) Metronomic therapy with cyclophosphamide and dexamethasone for prostate carcinoma. Cancer 98:1643–1648
24. Perry CM, McTavish D (1995) Estramustine phosphate sodium. A review of its pharmacodynamic and pharmacokinetic properties, and therapeutic efficacy in prostate cancer. Drugs Aging 7:49–74
25. Bracarda S, Tonato M, Rosi P et al (2000) Oral estramustine and cyclophosphamide in patients with metastatic hormone refractory prostate carcinoma: a phase II study. Cancer 88:1438–1444
26. Moore MJ, Osoba D, Murphy K et al (1994) Use of palliative endpoints to evaluate the effects of mitoxantrone and low-dose prednisone in patients with hormonally resistant prostate cancer. J Clin Oncol 12:689–694
27. Kantoff PW, Block C, Letvak L et al (1993) 14-Day continuous infusion of mitoxantrone in hormone-refractory metastatic adenocarcinoma of the prostate. Am J Clin Oncol 16:489–491
28. Osoba D, Tannock IF, Ernst DS, Neville AJ (1999) Health-related quality of life in men with metastatic prostate cancer treated with prednisone alone or mitoxantrone and prednisone. J Clin Oncol 17:1654–1663
29. Kantoff PW, Halabi S, Conaway M et al (1999) Hydrocortisone with or without mitoxantrone in men with hormone-refractory prostate cancer: results oft he Cancer and Leukemia Group B 9182 study. J Clin Oncol 17:2506–2513
30. Michaelson MD, Oudard S, Ou Y-C et al (2014) Randomized, placebo-controlled, phase III trial of sunitinib plus prednisone versus prednisone alone in progressive, metastatic, castration resistant prostate cancer. J Clin Oncol 32:76–82
31. Green AK, Corty RW, Wood WA et al (2015) Comparative effectiveness of mitoxantrone plus prednisone versus prednisone alone in metastatic castrate-resistant prostate cancer after docetaxel failure. Oncologist 20:516–522
32. Desai A, Mitchison TJ (1997) Microtubule polymerization dynamics. Annu Rev Cell Dev Biol 13:83–117
33. Cheetham P, Petrylak DP (2013) Tubulin-targeted agents including docetaxel and cabazitaxel. Cancer J 19:59–65
34. Gan L, Chen S, Wang Y et al (2009) Inhibition of the androgen receptor as a novel mechanism of taxol chemotherapy in prostate cancer. Cancer Res 69:8386–8394
35. Zhu ML, Horbinski CM, Garzotto M et al (2010) Tubulin-targeting chemotherapy impairs androgen receptor activity in prostate cancer. Cancer Res 70:7992–8002
36. Darshan MS, Loftus MS, Thadani-Mulero M et al (2011) Taxane-induced blockade to nuclear accumulation of the androgen receptor predicts clinical responses in metastatic prostate cancer. Cancer Res 71:6019–6029
37. Picus J, Schultz M (1999) Docetaxel (Taxotere) as monotherapy in the treatment of hormone-refractory prostate cancer: preliminary results. Semin Oncol 26:14–18
38. Friedland D, Cohen J, Miller R Jr et al (1999) A phase II trial of docetaxel (Taxotere) in hormone-refractory prostate cancer: correlation of antitumor effect to phosphorylation of Bcl-2. Semin Oncol 26:19–23
39. Berry W, Dakhil S, Gregurich MA, Asmar L (2001) Phase II trial of single-agent weekly docetaxel in hormone-refractory, symptomatic, metastatic carcinoma of the prostate. Semin Oncol 28:8–15
40. Berthold DR, Pond GR, Soban F et al (2008) Docetaxel plus prednisone or mitoxantrone plus prednisone for advanced prostate cancer: updated survival in the TAX 327 study. J Clin Oncol 26:242–245
41. Machiels JP, Mazzeo F, Clausse M et al (2008) Prospective randomized study comparing docetaxel, estramustine, and prednisone with docetaxel and prednisone in metastatic hormone-refractory prostate cancer. J Clin Oncol 26:5261–5268
42. Kelly WK, Halabi S, Carducci M et al (2012) randomized, double-blind, placebo-controlled phase III trial comparing docetaxel and prednisone with or without bevacizumab in men with metastatic castration-resistant prostate cancer: CALGB 90401. J Clin Oncol 30:1534–1540
43. Tannock IF, Fizazi K, Ivanov S et al (2013) Aflibercept versus placebo in combination with docetaxel and prednisone for treatment of men with metastatic castration-resistant prostate cancer (VENICE): a phase III, double-blind randomized trial. Lancet Oncol 14:760–768
44. Quinn DI, Tangen CM, Hussain M et al (2013) Docetaxel and atrasentan versus docetaxel and placebo for men with advanced castration-resistant prostate cancer (SWOG 20401): a randomized phase III trial. Lancet Oncol 14:893–900
45. Araujo JC, Mathev P, Armstrong AJ et al (2012) Dasatinib combined with docetaxel for castration-resistant prostate cancer: result from a phase I-II study. Cancer 118:63–71
46. Fizazi KS, Higano CS, Nelson JB et al (2013) Phase III, randomized, placebo-controlled study of docetaxel in combination with zibotentan in patient

with metastatic castration-resistant prostate cancer. J Clin Oncol 31:1740–1747
47. Chi KN, Higano CS, Blumenstein BA et al (2015) Phase III SYNERGY trial: Docetaxel +/- custirsen and overall survival in patients with metastatic castration-resistant prostate cancer and poor prognosis. J Clin Oncol 33(suppl; abstr 5009)
48. Recine F, Ceresoli GL, Baciarello G et al (2015) Improvement in survival and quality of life with new therapeutic agents in metastatic castration-resistant prostate cancer: comparison among the results. Q J Nucl Med Mol Imaging 59:400–410
49. Buonerba C, Palmieri G, Di Lorenzo G (2010) Docetaxel rechallenge in castration-resistant prostate cancer: scientific legitimacy of common clinical practice. Eur Urol 58:636–637
50. Di Lorenzo G, Buonerba C, Faiella A et al (2011) Phase II study of docetaxel re-treatment in docetaxel-pretreated castration-resistant prostate cancer. BJU Int 107:234–239
51. Oudard S, Kramer G, Caffo O et al (2015) Docetaxel rechallenge after an initial good response in patients with metastatic castration-resistant prostate cancer. BJU Int 115:744–752
52. Caffo O, Pappagallo G, Brugnara S et al (2012) Multiple rechallenges for castration-resistant prostate cancer patients responding to first-line docetaxel: assessment of clinical outcomes and predictive factors. Urology 79:644–649
53. Antonarakis ES, Lu C, Wang H et al (2014) AR-V7 and resistance to enzalutamide and abiraterone in prostate cancer. N Engl J Med 371:1028–1038
54. Antonarakis ES, Lu C, Luber B et al (2015) Androgen receptor splice-variant 7 and efficacy of taxane chemotherapy in patients with metastatic castration-resistant prostate cancer. JAMA Oncol 1:582–591
55. Onstenk W, Sienwerts AM, Kraan J et al (2015) Efficacy of cabazitaxel in castration-resistant prostate cancer is independent of the presence of AR-V7 in circulating tumor cells. Eur Urol 68:935–945
56. Yap TA, Pezaro CJ, de Bono JS (2012) Cabazitaxel in metastatic castration-resistant prostate cancer. Expert Rev Anticancer Ther 12:1129–1136
57. Seruga B, Ocana A, Tannock IF (2011) Drug resistance in metastatic castration-resistant prostate cancer. Nat Rev Clin Oncol 8:12–23
58. Tsao CK, Cutting E, Martin J, Oh WK (2014) The role of cabazitaxel in the treatment of metastatic castration-resistant prostate cancer. Ther Adv Urol 6:97–104
59. Mita AC, Denis LJ, Rowinsky EK et al (2009) Phase I and pharmacokinetic study of XRP6258 (RPR116258A), a novel taxane, administered as a 1-hour infusion every 3 weeks in patients with advanced solid tumors. Clin Cancer Res 15:723–730
60. Diéras V, Lortholary A, Laurence V et al (2013) Cabazitaxel in patients with advanced solid tumours: results of a phase I and pharmacokinetic study. Eur J Cancer 49:25–34
61. Pivot X, Koralewski P, Hidalgo J et al (2008) A multicenter phase II study of XRP6258 administered as a 1-h i.v. infusion every 3 weeks in taxane-resistant metastatic breast cancer patients. Ann Oncol 9:1547–1552
62. Villanueva C, Awada A, Campone M et al (2011) A multicentre dose-escalating study of cabazitaxel (XRP6258) in combination with capecitabine in patients with metastatic breast cancer progressing after anthracycline and taxane treatment: a phase I/II study. Eur J Cancer 47:1037–1045
63. Bahl A, Oudard S, Tombal B et al (2012) Impact of cabazitaxel on 2-year survival and palliation of tumour-related pain in men with metastatic castration-resistant prostate cancer treated in the TROPIC trial. Ann Oncol 24:2402–2408
64. Heidenreich A, Scholz HJ, Rogenhofer S et al (2013) Cabazitaxel plus prednisone for metastatic castration-resistant prostate cancer progressing after docetaxel: results from the German compassionate-use programme. Eur Urol 63:977–982
65. Castellano D, Antòn Aparicio LM, Esteban E et al (2014) Cabazitaxel for metastatic castration-resistant prostate cancer: safety data from the Spanish expanded access program. Expert Opin Drug Saf 13:1165–1173
66. Heidenreich A, Bracarda S, Mason M et al (2014) Safety of cabazitaxel in senior adults with metastatic castration-resistant prostate cancer: results of the European compassionate-use programme. Eur J Cancer 50:1090–1099
67. Bracarda S, Gernone A, Gasparro D et al (2014) Real-world cabazitaxel safety: the Italian early-access program in metastatic castration-resistant prostate cancer. Future Oncol 10:975–983
68. Bahl A, Masson S, Malik Z et al (2015) Final quality of life and safety data for patients with mCRPC treated with cabazitaxel in the UK Early Access Programme (EAP). BJU Int 16:880–887
69. Halabi S, Lin CY, Small EJ et al (2013) Prognostic model predicting metastatic castration-resistant prostate cancer survival in men treated with second-line chemotherapy. J Natl Cancer Inst 105:1729–1737
70. De Bono J, Hardy-Bessard A, Kim C et al (2016) Phase III non-inferiority study of cabazitaxel 20 mg/m2 versus 25 mg/m2 in patients with metastatic castration-resistant prostate cancer previously treated with docetaxel. J Clin Oncol 34(suppl; abstr 5008)
71. Sartor O, Oudard S, Sengelov L et al (2016) Cabazitaxel versus docetaxel in chemotherapy-naïve patients with metastatic castration-resistant prostate cancer: a three-arm Phase III study (FIRSTANA). J Clin Oncol 34(suppl; abstr 5006)
72. Regan MM, O'Donnell EK, Kelly WK et al (2010) Efficacy of carboplatin-taxane combinations in the management of castration-resistant prostate cancer: a pooled analysis of seven prospective clinical trials. Ann Oncol 21:312–318

73. Aparicio AM, Harzstark AL, Corn PG et al (2013) Platinum-based chemotherapy for variant castrate-resistant prostate cancer. Clin Cancer Res 19:3621–3630
74. Lee JL, Ahn JH, Choi MK et al (2014) Gemcitabine-oxaliplatin plus prednisolone is active in patients with castration-resistant prostate cancer for whom docetaxel-base chemotherapy failed. Br J Cancer 110:2472–2478
75. Sternberg CN, Petrylak DP, Sartor O et al (2009) Multinational, double-blind, phase III study of prednisone and either satraplatin or placebo in patients with castrate refractory prostate cancer progressing after prior chemotherapy: the SPARC trial. J Clin Oncol 27:5431–5438
76. Sternberg CN (2005) Satraplatin in the treatment of hormone-refractory prostate cancer. BJU Int 96:990–994
77. Kelland LR, Abel G, McKeage MJ et al (1993) Preclinical antitumor evaluation of bis-acetatoammine-dichloro-cyclohexylamine platinum (IV): an orally active platinum drug. Cancer Res 53:2581–2586
78. Shen MM, Abate-Shen C (2010) Molecular genetics of prostate cancer: new prospects for old challenges. Genes Dev 24:1967–2000
79. Grasso CS, Wu YM, Robinson DR et al (2012) The mutational landscape of lethal castrate resistant prostate cancer. Nature 487:239–243
80. Macconaill LE, Garraway LA (2010) Clinical implications of the cancer genome. J Clin Oncol 28:5219–5228
81. Stratton MR (2011) Exploring the genomes of cancer cells: progress and promise. Science 331:1553–1558
82. Farmer H, McCabe N, Lord CJ et al (2005) Targeting the DNA repair defect in BRCA mutant cells as a therapeutic strategy. Nature 434:917–921
83. Bryant HE, Schultz N, Thomas HD et al (2005) Specific killing of BRCA2-deficient tumours with inhibitors of poly(ADP-ribose) polymerase. Nature 434:913–917
84. Fong PC, Boss DS, Yap TA et al (2009) Inhibition of poly(ADP-ribose) polymerase in tumors from BRCA mutation carriers. N Engl J Med 361:123–134
85. Lord CJ, Ashworth A (2012) The DNA damage response and cancer therapy. Nature 481:287–294
86. Kaufman B, Shapira-Frommer R, Schmutzler RK et al (2015) Olaparib monotherapy in patients with advanced cancer and a germline BRCA1/2 mutation. J Clin Oncol 33:244–250
87. Docetaxel and carboplatin in treating patients with metastatic, hormone resistant prostate cancer containing inactivated genes in the BRCA 1/2 pathway (NCT02598895); www.clinicaltrials.gov. Accessed on 29th May 2016.
88. Moore SR, Reinberg Y, Zhang G (1992) Small cell carcinoma of prostate: effectiveness of hormonal versus chemotherapy. Urology 39:411–416
89. Papandreou CN, Daliani DD, Thall PF et al (2002) Results of a phase II study with doxorubicin, etoposide, and cisplatin in patients with fully characterized small-cell carcinoma of the prostate. J Clin Oncol 20:3072–3080
90. Beltran H, Tomlins S, Aparicio A et al (2014) Aggressive variants of castration-resistant prostate cancer. Clin Cancer Res 20:2846–2850
91. Beltran H, Prandi D, Mosquera JM et al (2016) Divergent clonal evolution of castration resistant neuroendocrine prostate cancer. Nat Med 22:298–305
92. Coleman RE (2001) Metastatic bone disease: clinical features, pathophysiology and treatment strategies. Cancer Treat Rev 27:165–176
93. Armstrong AJ, Garrett-Mayer E, Ou Yang YC et al (2007) Prostate-specific antigen and pain surrogacy analysis in metastatic hormone-refractory prostate cancer. J Clin Oncol 25:3965–3970
94. Berthold DR, Pond GR, Roessner M et al (2008) Treatment of hormone-refractory prostate cancer with docetaxel or mitoxantrone: relationships between prostate-specific antigen, pain, and quality of life response and survival in the TAX-327 study. Clin Cancer Res 14:2763–2767
95. James ND, Sydes MR, Clarke NW et al (2016) Addition of docetaxel, zoledronic acid, or both to first-line long-term hormone therapy in prostate cancer (STAMPEDE): survival results from an adaptive, multiarm, multistage platform randomized controlled trial. Lancet 387:1163–1177
96. Gravis G, Boher J-M, Joly F et al (2015) Androgen deprivation therapy (ADT) plus docetaxel versus ADT alone for hormone-naïve metastatic prostate cancer: long-term analysis of the GETUG-AFU-15 phase III trial. Eur Urol 70(2):256–262.
97. Sweeney CJ, Chen YH, Carducci M et al (2015) Chemohormonal therapy in metastatic hormone-sensitive prostate cancer. N Engl J Med 373:737–746
98. Sprenger C, Uo T, Plymate S (2015) Androgen receptor splice variant V7 (AR-V7) in circulating tumor cells: a coming of age for AR splice variants? Ann Oncol 26:1805–1807

12 Combinations of Hormonal Therapy and Chemotherapy

Giovanni Luca Ceresoli, Maria Bonomi, Maria Grazia Sauta, Elisa Zanardi, and Francesco Boccardo

12.1 Introduction

Prostate cancer (PC) is the second most frequently diagnosed cancer in men and the third leading cause of cancer death in male patients in the United States and Europe [1, 2]. It is a heterogeneous disease, with a complex natural history, whose growth is driven by androgens and androgen receptors [3]. In most cases, at least in countries where PSA screening is routinely used, patients have localized disease at presentation, even though de novo metastases can occur in a minority of cases [4–6]. In the United States, the proportion of PC patients presenting with metastatic disease at first diagnosis is 4–5 % [6, 7]. The incidence of up-front metastatic disease increases significantly in countries with poorer access to care [8]. Although localized PC may be successfully treated with radical prostatectomy and external beam radiation, many patients subsequently develop metastatic disease [9, 10]. Since its growth is driven by androgens, as initially observed by Huggins and Hodges in 1941 [11], androgen deprivation therapy (ADT) by medical or surgical castration is the standard treatment of hormone-naïve metastatic disease [12]. ADT is also widely used in intermediate and high-risk localized PC, as well as in locally advanced tumors [13]. The majority of patients are treated with medical castration with GnRH agonists or antagonists, which usually determines a profound PSA decline and a radiological and clinical benefit in most patients. However, essentially all patients experience progression to castration-resistant prostate cancer (CRPC) despite persisting low testosterone levels in around 1–2 years, and overall prognosis remains disappointing, although subsequent active treatments are available [4, 12]. The use of intermittent ADT [14, 15] or of combined androgen blockade with a combination of ADT with an androgen receptor antagonist such as bicalutamide [16, 17] has failed in delaying the onset of castration resistance [4, 12, 18].

G.L. Ceresoli (✉)
Department of Medical Oncology, Cliniche Humanitas Gavazzeni, Bergamo, Italy
e-mail: giovanni_luca.ceresoli@gavazzeni.it

M. Bonomi • M.G. Sauta
Department of Medical Oncology, Cliniche Humanitas Gavazzeni, Bergamo, Italy

E. Zanardi • F. Boccardo
Academic Unit of Medical Oncology, IRCCS AOU San Martino-IST (San Martino University Hospital and National Cancer Research Institute), Genoa, Italy

F. Bertoldo et al. (eds.), *Bone Metastases from Prostate Cancer*,
DOI 10.1007/978-3-319-42327-2_12

12.2 Rationale of Combining Chemotherapy and Hormonal Therapy

Hormone-sensitive cells may become castration resistant through two distinct, although not mutually exclusive, mechanisms: adaptation and clonal selection [19, 20] (Fig. 12.1). According to the adaptation model, primary PC is composed of homogeneous cells, and CRPC develops through genetic and epigenetic alterations of androgen-dependent cells. On the contrary, the clonal selection model proposes that primary PC cells are heterogeneous with respect to their androgen dependence; according to this theory, clones of castration-resistant cells exist "ab initio" and are selected by androgen depletion for their survival and proliferative advantages. This heterogeneity mimics the features of the normal prostatic gland, which contains three distinct epithelial cellular lineages with varying degrees of castration resistance: basal cells, luminal secretory cells, and neuroendocrine cells. They are supposed to originate from a common pool of prostate stem cells [21].

Preclinical studies with in vivo prostate cancer models have demonstrated that simultaneous androgen deprivation and chemotherapy are more effective than sequential treatment [22, 23]. The combination of chemotherapy with ADT has been first explored in metastatic CRPC. In the pivotal TAX327 trial, comparing docetaxel chemotherapy with mitoxantrone [24], and in the SWOG9916 trial, comparing the combination of docetaxel and estramustine with the same control arm [25], patients continued ADT throughout study treatment, to ensure continued androgen ablation. Medical castration was continued also in patients enrolled in the TROPIC trial, showing a survival improvement with cabazitaxel as compared to mitoxantrone in patients with disease progression during or after docetaxel-based chemotherapy [26]. On the contrary, in all these studies, at least 4 weeks had to have elapsed between the withdrawal of antiandrogens (6 weeks in the case of bicalutamide) and enrollment, so as to avoid the possibility of a confounding effect as a result of the response to antiandrogen withdrawal.

Early targeting of cells that survive hormonal therapy may potentially prevent the development of CRPC. The aim of these therapeutic strategies is the elimination of resistant cells at the time the tumor is apparently "androgen sensitive." More than 10 years ago, preclinical studies in mice had suggested that the earlier use of chemotherapy with taxanes (i.e., before the development of castration resistance) was therapeutically advantageous [22, 23].

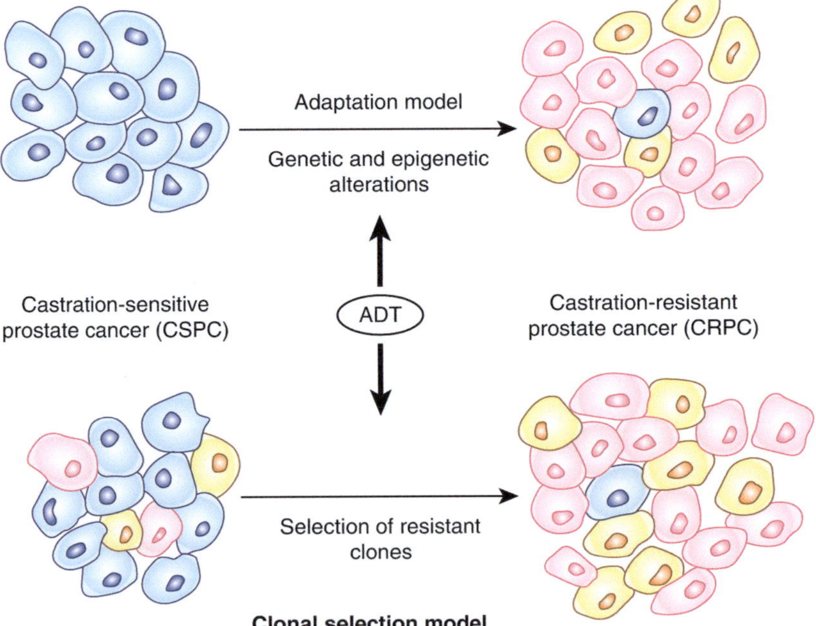

Fig. 12.1 Representation of two models of development of castration-resistant prostate cancer (CRPC) from castration-sensitive prostate cancer (CSPC). *ADT* androgen deprivation therapy. Androgen-dependent prostate cancer cells are represented in *blue*, androgen-resistant cells in *red* and *yellow*

On the other hand, more recent data have shown evidence of inhibition by taxanes of nuclear translocation of the androgen receptor. In vitro, exposure of PC cells to paclitaxel inhibited the translocation by targeting association of the androgen receptor with tubulin. Moreover, when tissue microarrays of PC patients treated with docetaxel were compared to those of docetaxel-untreated patients, a significant decrease in nuclear androgen receptor concentration was observed, paralleled by an increase in cytosolic expression [27].

12.3 Clinical Trials of Chemotherapy in Metastatic Castration-Sensitive Prostate Cancer

Based on this preclinical rationale, several trials have explored the use of combination therapy with ADT and chemotherapy, targeting both the androgen dependent and independent cells simultaneously, rather than waiting for CRPC to establish. In the past decades, several randomized trials had failed to demonstrate a survival improvement with this strategy [28–32]; however, these older trials were limited by the small sample size and by the use of drugs such as mitomycin C, estramustine phosphate, and weekly epirubicin, with no proven activity in PC. Following the results of the TAX327 study [24], docetaxel was extensively evaluated in combination with ADT in men with hormone-naïve metastatic PC, in the attempt to improve the duration and quality of patient survival. Three large randomized phase III trials evaluating the combination of docetaxel with ADT versus ADT alone in metastatic castration-sensitive PC (CSPC) have been recently reported (Table 12.1): the GETUG-AFU 15 study [33, 34], the CHAARTED trial [35], and the STAMPEDE study, a large phase III trial with multiple treatment arms evaluating multiple stages of PC [36, 37].

12.4 The GETUG-AFU 15 Trial

The GETUG-AFU 15 study was an open-label, randomized phase III study that assessed the addition of docetaxel to ADT in men with metastatic CSPC. Between October 2004 and December 2008, 385 patients were randomized from 30 centers (29 in France and 1 in Belgium) in a 1:1 ratio to receive ADT (orchiectomy or luteinizing hormone-releasing hormone agonists, alone or combined with nonsteroidal antiandrogens) or ADT plus docetaxel 75 mg/m^2 every 3 weeks for nine cycles [33, 34] (Table 12.1). Randomization was stratified according to treatment for primary PC, systemic therapy for biochemical relapse, and risk groups as defined by Glass et al. [38]. Glass risk groups had been developed within a large-scale randomized clinical trial comparing orchiectomy and flutamide to orchiectomy and placebo in CSPC patients. Risk factors included appendicular versus axial metastatic disease, Eastern Cooperative Oncology Group (ECOG) performance status 0 versus 1–3, PSA less than 65 versus 65 ng/ml or greater, and Gleason score less than 8 versus 8 or greater. Using these criteria three prognostic groups were developed, including a good (hazard ratio – HR-1), intermediate (HR 1.8), and poor (HR 2.8) group.

In GETUG-AFU 15 study, eligible patients had histologically confirmed adenocarcinoma of the prostate with radiologically proven metastases, were older than 18 years, and had a Karnofsky PS ≥70 %, a life expectancy of at least 3 months, and adequate hematological, hepatic, and renal function. The use of a short course of ADT was allowed for up to 2 months before study entry. The primary end point of the study was OS. Efficacy analyses were done by intention to treat. The original results of the study, after a median 50 months follow-up, were published in 2013 [33]; an updated long-term OS analysis with a median follow-up of 82.9 months was reported in 2015 [34]. The majority of patients enrolled in the study were metastatic at diagnosis (72 %), whereas the remaining patients had developed metastases following treatment of localized disease. A significant improvement in the predefined secondary end points of both biochemical and clinical progression-free survival (PFS) was reported for ADT plus docetaxel versus ADT alone. Namely, a 10-month improvement in median biochemical PFS was found (22.9 versus 12.9 months, HR

Table 12.1 Studies adding docetaxel to ADT in metastatic CSPC

	GETUG-15	CHAARTED	STAMPEDE (metastatic patients only[b])
N. of patients (ADT-docetaxel/ ADT)	385 (192/193)	790 (397/393)	1086 (724/362)
Median FU[a]	83 months	29 months	43 months
Median age[a]	64 years	63 years	65 years
De novo metastatic patients[a]	272 (71 %)	575 (73 %)	1037 (95 %)
Disease volume[a]			
High volume/risk	183 (48 %)	513 (65 %)	UK
Low volume/risk	202 (52 %)	277 (35 %)	UK
Visceral metastases[a]	51 (13 %)	123 (16 %)	UK
Bone metastases[a]			
Overall	311 (81 %)	UK	941 (87 %)
High volume for bone metastases only	177 (46 %)	389 (49 %)	UK
Gleason score ≥ 8[a]	216 (56 %)	484 (61 %)	70 %[b]
N. of planned docetaxel cycles	9	6	6
Grade ≥3 Toxicity (docetaxel arm)			
Neutropenia	32 %	12 %	12 %
Febrile neutropenia	7 %	6 %	12 %
Median OS (HR, 95 % CI; *p* value)			
Whole population	48.6 vs 62.1 months HR 0.88 (0.68–1.14) $p=0.3$	44.0 vs 57.6 months HR 0.61 (0.47–0.80) $p < 0.001$	45.0 vs 60.0 months HR 0.76 (0.62–0.92) $p=0.005$
High volume/risk	35.1 vs 39.8 months HR 0.78 (0.56–1.09) $p=0.1$	32.2 vs 49.2 months HR 0.60 (0.45–0.81) $P<0.001$	UK
Low volume/risk	83.4 months vs NR HR 1.02 (0.67–1.55) $p=0.9$	NR vs NR HR 0.60 (0.32–1.13) $p=0.11$	UK

ADT androgen deprivation therapy, *N* number, *OS* overall survival, *HR* hazard ratio, *CI* confidence intervals, *UK* unknown, and *NR* not reached

[a]Data refer to both arms (ADT and ADT/docetaxel) of each study

[a]Data of the STAMPEDE trial were reported only for metastatic patients enrolled in ADT and ADT/docetaxel arm

[b]Pooled data for metastatic and nonmetastatic patient

0.7, $p=0.0021$). However, no statistically significant difference in the primary end point of OS between the two treatment groups was observed: median OS was 60.9 (95 % CI 46.1–71.4) months in the ADT plus docetaxel versus 46.5 (95 % CI 39.1–60.6) months in the ADT-alone treatment arm (HR = 0.9; $p=0.44$). At the time of final analysis, all patients were retrospectively classified based on the tumor volume as defined per the CHAARTED study criteria (high volume defined as visceral metastases and/or four or more bone metastases with at least one outside the vertebral column and pelvis) [35]. In the overall population, the median OS was not significantly different between the two arms: 62.1 months (95 % CI, 49.5–73.7) in the ADT plus docetaxel arm and 48.6 months (95 % CI, 40.9–60.6) in the ADT arm (HR 0.88 [95 % CI, 0.68–1.14]; $p=0.3$). The OS of high-volume patients did not differ significantly according to the assigned treatment, with a median value of 39.8 (95 % CI 28.0–53.4) months for ADT plus docetaxel versus 35.1 (95 % CI 29.9–43.6) months in the ADT-alone treatment arm (HR: 0.78 [95 % CI, 0.56–1.09]; $p=0.14$). In patients with low-volume disease, median OS was not reached (NR; 95 % CI 69.5–NR) in the ADT plus docetaxel arm and 83.4 months (95 % CI

61.8–NR) in the ADT arm (HR: 1.02 [95 % CI 0.67–1.55]; $p=0.9$). The test of homogeneity of treatment effects among high- and low-volume subgroups did not reveal a significant difference between the estimated HRs in the two subgroups ($p=0.40$). Patients with metastatic disease after failure of local treatment had a significantly longer median OS than those with metastases at diagnosis (83.1 versus 46.5 months, HR: 1.57 [95 % CI, 1.09–2.26]; $p=0.015$). No survival difference was observed within each of these two groups according to treatment. Median time to subsequent treatment was longer in the ADT plus docetaxel arm: 28.1 versus 18.5 months, respectively. In the ADT arm, 127 of 149 patients (85 %) received docetaxel at progression (91 % in the high volume and 78 % in the low-volume subgroup). Other treatments administered after progression in a minority of patients were abiraterone acetate, enzalutamide, and cabazitaxel.

Serious adverse events were more common in the group given ADT plus docetaxel. The most frequent were neutropenia (21 %), febrile neutropenia (3 %), and abnormal liver function tests (2 %). Four treatment-related deaths (5 %) occurred in the ADT plus docetaxel group (two of which were neutropenia related); as a consequence, the data monitoring committee recommended prophylaxis with granulocyte colony-stimulating factor. After this recommendation, no further treatment-related deaths occurred. No serious adverse events were reported in the ADT-alone group.

12.4.1 The CHAARTED Trial

The CHAARTED trial also investigated the addition of docetaxel to ADT in metastatic hormone-sensitive disease [35]. In this trial 790 men with metastatic PC, enrolled between July 2006 and November 2012, were randomized 1:1 to receive ADT alone or ADT plus 75 mg/m^2 of docetaxel every 3 weeks for six cycles (Table 12.1). Premedication comprised oral dexamethasone 8 mg at 12 h, 3 h, and 1 h before docetaxel infusion; daily prednisone was not required. Randomization was allowed within 4 months of initiating ADT. Most patients enrolled in the study had metastases at diagnosis (75 %), and the remaining had developed metastases following treatment of local disease. Patients were stratified by volume of disease (high versus low), with high-volume disease defined as visceral metastases and/or four or more bone metastases with at least one beyond the pelvis and the axial skeleton. Other stratification factors included: age (≤70 versus >70 years), ECOG PS (0–1 versus 2), prior adjuvant ADT (>12 months or ≤12 months), and concurrent bisphosphonate or denosumab use (yes versus no). The primary end point was OS; secondary end points were PSA response (PSA <0.2 ng/ml at 6 and 12 months), time to clinical (radiographic or symptomatic) progression, time to CRPC (including biochemical progression), treatment tolerability, and quality of life. Patient characteristics were well balanced between the two arms. Median age was 64 years in the combination group and 63 years in the ADT-alone group. In both groups, approximately 70 % had an ECOG PS score of 0, approximately 65 % had high-volume disease, and 60 % had a Gleason score of 8 or higher. At a planned interim analysis, prespecified criteria for significance were met, and the data were released; the median follow-up was 28.9 months. The primary end point was met, with an improvement in the median OS of the whole study population of 13.6 months in the combined treatment arm (57.6 versus 44.0 months, HR 0.61, 95 % CI 0.47–0.80, $p<0.001$). In a subset analysis, the greatest difference in median OS between the two treatment arms (17 months) was observed in patients with high-volume disease. In this subgroup (514 patients), median OS was 49.2 months for patients treated with ADT plus docetaxel versus 32.2 months for those treated with ADT alone (HR 0.60, 95 % CI 0.45–0.81, $p<0.001$). The median OS was not reached at the time of the analysis in the cohort of patients with low-volume disease, with no statistically significant difference between the two treatment arms (HR 0.60, 95 % CI 0.32–1.13, $p=0.11$). The combination of ADT and docetaxel also met all the secondary end points. The median time to biochemical, symptomatic, or radiographic progression was

20.2 months in the combination group, as compared with 11.7 months in the ADT-alone group (HR 0.61, 95 % CI 0.51–0.72; *P*<0.001). PSA response (as defined above) at 12 months was 27.7 % in the combination group versus 16.8 % in the ADT-alone group (*P*<0.001). The reported toxicity in the combination arm was mild, with grade 3–4 neutropenia observed in 12.1 % of patients, and anemia, thrombocytopenia, and febrile neutropenia reported in 1.3 %, < 1 %, and 6.1 % of cases, respectively. Grade 3 peripheral neuropathy occurred in 1 % of patients. More than 85 % of patients completed all the six planned cycles of docetaxel, three quarters of them without dose modifications. One treatment-related death occurred in the docetaxel plus ADT arm; no deaths related to treatment toxicity were reported in the ADT-alone arm.

12.4.2 The STAMPEDE Trial

STAMPEDE is a large ongoing phase III trial with a multi-arm multistage design [36, 37]. Patients with high-risk locally advanced or metastatic prostate cancer, or with aggressively relapsing disease after initial therapy for local disease, and starting long-term ADT for the first time were enrolled. The study was opened to accrual in October 2008 in several centers in the United Kingdom and Switzerland. The hypothesis was that the early use of active therapies might give a large absolute benefit in OS, set as the primary study end point. Secondary outcome measures were failure-free survival (FFS), toxicity, quality of life, skeletal-related events (SREs), and cost effectiveness. FFS was defined as first of PSA failure, local or lymph node failure, distant metastases, and prostate cancer death. The first trial design included five research arms, but arms with celecoxib (ADT plus celecoxib and ADT plus celecoxib and zoledronic acid) were closed for lack of sufficient activity at a preplanned interim analysis [39]. The remaining original arms – ADT plus docetaxel, ADT plus zoledronic acid, and ADT plus the combination of docetaxel and zoledronic acid – successfully completed their recruitment throughout all interim stages in March 2013. An arm of abiraterone, prednisone, and ADT was introduced in November 2011, and its accrual was completed in January 2014 [40]. A new arm with radiotherapy, among newly diagnosed metastatic patients only, was introduced in January 2013, and another arm combining enzalutamide, abiraterone, and prednisone with ADT started in July 2014 [41]. The survival results for three research comparisons testing the addition of zoledronic acid, docetaxel, or both to ADT (considered as the control arm) in patients with M0 or M1 hormone-sensitive disease have been recently reported [37]. Patients were randomized 2:1:1:1 to standard ADT versus ADT plus docetaxel, zoledronic acid, or both, respectively. Age, stage, the presence of metastases, previous treatments, center, and the use of aspirin or non-steroid anti-inflammatory drugs were stratification factors. Docetaxel was given at 75 mg/mq every 3 weeks for six cycles with prednisolone 10 mg daily; zoledronic acid was administered at 4 mg every 3 weeks for six cycles (18 weeks), then every 4 weeks until 2 years. Primary end point of the study was OS. Overall, 2962 men were randomized to the four arms. Median age was 65 years (range 40–84), and 78 % of patients had ECOG PS 0. Most patients (61 %) had metastatic PC, in 85 % of cases with bone metastases. The remainder had either lymph node metastases with M0 status (15 %) or N0M0 disease (24 %). Radiotherapy was delivered in patients with N0M0 disease and was optional for men with N-positive M0 disease. With a median follow-up of 43 months, patients treated with ADT alone had a median OS of 71 months, and 5-year survival was 55 %. These data were the reference for each comparison of research groups with control. A statistically significant improvement in OS was reported in patients treated with ADT plus docetaxel, with a median OS of 81 months and a 5-year OS of 63 % (HR 0.78, 95 % CI 0.66–0.93; $p=0.006$). Similarly, patients treated with ADT plus docetaxel plus zoledronic acid had a longer median OS of 76 months and a 5-year OS of 60 % (HR 0.82, 95 % CI 0.69–0.97; $p=0.022$). On the contrary, no OS improvement was reported in the arm of patients treated with ADT plus zoledronic acid (HR 0.94, $p=0.45$). In a preplanned subset analysis, adding docetaxel to standard ADT showed significant OS improvement in patients with metastatic status but not in M0 patients; similar results were found in the subgroup of patients in which docetaxel and zoledronic acid were added to standard ADT. Namely, median OS of 362 metastatic patients treated with docetaxel plus ADT was 60 months as compared to 45 months of 724 metastatic patients treated with ADT alone, with an HR of 0.76 (95 % CI 0.62–0.92) and a $p=0.005$. FFS was significantly longer in patients receiving ADT plus docetaxel or ADT plus docetaxel and zole dronic acid. The effect of docetaxel on FFS was maintained in both metastatic and nonmetastatic patients. No effect on FFS was observed when adding zoledronic acid alone to ADT. Treatments used at progression included docetaxel in 41 % of patients enrolled in the standard arm; abiraterone acetate, enzalutamide, cabazitaxel, and radium 223 were equally distributed in the study arms. Grade 3–5 toxicity was more frequent in the docetaxel arms (52 % in docetaxel and docetaxel/zoledronic acid groups versus 32 % in the ADT arm). Febrile neutropenia rate was significantly higher in the docetaxel arms (14 % and 15 %, respectively, versus 1 % in the standard arm). In conclusion, addition of docetaxel to ADT improved OS in metastatic CSPC. Zoledronic acid did not improve OS. Addition of both agents to ADT improved OS but offered no obvious benefit over adding just docetaxel. According to the authors, docetaxel should be considered in routine practice for suitable men with newly diagnosed metastatic disease and also for selected men with high-risk nonmetastatic disease in view of substantial prolongation of FFS.

12.5 Comparison and Meta-analyses of the Trials

12.5.1 Critical Comparison

The GETUG-AFU 15, CHAARTED, and STAMPEDE trials have similar designs but several remarkable differences (Table 12.1). CHAARTED and STAMPEDE are notably larger in comparison to GETUG-AFU 15, which on the other hand has the longest follow-up. In all trials the reference arm was ADT considered as the standard of care in the hormone-naïve setting; in the experimental arms, docetaxel administered every 3 weeks at the dose of 75 mg/m^2 was added to ADT within 4 months at the latest from ADT start. The number of the planned docetaxel cycles differed among the studies: six in CHAARTED and STAMPEDE, up to nine in GETUG-AFU 15. In all the three studies, OS was the primary end point. CHAARTED and STAMPEDE trials showed a statistically significant improvement of OS in the combination arm, while no improvement was found in GETUG-AFU 15 study, despite a higher number of delivered chemotherapy cycles. Notably, PFS defined either as biochemical or clinical/radiological failure was significantly improved by the addition of docetaxel in all the trials. The effect of post-protocol therapy on OS in the two arms of the different trials should be further elucidated; treatment at progression was not planned, and also the availability of life-prolonging agents was different for CHAARTED and STAMPEDE trials as compared to GETUG-AFU 15, due to the different accrual times of the studies. The positive results of combined therapy in high-volume patients were not confirmed by the post hoc analysis of the GETUG-AFU 15 trial [34]. However, as acknowledged by the authors themselves, the study was underpowered to assess this end point.

12.5.2 Meta-analyses

Two meta-analyses of aggregate data of trials comparing ADT versus the combination of ADT and chemotherapy with docetaxel have been recently reported [42, 43]. In the first, published by Tucci et al. [42], a total of 2951 patients were included from the three above-discussed trials (GETUG-AFU 15, CHAARTED, and STAMPEDE). Other studies enrolling only M0 patients were excluded [44]. Overall, 2262 (61 %) patients were metastatic: 951 received docetaxel and ADT, while 1311 ADT alone. In metastatic patients, the addition of docetaxel was associated with improved OS (HR 0.73, 95 % CI 0.60–0.90, $p=0.002$). Also when the whole study population (2951 patients) was considered, the benefit of adding docetaxel remained significant (HR 0.74; 95 % CI 0.61–0.91; $p=0.003$). Although with limited statistical power, no significant interaction was demonstrated between the addition of docetaxel and the high or low volume of disease ($p=0.5$). The addition of docetaxel was also associated with improvement in PFS (in metastatic patients: HR 0.63, 95 % CI 0.57–0.70; $p<0.001$). The authors considered the OS improvement not only statistically but also clinically significant, due to a 27 % reduction in the risk of death; this reduction was up to 33 % in patients with high-volume disease. Of note, no relevant statistical heterogeneity was found among the three trials. Based on the result of their analysis, Tucci et al. suggested that the combination of chemotherapy and hormonal treatment should be considered in all fit patients with metastatic CSPC.

The second meta-analysis by Vale et al. [43] included all relevant randomized controlled trials (published, unpublished, and ongoing) comparing either ADT with or without docetaxel or ADT with or without bisphosphonates for patients with high-risk localized or metastatic CSPC. For each trial, HRs of the effects of docetaxel or bisphosphonates on OS and FFS (time from randomization to biochemical or clinical failure or death from any cause) were extracted and then combined. Five trials compared standard of care with or without docetaxel in patients with metastatic PC; only the results from three (CHAARTED, GETUG-AFU 15, STAMPEDE) of these trials (accounting for 93 % of all randomized patients) were available and suitable for analysis. The pooled analysis showed that the addition of docetaxel to standard of care improved OS, with an HR of 0.77 (95 % CI 0.68–0.87; $p<0.0001$) and an absolute improvement in 4-year OS of 9 % (95 % CI 5–14). Of note, docetaxel also improved FFS, with an HR of 0.64 (0.58–0.70; $p<0.0001$) translating into a reduction in absolute 4-year failure rates of 16 % (95 % CI 12–19). On the contrary, no benefit from the addition of docetaxel was evidenced in men with M0, locally advanced disease. Moreover, no improvement was shown with zoledronic acid in patients with both M1 and M0 disease. The authors concluded that the addition of docetaxel to ADT should be considered standard care for men with metastatic hormone-sensitive PC who are starting treatment for the first time.

12.5.3 Effect of Chemotherapy/Ormonotherapy on Skeletal-Related Events in CSPC

No specific analysis on the impact of addition of docetaxel to ADT on incidence and timing of skeletal-related events (SREs) was reported in GETUG-AFU 15 and CHAARTED trials. In the CHAARTED study, patients were stratified per planned use of agents approved for prevention of SREs (zoledronic acid and denosumab). The combination of chemotherapy with ADT was active in patients with skeletal involvement; in particular, subgroup analysis showed a survival improvement with docetaxel in high-volume patients with bone metastases alone (389 patients; HR 0.64, 95 % CI 0.46–0.89).

SREs were among the secondary end points of the STAMPEDE study [37]. Time to first SRE was improved in the docetaxel + ADT arm (HR 0.60, 95 % CI 0.48–0.74) and in docetaxel + zoledronic acid + ADT arm (HR 0.55, 95 % CI 0.44–0.69) but not in the zoledronic acid + ADT group. Mean time to skeletal-related event was 61.4 months in ADT only, 68 months in docetaxel + ADT, and 68.3 months in docetaxel + zoledronic acid + ADT arm.

12.6 Patient Selection for Up-Front Chemotherapy in Castration-Sensitive Metastatic PC

Although the above discussed trials and meta-analyses seem to show a clear benefit from the early use of chemotherapy with docetaxel in patients with metastatic hormone-sensitive PC, many important issues regarding patient selection for this therapeutic option remain open. It is clear, from everyday clinical practice, that this strategy does not fit all patients and is influenced by several individual factors including history, biology, and extent of the disease, age, performance status, and coexisting comorbidity.

Most patients in GETUG-AFU 15, CHAARTED, and STAMPEDE trials were metastatic at diagnosis (Table 12.1), ranging from 67 to 76 % in the different arms of the first two studies [33–35]. As reported before in this chapter, PC patients presenting with metastatic disease at first diagnosis in the United States and Western Europe account for 4–5 % of the total population [6, 7]. A Gleason score of 8 or higher was reported in the majority of enrolled patients in the three studies, ranging from 55 to 74 %. Median age was between 63 and 65 years. Patients older than 70 years, which are very common in clinical practice, were underrepresented. In the CHAARTED trial, subgroup analysis according to age confirmed docetaxel efficacy also in patients ≥70 years, but they represented only 23 % (178 of 790) of the total study population [35]. Moreover, elderly patients included in the three trials likely represent a selection bias, because they had to be fit enough to receive chemotherapy. As a consequence, the risk-benefit ratio of adding chemotherapy in CSPC might be unfavorable, for example, in elderly patients with a long-lasting, slowly progressing disease and low Gleason score, whereas in other patients, early chemotherapy could target in a timely manner ADT-resistant cell clones, avoiding rapid disease progression and deterioration of the patient toward a condition in which he would be too frail to receive chemotherapy. Apart from the obvious case of a man who is unfit for chemotherapy, a deeper knowledge of disease biology is needed to help the clinician in selecting the best treatment for each patient.

While for patients with metastatic CRPC several prognostic models have been proposed [45], suggesting also that metastatic site is an important predictor of OS [46], only few studies are available for metastatic CSPC. Recently, the Glass model developed in 2003 to define subgroups with good, intermediate, and poor prognosis was validated in the population of the GETUG-AFU 15 trial [47], with the aim to develop a more sensitive prognostic model. Potential prognostic factors were recorded: age, performance status, Gleason score, hemoglobin, PSA, alkaline phosphatase (ALP), lactate dehydrogenase (LDH), metastatic localization, body mass index, and pain. These factors were used to develop a new prognostic model. Before analysis, the data were split into learning and validation sets. The outcome was OS. ALP was the strongest prognostic factor in discriminating patients with good or poor prognosis. In the learning set, median OS in patients with normal and abnormal ALP was 69.1 and 33.6 months, and 5 years survival was 62.1 % and 23.2 %, respectively, with an HR of 3.11. The discriminatory ability of ALP was superior to that of the Glass risk model itself.

Several studies have analyzed the role of disease burden in metastatic PC, both in hormone-sensitive and in castration-resistant disease, with definition of volume comparable with that used in the CHAARTED trials. The results of these investigations have consistently demonstrated better survival outcomes in patients with low volume as compared to high volume disease. In patients with CSPC, the presence of a high metastatic burden (particularly in case of visceral metastases or appendicular skeletal involvement) is associated with a worse prognosis [48]. Patients enrolled in the CHAARTED trial were stratified according to the extent of metastatic disease (high versus low volume of disease), with high volume disease defined as visceral metastases and/or 4 or more sites of bone disease with at least one beyond the pelvis and the vertebral column [35]. This stratification was retrospectively applied to GETUG-AFU 15 patients [34]. Overall, high-volume patients were more represented in CHAARTED study, with 65 % of total patients as compared to 48 % in GETUG-15 trial. Data on disease volume are so far lacking for STAMPEDE study. Subgroup data of the CHAARTED trial have suggested that the benefit associated with concomitant administration of docetaxel with ADT was more pronounced in patients with high-volume disease than in patients with low-volume disease [35]. In their meta-analysis of the three trials, Tucci et al. [42] did not demonstrate a significant interaction between disease volume and treatment efficacy. Of note, in the CHAARTED trial the HR for death with ADT plus docetaxel in patients with low volume disease was 0.60 (95 % CI 0.32–1.13; $p=0.11$), the same reported for patients with high volume disease (0.60; 95 % CI 0.45–0.81; $p<0.001$). A longer follow-up with a higher number of events is needed to definitively establish the interaction between docetaxel efficacy and disease volume.

Although docetaxel is commonly used and its adverse events are well known and generally manageable, the toxicity of adding chemotherapy to ADT should be considered with caution. Neutropenia was the most threatening adverse event in all trials (Table 12.1); it was reported more commonly in the GETUG-15 study, with a higher rate of treatment discontinuation due to toxicity issues (20.3 % versus 12.5 % in the CHAARTED study), and a higher rate of toxic deaths in the chemotherapy arm (5 % versus 0.3 % for CHAARTED). Of note, a higher number of chemotherapy cycles were planned in GETUG-15, and myelotoxicity was likely underestimated in CHAARTED trial, as blood counts were not monitored routinely between cycles. The different (and probably under-reported) use of granulocyte colony-stimulating factors and discrepancies in the patient castration levels at the start of chemotherapy [49] may further explain the different toxicity profile of docetaxel in the three studies. Interestingly, in the STAMPEDE study the early excess in toxicity in the chemotherapy arm seemed to settle subsequently, with 1-year grade ≥3 toxicity of 10.1 % in the ADT plus docetaxel arm versus 9.7 % in the ADT alone arm [17]. Chemotherapy toxicity is often worse in the real-world population compared with the toxicity reported in clinical trials. As reported by Templeton et al. [50], survival of patients with metastatic prostate cancer treated in the same institution with docetaxel in routine practice was shorter than for men included in trials and was associated with more toxicity. Therefore, before considering the addition of docetaxel to ADT, several clinical factors (age, performance status, comorbidity, and concomitant medications) should be taken in account to reduce the risk of severe toxicity that could negatively affect quality of life and survival.

Conclusions

The last years have witnessed an impressive improvement in the knowledge of the biology of metastatic PC, and the rapid availability of several new active agents [4, 12]. The large randomized studies analyzed in this chapter, addressing the early use of docetaxel in combination with ADT in men with metastatic CSPC, have added complexity to this scenario. Overall, there is evidence that at least a subset of patients with metastatic CSPC may benefit from the combination of ADT with docetaxel as initial therapy. Clearly, this approach should not be proposed to all cases, because patients enrolled in GETUG-15, CHAARTED and STAMPEDE trials are not representative of the "real life" patients, who have often slowly progressing disease that develops distant metastases several years after diagnosis and local treatments. Furthermore, patients enrolled in these trials had a good performance status and were all fit for chemotherapy, and likely had less comorbidity than the average PC patient.

Several trials are ongoing to define the role of chemotherapy in earlier stages of disease, including high-risk localized PC and biochemical failure after local therapy. Other studies are also evaluating non-chemotherapy drugs like abiraterone or enzalutamide, and the role of local treatment of primary prostate cancer in patients with de novo metastatic disease. [51]

In summary, the available results from the above discussed trials support the use of early docetaxel combined with ADT in selected hormone-naïve metastatic PC patients. At present, early chemotherapy should be considered and discussed at least for men with high-volume

PC (according to CHAARTED definition) presenting with distant metastases at or soon after diagnosis, and who are judged to be fit to receive chemotherapy.

References

1. Siegel RL, Miller KD, Jemal A (2016) Cancer statistics, 2016.CA. Cancer J Clin 66:7–30
2. Ferlay J, Shin HR, Bray F et al (2010) Estimates of worldwide burden of cancer in 2008: GLOBOCAN 2008. Int J Cancer 127:2893–2917
3. Gundem G, Van Loo P, Kremeyer B et al (2015) The evolutionary history of lethal metastatic prostate cancer. Nature 520:353–357
4. Attard G, Parker C, Eeles RA et al (2016) Prostate cancer. Lancet 387:70–82
5. Wu JN, Fish KM, Evans CP et al (2014) No improvement noted in overall or cause-specific survival for men presenting with metastatic prostate cancer over a 20-year period. Cancer 120:818–823
6. Miller DC, Hazer KS, Stewart A et al (2003) Prostate carcinoma presentation, diagnosis and staging: an update from the National Cancer Data Base. Cancer 98:1169–1178
7. Ryan CJ, Elkin EP, Small EJ et al (2006) Reduced incidence of bony metastasis at initial prostate cancer diagnosis: data from CaPSURE. Urol Oncol 24:396–402
8. Center MM, Jemal A, Lortet-Tieulent J et al (2012) International variation in prostate cancer incidence and mortality rates. Eur Urol 61:1079–1092
9. Wilt TJ, Brawer MK, Jones KM et al (2012) Radical prostatectomy versus observation for localized prostate cancer. N Engl J Med 367:203–213
10. Wallis CJ, Saskin R, Choo R et al (2015) Surgery versus radiotherapy for clinically localized prostate cancer: a systematic review and meta-analysis. Eur Urol 70(1):21–30
11. Huggins C, Hodges CV (1941) Studies in prostate cancer. 1. The effect of castration of oestrogen and of androgen injection on serum phosphatases in metastatic carcinoma of the prostate. Cancer Res 1: 293–297
12. Gillessen S, Omlin A, Attard G et al (2016) Management of patients with advanced prostate cancer: recommendations of the St Gallen Advanced Prostate Cancer Consensus Conference (APCCC) 2015. Ann Oncol 26:1589–1604
13. D'Angelillo RM, Franco P, De Bari B et al (2015) Combination of androgen deprivation therapy and radiotherapy for localized prostate cancer in the contemporary era. Crit Rev Oncol Hematol 93:136–148
14. Hussain M, Tangen C, Higano C et al (2016) Evaluating intermittent androgen-deprivation therapy phase III clinical trials: the devil is in the details. J Clin Oncol 34:180–185
15. Magnan S, Zarychanski R, Pilote L et al (2015) Intermittent vs continuous androgen deprivation therapy for prostate cancer: a systematic review and meta-analysis. JAMA Oncol 1:1261–1269
16. Prostate Cancer Trialists' Collaborative Group (2000) Maximum androgen blockade in advanced prostate cancer: an overview of the randomised trials. Lancet 355:1491–1498
17. Samson DJ, Seidenfeld J, Schmitt B et al (2002) Systematic review and meta-analysis of monotherapy compared with combined androgen blockade for patients with advanced prostate carcinoma. Cancer 95:361–376
18. James ND, Spears MR, Clark NW et al (2015) Survival with newly diagnosed metastatic prostate cancer in the "Docetaxel Era": data from 917 patients in the control arm of the STAMPEDE trial (MRC PR08, CRUK/06/019). Eur Urol 67:1028–1038
19. Zong Y, Goldstein AS (2013) Adaptation or selection: mechanisms of castration-resistant prostate cancer. Nat Rev Urol 10:90–98
20. Ahmed M, Li LC (2013) Adaptation and clonal selection models of castration-resistant prostate cancer: current perspective. Int J Urol 20:362–371
21. Goldstein AS, Stoyanova T, Witte ON (2010) Primitive origins of prostate cancer: *in vivo* evidence for prostate-regenerating cells and prostate cancer-initiating cells. Mol Oncol 4:385–396
22. Eigl BJ, Eggener SE, Baybik J et al (2005) Timing is everything: preclinical evidence supporting simultaneous rather than sequential chemohormonal therapy for prostate cancer. Clin Cancer Res 11:4905–4911
23. Tang Y, Khan MA, Goloubeva O et al (2006) Docetaxel followed by castration improves outcomes in LNCaP prostate cancer-bearing severe combined immunodeficient mice. Clin Cancer Res 12:169–174
24. Tannock IF, de Wit R, Berry WR et al (2004) Docetaxel plus prednisone or mitoxantrone plus prednisone for advanced prostate cancer. N Engl J Med 351:1502–1512
25. Petrylak DP, Tangen CM, Hussain MHA et al (2004) Docetaxel and estramustine compared with mitoxantrone and prednisone for advanced refractory prostate cancer. N Engl J Med 351:1513–1520
26. de Bono JS, Oudard S, Ozguroglu M et al (2010) Prednisone plus cabazitaxel or mitoxantrone for metastatic castration-resistant prostate cancer progressing after docetaxel treatment: a randomised open-label trial. Lancet 376:1147–1154
27. Zhu ML, Horbinski CM, Garzotto M et al (2010) Tubulin-targeting chemotherapy impairs androgen receptor activity in prostate cancer. Cancer Res 70:7992–8002
28. De Reijke TM, Keuppens FL, Whelan P et al (1999) Orchiectomy and orchiectomy plus mitomycin C for metastatic prostate cancer in patient with poor prognosis: the final results of a European Organization for Research in Cancer Therapy Genitourinary Group Trial. J Urol 162:1658–1664

29. Janknegt RA, Boon TA, van de Beek C, Grob P (1997) Combined hormono/chemotherapy as primary treatment for metastatic prostate cancer: a randomized, multicenter study of orchiectomy alone versus orchiectomy plus estramustine phosphate. The Dutch Estracyt Study Group. Urology 49:411–420
30. Noguchi M, Noda S, Yoshida M et al (2004) Chemohormonal therapy as primary treatment for metastatic prostate cancer: a randomized study of estramustine phosphate plus luteinizing hormone-releasing hormone agonist versus flutamide plus luteinizing hormone-releasing hormone agonist. Int J Urol 11:103–109
31. Millikan RE, Wen S, Pagliaro LC et al (2008) Phase III trial of androgen ablation with or without three cycles of systemic chemotherapy for advanced prostate cancer. J Clin Oncol 26:5936–5942
32. Pummer K, Lehnert M, Stettner H, Hubmer G (1997) Randomized comparison of total androgen blockade alone versus combined with weekly epirubicin in advanced prostate cancer. Eur Urol 32:81–85
33. Gravis G, Fizazi K, Joly F et al (2013) Androgen-deprivation therapy alone or with docetaxel in non-castrate metastatic prostate cancer (GETUG-AFU 15): a randomised, open-label, phase 3 trial. Lancet Oncol 14:149–158
34. Gravis G, Boher J-M, Joly F et al (2016) Androgen deprivation therapy (ADT) plus docetaxel versus ADT alone for hormone-naïve metastatic prostate cancer: long-term analysis of the GETUG-AFU-15 phase III trial. Eur Urol 70(1):21–30
35. Sweeney CJ, Chen YH, Carducci M et al (2015) Chemohormonal therapy in metastatic hormone-sensitive prostate cancer. N Engl J Med 373:737–746
36. James ND, Sydes MR, Clarke NW et al (2008) STAMPEDE: systemic therapy for advancing or metastatic prostate cancer. A Multi-arm multi-Stage randomised controlled trial. Clin Oncol 20:577–581
37. James ND, Sydes MR, Clarke NW et al (2016) Addition of docetaxel, zoledronic acid, or both to first-line long-term hormone therapy in prostate cancer (STAMPEDE): survival results from an adaptive, multiarm, multistage platform randomized controlled trial. Lancet 387:1163–1177
38. Glass TR, Tangen CM, Crawford ED, Thompson I (2003) Metastatic carcinoma of the prostate: identifying prognostic groups using recursive partitioning. J Urol 169:164–169
39. James ND, Sydes MR, Mason MD et al (2012) Celecoxib plus hormone therapy versus hormone therapy alone for hormone-sensitive prostate cancer: first results from the STAMPEDE multiarm, multistage, randomized controlled trial. Lancet Oncol 13:549–558
40. Sydes MR, Parmar MK, Mason MD et al (2012) Flexible trial design in practice - stopping arms for lack-of-benefit and adding research arms mid-trial in STAMPEDE: a multi-arm multi-stage randomized controlled trial. Trials 13:168
41. Attard G, Sydes MR, Mason MD et al (2014) Combining enzalutamide with abiraterone, prednisone, and androgen deprivation therapy in the STAMPEDE trial. Eur Urol 66:799–802
42. Tucci M, Bertaglia V, Vignani F et al (2016) Addition of docetaxel to androgen deprivation therapy for patients with hormone-sensitive metastatic prostate cancer: a systematic review and meta-analysis. Eur Urol 69:563–573
43. Vale CL, Burdett S, Rydzewska LHM et al (2016) Addition of docetaxel or bisphosphonates to standard of care in men with localized or metastatic, hormone-sensitive prostate cancer: a systematic review and meta-analyses of aggregate data. Lancet Oncol 17:243–256
44. Fizazi K, Faivre L, Lesaunier F et al (2015) Androgen deprivation therapy plus docetaxel and estramustine versus androgen deprivation therapy alone for high-risk localized prostate cancer (GETUG 12): a phase 3 randomised controlled trial. Lancet Oncol 16:787–794
45. Halabi S, Lin CY, Kelly WK et al (2014) Updated prognostic model for predicting overall survival in first-line chemotherapy for patients with metastatic castration-resistant prostate cancer. J Clin Oncol 32:671–677
46. Halabi S, Kelly WK, Ma H et al (2016) Meta-analysis evaluating the impact of site of metastasis on overall survival in men with castration-resistant prostate cancer. J Clin Oncol 34:1652–1659
47. Gravis G, Boher JM, Fizazi K et al (2015) Prognostic factors for survival in non-castrate metastatic prostate cancer: validation of the Glass model and development of a novel simplified prognostic model. Eur Urol 68:196–204
48. Fizazi K, Jenkins C, Tannock IF (2015) Should docetaxel be standard of care for patients with metastatic hormone-sensitive prostate cancer? Pro and contra. Ann Oncol 26:1660–1667
49. Franke RM, Carducci MA, Rudek MA, et al (2010) Castration-dependent pharmacokinetics of docetaxel in patients with prostate cancer. J Clin Oncol 28: 4562–4567
50. Templeton AJ, Vera-Badillo FE, Wang L, et al (2013) Translating clinical trials to clinical practice: outcomes of men with metastatic castration resistant prostate cancer treated with docetaxel and prednisone in and out of clinical trials. Ann Oncol 24: 2972–2977
51. Fizazi K, Abrahamsson P-A, Ahlgren G, et al (2015) Achievements and perspectives in prostate cancer phase 3 trials from Genitourinary Research Groups in Europe: introducing the Prostate Cancer Consortium in Europe. Eur Urol 67:904–912

13 Surgery: Treatment of Oligometastatic Disease

Alessandro Luzzati, Gennaro Scotto, Giuseppe Perrucchini, and Carmine Zoccali

The treatment of the patient with bone metastases from prostate cancer is usually based on medical and radiation therapy [1–6]. Nevertheless, sometimes indication for surgery is present with:

- "Curative" aim: in case of solitary metastasis, onset after several years from the extirpation of the primary tumor in a healthy patient. In this case, surgery should extirpate the metastasis obtaining a wide margin.
- Palliative aim: in multimetastatic patient in case of
  - Impending and already-occurred fracture: quite rare indication considering that prostate metastasis is usually osteoblastic
  - Pain lesion
  - Spinal cord compression

The techniques can be classified in two main groups:

- Resections techniques, where a wide margin is aimed
- Stabilization technique, with an exclusively biomechanical value

A. Luzzati (✉) • G. Scotto • G. Perrucchini
Oncological and Reconstructive Center, I.R.C.C.S. Istituto Ortopedico Galeazzi, Milan, Italy
e-mail: alessandro.luzzati@gmail.com

C. Zoccali
Oncological Orthopedics Unit, Regina Elena National Cancer Institute, Rome, Italy

They will be progressively shown basing on the bone segment where they are applied.

13.1 Vertebral Metastases Techniques

Approximately 70 % of all bone metastases are located in the spine, most frequently involved in the thoracic vertebras (60–70 %), followed by lumbar (15–30 %), and more rarely, cervical (less than 10 %). About half of metastatic spine patients experience multiple level lesions [7, 8].

To identify the best approach, the patient survival has to be estimated; in literature several scores are available [9], but, even if it underwent a recent criticism [10], the most used is the modified Tokuhashi score [11]. The authors individuated six parameters, including general condition, extraspinal bone metastasis, number of metastasis in the vertebral body, visceral metastasis, primary site, and severity of cord palsy. For each parameter a value between 0 and 2 is assigned, but for primary site, a value between 0 and 5 is assigned. Based on the total score, the patient is designated to one of three possible survival classes:

- Group I (score 0–8): survival inferior to 6 months
- Group II (score 9–11): survival inferior to 12 months
- Group III (score 12–15): survival superior to 12 months

F. Bertoldo et al. (eds.), *Bone Metastases from Prostate Cancer*,
DOI 10.1007/978-3-319-42327-2_13

Tokuhashi suggested conservative or palliative treatment for patients in groups I and II, with multiple vertebral lesions. Excisional surgery was suggested for group III and patients in group II with single spinal metastases.

In case of prostate metastasis, the value to assign to primary site is 5 (?) because of its favorable intrinsic prognosis.

Drzymalski et al. [12], in a study on 333 patients affected by spinal metastasis, evidenced as the median survival after diagnosis of spinal metastasis was 24 months, but among the 28 patients with a solitary vertebral metastasis, the median survival was 55.9.

A higher prostate-specific antigen (PSA) level at diagnosis of metastasis, the presence of additional metastasis at diagnosis of spinal metastasis, and a long free of disease time between the diagnosis of prostate cancer and spinal metastasis resulted as independent prognostic factors ($p=0.0001$).

13.1.1 En Bloc Vertebrectomy

En bloc vertebrectomy is a high-demanding surgery with a high complication rate so indication has to be reserved just for selected cases [9]. It should be performed in case of solitary lesion, occurred in healthy patient at several years from the extirpation of the primary tumor.

Surgery is usually performed by a posterior approach for the dorsal spine and upper lumbar spine, whereas a preparatory anterior approach is advisable for lower lumbar levels to divide vascular bundles from the mass and the near-spine elements (Fig. 13.1).

Cervical en bloc vertebrectomy is technically more difficult so no case is evident in literature for metastatic patients.

13.1.2 Stabilization and Intralesional Surgery (Curettage)

In case of risk of fracture, or in case of spinal cord compression, patients enrolled in group II of Tokuhashi (intermediate survival) decompression and/or stabilization could be a good solution.

In 2012, Crnalic et al. [13] identified a new specific score for patient with cord compression from prostate cancer; the items include hormone status of prostate cancer, Karnofsky performance status, evidence of visceral metastasis, and preoperative serum prostate-specific antigen (PSA). They identified three specific prognostic groups corresponding to different score:

- Group A (score 0–1), with a median survival of 3 months
- Group B (score 2–4), with a median survival of 16 months
- Group C (score 5–6), where more the half part of the patients were alive at publication of their experience

Patients with a score higher than 2 are more suitable to undergo surgery in case of spinal cord compression.

Stabilization alone is rare, considering the high frequency of osteoblastic lesions; nevertheless it can be fundamental in case of spinal cord compression; indeed, the following decompression can cause an iatrogenic instability.

Decompression can be performed both from anterior and posterior approach basing on the metastasis-specific localization, the spine level, and the surgeon expertise. In the thoracic spine, decompression should be performed from an anterior approach because the presence of the spinal cord could make difficult and effective decompression from a midline posterior access; nevertheless, cutting roots could be useful to have access to the vertebral body from behind.

At lumbar levels the presence of cauda equina allows an easier access to the anterior metastatic bodies.

Posterior stabilization is the most commune; it is performed by posterior midline incision or also by minimally invasive approach consisting in little incisions corresponding to the pedicles necessary for the screw insertion through the pedicle [14].

Several instrumentations are commercially available, but nowadays carbon fiber-reinforced rods should be preferred [15]. Indeed, they should allow a more effective adjuvant radiotherapy because it is characterized by a lower level of artifacts.

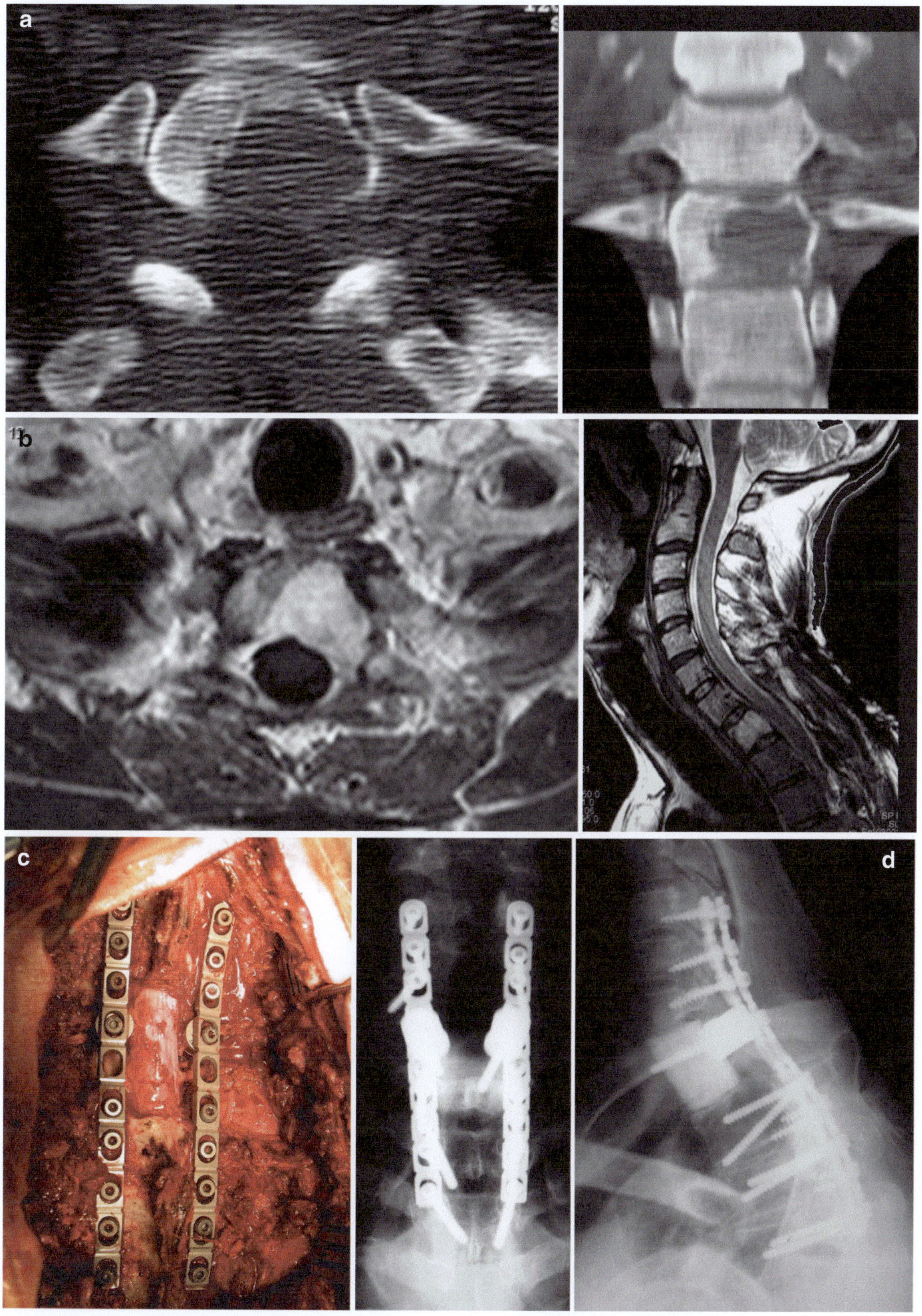

Fig. 13.1 A D1 solitary osteolytic metastasis; the 56-year- old patient underwent en bloc vertebrectomy and reconstruction with homoplastic diaphysis segment filled with the autoplastic morcellized bone, plates, and screws; (**a**) preoperative CT scan showing an osteolytic lesion in the D1 vertebral body, (**b**) preoperative MRI, (**c**) intraoperative imaging showing posterior stabilization, and (**d**) a 2-year follow-up X-ray

The artifacts at CT scan blind some areas in the surrounding tissue, introducing diffraction and refraction phenomena, so the actual dose administered to the tissues becomes unpredictable.

Anterior stabilization can be done with a body cage alone or with anterior plating and screws; also in those cases, carbon fiber cages should be preferred [16, 17].

13.1.3 Augmentation Technique

Cement plasty (Kyphoplasty, vertebroplasty, vesselplasty): these techniques are very commune in osteoporotic fractures; nevertheless they can have indication also in metastatic lesion.

In case of metastatic spinal fracture, they can be able to stabilize it in a minimally invasive way, even if attention has to be paid for possible posterior cement or tumor migration.

Indeed, spine metastasis from prostate cancer difficultly causes body fracture, but they can cause important not responsive pain that can be effectively treated with these techniques [18, 19].

The procedure can be performed by monoportal or biportal transpedicular approach basing on the specific necessity of stabilization; the integrity of the posterior body wall is essential for safety performing the procedure (Fig. 13.2).

13.2 Femoral Metastases Techniques

Proximal femur is the most commune site of metastasis, after the spine [20].

Even if the treatment of these lesions should not modify directly the survival from a biological/oncological point of view, the patient constricted to bed because of risk of fracture is exposed to complications that could interfere with medical therapies decreasing survival [21, 22].

Otherwise survival estimation is important as in the other sites for the best therapeutic strategy, but in case of metastases located in the limbs and moreover in the proximal femur, an important problem is to value the fracture risk [23].

Several systems are available, but the most used is the Mirel's classification [24]; it identifies four items: location of the metastasis, its nature and radiographic appearance, its size related to the diameter of the entire segment, and the presence of pain.

Each item is scaled from 1 to 3.

When the total score is 7 or less, observation and radiation therapy is advisable; when it is 9 or more, prophylactic fixation is suggested; if the score is 8, the indication is uncertain, and it should be valued basing on clinical conditions as well.

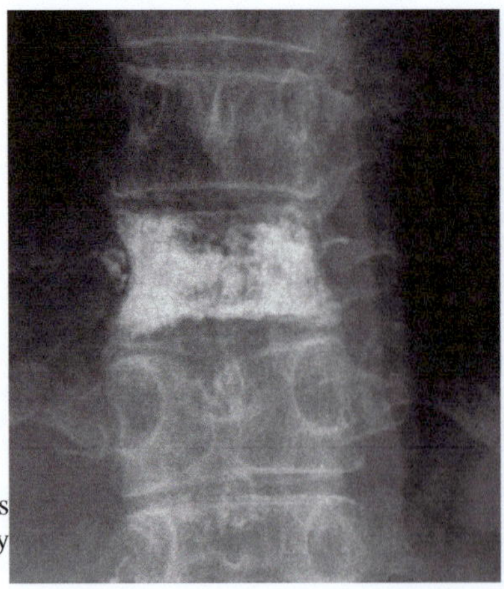

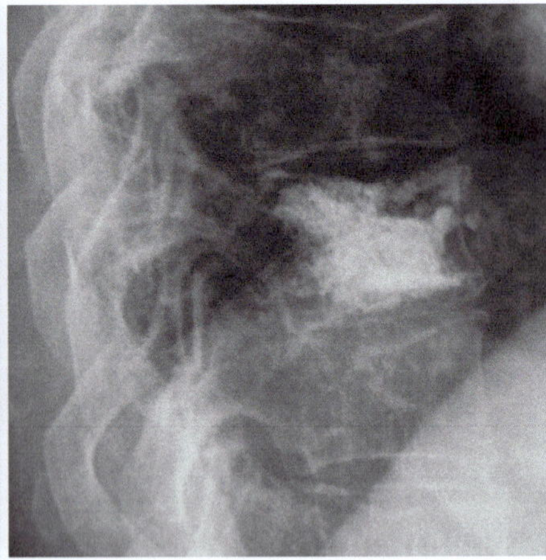

Fig. 13.2 A percutaneous vertebroplasty performed by biportal approach

	1	2	3
Location	Upper extremity	Lower extremity	Intertrochanteric
Radiographic appearance	Blastic	Mixed	Lytic
Size	<1/3	1/3–2/3	>2/3
Pain	Mild	Moderate	Severe and functional

The metastasis of prostate cancer is usually osteoblastic so surgical indication is usually less frequent than metastases from other primitive tumors.

13.2.1 Proximal Femur Resection and Prosthesis Reconstruction

In case of solitary lesion, in a healthy patient after several years from the primary tumor eradication, wide surgery has to be preferred. This means performing a resection of the proximal part of the femur which is extended distally about 2 cm distally to the inferior edge of the disease.

Reconstruction is performed with a modular prosthesis which is assembled to reach the resection size [25–27]; the intramedullary stem should be as long as possible to reinforce the entire femur, stabilizing the segment also in case of further distal metastasis onset. When the greater and the lower trochanters are not involved, they should be spared to maintain the muscular insertion (Fig. 13.3). The psoas muscle is the most important stabilizer.

An ideal modular prosthesis should allow a minimal resection, arming the entire femur when necessary; it should be cemented to assure the grip even in case of further metastasis.

Resection has to be preferred also in case of multimetastatic patients when the disease extends also in the head and femoral neck; intramedullary nailing should complicate with proximal screws cut out.

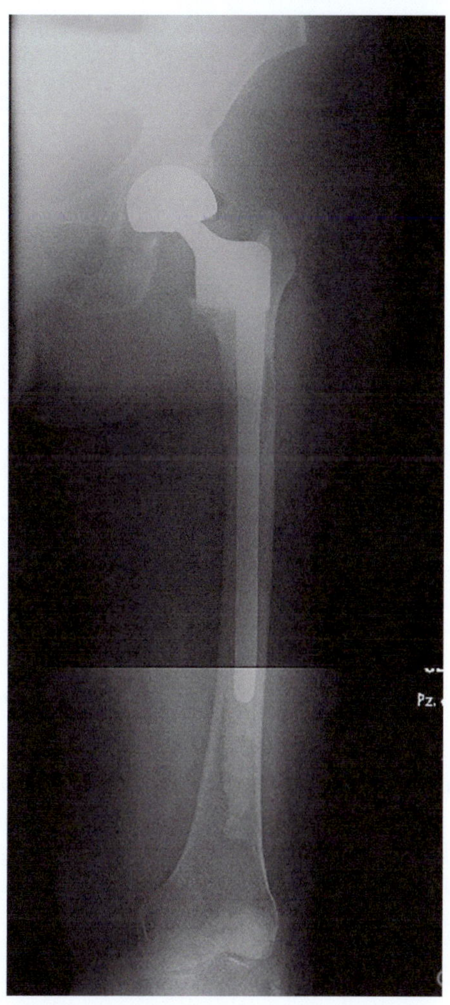

Fig. 13.3 A postoperative X-ray showing a hip prosthesis where the greater and lower trochanters and their muscular insertions were spared

13.2.2 Diaphysis Resection and Reconstruction

The indication to resection in the diaphysis is the same of that of the proximal femur. Obviously it is very rare. Reconstruction can be performed with a diaphyseal prosthesis (Fig. 13.4) or a homologous diaphysis filled with cement and stabilized with plate and screws [28].

13.2.3 Intramedullary Stabilization

Intramedullary stabilization is the mainstay treatment in case of fractures or impeding fractures of

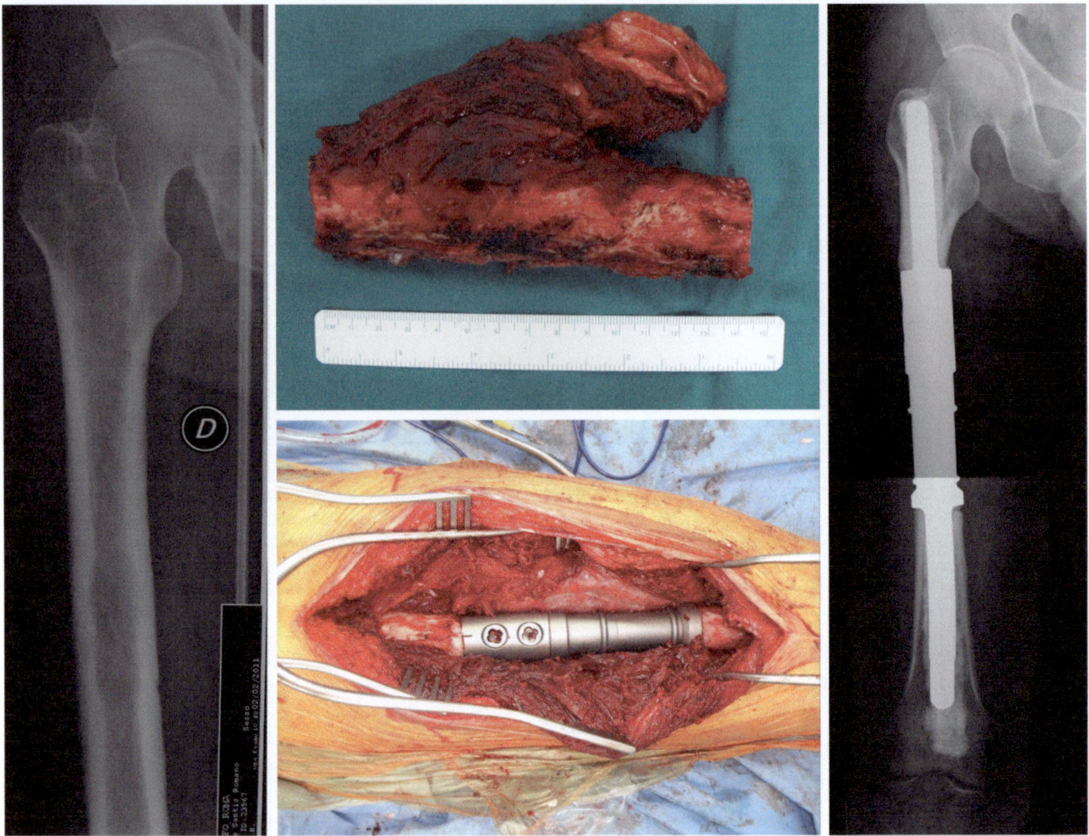

Fig. 13.4 A solitary lesion of the femur diaphysis *on the left*; in the upper center figure the resected specimen and in the lower center picture a diaphyseal prosthesis; *on the right* the postoperative X-ray

lesions located from the trochanteric area until the distal diaphysis in multimetastatic patient [29]. Surgery aims to allow weight bearing as soon as possible so that the patient can undergo chemotherapy.

The nail must be always long and stabilizes the entire femur; it has to be distally locked, and a cervical screw must be always present even in case of diaphyseal metastasis considering the high frequency of femoral neck lesions: the screw in the femoral head will stabilize the femur also in case of successive metastasis (Fig. 13.5) even if a recent study sustains that it is not always necessary [30].

Intramedullary nailing has exclusively a biomechanical role; the treatment has to be completed by adjuvant radiotherapy; in case of not radiosensitive tumors, a wide resection could be indicated also in multimetastatic patients because of the inefficiency of adjuvant therapy.

Considering that, carbon fiber-reinforced nails are to be preferred in case of diaphyseal metastasis (Fig. 13.6); unfortunately, a carbon fiber nail with a cephalic screw is now not commercially available.

Also other cytoreductive technique can be associated as cryotherapy, radio-frequency thermoablation, or embolization [31]. Weight bearing has to be valued for every specific case.

13.2.4 Distal Femur Resection and Prosthesis Reconstruction

When metastasis is located in the distal part of the femur, where it is not possible to stabilize the

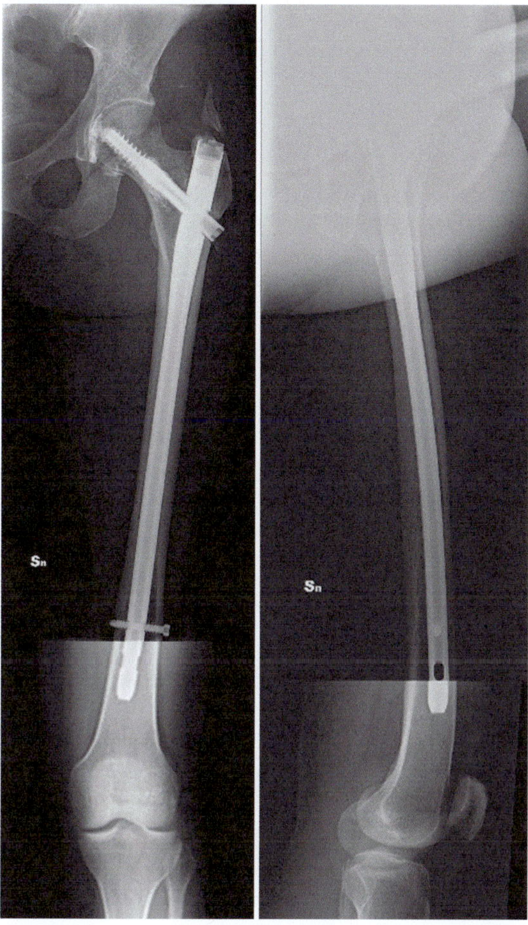

Fig. 13.5 In intramedullary nailing for an impending fracture of the proximal femur. The proximal neck screw and the extension for all the femur protect the patient in case of further metastasis as well

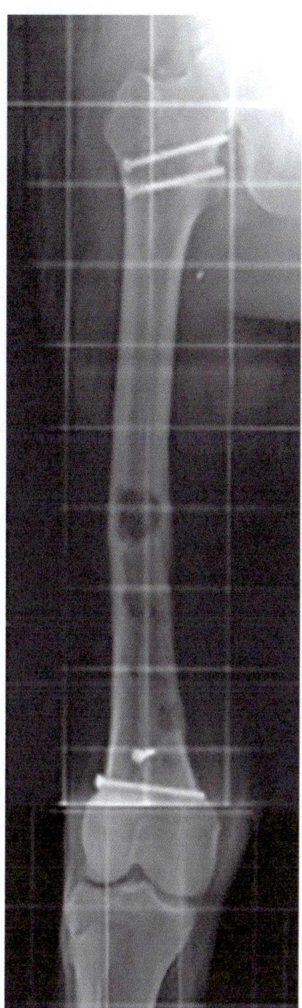

Fig. 13.6 A carbon fiber nail inserted in an impending fracture

segment with an intramedullary nailing, resection and prosthesis reconstruction is necessary. Nevertheless indication is very rare.

13.3 Tibial Metastases Techniques

13.3.1 Proximal Tibial Resection and Prosthesis Reconstruction

Rarely, in case of lesions located in the proximal part of the tibia, resection and prosthesis reconstruction can be indicated, moreover in case of single metastasis.

In case of multimetastatic disease, minimally invasive technique as cement augmentation could be preferred to allow weight bearing with a minimal impact.

13.3.2 Intramedullary Stabilization

Intramedullary stabilization is the most frequent operation performed on the metastatic tibia [32]. As in the femur, the nail has to be long and locked distally (Fig. 13.7). Weight bearing has to be valued for every specific case.

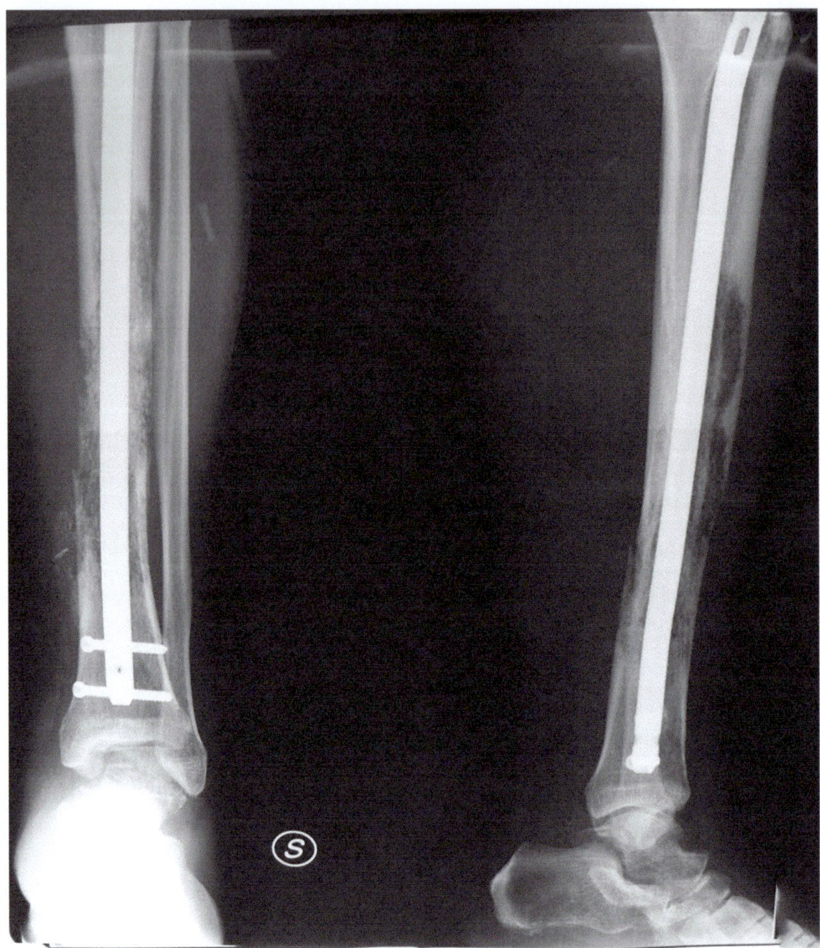

Fig. 13.7 A locked tibial nail for an extensive diaphyseal prostate metastasis

13.4 Humerus Metastases Techniques

Indications for surgery in superior limbs are very rare in prostate cancer metastases because the risk of fracture is very low, because of the lower load than inferior limbs, and because of the osteoblastic nature of the lesions [33].

13.4.1 Proximal Humerus Resection and Prosthesis Reconstruction

In case of solitary lesion of the proximal femur, onset after years from the primary tumor eradication in a healthy patient, wide resection and prosthesis reconstruction is indicated (Fig. 13.8).

The reconstruction possibilities are two: the standard prosthesis and the inverted (?) prosthesis. In the first case, the prosthesis mimics the normal anatomy; in the inverted prosthesis, the concave surface is on the humeral part, whereas the convex side is on the scapular side. The second one is preferred when it is possible to spare the deltoid muscle and circumflex nerve so that abduction could be still possible even after wide resection [34].

13.4.2 Diaphysis Resection and Reconstruction

Indication of wide resection in humeral diaphysis is the same with that in the proximal humerus.

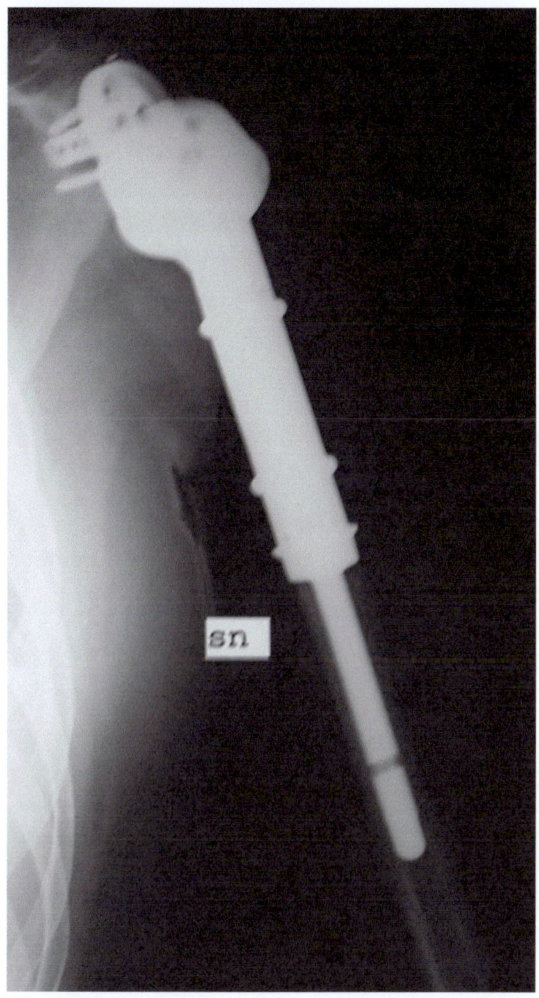

Fig. 13.8 Postoperative X-ray showing reverse prosthesis reconstruction after proximal humerus resection

Reconstruction can be performed with diaphyseal prosthesis or by homograft.

13.4.3 Intramedullary Stabilization

Lesion located in the proximal humerus and in the diaphysis in multimetastatic patients can be treated by intramedullary nailing (Fig. 13.9) [35].

Nevertheless, indication is very rare in prostate cancer, especially considering the prevalent osteoblastic nature of the lesions. Several nailing systems are commercially available; in the humerus, besides carbon-fiber nails is available also a liquid nailing system constituted by a monomer which becomes hard when exposed to UV light; then it can be drilled and screwed to stabilize fracture and impending fracture, allowing adjuvant radiotherapy (Fig. 13.10) [36].

13.5 Scapular Metastases

Scapular metastases from prostate cancer are quite commune. In case of solitary lesions, indication for wide resection has to be valued basing on clinical conditions. In multimetastatic patient no risk of fracture is present, so minimally invasive techniques should be preferred; sometimes, a partial or a total scapulectomy can be indicated also in multimetastatic patients, for big size lesion at risk for skin ulceration.

Reconstruction is not always performed, moreover in case of total scapulectomy when rotatory cuff muscles are not preserved (Fig. 13.11).

No modular prosthesis is commercially available so reconstruction has to be performed using homograft or custom-made [37].

13.6 Pelvic Metastases Techniques

The pelvis is a frequent site for metastasis, but usually they do not require surgical treatment because they are often stable, mostly in case of prostate metastases.

Indications for resection have to be valued case by case considering that resection surgery can be very difficult in case of lesions located in the acetabular area but quite easy if located in the wings. Solitary lesion onset in a healthy patient several years after resection could undergo wide resection.

In case of osteolytic metastasis in the acetabular roof, minimally invasive cement augmentation could be helpful to allow an early weight bearing (Fig. 13.12) [38, 39].

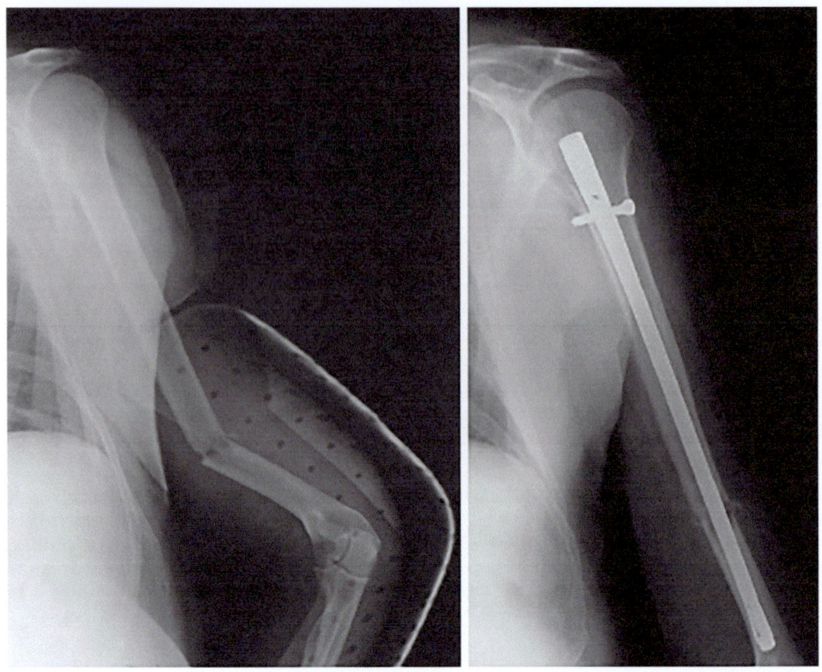

Fig. 13.9 Postoperative X-ray showing intramedullary humerus stabilization

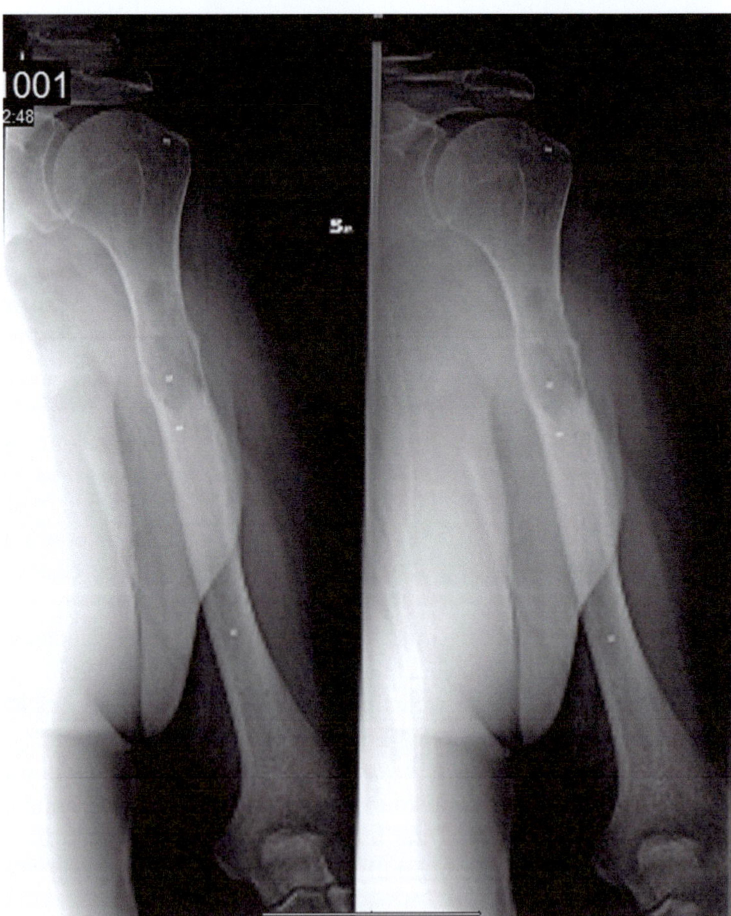

Fig. 13.10 A liquid nail used to stabilize an impending fracture of the humerus; a soft shell is inserted inside the medullary canal, then it is filled with a monomer: the exposition to a UV light causes polymerization and its hardening

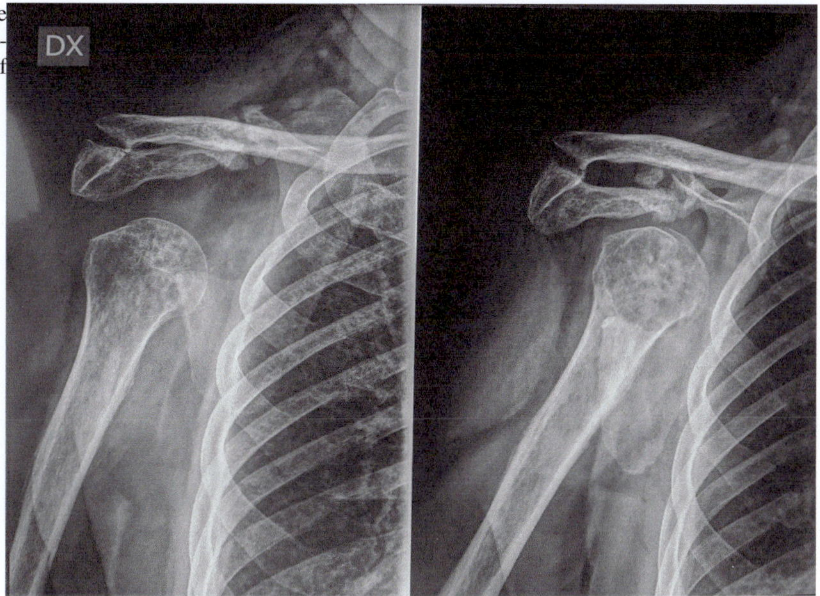

Fig. 13.11 A postopera-tive X-ray after partial scapulectomy for solitary metastasis of prostate cancer

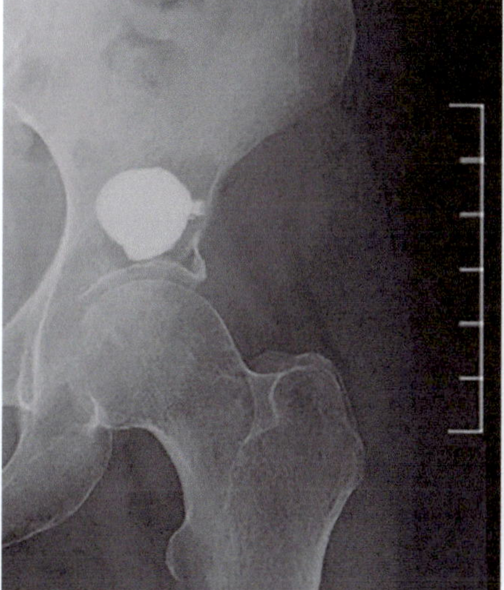

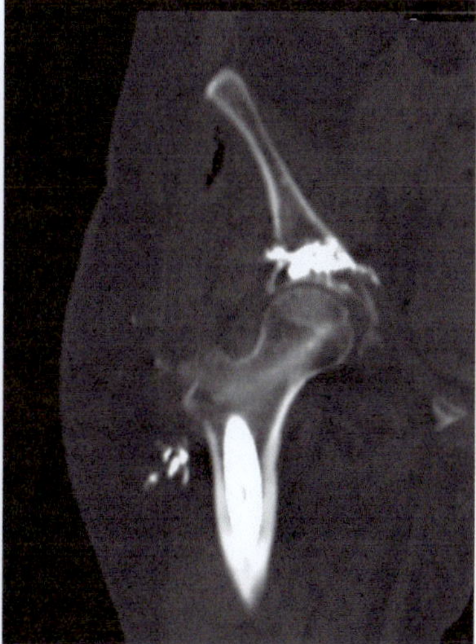

Fig. 13.12 On the left is an acetabuloplasty performing with a system which partially maintains inside the cement; on the right the direct filling of the acetabular is in the roof

13.7 Complications

13.7.1 Bone Explosion (During Intramedullary Stabilization)

The bone affected by prostate cancer metastasis is harder than normal but less elastic as well. In case of intramedullary stabilization, particular attention has to be paid during the reaming; indeed, the nail should be inserted inside the femur without effort. Hammering the nail can cause the femur fracture, as shown in the picture (Fig. 13.13); wiring the fracture is useless because it will hardly heal. A nail removal, resection of the proximal femur, and prosthesis reconstruction were then scheduled.

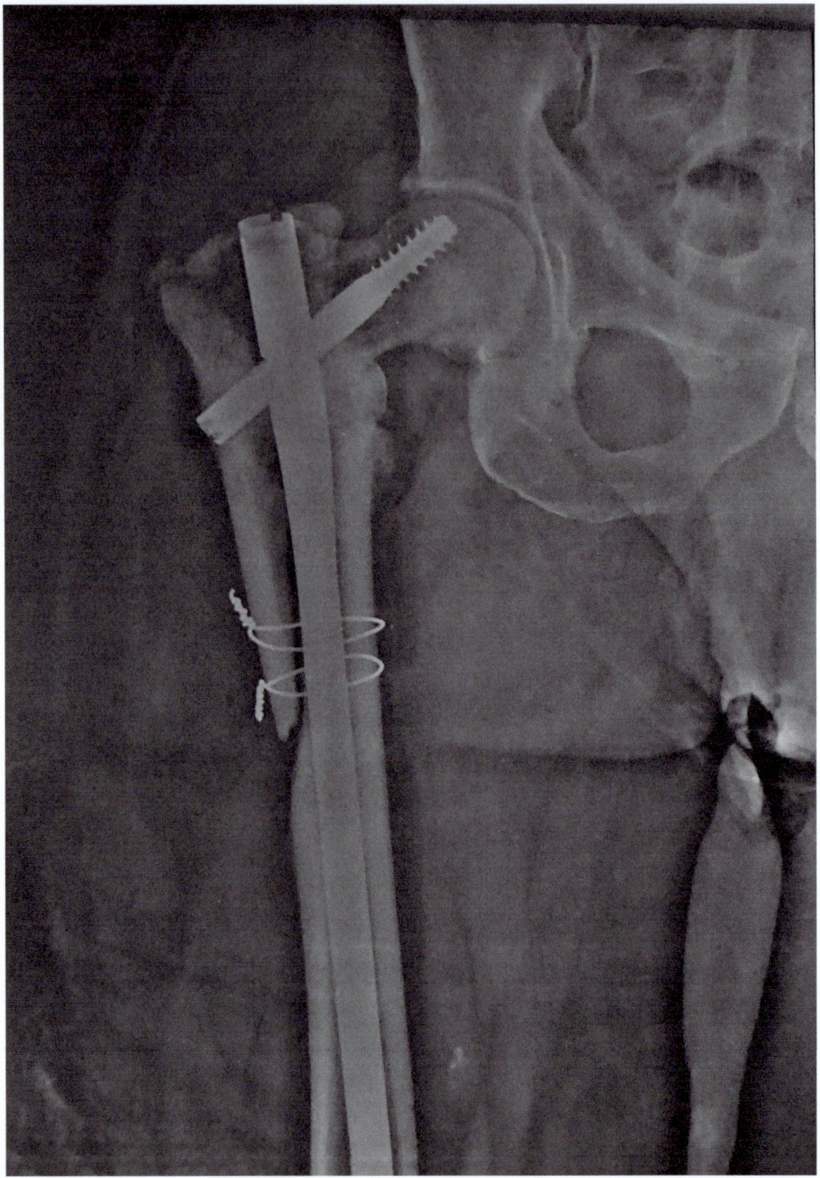

Fig. 13.13 A failure surgery. In this case the nail was hammered inside the medullary canal, but this caused its explosion; the surgeon unsuccessfully tried to stabilize it with wiring. The patient has to undergo further surgery of resection and prosthesis reconstruction

13.7.2 Corticalization of the Trabecular Bone (Cutter Rupture) (Fig. 13.14)

Prostate metastases are osteoblastic in most cases; it is not rare to see total or subtotal substitution of a segment as shown in the following picture. Cutting and drilling the bone can be very difficult, and a right strategy has to be valued every time before surgery. In the last square, it is possible to note the cutter broken inside the medullary corticalized (Fig. 13.14). In that case a little fenestration was done in the femur for its removal.

13.8 Adjuvant Techniques

The minimally invasive cytoreduction techniques play an important role in case of prostate cancer, because in most cases, no mechanical instability is present, and they can guarantee a good effect, particularly on the pain.

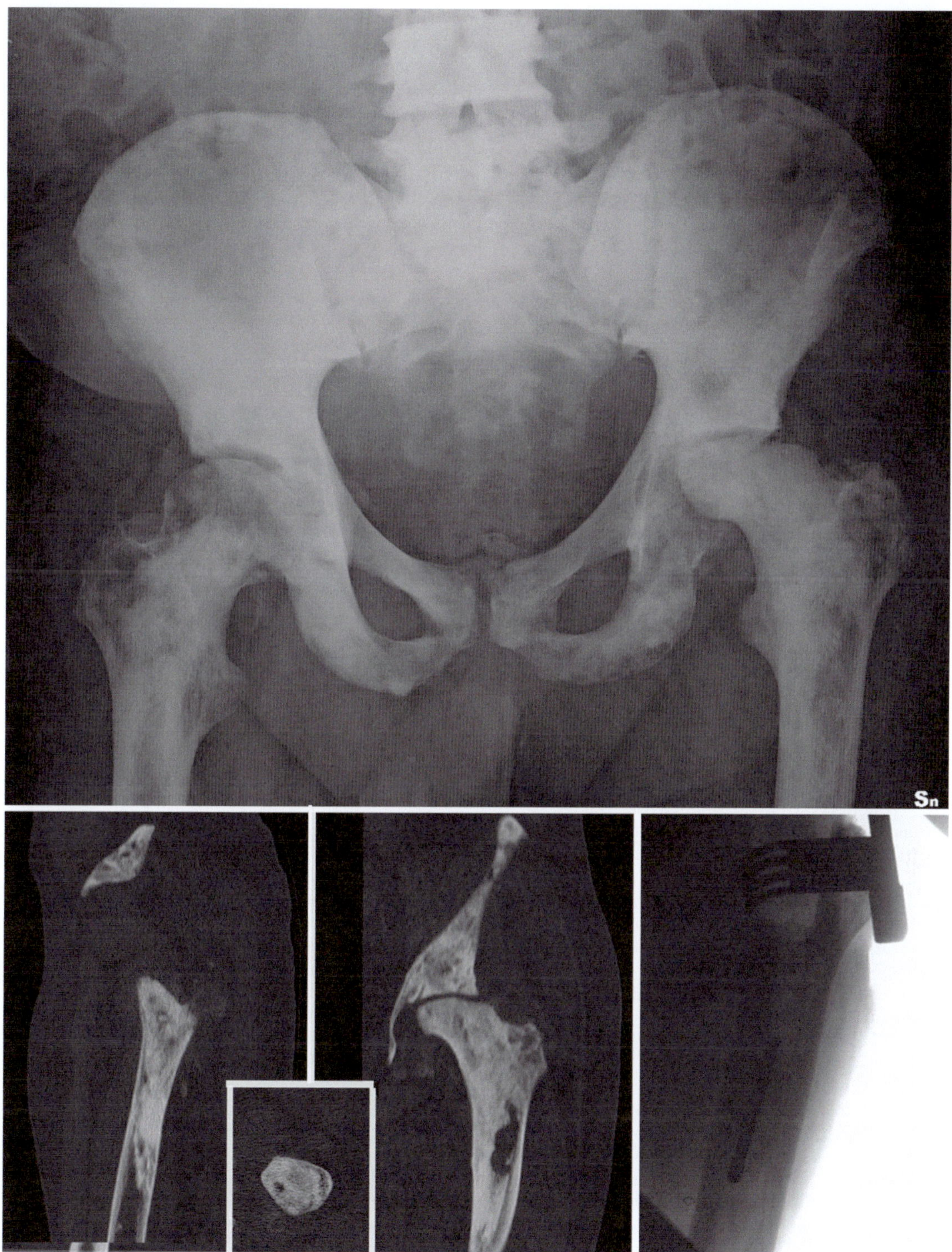

Fig. 13.14 A subtotal substitution of the normal bone from prostate cancer metastases. In this case, resection was performed just for mechanical problem, but the medullary drilling was problematic because of the hardness of the segment so that the cutter broke inside

Cryotherapy and radio-frequency thermoablation are probably the most commune; they are less invasive, and the treatment can be completed with adjuvant radiotherapy [31].

References

1. Westhoff PG, de Graeff A, Monninkhof EM, Pomp J, van Vulpen M, Leer JW, Marijnen CA, van der Linden YM, Dutch Bone Metastasis Study Group (2015) Quality of life in relation to pain response to radiation therapy for painful bone metastases. Int J Radiat Oncol Biol Phys 93(3):694–701
2. Conde Moreno AJ, Ferrer Albiach C, Muelas Soria R, González Vidal V, García Gómez R, Albert AM (2014) Oligometastases in prostate cancer: restaging stage IV cancers and new radiotherapy options. Radiat Oncol 9:258
3. Smith MR, Saad F, Oudard S, Shore N, Fizazi K, Sieber P, Tombal B, Damiao R, Marx G, Miller K, Van Veldhuizen P, Morote J, Ye Z, Dansey R, Goessl C (2013) Denosumab and bone metastasis-free survival in men with nonmetastatic castration-resistant prostate cancer: exploratory analyses by baseline prostate-specific antigen doubling time. J Clin Oncol 31(30):3800–3806
4. Gül G, Sendur MA, Aksoy S, Sever AR, Altundag K (2016) A comprehensive review of denosumab for bone metastasis in patients with solid tumors. Curr Med Res Opin 32(1):133–145
5. Vignani F, Bertaglia V, Buttigliero C, Tucci M, Scagliotti GV, Di Maio M (2016) Skeletal metastases and impact of anticancer and bone-targeted agents in patients with castration-resistant prostate cancer. Cancer Treat Rev 44:61–73
6. Singh T, Kaur V, Kumar M, Kaur P, Murthy RS, Rawal RK (2015) The critical role of bisphosphonates to target bone cancer metastasis: an overview. J Drug Target 23(1):1–15
7. Delank KS, Wendtner C, Eich HT, Eysel P (2011) The treatment of spinal metastases. Dtsch Arzt Int 108:71–U27
8. Bartels RHMA, van der Linden YM, van der Graaf WTA (2008) Spinal extradural metastasis: review of current treatment options. CA Cancer J Clinicians 58:245–259
9. Tomita K, Kawahara N, Kobayashi T, Yoshida A, Murakami H, Akamaru T (2001) Surgical strategy for spinal metastases. Spine (Phila Pa 1976) 26(3):298–306
10. Zoccali C, Skoch J, Walter CM, Torabi M, Borgstrom M, Baaj AA (2015) The Tokuhashi score: effectiveness and pitfalls. Eur Spine J 1
11. Tokuhashi Y, Matsuzaki H, Oda H, Oshima M, Ryu J (2005) A revised scoring system for preoperative evaluation of metastatic spine tumor prognosis. Spine (Phila Pa 1976) 30(19):2186–2191
12. Drzymalski DM, Oh WK, Werner L, Regan MM, Kantoff P, Tuli S (2010) Predictors of survival in patients with prostate cancer and spinal metastasis. Presented at the 2009 Joint Spine Section Meeting. Clinical article. J Neurosurg Spine 13(6):789–794
13. Crnalic S, Löfvenberg R, Bergh A, Widmark A, Hildingsson C (2012) Predicting survival for surgery of metastatic spinal cord compression in prostate cancer: a new score. Spine (Phila Pa 1976) 37(26): 2168–2176
14. Rao PJ, Thayaparan GK, Fairhall JM, Mobbs RJ (2014) Minimally invasive percutaneous fixation techniques for metastatic spinal disease. Orthop Surg 6(3):187–195
15. Weimin H, Zhengqi C, Ruoxian S, Ke Z, Xiuchun Y (2016) Non-fusion procedure using PEEK rod systems for lumbar degenerative diseases: clinical experience with a 2-year follow-up. BMC Musculoskelet Disord 17:53
16. Heary RF, Kheterpal A, Mammis A, Kumar S (2011) Stackable carbon fiber cages for thoracolumbar interbody fusion after corpectomy: long-term outcome analysis. Neurosurgery 68(3):810–818
17. Disch AC, Schaser KD, Melcher I, Luzzati A, Feraboli F, Schmoelz W (2008) En bloc spondylectomy reconstructions in a biomechanical in-vitro study. Eur Spine J 17(5):715–725
18. Farrokhi M, Nouraei H, Kiani A (2012) The efficacy of percutaneous vertebroplasty in pain relief in patients with pathological vertebral fractures due to metastatic spinal tumors. Iran Red Crescent Med J 14(9):523–530
19. Cheung G, Chow E, Holden L et al (2006) Percutaneous vertebroplasty in patients with intractable pain from osteoporotic or metastatic fractures: a prospective study using quality-of-life assessment. Can Assoc Radiol J 57(1):13–21
20. Campanacci M (1999) Bone and soft tissue tumors. Springer, Wien/New York
21. Zacherl M, Gruber G, Glehr M, Ofner-Kopeinig P, Radl R, Greitbauer M, Vecsei V, Windhager R (2011) Surgery for pathological proximal femoral fractures, excluding femoral head and neck fractures: resection vs. stabilisation. Int Orthop 35(10):1537–1543
22. Camnasio F, Scotti C, Peretti GM, Fontana F, Fraschini G (2008) Prosthetic joint replacement for long bone metastases: analysis of 154 cases. Arch Orthop Trauma Surg 128(8):787–793
23. Mavrogenis AF, Pala E, Romagnoli C, Romantini M, Calabro T, Ruggieri P (2012) Survival analysis of patients with femoral metastases. J Surg Oncol 105(2):135–141
24. Mirels H. Metastatic disease in long bones: a proposed scoring system for diagnosing impending pathologic fractures. 1989. Clin Orthop Relat Res. 2003;(415 Suppl):S4–13.
25. Guzik G (2016) Results of the treatment of bone metastases with modular prosthetic replacement-analysis of 67 patients. J Orthop Surg Res 11(1):20

26. Henrichs MP, Krebs J, Gosheger G, Streitbuerger A, Nottrott M, Sauer T, Hoell S, Singh G, Hardes J (2014) Modular tumor endoprostheses in surgical palliation of long-bone metastases: a reduction in tumor burden and a durable reconstruction. World J Surg Oncol 12:330
27. Chandrasekar CR, Grimer RJ, Carter SR, Tillman RM, Abudu A, Buckley L (2009) Modular endoprosthetic replacement for tumours of the proximal femur. J Bone Joint Surg Br 91(1):108–112
28. Benevenia J, Kirchner R, Patterson F, Beebe K, Wirtz DC, Rivero S, Palma M, Friedrich MJ (2015) Outcomes of a Modular Intercalary Endoprosthesis as Treatment for Segmental Defects of the Femur, Tibia, and Humerus. Clin Orthop Relat Res 474(2):539–548
29. Fasano FJ Jr, Olysav DJ, Stauffer ES (1988) Intramedullary stabilization of neoplastic destructive disease involving the subtrochanteric region of the femur. Orthopedics 11(12):1699–1704
30. Moon B, Lin P, Satcher R, Bird J, Lewis V (2015) Intramedullary nailing of femoral diaphyseal metastases: is it necessary to protect the femoral neck? Clin Orthop Relat Res 473(4):1499–1502. doi:10.1007/s11999-014-4064-1
31. Di Francesco A, Flamini S, Zugaro L, Zoccali C (2012) Preoperative radiofrequency ablation in painful osteolytic long bone metastases. Acta Orthop Belg 78(4):523–530
32. De Geeter K, Reynders P, Samson I, Broos PL (2001) Metastatic fractures of the tibia. Acta Orthop Belg 67(1):54–59
33. Schwabe P, Ruppert M, Tsitsilonis S, Melcher I, Schaser KD, Märdian S (2014) Surgical management and outcome of skeletal metastatic disease of the humerus. Acta Chir Orthop Traumatol Cech 81(6):365–370
34. Subhadrabandhu S, Takeuchi A, Yamamoto N, Shirai T, Nishida H, Hayashi K, Miwa S, Tsuchiya H (2015) Frozen autograft-prosthesis composite reconstruction in malignant bone tumors. Orthopedics 38(10): e911–e918
35. Laitinen M, Nieminen J, Pakarinen TK (2011) Treatment of pathological humerus shaft fractures with intramedullary nails with or without cement fixation. Arch Orthop Trauma Surg 131(4):503–508
36. Zani BG, Baird R, Stanley JR, Markham PM, Wilke M, Zeiter S, Beck A, Nehrbass D, Kopia GA, Edelman ER, Rabiner R (2016) Evaluation of an intramedullary bone stabilization system using a light-curable monomer in sheep. J Biomed Mater Res B Appl Biomater 104(2):291–299
37. Capanna R, Totti F, Van der Geest IC, Müller DA (2015) Scapular allograft reconstruction after total scapulectomy: surgical technique and functional results. J Shoulder Elbow Surg 24(8):e203–e211
38. Colman MW, Karim SM, Hirsch JA, Yoo AJ, Schwab JH, Hornicek FJ, Raskin KA (2015) Percutaneous acetabuloplasty compared with open reconstruction for extensive periacetabular carcinoma metastases. J Arthroplasty 30(9):1586–1591
39. Zhang J, Yang Z, Wang J, Wang J, Liu P, Sun H, Li K, Yang Y (2012) Study of treatment using percutaneous acetabuloplasty and interstitial implantation of (125)I seeds for patients with metastatic periacetabular tumors. World J Surg Oncol 10:250

14 Bone Metastases from Prostate Cancer: Radiotherapy

Barbara Avuzzi and Riccardo Valdagni

14.1 Introduction

Radiotherapy is an effective treatment in patients with prostate cancer and metastatic bone disease. It has been in use for about a century, since radium has been found efficacious in the treatment of cancer. At the end of the 1960s, with the growth of high-energy radiation units, modern techniques of external beam irradiation (external beam radiation therapy (EBRT)) started to be routinely used. In subsequent years, technological evolution enabled the development of highly sophisticated treatment techniques, evolving from two-dimensional (2D) radiotherapy to three-dimensional conformal radiation therapy (3D-CRT) and, in the last two decades, to intensity-modulated radiation therapy (IMRT). IMRT main benefit is linked to the possibility to modulate the fluence of the beams, allowing an optimal dose distribution and enabling to irradiate structures with highly irregular shape close to critical organs [1, 2]. More recently, with the development of volumetric-modulated arc therapy (VMAT), an additional advantage in target volume coverage and normal tissue sparing has been reached, with a reduced treatment delivery time compared with IMRT [3, 4]. These techniques concur to improve tumor control and to reduce toxicity in the surrounding healthy tissues.

Radiotherapy evolution has had a relevant impact in the management of patients with bone metastases, developing from treatments with solely palliative aim (pain relief and skeletal event prevention) using traditional techniques (2D – 3D – hemibody irradiation) to more aggressive treatments whose purpose is to locally control metastatic sites and to try to improve survival. More sophisticated techniques, such as image-guided radiotherapy (IGRT), which makes use of imaging to improve the precision and accuracy of treatment delivery during radiation treatments, and stereotactic body radiotherapy (SBRT), with prescription and delivery of high radiation doses, are now part of the multimodal management of oligometastatic patients [5–8] (Figs. 14.1 and 14.2).

B. Avuzzi (✉)
Division of Radiation Oncology 1, Fondazione IRCCS Istituto Nazionale dei Tumori, via G. Venezian 1, Milan 20133, Italy

Prostate Cancer Program, Fondazione IRCCS Istituto Nazionale dei Tumori, Milan, Italy
e-mail: barbara.avuzzi@istitutotumori.mi.it

R. Valdagni
Division of Radiation Oncology 1, Fondazione IRCCS Istituto Nazionale dei Tumori, via G. Venezian 1, Milan 20133, Italy

Department of Diagnostic Imaging and Radiotherapy, Università degli Studi di Milano, Milan, Italy

Prostate Cancer Program, Fondazione IRCCS Istituto Nazionale dei Tumori, Milan, Italy

F. Bertoldo et al. (eds.), *Bone Metastases from Prostate Cancer*,
DOI 10.1007/978-3-319-42327-2_14

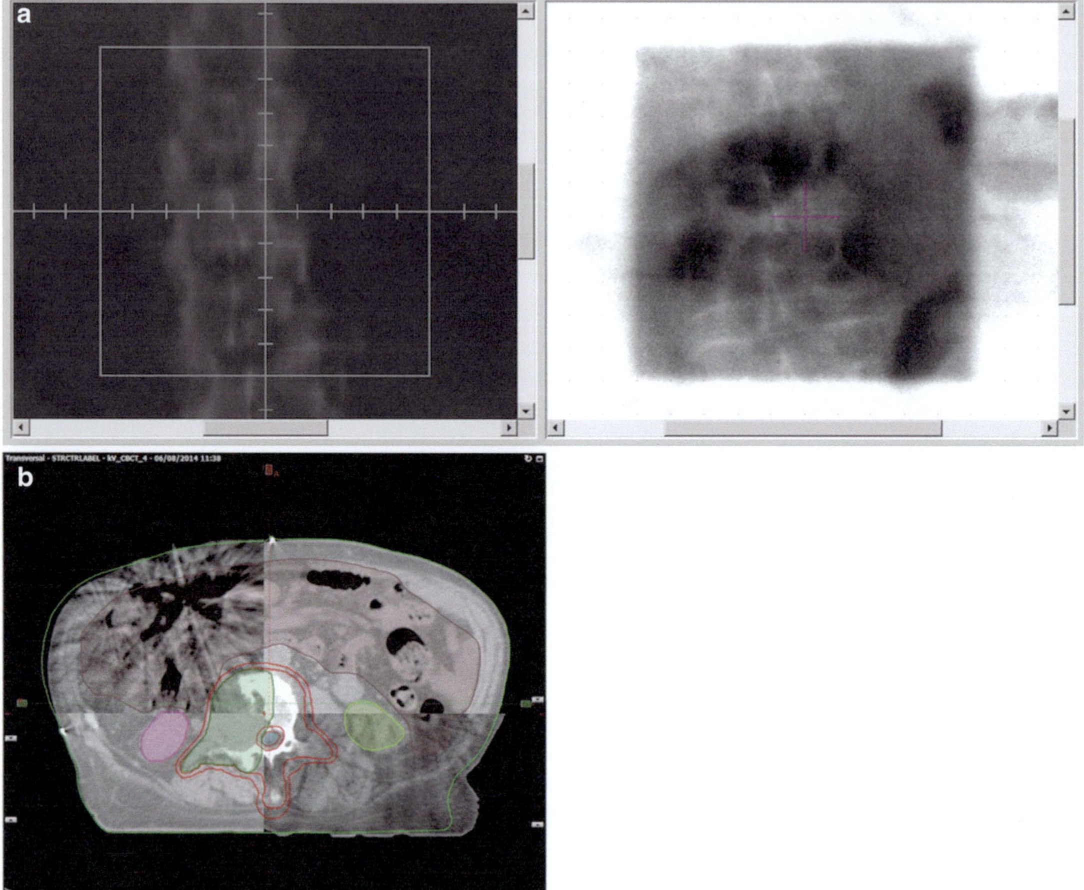

Fig. 14.1 Treatment delivery using portal imaging with digitally reconstructed radiograph (DRR) (**a**) and cone beam CT (**b**) to improve target visibility

14.2 External Beam Radiotherapy

Prostate cancer has a tropism for bone, which is frequently the first site of metastatic dissemination [9]. More than 80 % of men with prostate cancer have a radiological evidence of bone involvement, and skeletal complications are the major causes of comorbidity in these patients. According to the natural history of the disease, bone metastases are in general initially asymptomatic. Approximately 40 % of patients will be then affected by bone pain, 20 % will experience a pathologic fracture, and 5 % will develop a spinal cord compression [10]. EBRT has a crucial role in the treatment of bone metastases, particularly in symptomatic states of the disease. The primary goals of EBRT in these scenarios are as follows: palliation of pain, prevention of skeletal events (pathological fractures and spinal cord compressions), and reversion of neurological impairment due to compression of spinal cord or spinal nerves.

Studies conducted in these settings were essentially focused on the definition of optimal prescription of dose, on the effect of different dose schedules comparing both radiotherapy in single-fraction and multiple-fraction regimens,

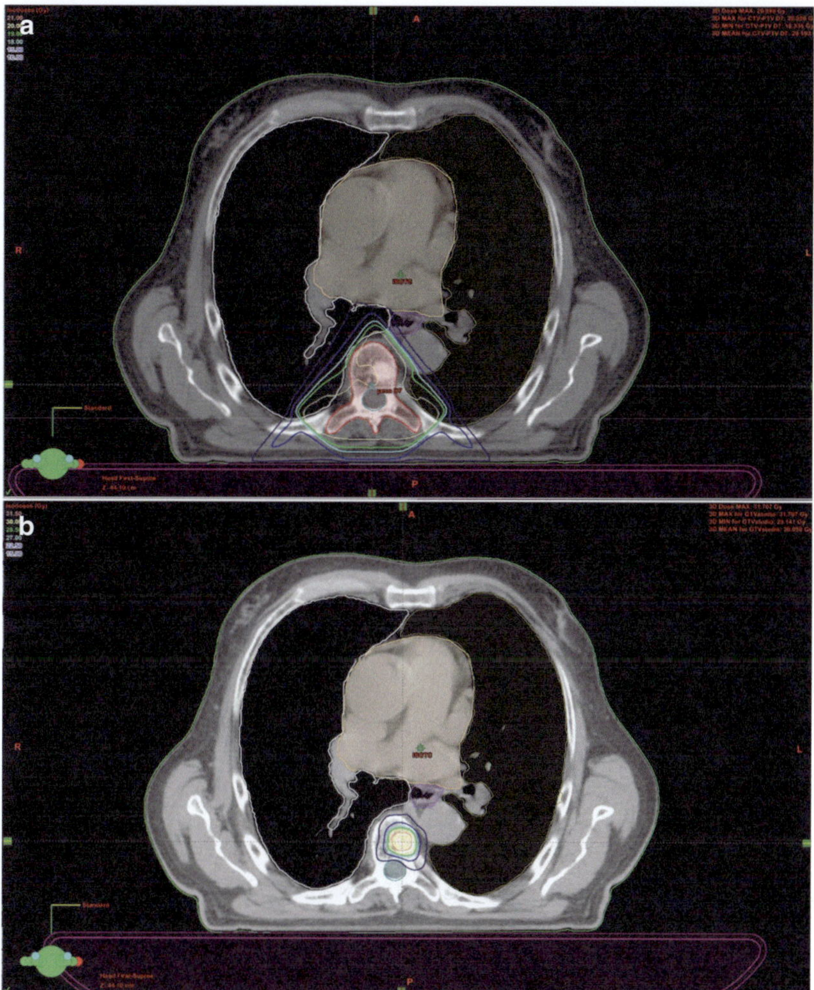

Fig. 14.2 Comparison between conventional planning with 3D-CRT (20 Gy/5 fractions) (**a**) and SBRT treatment with VMAT (30 Gy/3 fractions) (**b**) in a single vertebral metastatic localization

on the duration of pain relief, on the necessity and safety of re-treatment, and on management of metastatic spinal cord compression.

The association of zoledronic acid to androgen deprivation in patients with more aggressive diseases could have a potential role in the prevention of metastatic bone progression in the context of an integrate multimodal radiation treatment [11]. Preliminary results from the TROG 03.04 RADAR trial showed an advantage in biochemical control in patients with Gleason score 8–10 undergoing radical radiotherapy and long-term androgen deprivation therapy plus zoledronic acid [11]. This topic opens up a future perspective in the radiotherapy combinations and will not be further discussed in this chapter.

14.2.1 Radiation Dose and Fractionation

Radiation schedules in EBRT have been widely evaluated in several randomized and nonrandomized studies, all comparing single fraction with different multifractionated regimens.

The Bone Pain Trial Working Party published one of the three largest randomized trials (Table 14.1) of single versus multiple-fraction palliative EBRT [12]. Seven hundred and sixty-five patients were randomized to receive 8 Gy in one fraction vs. multifractionated regimen (20 Gy/5 fractions or 30 Gy/10 fractions). Primary endpoint was pain relief. With an overall survival of 44 % at 12 months, there were no

Table 14.1 Summary of studies on SBRT in bone metastases from prostate cancer

Author	Year	Number of patients	Dose/fractionation	Primary disease	Overall response rate	Re-treatment rate
Bone Pain Trial Working Party [12]	1999	761	8 Gy/1 (*n*=383) 20 Gy/5 or 30 Gy/10 (*n*=378)	Breast (36 %) Prostate (33 %) Lung (13 %) Other (16 %) Unknown (2 %)	78 % (no differences between two groups)	23 % (8 Gy/1) 10 % (20 Gy/5–30 Gy/10)
Steenland et al. (Dutch Bone Metastasis Study) [13]	1999	1171	8 Gy/1 (*n*=585) 4 Gy/6 (*n*=586)	Breast (39 %) Prostate (23 %) Lung (25 %) Other locations (13 %)	71 % (No differences between two groups)	25 % (8 Gy/1) 7 % (4 Gy/6)
Hartsell et al. [14]	2005	898	8 Gy/1 (*n*=455) 30 Gy/10 (*n*=443)	N.R.	66 % (no differences between two groups)	18 % (8 Gy/1) 9 % (30 Gy/10)

mts metastases, *ADT-FS* androgen deprivation therapy-free survival, *LC* local control, *DPFS* distant progression-free survival

differences between the two groups in time of pain response, pain relief, and first improvement of pain. Re-treatment rate was twofold in single-fraction group, with the same probability of pain relief after re-treatment in both groups. No differences in toxicities, spinal cord compression, or pathological fracture between single-fraction and multifractionated schedules were seen [12]. The Dutch Bone Metastasis Study had as primary goal the evaluation of efficacy of single-fraction 8 Gy compared to 4 Gy×6 fractions [13]. One thousand one hundred seventy-one patients were randomized to the two treatment schedules. Median survival was 7 months. Seventy-one percent of patients had pain relief at some time during the first year, and the two treatment schedules were equivalent in terms of palliation. Re-treatment rate was 16 % and was four times greater for single fraction; an acceptable pain relief was achieved. More pathological fractures were observed in single-fraction group, although the absolute percentage was low (3 %). No differences in treatment-related toxicities were found [13]. A subsequent analysis of the same study excluding re-treated patients confirmed that single fraction of 8 Gy was equally effective as 30 Gy in ten fractions. It was pointed out that response to initial treatment depended on the primary site of disease. Patients with prostate cancer had the lowest success rate, while patients with breast cancer had the highest percentages of response. Furthermore, re-treatment was found to be the most beneficial in patients treated with single fraction than in patients treated with multiple fractions [14]. Hartsell et al. published the results of a phase III trial, conducted by the Radiation Therapy Oncology Group (RTOG) and the North Central Cancer Treatment Group (NCCTG), including patients with breast and prostate cancer bone metastases [15]. Eight hundred ninety-eight patients were randomly assigned to receive 8 Gy in one fraction or 30 Gy in ten fractions. Complete or partial improvement of pain was observed in 66 % of patients after 3 months from randomization. No differences in response rate were found between the two groups. Re-treatment rate was twice in 8 Gy arm compared to 30 Gy arm (18 % vs 9 %). Grade 2–4 acute toxicity was more frequent in multifractionated group than in single-fraction group (17 % vs. 10 %). Late toxicity was rare [15].

All published randomized trials were analyzed in a series of comprehensive meta-analysis [16–18], the most recent including 5263 patients enrolled in 25 randomized controlled trial [19]. Results showed that single- and multiple-fraction regimens provided similar complete and overall response rates. Pathological fractures rate was equal in both groups, while the reduction of spinal cord compression trended in favor of multiple fractions, without statistical significativity. The re-treatment rate was 2.6-fold greater in single-fraction arm. No differences in acute toxicities were seen between the two groups. A subanalysis of patients with neuropathic pain enrolled in a randomized trial published by Roos et al. was also performed, showing that single fraction of 8 Gy was less effective than a multifractionated regimen of 20 Gy in five fractions, without reaching statistical significance [19, 20].

The optimal dose of single fraction able to achieve pain relief without significant side effects is currently unknown. Dennis et al. in a systematic review analyzed single-fraction arms in 24 randomized trials including 3233 patients [21]. The most widely prescribed dose was 8 Gy (84 % of the patients, $n=2717$). The other delivered doses were 4 Gy ($n=246$), 5 Gy ($n=14$), 6 Gy ($n=108$), and 10 Gy ($n=134$). Only three of considered trials directly compared single-fraction arms with an advantage in pain response of 8 Gy vs. 4 Gy and a non-superior response of 8 Gy vs. 6 Gy. Authors concluded that defining the single fraction of 8 Gy as the optimal dose is still an open question, and future clinical trials should directly compare doses and radiation techniques [21].

Despite the results of randomized studies that showed equal efficacy in pain relief between single fraction and multiple fractions in uncomplicated bone metastases, a reluctance to employing single fraction was highlighted in the radiation oncology community [22]. A survey to assess pattern of practice on 962 members of three radiation oncology professional organizations (ASTRO, American Society for Radiation Oncology; CARO, Canadian Association of Radiation Oncology; Royal Australian and New Zealand College of Radiologist) was conducted. Five hypothetical cases of bone metastases from different primary cancers (breast, lung, or prostate) were proposed. The responses of surveyed physicians included 101 different treatment schedules (range, 3 Gy/1 fraction to 60 Gy/2 fractions; median dose 30 Gy/10 fractions). Most radiation oncologist continued to prescribe multifractionated schedules. A prescription trend versus single-fraction radiotherapy was seen as a function of country of training (Canada and Europe vs. the United States) and location of practice (university or academic centers vs. private institutions) [22]. A recent review published by Popovic et al. [23] analyzed results derived from international surveys administered to radiation oncologist examining actual prescription practice for painful metastases. Considering the most recent patient data, there was not an increasing trend of prescription of single-fraction dose in function of treatment year in uncomplicated bone metastases. Geographical differences were found; Canadian physicians were more readily prescribing single fraction than physicians from the United Kingdom or Norway. Authors concluded that, despite clinical evidence, there was a global reluctance in the prescription of single fraction. Many factors influenced this trend and were related to radiation oncologist preferences, patients, radiotherapy centers, and personal beliefs [23].

14.2.2 Reirradiation

In patients with bone metastases, radiotherapy has a role in palliation of pain, even in a re-treatment setting. Re-treatment rates are about 8 % in patients previously irradiated with multifractionated radiotherapy and 20 % in patients treated with single fraction [19].

New and more sophisticated therapies and improvements in supportive care resulted in increased survival of patients, leading to the need to receive further radiation treatments [24].

Reirradiation can be considered in three different settings: (1) no pain relief or progression of pain after a first course of radiation, (2) partial response to initial treatment and the need to achieving further pain reduction, and (3) partial or complete response to initial radiotherapy and subsequent pain progression [25].

Available studies on reirradiation were analyzed in a systematic review conducted by Wong et al. [26], updating a previously review of Huisman et al. [27]. Fifteen articles with an evaluable population of 645 patients were considered. Overall response rate to reirradiation was 68 %, with 20 % of patients experiencing a complete response to the treatment. Patients who had a previous complete response to radiotherapy were more likely to achieve a complete and more durable pain response upon re-treatment than patients with initial partial response. Toxicities were not consistently reported; however, no grade 3 or 4 toxicity, pathological fractures, and spinal cord compression were recorded [26].

A consensus on when performing reirradiation after a first course of radiotherapy hasn't been reached yet [28]; in a survey conducted by the International Bone Consensus Working Party, the majority of radiation oncologist considered for reirradiation a time period beginning 4 weeks after completion of the initial treatment course [28, 29].

Available data are not conclusive to define optimal dose and fractionation when a reirradiation is needed. The ASTRO evidence-based guidelines on palliative radiotherapy for bone metastases recommend to treat patients within the already available clinical data on doses and fractionation schedules [30]. Chow et al. published the results of a randomized trial, aiming to compare two different dose fractionation schedules (8 Gy in one fraction versus 20 Gy in multiple fractions) in patients undergoing a repeated radiotherapy. Four hundred and twenty-five patients were assigned to each treatment group. Primary endpoint was overall pain response at 2 months (complete and partial response were included). No differences were seen between the two groups in pain relief and in freedom of pain progression. No cases of radiation myelitis were reported. Authors concluded that repeated radiation therapy was effective, irrespective to the adopted treatment schedule. Forty-eight percent of all patients had a reduction of pain in re-treated sites, and 68 % of patients reported an improved quality-of-life pain score. Eight Gy seemed to be non-inferior to multifractionated schedule, but it wasn't excluded that a small proportion of patients could benefit more from multiple fractions [31]. Available clinical data were also analyzed with the aim of building a prognostic model, considering different risk groups to predict survival in patients requiring reirradiation for painful bone metastases. Authors recommend the use of 8 Gy in single fraction in the worst group identified in their survival model (low Karnofsky performance status score and more aggressive primary cancer site, such as the lung) [32].

14.2.3 EBRT in Management of Spinal Cord Compression or Pathological Fractures

Metastatic spinal cord compression (MSCC) is an oncologic emergency and may cause paralysis, sensory loss, and sphincter incontinence, if left untreated [33, 34]. EBRT is generally the treatment of choice for MSCC. Two randomized phase III multicenter Italian trials were conducted with the aim of defining the most effective radiation schedule in patients with MSCC and short life expectancy [35, 36]. The first compared a short-course radiotherapy (8 Gy × 2 days) with a split-course regimen (5 Gy × 3, 3 Gy × 5). Two hundred and seventy-six patients were randomized to the two different schedules. Pain relief was achieved in 56.9 % of patients, and no significant difference in response rate or survival was found. Toxicity was similar and acceptable in both radiation schemes. Authors concluded that a short-course regimen could be the best and more convenient choice for patients with MSCC and short life expectancy [35]. On the premise of the first trial, the second randomized study started with the aim to define whether, in the same category of patients, 8 Gy in single fraction was effective as 8 Gy in two fractions. Three hundred and three patients were enrolled. Results showed no differences in response rates for back pain, motor function, and sphincter control between the two treatment arms. Pain relief was achieved in 53 % of patients. Tolerance to both regimens was good and, after a median follow-up of 31 months, no myelopathy was registered [36]. Among 579 patients enrolled in the two randomized trials, Maranzano et al. analyzed the outcomes of patients undergoing reirradiation for local relapse. Only 50 % of the 24 relapsed patients were re-treated, and different re-treatment schedules were used. Patient walking capacity before reirradiation was a predictor of functional outcome, and no case of myelopathy was recorded [37].

Rades et al. published the results of a prospective study comparing local control of short-course (8 Gy x1 or 5 Gy×4) and long-course radiotherapy (3 Gy×10 or 2.5 Gy×15 or 2 Gy×20) in patients with MSCC and long life expectancy [38]. Primary endpoint was local control. Motor function and survival were analyzed as secondary focuses of interest. Results showed, on 265 patients included in the study, a significantly better local control after long-course radiotherapy than after short-course radiotherapy (81 % vs. 61 %, $p=0.0005$). Radiation schedule had no significant impact on functional outcomes or overall survival. Acute toxicity was moderate and no cases of myelopathy were recorded. Authors concluded that patients with a relatively favorable survival prognosis might have higher risk for local relapse and benefit from long-course radiotherapy, while patients with a poor expected survival appeared adequately treated with short-course radiotherapy [38]. EBRT can also be combined with decompressive surgical resection in selected patients. Patchell et al. [39] analyzed functional outcomes in 101 patients with MSCC randomized to receive decompressive surgery followed by radiotherapy or radiotherapy alone. Surgical group outcome was significantly better than radiotherapy group in ability to walk after treatment (84 % vs. 57 %, respectively). Surgery plus radiotherapy allowed to most patients to remain ambulatory since dead and reduced the use of corticosteroids and opioid. Combined treatment also had an impact on overall survival. The trial was stopped early because of the superiority of surgical treatment outcomes. However, this approach should be proposed in selected patients; very radiosensitive tumors, multiple areas of spinal cord compression, or total paraplegia for more than 48 h were exclusion criteria from the trial [39]. A subsequent analysis of this study showed that age was a relevant variable in predicting ambulatory preservation and survival. In patients ≥65 years, there were no difference in outcome between EBRT alone and surgery followed by EBRT [40].

The role of postoperative radiotherapy in patients with metastatic pathological fractures underwent to orthopedic stabilization was reported in a retrospective study published by Towsend et al [41]. Thirty-five of a total of 64 patients had combined treatment (surgery plus radiation). Functional status was significantly better in patients treated with surgery and radiation than with surgery alone (53 % vs. 11.5 %, respectively), suggesting the benefit of radiotherapy in this setting [41]. In a more recent retrospective study, Wolanczyk et al. reported the outcome of 72 patients undergoing surgical stabilization for complete or impending pathologic fractures and subsequently treated with EBRT with or without zoledronic acid (43 % and 44 % of patients, respectively) or zoledronic acid alone (13 % of patients) [42]. Median overall survival time was 14 months, and median prescribed dose was 30 Gy (30–40 Gy/2–3 Gy per fraction). Local progression, pain progression, and need for re-treatment (surgery or EBRT) were analyzed. Local tumor progression was 7 % and 9 %, respectively, in irradiated patients with or without zoledronic acid and 44 % in patients treated with zoledronic acid alone ($p=0.02$). Local pain progression was 16 %, 19 %, and 44 % in the same groups, respectively ($p=0.011$). No difference was seen in re-treatment rate between the different groups. Authors concluded confirming the efficacy and the need of postoperative EBRT after orthopedic stabilization for metastatic bone disease [42].

14.3 Hemibody Irradiation

In the past years, hemibody irradiation (HBI) was often used for the treatment of widespread, symptomatic, metastatic bone disease from different types of cancers, prostate included.

Since 1970s, this technique evolved for palliation of uncontrolled pain in patients with a massive bone involvement, with the advantage of treating many sites fast and simultaneously.

The response rates were similar to those of the irradiation with local fields, but pain relief was more rapid, occurring often after 48 h from irradiation [43–47].

HBI can be delivered with different field sizes and different patient positions. Three different types of field arrangements were more frequently described: upper half-body irradiation (UBHI) from the top of the head to the level of the iliac crest (L4-L5 interface), lower half-body irradiation (LHBI) from iliac crest to the ankles, and midportion-body irradiation (MBI) from the top of the diaphragm to the bottom of the obturator foramen [48].

Consensually with the development of this technique, the Radiation Therapy Oncology Group began a series of studies in order to evaluate the efficacy and safety of this treatment. RTOG 78-10 showed that a single fraction of HBI was effective, with pain relief in 73 % of patients, and identified as safest doses 6 Gy for UBHI and 8 Gy for LHBI and MBI. Increased toxicity was seen with higher doses without clinical benefit [46, 49].

RTOG 82-06 explored the possibility that HBI added to irradiation with local fields had an effect on occult disease with a delay of appearance of new metastases and a decrease of the frequency of further treatments. Patients were randomized to receive the standard palliative treatment (3 Gy × 10 fractions) with or without HBI. The results demonstrated an advantage for the HBI group in time-to-disease progression (35 % for local + HBI vs. 46 % in local only) and time-to-new disease at 1 year (50 % for local + HBI vs. 68 % in local only), without having an impact on overall survival. The maximum benefit was observed in breast and prostate cancer, but an increased toxicity was recorded with the use of HBI [50].

RTOG 88-22 protocol started with the aim to evaluate fractionated HBI; the results showed a modest improvement in reduction of local failure in the fractionated schedule, with a maximum tolerated dose of 17.5 Gy (2.5 Gy per fraction). It was concluded that single high-dose HBI was as effective as fractionated HBI. The major dose limiting toxicity was hematological (thromboleukopenia) [51].

The main problem with respect to HBI, even when it's carried out in single fraction, is the need of hospitalization or close monitoring due to the necessity of premedication with steroids, hydration, and antiemetics administration to prevent acute toxicity, particularly in the treatment of upper body. The majority of treated patients experiences gastrointestinal toxicity such as nausea and vomiting, particularly in the first hours after the irradiation, and diarrhea lasting 3–7 days. All symptoms are transient. Hematological toxicity has a peak at 2 weeks but disappears after 4–6 weeks from the HBI exposure and rarely needs blood transfusion. Radiation pneumonitis is rare if lung dose is lower than 7 Gy [43, 46, 47].

Modified fields were used over the years, with the aim of reducing toxicity. Bashir et al reported a 10-year experience of palliative treatments with modified HBI for metastatic carcinoma of the prostate, excluding the skull and the lower leg from treatment fields; the results showed a successful outcome with pain response and reduction of analgesic intake. The treatment was easier, with a simplified setup, and patients were protected from unnecessary distressing toxicities such as alopecia, dry mouth, and parotitis [52]. A randomized phase III trial of the International Atomic Energy Agency (IAEA) aimed to find the most effective and efficient method to deliver HBI. Three different fractionation schedules were used: 15 Gy in five fractions over 5 days, 8 Gy in two fractions over 1 day, and 12 Gy in four fractions over 2 days. Pain relief was seen in 91 % of patients; toxicity was acceptable: moderate in 50 % of the patients, absent in 41 %, and severe only in 12 %. The study highlighted that all primary tumors responded to all prescribed schedules with the exception of prostate cancer, for which 15 Gy over 5 days was the most effective schedule [53].

Despite HBI offers the possibility of treating multiple metastases with rapid pain relief, treatment-related morbidity can be significant compared to the irradiation with local fields, and the majority of patients requires anyway a re-treatment at 1 year [50, 54]. Over the years, this technique has been gradually abandoned.

14.4 Stereotactic Body Radiotherapy

Diagnostic advances and improvements of radiological techniques have enabled the detection of metastatic disease at an early stage, with evidence of single or limited distant localization of primary cancer, defined as oligometastases. The term oligometastases, first coined by Hellmann and Weichselbaum in 1995, describes a state of metastatic disease amenable to potentially curable local therapy [55]. Local treatments of oligometastatic disease, including surgical resection, radiofrequency, cryoablation, and radiotherapy, have been widely investigated for different types of cancers, such as liver localization or lung metastases, with the purpose of improving long-term disease control and obtaining an impact on overall survival [56–58].

Stereotactic body radiation therapy (SBRT) is a highly precise external beam radiation technique able to deliver high radiation doses to small volumes and is an effective treatment in the management of oligometastatic patients. SBRT is constantly evolving, and a variety of systems for dose delivering, which include different available technologies, are provided: standard linac machines, Novalis Brainlab, and Accuray CyberKnife, among many others. Megavoltage photons or protons [59] can be used for SBRT with different radiation techniques (multiple static beams, rotational fields of varying degrees of complexity with or without beam intensity modulation). First introduced in the context of intracranial stereotactic radiosurgery is now known that SBRT may improve local tumor control in different extracranial organs with a reduction of treatment-related toxicities [60, 61]. The primary goal of this treatment is indeed to ensure a high-dose delivery to the tumor with a steep dose falloff gradient to the surrounding healthy tissues [62]. Dose gradient allows a maximization of tumor control with a minimization of normal tissue exposure and with a potential reduction of radiation-induced side effects. Image-guided radiation therapy (IGRT), as previously described, ensures a high level of precision of dose delivering with daily image guidance [63, 64]. SBRT can be delivered as a single high-dose fraction or may be fractionated into several sessions using larger daily doses than normally fractionated radiotherapy [62].

Emerging data indicate that patients with limited metastatic localization from different types of cancer get a better local disease control and may experience an improvement in disease-free survival, when treated with SBRT [65–67].

There are no randomized studies investigating the different aspects of SBRT in the management of bone metastases; several published data have shown that SBRT is safe and effective, even in spinal metastatic localizations, due to its ability of delivering high radiation doses to the bone, with spinal cord sparing. Despite dataset differed in the numbers of patients, primary cancer, and prescribed doses, local control ranged from 87 to 96 % with sporadic reports of radiation-induced myelopathy [68]. Pattern of local recurrence after single-dose SBRT for spinal metastases is less than 5 % [69].

Several retrospective and some prospective studies have been published with the aim of defining local control, pain relief, acute and late toxicities, optimal doses, and fractionation schedules. Published data concern the role of SBRT in unirradiated lesions, in re-treatments, and in the postoperative setting (bone resection, laminectomy, or vertebroplasty).

14.4.1 Unirradiated and Reirradiated Patients: Mixed Cases

Chang et al. in 2004 in a phase I clinical trial, reported on 15 patients treated with SBRT (30 Gy/5 fractions) [70]. Authors concluded that SBRT, with computed tomographic image guidance, was a feasible and highly precise technique for the treatment of spinal metastases, with no reported neurological toxicity at median follow-up of 9 months [70].

From Pittsburg University, Gerszten et al. [71] reported the results of a prospective longitudinal study on a cohort of 500 spinal metastases in 393 patients treated with CyberKnife; dose prescription ranged from 12.5 to 25 Gy in a single fraction. Sixty-nine percent of lesions had received previous radiotherapy. Spinal radiosurgery was found to be highly effective in pain relief, with a long-term pain control in 86 % of treated patients and local disease control in 88 % of the cases. No cases of myelopathy were recorded [71].

RTOG 0631 phase II/III study aimed to evaluate feasibility and safety of a more intensive dose of SBRT in patients with localized spine metastases in a cooperative group setting. Dose prescription was 16 Gy in one fraction. Forty-four patients were fit for analysis and grade 1–2 toxicity was seen in 11 patients; grade 3 toxicity was recorded only in one case, with no evidence of grade 4–5 toxicities [72].

Wang et al. in a prospective phase I–II study on 165 patients with non-cord-compressing spinal metastases treated with SBRT (27–30 Gy/3 fractions) showed a significant pain reduction during the 6 months post-SBRT, without acute and late spinal cord toxicities [73].

On a case series of 121 patients with less than five metastatic localizations in different organs (bone, lung, liver, lymph nodes, brain, pelvis), Milano et al. observed that none of bone lesions recurred after SBRT in long-term survival patients and the only case of grade 3 toxicity was not related with bone irradiation [66]. A recent report of Moussazadeh et al. [74] assessed tumor control and toxicity in patients with at least 5-year follow-up after 24 Gy of single-fraction SBRT to spinal localization. Thirty-one patients with 36 treated segments were followed for a median of 6.1 years. Three treatment failures occurred at a median follow-up of 48.6 months, two in the radiation field and one on treatment margin. To note that 13 treated sites (36.1 %) in 12 patients demonstrated progressive vertebral body collapse at a median of 25.7 months, 14 % became symptomatic and required medical intervention [74].

An optimal dose prescription has not been yet defined in previously unirradiated bone metastases. A report of Greco et al. on 126 metastatic sites treated with single-dose SBRT found that prescribed dose (>22 Gy) was predictive of local control [75]. Similar results were previously published by Yamada et al. in a study on 103 spinal metastases treated with single-fraction SBRT at a median dose of 24 Gy [76].

Dosimetric analysis performed on patients treated with SBRT found that 10 Gy to a maximum point is safe for single-fraction SBRT and a normalized 2-Gy-equivalent biological equivalent dose (BED*) of 30–35 $Gy_{2/2}$ to the thecal sac is correlated with a low risk of radiation myelopathy [77].

*BED (biologically effective dose of a given schedule) is the total dose required to give the same log cell kill as the schedule being studied. Calculation of the biologically effective dose is based on linear quadratic cell survival in radiobiology. It aims to indicate quantitatively the biological effect of any radiotherapy treatment, taking account of changes in dose per fraction or dose rate, total dose, and overall time. Calculation of BED takes into account alpha/beta for the given tissue and the endpoint of interest (describing the prevalence of single-hit cell inactivation versus double-hit cell inactivations, differences for acute and late endpoints), the recovery time of the tissue, the proliferation rate, the kickoff time for repopulation, and the correction term for dose accumulation/day [78].

14.4.2 Reirradiation

In the presence of progression of spinal metastases after conventionally fractionated EBRT treatment, options depend on the toxicity to the spinal cord. For these patients, stereotactic radiotherapy techniques could be the treatment of choice. A series of study have considered the impact of SBRT after conventional EBRT in terms of local control and neurological toxicities. In a set of five previously irradiated patients, Hamilton et al. reported the first preliminary experience on re-treatment with a single fraction of SBRT (8–10 Gy), achieving a local control of 100 % at 6 months, without evidence of vertebral collapse [79]. In their preliminary feasibility report, Ryu et al. treated ten patients with EBRT (25 Gy/ 10 fractions) plus a single-fraction planned SBRT boost of 6–8 Gy, with no relevant toxicity at 6 months of follow-up and varying degrees of pain relief in all patients [80]. Similar results were seen in 18 patients re-treated with stereotactic technique and fractionated 3D-EBRT or IMRT in Heidelberg experience [81]. Sahgal et al. reported their results on 37 reirradiated spine lesions with 24 Gy/3 fractions, with an effective tumor control (31 of 37 reirradiated tumors), and without cases of radiation-induced myelopathy at 6 months of follow-up [82]. A review of the same author on re-treated patients with myelopathy defines as a safe total maximum normalized dose to the thecal sac less than 70 $Gy_{2/2}$ and an SBRT thecal sac re-treatment maximum normalized dose not exceeding 25 $Gy_{2/2}$, with a minimum time interval to reirradiation of at least 5 months [83]. Thibault et al. [84] retrospectively evaluated a retreatment with SBRT in 40 patients with 56 irradiated spinal segments failed after a first course of SBRT; 42.9 % of the segments had been initially irradiated with conventional EBRT too. Prescribed median re-treatment dose was 30 Gy in four fractions. Surgery was performed before a second course of SBRT in case of neurological symptoms or mechanical instability; no vertebral compression fractures were observed in 19 of 56 non-operated metastatic segments, and no cases of myelopathy were seen in all patients, with a median follow-up time of 6.8 months. Local control rate was 77 % [84].

14.4.3 Postoperative SBRT

Few data have been published about the use of SBRT in patients undergoing surgery for neurological problems related to vertebral metastases. On a series of 18 postoperative patients who received SBRT on residual spinal tumor, Rock et al. [85] reported neurological stability and an improvement of preoperative neurological deficit in 92 % and 62 % of cases, respectively. Thirty-three percent of patients had complete resolution of pain. Only one patient showed a neurological deterioration after radiation, due to rapid disease progression. Dose prescription ranged from 6 to 16 Gy. No significant morbidities were described [85]. Gertszten et al. prospectively evaluated 20 patients with symptomatic pathological compression fractures undergoing surgical spinal stabilization. All patients were treated with kyphoplasty and subsequently with a single-fraction SBRT (mean time after surgery was 12 days) performed with CyberKnife. Mean dose prescription was 18 Gy (16–20 Gy). Long-term pain relief was seen in 92 % of patients without evidence of radiation-induced spinal cord damage [86].

14.4.4 SBRT in Bone Metastases from Prostate Cancer

There is an increasing evidence that oligometastatic prostate cancer has a better prognosis compared with more extensive disease [87, 88]. In a retrospective analysis on 369 patients radically treated for prostate cancer at University of Rochester, Singh et al. found, among the 74 patients who developed bone metastases, a significantly better survival in the presence of ≤5 bone lesions than in the presence of >5 lesions [87]. Schweizer et al. reporting on 450 men with PSA-recurrent prostate cancer after radical prostatectomy showed that, in a multivariable model, the number of metastases at first presentation (≤3 vs ≥4) was associated with overall survival [88]. Ost et al. [89] tried to identify prognostic factors related to prostate cancer specific-survival (PCSS) retrospectively analyzing 80 patients who had developed non-castration-resistant metastases (nodal, skeletal, and/or visceral). In multivariate analysis PSA doubling time (PSA DT) >3 months, the pattern of metastatic spread (node or axial skeleton involvement) and the presence of one metastasis versus more than one localization were associated with an improved PCSS [89]. Different clinical outcomes between localized and widespread disease imply that the early detection of metastases and the proper selection of patients to more aggressive local treatment could play a crucial role in the management of these patients.

Berkovich et al. at Ghent University Hospital investigated whether repeated SBRT of oligometastatic disease was able to delay the onset of palliative androgen deprivation therapy (ADT) [90]. Twenty-four patients with a biochemical recurrence after treatment with curative intent (surgery, radiotherapy, or both) and with a diagnosis of ≤3 synchronous asymptomatic metastases detected with positron emission tomography were treated with a SBRT schedule of 50 Gy in ten fractions. Primary endpoint of the study was androgen deprivation therapy-free survival (ADT-FS), defined as the time between the first day of SBRT and the initiation of ADT. Patients started hormone therapy if PSA level was greater than 50 ng/mL or if the number of metastases was greater than three. Twenty-nine lesions (lymph node or bone metastases) were treated, without infield recurrences recorded at 2-year follow-up and clinical progression-free survival was 42 %. Ten patients started ADT, with a median ADT-FS of 38 months; 11 and 3 patients, respectively, required a second and third salvage re-treatment with SBRT due to metachronous low-volume metastatic disease. No grade 3 toxicity was observed [90]. An update of this study was published by Decaestecker et al., including 50 patients with 70 metastatic lesions. In 15 patients, a different irradiation schedule of 30 Gy in three fractions was used due to logistic advantages. Local control was 100 %, without grade 3 toxicity. In 50 % of patients, palliative ADT was postponed by at least 2 years [91].

Muacevic et al. [92] published data on 40 patients prospectively enrolled and treated 64 metastatic bone lesions with a single fraction of SBRT (mean dose 20.2 Gy). Patients were considered for SBRT regardless of their hormone therapy responsiveness. At a mean follow-up of 14 months, local tumor control rate was 95.5 %, and a significant decrease of PSA following treatment was observed. Only one case of progressive neurological deficit was documented [92]. Amhed et al. [93] reported outcomes and toxicity in 17 patients treated on 21 metastatic lesions with a single fraction of SBRT (median dose 20 Gy). Eleven patients had hormone-refractory disease. Local control was 100 % without case of grade ≥3 toxicity [93].

A multi-institutional study published by Ost et al. [94] focused on SBRT in 119 patients with three or fewer metastases from prostate cancer, treatment naïve. One hundred sixty-three localizations (bone, lymph node, or viscera) were irradiated with SBRT at different biologically effective dose (BED) with the aim of estimate distant progression-free survival (DPFS) and local progression-free survival (LPFS). The metastatic sites were treated with four different BEDs: 80–99 ($n=29$), 100–119 ($n=20$), 120–139 ($n=66$), and $e>140$ ($n=4$). Median DPFS was 21 months, and the median time from first SBRT to the start of ADT was 28 months. They found that a lower radiation dose predicted for high local recurrence rate with a 3-year LPFS of 79 % for patients treated with a BED ≤100 Gy versus 99 % for patients treated with >100 Gy. No toxicity of grade ≥3 was observed [94].

Recently, Pasqualetti et al. [95] reported on a case series of 29 patients with 45 oligometastatic localizations (defined as ≤3 synchronous lesions) detected with fluoromethyl choline ([18 F] FMCH) PET/CT and treated with repeated salvage SBRT until disease progression (development of >3 active synchronous metastases). Lymph node localizations and bone localization were 55.5 % and 45.5 %, respectively. Twenty-four Gy in one fraction or 27 Gy in three fractions were prescribed. Local control was 100 %, and after a median follow-up of 11.5 months, 15/29 patients achieved a PSA control with a single course of SBRT [95]. The main studies on the treatments of oligometastatic patients are reported in Table 14.2.

A phase II randomized study comparing surveillance versus metastasis-directed therapy (surgery or SBRT) followed by surveillance in oligometastatic prostate cancer is currently open to recruitment. Patients are stratified according to the location of metastases (node vs bone metastases) and PSA DT (≤3 vs. >3). “Active” surveillance consists of three monthly PSA testing and repetition of imaging at PSA progression. Androgen deprivation therapy-free survival (ADT-FS) is the primary endpoint, and ADT will be started in both arms in case of progression of metastatic disease (>3 lesions), local progression, or symptoms [96].

In spite of the limited follow-up available, many reports suggest that stereotactic body radiotherapy is an effective and safe treatment for metastatic prostate cancer. Diagnostic improvement and results of ongoing trials will further clarify the role of SBRT in this setting.

Table 14.2 Summary of the three largest randomized trials comparing single versus multiple fractions in palliative EBRT

Author	Year	N° of pts/N° of months	Site of months	N° of mts	Dose/fractionation	Primary endpoint	Results	Follow-up (months)	Toxicity
Berkovic [91]	2013	24/29	Bone/lymph nodes	≤3	50 Gy/10	ADT-FS	ADT-FS 82 %–1 year 54 %–2 years LC 100 %	24 (median)	No tox ≥ grade 3
Decaestecker [92]	2014	50/70	Bone/lymph nodes/ viscera	≤3	50 Gy/10 30 Gy/3	ADT-FS	ADT-FS 50 %–2 years LC 100 %	24 (median)	No tox ≥ grade 3
Muacevic [93]	2011	40/64	Bone	≤2	16.5–22 Gy (mean 20.2 Gy)/1	Safety and feasibility	LC 95.5 %	14 (mean)	One case of progressive neurological deficit
Amhed [94]	2013	17/21	Bone/lymph nodes/ viscera	≤5	8–24 Gy (mean 20 Gy)/1	Outcome and Toxicity	LC 100 %	6 (median)	No tox ≥ grade 3
Ost [95]	2015	119/163	Bone/lymph nodes/ viscera	≤3	BED 80–99 Gy 120–139 Gy >140 Gy	DPFS	DPFS Median: 21 months 31 %–3 years 15 %–5 years	36 (median)	No tox ≥ grade 3
Pasqualetti [96]	2016	29/45	Bone/lymph nodes	≤3	24 Gy/1 27 Gy/3	ADT-FS	ADT-FS Median: 39.7 months LC 100 %	11.5 (median)	No tox ≥ grade 2

References

1. Webb S (2003) The physical basis of IMRT and inverse planning. Br J Radiol 76(910):678–689
2. Intensity Modulated Radiation Therapy Collaborative Working Group (2001) Intensity-modulated radiotherapy: current status and issues of interest. Int J Radiat Oncol Biol Phys 51(4):880–914
3. Otto K (2008) Volumetric modulated arc therapy: IMRT in a single gantry arc. Med Phys 35(1): 310–317
4. Teoh M, Clark CH, Wood K, Whitaker S, Nisbet A (2011) Volumetric modulated arc therapy: a review of current literature and clinical use in practice. Br J Radiol 84(1007):967–996
5. Baumann M, Krause M, Overgaard J, Debus J, Bentzen SM, Daartz J, Richter C, Zips D, Bortfeld T (2016) Radiation oncology in the era of precision medicine. Nat Rev Cancer 16(4):234–249
6. Lo SS, Fakiris AJ, Chang EL, Mayr NA, Wang JZ, Papiez L, Teh BS, McGarry RC, Cardenes HR, Timmerman RD (2010) Stereotactic body radiation therapy: a novel treatment modality. Nat Rev Clin Oncol 7(1):44–54
7. Dawson LA, Jaffray DA (2007) Advances in image-guided radiation therapy. J Clin Oncol 25(8): 938–946
8. Martin AG, Thomas SJ, Harden SV, Burnet NG (2015) Evaluating competing and emerging technologies for stereotactic body radiotherapy and other advanced radiotherapy techniques. Clin Oncol (R Coll Radiol) 27(5):251–259
9. Bubendorf L, Schöpfer A, Wagner U, Sauter G, Moch H, Willi N, Gasser TC, Mihatsch MJ (2000) Metastatic patterns of prostate cancer: an autopsy study of 1,589 patients. Hum Pathol 31(5):578–583
10. Bhattasali O, Chen LN, Tong M, Lei S, Collins BT, Krishnan P, Kalhorn C, Lynch JH, Suy S, Dritschilo A, Dawson NA, Collins SP (2013) Rationale for stereotactic body radiation therapy in treating patients with oligometastatic hormone-naïve prostate cancer. Front Oncol 3:293
11. Denham JW, Joseph D, Lamb DS, Spry NA, Duchesne G, Matthews J, Atkinson C, Tai KH, Christie D, Kenny L, Turner S, Gogna NK, Diamond T, Delahunt B, Oldmeadow C, Attia J, Steigler A (2014) Short-term androgen suppression and radiotherapy versus intermediate-term androgen suppression and radiotherapy, with or without zoledronic acid, in men with locally advanced prostate cancer (TROG 03.04 RADAR): an open-label, randomised, phase 3 factorial trial. Lancet Oncol 15(10):1076–1089
12. 8 Gy single fraction radiotherapy for the treatment of metastatic skeletal pain: randomised comparison with a multifraction schedule over 12 months of patient follow-up. (1999) Bone Pain Trial Working Party. Radiother Oncol 52(2):111–121
13. Steenland E, Leer JW, van Houwelingen H, Post WJ, van den Hout WB, Kievit J, de Haes H, Martijn H, Oei B, Vonk E, van der Steen-Banasik E, Wiggenraad RG, Hoogenhout J, Wárlám-Rodenhuis C, van Tienhoven G, Wanders R, Pomp J, van Reijn M, van Mierlo I, Rutten E (1999) The effect of a single fraction compared to multiple fractions on painful bone metastases: a global analysis of the Dutch Bone Metastasis Study. Radiother Oncol 52(2):101–109
14. van der Linden YM, Lok JJ, Steenland E, Martijn H, van Houwelingen H, Marijnen CA, Leer JW, Dutch Bone Metastasis Study Group (2004) Single fraction radiotherapy is efficacious: a further analysis of the Dutch Bone Metastasis Study controlling for the influence of retreatment. Int J Radiat Oncol Biol Phys 59(2):528–537
15. Hartsell WF, Scott CB, Bruner DW, Scarantino CW, Ivker RA, Roach M 3rd, Suh JH, Demas WF, Movsas B, Petersen IA, Konski AA, Cleeland CS, Janjan NA, DeSilvio M (2005) Randomized trial of short- versus long-course radiotherapy for palliation of painful bone metastases. J Natl Cancer Inst 97(11):798–804
16. Sze WM, Shelley MD, Held I, Wilt TJ, Mason MD (2003) Palliation of metastatic bone pain: single fraction versus multifraction radiotherapy--a systematic review of randomised trials. Clin Oncol (R Coll Radiol) 15(6):345–352
17. Wu JS, Wong R, Johnston M, Bezjak A, Whelan A, Cancer Care Ontario Practice Guidelines Initiative Supportive Care Group (2003) Meta-analysis of dose-fractionation radiotherapy trials for the palliation of painful bone metastases. Int J Radiat Oncol Biol Phys 55(3):594–605
18. Chow E, Harris K, Fan G, Tsao M, Sze WM (2007) Palliative radiotherapy trials for bone metastases: a systematic review. J Clin Oncol 25(11):1423–1436
19. Chow E, Zeng L, Salvo N, Dennis K, Tsao M, Lutz S (2012) Update on the systematic review of palliative radiotherapy trials for bone metastases. Clin Oncol (R Coll Radiol) 24(2):112–124
20. Roos DE, Turner SL, O'Brien PC, Smith JG, Spry NA, Burmeister BH, Hoskin PJ, Ball DL, Trans-Tasman Radiation Oncology Group, TROG 96.05 (2005) Randomized trial of 8 Gy in 1 versus 20 Gy in 5 fractions of radiotherapy for neuropathic pain due to bone metastases (Trans-Tasman Radiation Oncology Group, TROG 96.05). Radiother Oncol 75(1):54–63
21. Dennis K, Makhani L, Zeng L, Lam H, Chow E (2013) Single fraction conventional external beam radiation therapy for bone metastases: a systematic review of randomised controlled trials. Radiother Oncol 106(1):5–14
22. Fairchild A, Barnes E, Ghosh S, Ben-Josef E, Roos D, Hartsell W, Holt T, Wu J, Janjan N, Chow E (2009) International patterns of practice in palliative radiotherapy for painful bone metastases: evidence-based practice? Int J Radiat Oncol Biol Phys 75(5): 1501–1510
23. Popovic M, den Hartogh M, Zhang L, Poon M, Lam H, Bedard G, Pulenzas N, Lechner B, Chow E (2014) Review of international patterns of practice for the

treatment of painful bone metastases with palliative radiotherapy from 1993 to 2013. Radiother Oncol 111(1):11–17

24. Chow E, Hoskin PJ, Wu J, Roos D, van der Linden Y, Hartsell W, Vieth R, Wilson C, Pater J (2006) A phase III international randomised trial comparing single with multiple fractions for re-irradiation of painful bone metastases: National Cancer Institute of Canada Clinical Trials Group (NCIC CTG) SC 20. Clin Oncol (R Coll Radiol) 18(2):125–128
25. Chow E, Wu JS, Hoskin P, Coia LR, Bentzen SM, Blitzer PH (2002) International consensus on palliative radiotherapy endpoints for future clinical trials in bone metastases. Radiother Oncol 64(3): 275–280
26. Wong E, Hoskin P, Bedard G, Poon M, Zeng L, Lam H, Vulpe H, Tsao M, Pulenzas N, Chow E (2014) Re-irradiation for painful bone metastases: a systematic review. Radiother Oncol 110(1):61–70
27. Huisman M, van den Bosch MA, Wijlemans JW, van Vulpen M, van der Linden YM, Verkooijen HM (2012) Effectiveness of reirradiation for painful bone metastases: a systematic review and meta-analysis. Int J Radiat Oncol Biol Phys 84(1):8–14
28. International Bone Metastases Consensus Working Party (2001) International bone metastases consensus on endpoint measurements for future clinical trials: proceedings of the first survey and meeting (work in progress) International Bone Metastases Consensus Working Party. Clin Oncol (R Coll Radiol) 13(2):82–84
29. Chow E, Hoskin P, Mitera G, Zeng L, Lutz S, Roos D, Hahn C, van der Linden Y, Hartsell W, Kumar E, International Bone Metastases Consensus Working Party (2012) Update of the international consensus on palliative radiotherapy endpoints for future clinical trials in bone metastases. Int J Radiat Oncol Biol Phys 82(5):1730–1737
30. Lutz S, Berk L, Chang E, Chow E, Hahn C, Hoskin P, Howell D, Konski A, Kachnic L, Lo S, Sahgal A, Silverman L, von Gunten C, Mendel E, Vassil A, Bruner DW, Hartsell W, American Society for Radiation Oncology (ASTRO) (2011) Palliative radiotherapy for bone metastases: an ASTRO evidence-based guideline. Int J Radiat Oncol Biol Phys 79(4):965–976
31. Chow E, van der Linden YM, Roos D, Hartsell WF, Hoskin P, Wu JS, Brundage MD, Nabid A, Tissing-Tan CJ, Oei B, Babington S, Demas WF, Wilson CF, Meyer RM, Chen BE, Wong RK (2014) Single versus multiple fractions of repeat radiation for painful bone metastases: a randomised, controlled, non-inferiority trial. Lancet Oncol 15(2):164–171
32. Chow E, Ding K, Parulekar WR, Wong RK, van der Linden YM, Roos D, Hartsell WF, Hoskin P, Wu JS, Nabid A, Leer JW, Vonk E, Babington S, Demas WF, Wilson CF, Brundage M, Zhu L, Meyer RM. Predictive model for survival in patients having repeat radiation treatment for painful bone metastases. Radiother Oncol. 2016;118(3):547–51.
33. Byrne TN (1992) Spinal cord compression from epidural metastases. N Engl J Med 327(9):614–619
34. Prasad D, Schiff D (2005) Malignant spinal-cord compression. Lancet Oncol 6(1):15–24
35. Maranzano E, Bellavita R, Rossi R, De Angelis V, Frattegiani A, Bagnoli R, Mignogna M, Beneventi S, Lupattelli M, Ponticelli P, Biti GP, Latini P (2005) Short-course versus split-course radiotherapy in metastatic spinal cord compression: results of a phase III, randomized, multicenter trial. J Clin Oncol 23(15):3358–3365
36. Maranzano E, Trippa F, Casale M, Costantini S, Lupattelli M, Bellavita R, Marafioti L, Pergolizzi S, Santacaterina A, Mignogna M, Silvano G, Fusco V (2009) 8Gy single-dose radiotherapy is effective in metastatic spinal cord compression: results of a phase III randomized multicentre Italian trial. Radiother Oncol 93(2):174–179
37. Maranzano E, Trippa F, Casale M, Anselmo P, Rossi R (2011) Reirradiation of metastatic spinal cord compression: definitive results of two randomized trials. Radiother Oncol 98(2):234–237
38. Rades D, Lange M, Veninga T, Stalpers LJ, Bajrovic A, Adamietz IA, Rudat V, Schild SE (2011) Final results of a prospective study comparing the local control of short-course and long-course radiotherapy for metastatic spinal cord compression. Int J Radiat Oncol Biol Phys 79(2):524–530
39. Patchell RA, Tibbs PA, Regine WF, Payne R, Saris S, Kryscio RJ, Mohiuddin M, Young B (2005) Direct decompressive surgical resection in the treatment of spinal cord compression caused by metastatic cancer: a randomised trial. Lancet 366(9486):643–648
40. Chi JH, Gokaslan Z, McCormick P, Tibbs PA, Kryscio RJ, Patchell RA (2009) Selecting treatment for patients with malignant epidural spinal cord compression-does age matter?: results from a randomized clinical trial. Spine (Phila Pa 1976) 34(5):431–435
41. Townsend PW, Smalley SR, Cozad SC, Rosenthal HG, Hassanein RE (1995) Role of postoperative radiation therapy after stabilization of fractures caused by metastatic disease. Int J Radiat Oncol Biol Phys 31(1):43–49
42. Wolanczyk MJ, Fakhrian K, Adamietz IA (2016) Radiotherapy, bisphosphonates and surgical stabilization of complete or impending pathologic fractures in patients with metastatic bone disease. J Cancer Educ 7(1):121–124
43. Rowland CG, Bullimore JA, Smith PJ, Roberts JB (1981) Half-body irradiation in the treatment of metastatic prostatic carcinoma. Br J Urol 53(6):628–629
44. Qasim MM (1981) Half body irradiation (HBI) in metastatic carcinomas. Clin Radiol 32(2):215–219
45. Salazar OM, Scarantino CW (1997) Theoretical and practical uses of elective systemic (half-body) irradiation after 20 years of experimental designs. Int J Radiat Oncol Biol Phys 39(4):907–913
46. Salazar OM, Rubin P, Hendrickson FR, Komaki R, Poulter C, Newall J, Asbell SO, Mohiuddin M, Van Ess J (1986) Single-dose half-body irradiation for palliation of multiple bone metastases from solid tumors.

Final Radiation Therapy Oncology Group report. Cancer 58(1):29–36

47. Berg RS, Yilmaz MK, Høyer M, Keldsen N, Nielsen OS, Ewertz M (2009) Half body irradiation of patients with multiple bone metastases: a phase II trial. Acta Oncol 48(4):556–561
48. Salazar OM, DaMotta NW, Bridgman SM, Cardiges NM, Slawson RG (1996) Fractionated half-body irradiation for pain palliation in widely metastatic cancers: comparison with single dose. Int J Radiat Oncol Biol Phys 36(1):49–60
49. Fitzpatrick PJ, Rider WD (1976) Half body radiotherapy. Int J Radiat Oncol Biol Phys 1(3–4):197–207
50. Poulter CA, Cosmatos D, Rubin P, Urtasun R, Cooper JS, Kuske RR, Hornback N, Coughlin C, Weigensberg I, Rotman M (1992) A report of RTOG 8206: a phase III study of whether the addition of single dose hemibody irradiation to standard fractionated local field irradiation is more effective than local field irradiation alone in the treatment of symptomatic osseous metastases. Int J Radiat Oncol Biol Phys 23(1):207–214
51. Scarantino CW, Caplan R, Rotman M, Coughlin C, Demas W, Delrowe J (1996) A phase I/II study to evaluate the effect of fractionated hemibody irradiation in the treatment of osseous metastases-RTOG 88-22. Int J Radiat Oncol Biol Phys 36(1):37–48
52. Bashir FA, Parry JM, Windsor PM (2008) Use of a modified hemi-body irradiation technique for metastatic carcinoma of the prostate: report of a 10-year experience. Clin Oncol (R Coll Radiol) 20(8):591–598
53. Salazar OM, Sandhu T, da Motta NW, Escutia MA, Lanzós-Gonzales E, Mouelle-Sone A, Moscol A, Zaharia M, Zaman S (2001) Fractionated half-body irradiation (HBI) for the rapid palliation of widespread, symptomatic, metastatic bone disease: a randomized Phase III trial of the International Atomic Energy Agency (IAEA). Int J Radiat Oncol Biol Phys 50(3):765–775
54. Lin A, Ray ME (2006) Targeted and systemic radiotherapy in the treatment of bone metastasis. Cancer Metastasis Rev 25(4):669–675
55. Hellman S, Weichselbaum RR (1995) Oligometastases. J Clin Oncol 13(1):8–10
56. Timmerman RD, Bizekis CS, Pass HI, Fong Y, Dupuy DE, Dawson LA, Lu D (2009) Local surgical, ablative, and radiation treatment of metastases. CA Cancer J Clin 59(3):145–170
57. Weichselbaum RR, Hellman S (2011) Oligometastases revisited. Nat Rev Clin Oncol 8(6):378–382
58. Rubin P, Brasacchio R, Katz A (2006) Solitary metastases: illusion versus reality. Semin Radiat Oncol 16(2):120–130
59. Bert C, Durante M (2014) Particle radiosurgery: a new frontier of physics in medicine. Phys Med 30(5):535–538
60. Timmerman RD, Kavanagh BD, Cho LC, Papiez L, Xing L (2007) Stereotactic body radiation therapy in multiple organ sites. J Clin Oncol 25(8):947–952
61. Timmerman RD, Herman J, Cho LC (2014) Emergence of stereotactic body radiation therapy and its impact on current and future clinical practice. J Clin Oncol 32(26):2847–2854
62. Potters L, Kavanagh B, Galvin JM, Hevezi JM, Janjan NA, Larson DA, Mehta MP, Ryu S, Steinberg M, Timmerman R, Welsh JS, Rosenthal SA, American Society for Therapeutic Radiology and Oncology; American College of Radiology (2010) American Society for Therapeutic Radiology and Oncology (ASTRO) and American College of Radiology (ACR) practice guideline for the performance of stereotactic body radiation therapy. Int J Radiat Oncol Biol Phys 76(2):326–332
63. Boda-Heggemann J, Lohr F, Wenz F, Flentje M, Guckenberger M (2011) kV cone-beam CT-based IGRT: a clinical review. Strahlenther Onkol 187(5):284–291
64. Potters L, Gaspar LE, Kavanagh B, Galvin JM, Hartford AC, Hevezi JM, Kupelian PA, Mohiden N, Samuels MA, Timmerman R, Tripuraneni P, Vlachaki MT, Xing L, Rosenthal SA, American Society for Therapeutic Radiology and Oncology; American College of Radiology (2010) American Society for Therapeutic Radiology and Oncology (ASTRO) and American College of Radiology (ACR) practice guidelines for image-guided radiation therapy (IGRT). Int J Radiat Oncol Biol Phys 76(2):319–325
65. Alongi F, Arcangeli S, Filippi AR, Ricardi U, Scorsetti M (2012) Review and uses of stereotactic body radiation therapy for oligometastases. Oncologist 17(8):1100–1107
66. Milano MT, Katz AW, Zhang H, Okunieff P (2012) Oligometastases treated with stereotactic body radiotherapy: long-term follow-up of prospective study. Int J Radiat Oncol Biol Phys 83(3):878–886
67. Tree AC, Khoo VS, Eeles RA, Ahmed M, Dearnaley DP, Hawkins MA, Huddart RA, Nutting CM, Ostler PJ, van As NJ (2013) Stereotactic body radiotherapy for oligometastases. Lancet Oncol 14(1):e28–e37
68. Sahgal A, Larson DA, Chang EL (2008) Stereotactic body radiosurgery for spinal metastases: a critical review. Int J Radiat Oncol Biol Phys 71(3):652–665
69. Ryu S, Rock J, Rosenblum M, Kim JH (2004) Patterns of failure after single-dose radiosurgery for spinal metastasis. J Neurosurg 101(Suppl 3):402–405
70. Chang EL, Shiu AS, Lii MF, Rhines LD, Mendel E, Mahajan A, Weinberg JS, Mathews LA, Brown BW, Maor MH, Cox JD (2004) Phase I clinical evaluation of near-simultaneous computed tomographic image-guided stereotactic body radiotherapy for spinal metastases. Int J Radiat Oncol Biol Phys 59(5):1288–1294
71. Gerszten PC, Burton SA, Ozhasoglu C, Welch WC (2007) Radiosurgery for spinal metastases: clinical experience in 500 cases from a single institution. Spine (Phila Pa 1976) 32(2):193–199
72. Ryu S, Pugh SL, Gerszten PC, Yin FF, Timmerman RD, Hitchcock YJ, Movsas B, Kanner AA, Berk LB, Followill DS, Kachnic LA (2014) RTOG 0631 phase 2/3 study of image guided stereotactic radiosurgery for localized (1-3) spine metastases: phase 2 results. Pract Radiat Oncol 4(2):76–81
73. Wang XS, Rhines LD, Shiu AS, Yang JN, Selek U, Gning I, Liu P, Allen PK, Azeem SS, Brown PD,

Sharp HJ, Weksberg DC, Cleeland CS, Chang EL (2012) Stereotactic body radiation therapy for management of spinal metastases in patients without spinal cord compression: a phase 1-2 trial. Lancet Oncol 13(4):395–402

74. Moussazadeh N, Lis E, Katsoulakis E, Kahn S, Svoboda M, DiStefano NM, McLaughlin L, Bilsky MH, Yamada Y, Laufer I (2015) Five-year outcomes of high-dose single-fraction spinal stereotactic radiosurgery. Int J Radiat Oncol Biol Phys 93(2):361–367
75. Greco C, Zelefsky MJ, Lovelock M, Fuks Z, Hunt M, Rosenzweig K, Zatcky J, Kim B, Yamada Y (2011) Predictors of local control after single-dose stereotactic image-guided intensity-modulated radiotherapy for extracranial metastases. Int J Radiat Oncol Biol Phys 79(4):1151–1157
76. Yamada Y, Bilsky MH, Lovelock DM, Venkatraman ES, Toner S, Johnson J, Zatcky J, Zelefsky MJ, Fuks Z (2008) High-dose, single-fraction image-guided intensity-modulated radiotherapy for metastatic spinal lesions. Int J Radiat Oncol Biol Phys 71(2): 484–490
77. Sahgal A, Ma L, Gibbs I, Gerszten PC, Ryu S, Soltys S, Weinberg V, Wong S, Chang E, Fowler J, Larson DA (2010) Spinal cord tolerance for stereotactic body radiotherapy. Int J Radiat Oncol Biol Phys 77(2): 548–553
78. Fowler JF (2010) 21 years of biologically effective dose. Br J Radiol 83(991):554–568
79. Hamilton AJ, Lulu BA, Fosmire H, Stea B, Cassady JR (1995) Preliminary clinical experience with linear accelerator-based spinal stereotactic radiosurgery. Neurosurgery 36(2):311–319
80. Ryu S, Fang Yin F, Rock J, Zhu J, Chu A, Kagan E, Rogers L, Ajlouni M, Rosenblum M, Kim JH (2003) Image-guided and intensity-modulated radiosurgery for patients with spinal metastasis. Cancer 97(8): 2013–2018
81. Milker-Zabel S, Zabel A, Thilmann C, Schlegel W, Wannenmacher M, Debus J (2003) Clinical results of retreatment of vertebral bone metastases by stereotactic conformal radiotherapy and intensity-modulated radiotherapy. Int J Radiat Oncol Biol Phys 55(1): 162–167
82. Sahgal A, Ames C, Chou D, Ma L, Huang K, Xu W, Chin C, Weinberg V, Chuang C, Weinstein P, Larson DA (2009) Stereotactic body radiotherapy is effective salvage therapy for patients with prior radiation of spinal metastases. Int J Radiat Oncol Biol Phys 74(3):723–731
83. Sahgal A, Ma L, Weinberg V, Gibbs IC, Chao S, Chang UK, Werner-Wasik M, Angelov L, Chang EL, Sohn MJ, Soltys SG, Létourneau D, Ryu S, Gerszten PC, Fowler J, Wong CS, Larson DA (2012) Reirradiation human spinal cord tolerance for stereotactic body radiotherapy. Int J Radiat Oncol Biol Phys 82(1):107–116
84. Thibault I, Campbell M, Tseng CL, Atenafu EG, Letourneau D, Yu E, Cho BC, Lee YK, Fehlings MG, Sahgal A (2015) Salvage Stereotactic Body Radiotherapy (SBRT) following in-field failure of initial SBRT for spinal metastases. Int J Radiat Oncol Biol Phys 93(2):353–360
85. Rock JP, Ryu S, Shukairy MS, Yin FF, Sharif A, Schreiber F, Abdulhak M, Kim JH, Rosenblum ML (2006) Postoperative radiosurgery for malignant spinal tumors. Neurosurgery 58(5):891–898; discussion 891–898
86. Gerszten PC, Germanwala A, Burton SA, Welch WC, Ozhasoglu C, Vogel WJ (2005) Combination kyphoplasty and spinal radiosurgery: a new treatment paradigm for pathological fractures. J Neurosurg Spine 3(4):296–301
87. Singh D, Yi WS, Brasacchio RA, Muhs AG, Smudzin T, Williams JP, Messing E, Okunieff P (2004) Is there a favorable subset of patients with prostate cancer who develop oligometastases? Int J Radiat Oncol Biol Phys 58(1):3–10
88. Schweizer MT, Zhou XC, Wang H, Yang T, Shaukat F, Partin AW, Eisenberger MA, Antonarakis ES (2013) Metastasis-free survival is associated with overall survival in men with PSA-recurrent prostate cancer treated with deferred androgen deprivation therapy. Ann Oncol 24(11):2881–2886
89. Ost P, Decaestecker K, Lambert B, Fonteyne V, Delrue L, Lumen N, Ameye F, De Meerleer G (2014) Prognostic factors influencing prostate cancer-specific survival in non-castrate patients with metastatic prostate cancer. Prostate 74(3): 297–305
90. Berkovic P, De Meerleer G, Delrue L, Lambert B, Fonteyne V, Lumen N, Decaestecker K, Villeirs G, Vuye P, Ost P (2013) Salvage stereotactic body radiotherapy for patients with limited prostate cancer metastases: deferring androgen deprivation therapy. Clin Genitourin Cancer 11(1):27–32
91. Decaestecker K, De Meerleer G, Lambert B, Delrue L, Fonteyne V, Claeys T, De Vos F, Huysse W, Hautekiet A, Maes G, Ost P (2014) Repeated stereotactic body radiotherapy for oligometastatic prostate cancer recurrence. Radiat Oncol 9:135
92. Muacevic A, Kufeld M, Rist C, Wowra B, Stief C, Staehler M (2013) Safety and feasibility of image-guided robotic radiosurgery for patients with limited bone metastases of prostate cancer. Urol Oncol 31(4):455–460
93. Ahmed KA, Barney BM, Davis BJ, Park SS, Kwon ED, Olivier KR (2013) Stereotactic body radiation therapy in the treatment of oligometastatic prostate cancer. Front Oncol 2:215
94. Ost P, Jereczek-Fossa BA, As NV, Zilli T, Muacevic A, Olivier K, Henderson D, Casamassima F, Orecchia R, Surgo A, Brown L, Tree A, Miralbell R, De Meerleer G (2016) Progression-free survival following stereotactic body radiotherapy for oligometastatic prostate cancer treatment-naive recurrence: a multi-institutional analysis. Eur Urol 69(1):9–12
95. Pasqualetti F, Panichi M, Sainato A, Matteucci F, Galli L, Cocuzza P, Ferrazza P, Coraggio G,

Pasqualetti G, Derosa L, Sollini M, Mannelli L, Ortori S, Monzani F, Ricci S, Greco C, Fabrini MG, Erba PA (2016) [(18)F]Choline PET/CT and stereotactic body radiotherapy on treatment decision making of oligometastatic prostate cancer patients: preliminary results. Radiat Oncol 11(1):9

96. Decaestecker K, De Meerleer G, Ameye F, Fonteyne V, Lambert B, Joniau S, Delrue L, Billiet I, Duthoy W, Junius S, Huysse W, Lumen N, Ost P (2014) Surveillance or metastasis-directed Therapy for Oligometastatic Prostate cancer recurrence (STOMP): study protocol for a randomized phase II trial. BMC Cancer 14:671

15 Bone-Targeted Agents

Daniele Santini, Carla Ripamonti, Alice Zoccoli, Michele Iuliani, Marco Fioramonti, Giulia Ribelli, and Francesco Pantano

In the last two decades, bisphosphonates and denosumab have been instrumental in the treatment of patients suffering with prostatic cancer bone metastases [17]. Recently abiraterone and enzalutamide have demonstrated potential beneficial effects on bone metabolism delaying and reducing skeletal complications. Even with recent improvements in medical treatment of skeletal metastases in prostate cancer, the development of effective and precise therapies aimed to improve patients' prognosis and quality of life remains a clinical challenge.

15.1 Bisphosphonates

Bisphosphonates are well established as successful agents for the management of osteoporosis as well as bone metastases in patients with solid cancer and multiple myeloma [38].

Bisphosphonates are analogues of pyrophosphate with a strong affinity for divalent metal ions, such as calcium ions, and for the skeleton. Indeed bisphosphonates are incorporated into bone matrix by binding to exposed hydroxyapatite crystals that provide a barrier to osteoclast-mediated bone resorption and have direct inhibitory effects on osteoblasts. In particular, bisphosphonates are embedded in bone at active remodeling sites, are released in the acidic environment of the resorption lacunae under active osteoclasts, and are taken up by them. There are two classes of bisphosphonates, non-nitrogen-containing and nitrogen-containing bisphosphonates (N-BPs). The nitrogen-containing bisphosphonates (alendronate, ibandronate, pamidronate, risedronate, and zoledronic acid) are more potent osteoclast inhibitors than are non-nitrogen-containing bisphosphonates (e.g., clodronate, etidronate, and tiludronate) [28]. Moreover, nitrogen-containing bisphosphonates inhibit farnesyl pyrophosphatase, an enzyme responsible for the prenylation of GTPases that are essential for osteoclast function, structural integrity, and the prevention of apoptosis [28, 31, 56]. The inhibition of farnesyl pyrophosphatase also results in the accumulation of isopentenyl diphosphate that is incorporated into a cytotoxic nucleotide metabolite, ApppI [31]. Therefore, bisphosphonates affect osteoclast differentiation and maturation and thereby act as potent inhibitors of bone resorption (Fig. 15.1). Preclinical evidence demonstrated that bisphosphonates do not affect only the bone microenvironment but have also a direct effect on macrophages, gamma

D. Santini (✉) • A. Zoccoli • M. Iuliani
M. Fioramonti • G. Ribelli • F. Pantano
Department of Medical Oncology, Campus Bio-Medico University of Rome, Rome, Italy
e-mail: D.Santini@unicampus.it

C. Ripamonti
Supportive Care in Cancer Unit, Fondazione IRCCS, Istituto Nazionale dei Tumori, Milan, Italy

F. Bertoldo et al. (eds.), *Bone Metastases from Prostate Cancer*,
DOI 10.1007/978-3-319-42327-2_15

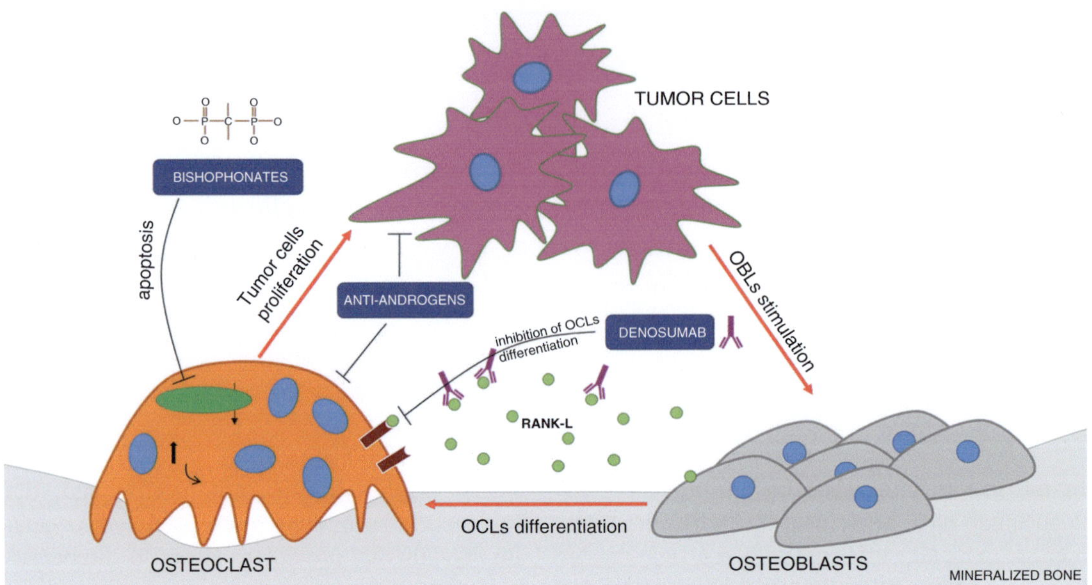

Fig 15.1 Mechanism of action of bisphosphonate, denosumab, and anti-androgen on the bone metastases "vicious cycle." *OCLs* osteoclasts, *OBLs* osteoblasts

delta T cells, osteoblasts, and cancer cells showing antitumor and/or antiangiogenic effects [6].

The efficacy of bisphosphonate treatment on patients with bone metastatic cancer depends on the specific bisphosphonate and on the administered doses (Table 15.1). In a combined analysis of two placebo-controlled studies of 378 men with metastatic prostate cancer, pamidronate (90 mg every 3–4 weeks) failed to demonstrate a significant overall treatment benefit compared to placebo in terms of reduction of SREs and palliation of bone pain [50]. In particular, Small et al. did not observe sustained or significant differences between the pamidronate and placebo groups for self-reported pain, analgesic use, or mobility [50]. In a double-blind placebo-controlled randomized trial, clodronate did not improve bone progression-free survival (BPFS) among men with bone metastases from prostate cancer. Heidenreich A et al. showed that clodronate treatment (300 mg for 8 days) of painful osseous metastases due to hormone-refractory prostate cancer resulted in a significant pain decrease with a concomitant reduction in the daily consumption of analgesics in 75 % of patients [16]. Similarly, ibandronate (6 mg over 1 h each day for 3 days followed by a single infusion of 6 mg every 4 weeks) showed a significant improvement in bone pain in patients with hormone-refractory prostate cancer and bone metastases [15]. Zoledronic acid is the most potent bisphosphonate currently used in men with bone metastatic prostate cancer that has progressed after initial hormone therapy. The benefit of zoledronic acid (4 mg every 3 weeks) was demonstrated in a randomized, placebo-controlled trial in patients with hormone-refractory metastatic prostate carcinoma. This study showed a significant reduction in the frequency of SREs, a longer median time to develop SREs, and lower pain and analgesic scores [44]. In particular, a greater proportion of patients who received placebo had SREs than those who received zoledronic acid at 4 mg (44.2 % versus 33.2 %); median time to first SRE was 321 days for patients who received placebo and was not reached for patients who received zoledronic acid at 4 mg. In a subsequent placebo-controlled randomized clinical trial, zoledronic acid reduced the incidence of SREs (38 % versus 49 % for the placebo group) in men with hormone-refractory metastatic prostate cancer. Moreover, zoledronic acid increased the median time to the first SRE (488 days versus 321 days in the placebo group)

Table 15.1 Summary of main randomized controlled trials evaluating in men with prostate cancer

N° of patients/primary cancer	Scheduling	Study	Results	References
Clodronate				
Hormone refractory metastatic prostate cancer	3 mg i.v. for 8 days	Open, uncontrolled study	Significant decrease in bone pain score in 75 % of patients ($p <$ 0.001)	8
Ibandronate				
Hormone refractory metastatic prostate cancer	6 mg i.v. on days 1-3 then 6 mg every 4 weeks	Open, uncontrolled study	92 % of patients had significant pain reduction, and 39 % of patients were completely pain free	9
Pamidronate				
Hormone refractory metastatic prostate cancer	90 mg i.v. every 3 weeks for 27 weeks	Double-bind, placebo-controlled trial	No significant or sustained effect o pain score	7
Zoledronic acid				
Hormone refractory metastatic prostate cancer	4 or 8 mg i.v every 3 weeks for 15 months	Double-bind, placebo-controlled trail	SRE incidence reduction (44.2 % placebo group vs 33.2 % ZA group) and significant decrease in bone pain and analgesic use	10
Hormone refractory metastatic prostate cancer	4 or 8 mg i.v every 3 weeks for 15 months	Double-bind, placebo-controlled trail	SRE incidence reduction (38 % placebo group vs 49 % ZA group) and median time to first SRE increase (321 days placebo group vs 488 days ZA group)	11
Nonmetastatic prostate cancer	4 mg i.v. every 6 months	Randomized placebo-controlled trial	BMD improvement in ZA group compared to placebo: lumbar spine (6 % vs 5 %), left total hip (1 % vs 8 %) and left femoral neck (3 % vs 8 %)	12
Nonmetastaticprostate cancer	4 mg i.v. only in day 1	Randomized controlled trial	BMD improvement in ZA group compared to placebo in lumbar spine and in total hip	13
Nonmetastatic prostate cancer	4 mg i.v. every 3 months	Randomized controlled trial	BMD improvement in ZA group compared to placebo in lumbar spine, femoral neck, and in trochanter and total hip	14

(continued)

Table 15.1 (continued)

N° of patients/primary cancer	Scheduling	Study	Results	References
High-risk, locally advanced, metastatic or recurrent prostate cancer	4 mg for six 3-weekly cycles, then 4-weekly in combination with docetaxel 75 mg/ml (six 3-weekly cycles) + prednisolone 10 mg daily	Randomized controlled trial	No improvement in overall survival in ZA group or delay in SRE	15
Castration-sensitive metastatic prostate cancer	4 mg i.v. every 4 weeks	Double-bind, placebo-controlled trial	Early ZA treatment did not increase time to first SRE (median time 31 months in ZA group vs 29,8 months in placebo group)	16

ZA zoledronic acid, *BMD* bone mineral density, *SRE* skeletal-related event

and reduced the ongoing risk of SREs by 36% compared with placebo [45]. Further evidence of zoledronic acid efficacy in preventing bone fractures was demonstrated in a randomized phase III trial (RTOG 0518) in patients with high-grade and/or locally advanced, nonmetastatic prostate adenocarcinoma receiving luteinizing hormone-releasing hormone (LHRH) agonist and radiotherapy (RT). Data showed that zoledronic acid treatment was associated with improved bone mineral density (BMD) [21]. Similar results were obtained in another study that showed an increase in BMD and a durable suppression of serum N-telopeptide levels for 12 months in men receiving a gonadotropin-releasing hormone (GnRH) agonist in combination with zoledronic acid [29].

In the adjuvant setting of hormone-sensitive prostate cancer, zoledronic acid can be given to prevent and treat tumor therapy-induced bone loss. A randomized phase III trial demonstrated that this agent increased bone density in patients with nonmetastatic prostate cancer receiving androgen deprivation therapy (ADT) [51]. Data showed that lumbar spine bone mineral density increased 5.6% from baseline in 1 year in the zoledronic acid group and decreased 2.2% in the placebo group (mean difference 7.8%). Bone mineral density significantly increased from baseline also in the femoral neck, trochanter, and total hip [51]. Currently, the key question is what is the role of zoledronic acid in hormone-sensitive prostate cancer? In the STAMPEDE trial, the addition of zoledronic acid to docetaxel did not improve survival outcomes or delay the SRE incidence [20]. In the CALGB/ALLIANCE 90202 study comparing early treatment in hormone-sensitive prostate cancer versus delayed treatment in castration-resistant prostate cancer (CRPC), no difference in SRE-free survival and no change in survival outcomes were noted. Thus, zoledronic acid did not improve SRE in hormone-sensitive disease (median time to first SRE was 31.9 months in the zoledronic acid group and 29.8 months in the placebo group) [53].

15.2 Denosumab

Bone metabolism is a dynamic process that balances bone formation and bone resorption. Bone resorption is performed by active osteoclasts, while bone formation implies inhibition of bone-resorbing activity and stimulation of osteoblast bone deposition [25]. The receptor activators of nuclear factor-kappaB ligand (RANKL)/RANK/osteoprotegerin (OPG) are members of the TNF and TNF-receptor superfamily and act as essential mediators of OCL formation, function, and survival. RANKL normally secreted by osteoblast binds to its receptor RANK, which is expressed by precursors and mature osteoclasts, stimulating bone resorption activity; in contrast, OPG, the decoy receptor for RANKL, prevents osteoclast activation [10]. In addition to its role as a regulator of bone remodeling, the RANKL/RANK/OPG network also has a key role in osteolytic bone metastasis [10]. The morphometric analysis of immunohistochemical staining showed that RANK, OPG, and RANKL were not significantly expressed in hyperplastic prostate, while their expression levels were increased 50, 45, and 52.5 %, respectively, in prostate cancer tissue [23]. Understanding the molecular mechanisms that trigger the vicious cycle of bone metastases has provided potential targets such as the RANKL/RANK pathway. It has proven to be an effective target for translational research due to its central role in the cascade of events leading to metastatic bone disease. Indeed it has been demonstrated that RANK expression level in the primary tumor correlated with the occurrence of bone metastases, and RANK-expressing cancer could be found in up to 80 % of bone metastases originating from solid tumors [27, 47], suggesting that RANK enables cancer cells to migrate to bone where RANKL is abundantly expressed by osteoblasts. Furthermore, RANKL was also able to directly induce prostate cancer cell proliferation increasing this vicious cycle [30] (Fig. 15.1). Recent evidence suggests an important role for RANKL/RANK in the immune system including in lymph node development, lymphocyte differentiation, dendritic cell survival, T-cell activation, and tolerance induction.

Denosumab (AMG162) is a human noncytotoxic IgG2 monoclonal antibody with an extremely high affinity and specificity for human RANKL. It is approved for the treatment of osteoporosis, cancer treatment-induced bone loss, bone metastases, and other skeletal pathologies mediated by osteoclasts [22]. Several clinical trials demonstrated the ability of denosumab to prevent the development of bone metastasis in high-risk prostate cancer patients (Table 15.2).

In a randomized double-blind phase III study of castration-resistant prostate cancer patients with bone metastases, the median time to first SRE for the denosumab arm was significantly prolonged (21 months) compared to the zoledronic acid arm (17 months) with no improvement in OS or progression of disease [12]. In particular, 1904 patients were randomly assigned to treatment, of whom 951 received zoledronic acid and 950 received denosumab. Denosumab significantly delayed the time to first on-study skeletal-related event by 18 % compared with zoledronic acid, with a between-group difference of 3.6 months. Overall survival and investigator-reported disease progression were not significantly different between treatment groups [12]. In another phase III trial, 1432 men with nonmetastatic castration-resistant prostate cancer were randomly assigned to denosumab or placebo. Denosumab increased the time to development of first bone metastasis by a median of 4.2 months compared with placebo, in a population of men deemed to be at high risk for the development of metastatic disease (baseline PSA value ≥8.0 ng/mL and/or PSA doubling time (PSADT) ≤10.0 months). No difference in OS was noted (median 44 versus 45 months; HR, 1.01) [55]. To determine the efficacy of denosumab in men at greatest risk for bone metastases, the researchers evaluated bone-metastasis-free survival (BMFS) in a subset of men with PSADT ≤6 months. Median BMFS in the placebo group of men with PSADT ≤6 months was 6.5 months shorter than for the placebo group (18.7 months versus 25.2 months) [55].

It has been demonstrated that denosumab prevented bone loss in men at high risk for fractures receiving ADT for nonmetastatic prostate cancer [52, 54]. In a phase III study, it was found that denosumab is able to decrease the incidence of new vertebral fractures at 12, 24, and 36 months. The cumulative incidence of new vertebral fractures at 36 months was 3.9 % in the placebo group and 1.5 % in the denosumab group with a significant decrease of 62 %. This drop was significant even at 12 months (1.9 for placebo versus 0.3 for denosumab) and 24 months (3.3 for placebo versus 1.0 for denosumab) [52, 54].

Table 15.2 Summary of main randomized controlled trials evaluating denosumab in men with prostate cancer

N° of patients/primary cancer	Scheduling	Study	Results	References
Denosumab				
Bone metastatic castration resistant prostate cancer	120 mg subcutaneous denosumab plus intravenous placebo, or 4 mg intravenous zoledronic acid plus subcutaneous placebo every 4 weeks	Multicenter, double-blind study, randomized	Median time to first SRE was 20.7 months with denosumab compared with 17.1 months with zoledronic acid	24
Nonmetastatic castration resistant prostate cancer	Denosumab 120 mg or subcutaneous placebo every 4 weeks	Double-blind, randomized, placebo-controlled study	Denosumab significantly increased bone-metastasis-free survival by a median of 4.2 months compared with placebo	25
Nonmetastatic hormone-sensitive prostate cancer receiving androgen-deprivation therapy (ADT)	Denosumab at a dose of 60 mg subcutaneously every 6 months or placebo	Double-bind, multicenter study	BMD of the lumbar spine had increased by 5.6 % in the denosumab group as compared with a loss of 1.0 % in the placebo group	26

BMD bone mineral density, *SRE* skeletal-related event

15.3 Safety of Bone Target Therapies

One of the most commonly reported adverse events related to bisphosphonates and denosumab treatment is hypocalcemia that is most often asymptomatic with these agents [17]. In particular, hypocalcemia occurred more frequently with denosumab than with zoledronic acid as shown in the phase III trial in patients with CRPC and bone metastases (13 % versus 6 %, $p<0.0001$) [12]. In an integrated analysis of 5723 patients from three randomized phase III trials, the safety profile for denosumab was better than for zoledronic acid, demonstrating no effect on renal function and no need for dose adjustment or renal monitoring [24]. In patients receiving zoledronic acid, the incidence of hypocalcemia was lower than in patients receiving denosumab (1.3 % versus 3.1 % for grade 3 or grade 4 toxicities), though most cases were asymptomatic [24]. Thus, repletion of vitamin D levels before and during the therapy and monitoring of calcium levels during therapy are recommended in the prescribing information of denosumab [18].

15.4 Osteonecrosis of the Jaw (ONJ)

Osteonecrosis of the jaw (ONJ) is a relatively uncommon but potentially serious adverse event reported in patients treated with antiresorptive agents such as bisphosphonates (BPs) and the RANKL inhibitor denosumab [43]. The reported incidence of ONJ is 1.2–9.9 % (mostly derived from retrospective analyses) with pooled risk estimated incidence, in BPs users of 2.4 % [37]. In RCTs comparing zoledronic acid and denosumab in 5677 patients who underwent screening dental procedure, 89 ONJ cases were reported, of which 52 are in the denosumab group [43]. ONJ was defined as the persistence of exposed bone in the oral cavity, despite an adequate treatment for

6 weeks, without local evidence of malignancy and no prior RT to the affected region [41]. However, ONJ may present with the nonexposed variant of ONJ. Recently Fedele et al. [11] performed a secondary analysis of data from MISSION, a cross-sectional study of a large population of patients with bisphosphonate-associated ONJ recruited in 13 European centers [3]. A total of 886 consecutive patients were recruited and 799 were studied after data cleaning. Of these, 607 (76 %) were diagnosed according to the traditional definition. Diagnosis in the remaining 192 (24 %) could not be adjudicated as they had several abnormal features relating to the jaws but no visible necrotic bone. The groups were similar for most of the phenotypic variables tested. Thus the authors showed that the use of the traditional definition may result in one quarter of patients remaining undiagnosed. The American Association of Oral and Maxillofacial Surgeons (AAOMS) recommend the term medical-related osteonecrosis of the jaw (MRONJ) as preferred [39] because of the recognition of jaw necrosis as a complication of other drugs including the RANK ligand inhibitor denosumab and antiangiogenic agents. Table 15.1 shows the MRONJ staging [39]. Among the risk factors, we must consider the presence of chronic periodontal pathologies; poor oral hygiene; use, duration, and type of BP therapy or denosumab; oral infections; dental caries; tooth extractions; use of dental appliances; denture traumatisms; fractures; invasive dental surgery during the course of BP therapy; concurrent disease (e.g., diabetes, peripheral vasculopathy); and presence of anemia [39, 41]. In a retrospective study on 567 cases with ONJ, [57] found that, in 205 of them (36.2 %), no invasive procedure was performed. MRONJ is linked to concomitant use of different drugs such as chemotherapy, antiretrovirals, steroids, thalidomide, bevacizumab, docetaxel, TKI sunitinib or sorafenib, and anthracyclines [5]. The role of genetic factors is receiving increased attention [32].

ONJ may be asymptomatic for weeks or months. Lesions become symptomatic when there is associated inflammation of surrounding soft tissues, infection, and loosening of teeth drainage and when exposed bone produces trauma to adjacent soft tissues (cutaneous fistula, mucosal fistula, bone exposed through the skin). Preventive dental measures, after dental screening examination [1, 7, 40, 41, 59], are advocated to reduce the ONJ incidence [9, 29, 37] due to their efficacy in patients with bone metastases. Active oral infections should be treated, and sites at high risk for infection should be eliminated. Oral care should be provided by a dentist or dental professional who is familiar with cancer therapy. Patient education on the importance of oral hygiene, the regular dental evaluation, and the risk of ONJ is paramount. Treatment of MRONJ is based on a conservative therapy with limited debridement, oral antibiotics, oral rinsed with chlorhexidine or hydrogen peroxide, antibacterial mouth rinse, and pain control. Major surgery is indicated after the formation of necrotic bone sequestrum. Total sequestration of necrotic bone was obtained in ten patients with ONJ lesions ≤2.5 cm treated with topical application of an oil suspension enriched with medical 03 gas after the failure of various cycles of antibiotics [35]. No patient required surgical intervention. In another open-label prospective study, [36] evaluated the efficacy and tolerability of medical ozone (03) treatment delivered as gas insufflation on each ONJ lesion >2.5 cm developed in 24 patients treated with zoledronic acid after failure of various antibiotics. Six patients had the sequestrum and spontaneous expulsion of the necrotic bone followed by oral mucosa re-epithelization. In 12 patients with the largest and deeper ONJ lesions, 03 gas therapy produced the sequestrum of the necrotic bone after 10–38 insufflations; surgery was necessary to remove it in 11 patients. Removal was possible without the resection of healthy mandible edge because of the presence of bone sequestrum. No adverse event was reported and no ONJ relapse appeared. There are reports that low-level laser therapy improves healing and symptoms related to ONJ [49, 58]. Future research is required to better understand the individualized treatment of ONJ in cancer patients as well as in patients with osteoporosis.

American Association of Oral and Maxillofacial Surgeons (AAOMS) medication-related ONJ (MRONJ) staging

ONJ staging	Characteristics
At risk	No apparent necrotic bone in patients who have been treated with antiresorptive therapy
Stage 0	No clinical evidence of necrotic bone, but nonspecific clinical findings, radiographic changes and symptoms
Stage 1	Exposed and necrotic bone, or fistulae that probes to bone, in asymptomatic patients without evidence of infection
Stage 2	Exposed and necrotic bone, or fistulae that probes to bone, associated with infection as evidenced by pain and erythema in region of exposed bone ± purulent drainage
Stage 3	Exposed and necrotic bone or a fistula that probes to bone in patients with pain, infection, and 1+ complication*

*Exposed and necrotic bone extending beyond the region of alveolar bone resulting in pathologic fracture, extraoral fistula, oral antral/oral nasal communication, or osteolysis extending to the inferior border of the mandible or the sinus floor.

Ruggiero SL, et al. J Oral Maxillofac Surg 2014;72:1938–56.

15.5 Other Molecules

Several molecules that are under intensive clinical testing on humans, although they target directly the tumor cell and not the bone microenvironment, have demonstrated over an improved survival, of being able to modify the natural history of bone metastases, resulting in a delay of the occurrence of SRE, a reduction of bone pain, and an improvement in quality of life. These therapeutic options include abiraterone and enzalutamide.

15.5.1 Abiraterone

Abiraterone acetate (ABI) (Zytiga, Janssen) is a selective inhibitor of androgen biosynthesis; it acts potently and irreversibly blocks Cyp17 resulting in virtually undetectable serum and intratumoral androgen production in the adrenals, testes, and prostate cancer cells [2, 33]. ABI is currently approved in both pre- and post-docetaxel setting of mCRPC.

In phase III studies in metastatic castration-resistant prostate cancer (mCRPC) patients, it was demonstrated that ABI treatment is associated not only with a significant survival advantage in both chemotherapy-naive and chemotherapy-treated patients but also, in docetaxel treated patients, with a better pain control from skeletal metastases and a delay in time to development SREs and in radiological skeletal progression [7, 13, 14, 26, 42].

In particular, in the pivotal study COU-301, involving patients with metastatic castration-resistant prostate cancer who previously received chemotherapy, De Bono showed an improvement in overall survival in the abiraterone with prednisone arm (14.8 months) versus the prednisone-only treated patients' group (10.9 months), with a 35 % reduction in the risk of death in the abiraterone arm [8]. In addition, abiraterone acetate and prednisone offer effective pain relief, delayed pain progression, and prevention of skeletal-related events compared with prednisone alone. Indeed, 25 % of patients developed a skeletal event in 9.9 months when treated with abiraterone and 4.9 months with placebo, and the median time to occurrence of first SRE was 25.0 months with abiraterone compared to 20.3 months with placebo [7, 13, 14]. In addition, in patients with clinically significant pain at baseline, abiraterone acetate and prednisone offer effective pain relief and delayed pain progression. Indeed, in patients with significant pain at baseline, abiraterone acetate and prednisone obtained a more significative palliation in 157 of 349 (45.0 %) of patients versus 47 of 163 (28.8 %) in those who did not receive abiraterone and faster palliation (median time to palliation 5.6 months versus 13.7 months) of pain intensity than did prednisone only [26].

In the COU-302 trial, abiraterone acetate plus prednisone before docetaxel was shown to yield a significant improvement in radiographic progression-free survival associated with a trend toward improved overall survival [42].

An interim analysis of the COU-302 study confirmed that patients treated with abiraterone showed a statistically significant improvement in rPFS (HR 0.52; $p< 0.0001$). The overall survival (OS) analysis favored abiraterone over prednisone alone (median 35.3 versus 30.1 months), and the OS benefit of abiraterone was supported in an exploratory multivariate analysis (HR 0.74; $p=0.0017$) that adjusted for baseline prognostic factor. In addition, analyses of prespecified measures of patient-reported outcomes confirmed that abiraterone treatment delayed pain progression and deterioration in functional status compared with prednisone alone [34].

Finally a more recent post hoc analysis [46] of study COU-AA-302 demonstrated that treatment with abiraterone acetate and prednisone with concomitant bone-targeted therapy (BTT; zoledronic acid (93 %), denosumab (6 %), and other BTTs (1 %)) for treatment of bone metastases was safe and well tolerated and that the efficacy of abiraterone is maintained with concomitant BTT, with a possible added benefit of delaying the need for opiates to control pain. In this analysis, the comparisons among all patient groups favored abiraterone over prednisone alone, and concomitant BTT was associated with increased effectiveness of abiraterone regarding clinical outcomes. In particular, among patients treated with abiraterone, BTT was associated with a longer time to ECOG PS deterioration. Abiraterone in combination with BTT, compared with prednisone with BTT, delayed the median time to deterioration in ECOG PS by 3.9 months. These findings confirm the efficacy of abiraterone plus BTT combination in clinical practice. In conclusion, it is reasonable to speculate that the ABI effects on metastatic bone disease may be secondary to a systemic control of the disease due to a direct antitumor effect that, in turn, leads to a decrease of cancer cells/OCLs/OBLs vicious circle or, alternatively, to a specific action directed to bone microenvironment [19] (Fig. 15.1).

15.5.2 Enzalutamide

Other new drugs are being tested in metastatic prostate cancer with potential therapeutic effect even on bone metastases (enzalutamide, cabozantinib, etc.). In particular, enzalutamide (formerly MDV3100, trade name XTANDI™, Astellas) is a latest-generation drug able to bind the androgen receptor, to prevent its translocation within the nucleus and its deregulatory function on DNA, and currently approved for the treatment of adult men with metastatic castration-resistant prostate cancer (mCRPC).

The AFFIRM study evaluated enzalutamide in men with mCRPC who had previously received docetaxel [13, 14, 48]. This trial has demonstrated that enzalutamide increases survival with a median of 18.4 months versus 13.6 months in the placebo group.

A subanalysis of AFFIRM trial [13, 14] focused on the effect of enzalutamide versus placebo on SRE, pain, and QOL. The subanalysis showed that enzalutamide significantly retard SREs with delayed time to the first SRE at 16.7 months versus 13.3 months in those who received placebo, representing a 31 % reduction in risk of SRE ($P=.0001$). The distribution of first SRE showed a generally favorable effect of enzalutamide, with fewer patients experiencing radiation to the bone (20 % for enzalutamide versus 25 % for placebo) and spinal cord compression (6 % versus 8 %), but about 4 % in each group experiencing pathological fracture. In addition, all parameters of pain palliation, including time to pain progression, mean reduction in pain intensity, and reduction in pain interference with daily activity, were all in favor of the enzalutamide compared to the placebo arm.

More recently, the mCRPC chemo-naive patients were investigated in a new phase III trial; the PREVAIL trial aimed to evaluate enzalutamide in men with chemo-naïve mCRPC that had progressed despite the use of androgen deprivation therapy (ADT) (luteinizing hormone-releasing hormone analogue or orchiectomy) [4]. The study demonstrated a statistically significant delay in the growth or spread of metastatic prostate cancer, a reduction in the risk of death, and a delay of the time to initiation of chemotherapy compared with the placebo arm. More in detail, the results showed a reduction of risk of radiographic progression or death by 81 % (HR = 0.19; $p < 0.0001$), compared with placebo and a rate of radiographic progression-free survival at 12 months of follow-up of 65 % among patients treated with enzalutamide versus 14 % among patients receiving placebo.

The secondary endpoint of the study included the time until the initiation of cytotoxic chemotherapy, the time until the first skeletal-related event, the best overall soft-tissue response, the time until PSA progression, and a decline in the PSA level of 50 % or more from baseline; the results showed the superiority of enzalutamide over placebo with respect to all the prespecified endpoints. The median time until the initiation of cytotoxic chemotherapy was 28 months in the enzalutamide group versus 10.8 months in the placebo group. Treatment with enzalutamide also resulted in a reduction in the risk of a first SRE; indeed at a median of approximately 31 months, the SRE occurred in 32 % of patients in the enzalutamide group and in 37 % in the placebo group.

Enzalutamide was also superior to placebo with respect to the time until a decline in the quality of life. The median time until a quality-of-life deterioration, as measured on the FACT-P scale, was 11.3 months in the enzalutamide group and 5.6 months in the placebo group.

References

1. Advisory Task Force on Bisphosphonate-Related Osteonecrosis of the Jaws, American Association of Oral and Maxillofacial Surgeons (2007) American Association of Oral and Maxillofacial Surgeons position paper on bisphosphonate-related osteonecrosis of the jaws. J Oral Maxillofac Surg 65:369–376
2. Barrie SE, Potter GA, Goddard PM et al (1994) Pharmacology of novel steroidal inhibitors of cytochrome P450(17) alpha (17 alpha-hydroxylase/C17-20 lyase). J Steroid Biochem Mol Biol 50:267–273
3. Bedogni A, Fedele S, Bedogni G et al (2014) Staging of jaw osteonecrosis requires computed tomography for accurate definition of the extent of bony disease. Br J Maxillofac Surg 52:603–608
4. Beer T, Armstrong A, Rathkopf D et al (2014) Enzalutamide in metastatic prostate cancer before chemotherapy. N Engl J Med 371:424–433
5. Berenson JR, Stopeck AT. Medication-related osteonecrosis of the jaw in patients with cancer. http://www.uptodate.com/contents/medication-related-osteonecrosis-ofthe jaw-in-patients-with-cancer. Accessed on 28 Jan 2016
6. Coleman R, Gnant M, Morgan G et al (2012) Effects of bone-targeted agents on cancer progression and mortality. J Natl Cancer Inst 104:1059–1067
7. Damato K, Gralow J, Hoff A et al (2005) Expert panel recommendations for the prevention, diagnosis, and treatment of osteonecrosis of the jaws. LDA J 64: 21–24
8. De Bono JS, Logothetis CJ, Molina A et al (2011) Abiraterone and increased survival in metastatic prostate cancer. N Engl J Med 364:1995–2005
9. Dimopoulos MA, Kastritis E, Bamia C et al (2009) Reduction of osteonecrosis of the jaw (ONJ) after implementation of preventive measures in patients with multiple myeloma treated with zoledronic acid. Ann Oncol 20:117–120
10. Dougall WC, Chaisson M (2006) The RANK/RANKL/OPG triad in cancer-induced bone diseases. Cancer Metastasis Rev 25:541–549
11. Fedele S, Bedogni G, Scoletta M et al (2015) Up to a quarter of patients with osteonecrosis of the jaw associated with antiresorptive agents remain undiagnosed. Br J Oral Maxillofac Surg 53:13–17
12. Fizazi K, Carducci M, Smith M et al (2011) Denosumab versus zoledronic acid for treatment of bone metastases in men with castration-resistant prostate cancer: a randomised, double-blind study. Lancet 377:813–822
13. Fizazi K, Scher HI, Molina A et al (2012) Abiraterone acetate for treatment of metastatic castration-resistant prostate cancer: final overall survival analysis of the COU-AA-301 randomised, double-blind, placebo-controlled phase 3 study. Lancet Oncol 13:983–992
14. Fizazi K, Scher HI, Saad F et al (2012) Impact of Enzalutamide, an androgen receptor signaling inhibitor, on time to first skeletal related event (SRE) and

pain in the phase 3 AFFIRM Study. Ann Oncol 23 abstract 8960
15. Heidenreich A, Elert A, Hofmann R (2002) Ibandronate in the treatment of prostate cancer associated painful osseous metastases. Prostate Cancer Prostatic Dis 5:231–235
16. Heidenreich A, Hofmann R, Engelmann UH (2001) The use of bisphosphonate for the palliative treatment of painful bone metastasis due to hormone refractory prostate cancer. J Urol 165:136–140
17. Horwich A, Parker C, de Reijke T et al (2013) Prostate cancer: ESMO Clinical Practice Guidelines for diagnosis, treatment and follow-up. Ann Oncol 24: 106–114
18. Iranikhah M, Stricker S, Freeman MK (2014) Future of bisphosphonates and denosumab for men with advanced prostate cancer. Cancer Manag Res 6: 217–224
19. Iuliani M, Pantano F, Buttigliero C et al (2015) Biological and clinical effects of abiraterone on anti-resorptive and anabolic activity in bone microenvironment. Oncotarget 6:12520–12528
20. James ND, Sydes MR, Clarke NW et al (2015) STAMPEDE investigators. Addition of docetaxel, zoledronic acid, or both to first-line long-term hormone therapy in prostate cancer (STAMPEDE): survival results from an adaptive, multiarm, multistage, platform randomised controlled trial. Lancet 387(10024):1163–1177
21. Kachnic LA, Pugh SL, Tai P et al (2013) RTOG 0518: randomized phase III trial to evaluate zoledronic acid for prevention of osteoporosis and associated fractures in prostate cancer patients. Prostate Cancer Prostatic Dis 16:382–386
22. Lacey DL, Boyle WJ, Simonet WS et al (2012) Bench to bedside: elucidation of the OPG-RANK-RANKL pathway and the development of denosumab. Nat Rev Drug Discov 11:401–419
23. Li X, Liu Y, Wu B et al (2014) Potential role of the OPG/RANK/RANKL axis in prostate cancer invasion and bone metastasis. Oncol Rep 32:2605–2611
24. Lipton A, Fizazi K, Stopeck AT et al (2012) Superiority of denosumab to zoledronic acid for prevention of skeletal-related events: a combined analysis of 3 pivotal, randomised, phase 3 trials. Eur J Cancer 48:3082–3092
25. Liu XH, Kirschenbaum A, Yao S et al (2005) Cross-talk between the interleukin-6 and prostaglandin E(2) signaling systems results in enhancement of osteoclastogenesis through effects on the osteoprotegerin/receptor activator of nuclear factor-{kappa}B (RANK) ligand/RANK system. Endocrinology 146:1991–1998
26. Logothetis CJ, Basch E, Molina A et al (2012) Effect of abiraterone acetate and prednisone compared with placebo and prednisone on pain control and skeletal-related events in patients with metastatic castration-resistant prostate cancer: exploratory analysis of data from the COU-AA-301 randomised trial. Lancet Oncol 13:1210–1217
27. Loser K, Mehling A, Loeser S et al (2006) Epidermal RANKL controls regulatory T-cell numbers via activation of dendritic cells. Nat Med 12:1372–1379
28. Luckman SP, Hughes DE, Coxon FP et al (1998) Nitrogen-containing bisphosphonates inhibit the mevalonate pathway and prevent post-translational prenylation of GTP-binding proteins, including Ras. J Bone Miner Res 13:581–589
29. Michaelson MD, Kaufman DS, Lee H et al (2007) Randomized controlled trial of annual zoledronic acid to prevent gonadotropin-releasing hormone agonist-induced bone loss in men with prostate cancer. J Clin Oncol 25(9):1038–1042
30. Miller RE, Roudier M, Jones J et al (2008) RANK ligand inhibition plus docetaxel improves survival and reduces tumor burden in a murine model of prostate cancer bone metastasis. Mol Cancer Ther 7(7): 2160–2169
31. Mönkkönen H, Auriola S, Lehenkari P et al (2006) A new endogenous ATP analog (ApppI) inhibits the mitochondrial adenine nucleotide translocase (ANT) and is responsible for the apoptosis induced by nitrogen-containing bisphosphonates. Br J Pharmacol 147:437–445
32. Nicoletti P, Cartsos VM, Palaska PK et al (2012) Genomewide pharmacogenetics of bisphosphonate-induced osteonecrosis of the jaw: the role of RBMS3. Oncologist 17:279
33. O'Donnell A, Judson I, Dowsett M et al (2004) Hormonal impact of the 17alpha-hydroxylase/C(17,20)-lyase inhibitor abiraterone acetate (CB7630) in patients with prostate cancer. Br J Cancer 90:2317–2325
34. Rathkopf DE, Smith MR, de Bono JS et al (2014) Updated interim efficacy analysis and long-term safety of abiraterone acetate in metastatic castration-resistant prostate cancer patients without prior chemotherapy (COU-AA-302). Eur Urol 66:815–825
35. Ripamonti CI, Cislaghi E, Mariani L et al (2011) Efficacy and safety of medical ozone (03) delivered in oil suspension applications for the treatment of osteonecrosis of the jaw in patients with bone metastases treated with bisphosphonates: Preliminary results of a phase I-II study. Oral Oncol 47:185–190
36. Ripamonti CI, Maniezzo M, Boldini S et al (2012) Efficacy and tolerability of medical ozone gas insufflations in patients with osteonecrosis of the jaw treated with bisphosphonates-Preliminary data. Med Ozone Gas Insufflat Treat ONJ Lesions J Bone Oncol 1:81–87
37. Ripamonti CI, Maniezzo M, Campa T et al (2009) Decreased occurrence of osteonecrosis of the jaw after implementation of dental preventive measures in solid tumor patients with bone metastases treated with bisphosphonates. The experience of the National Cancer Institute of Milano. Ann Oncol 20(1):137–145
38. Roelofs AJ, Thompson K, Gordon S et al (2006) Molecular mechanisms of action of bisphosphonates: current status. Clin Cancer Res 12:6222s–6230s

39. Ruggiero RL et al (2014) American association of oral and maxillofacial surgeons position paper on medication-related osteonecrosis of the jaw-2014 update. J Oral Maxillofac Surg 72/10:1938–1956
40. Ruggiero S, Gralow J, Marx RE et al (2006) Practical guidelines for the prevention, diagnosis, and treatment of osteonecrosis of the jaw in patients with cancer. J Oncol Pract 2(1):7–14
41. Ruggiero SL, Dodson TB, Assael LA et al (2009) American Association of oral and maxillofacial surgeons position paper on bisphosphonate-related osteonecrosis of the jaw-2009 update. J Oral Maxillofac Surg 67(Suppl 5):2–12
42. Ryan CJ, Smith MR, de Bono JS et al (2013) Abiraterone in metastatic prostate cancer without previous chemotherapy. N Engl J Med 368:138–148
43. Saad F, Brown JE, Poznack V et al (2012) Incidence, risk factors, and outcome of osteonecrosis of the jaw: integrated analysis from three blinded active-controlled phase III trials in cancer patients with bone metastases. Ann Oncol 23:1341–1347
44. Saad F, Gleason DM, Murray R et al (2002) A randomized, placebo-controlled trial of zoledronic acid in patients with hormone refractory metastatic prostate carcinoma. J Natl Cancer Inst 94(19):1458–1468
45. Saad F, Gleason DM, Murray R et al (2004) Long term efficacy of zoledronic acid for the prevention of skeletal complications in patients with metastatic hormone refractory prostate carcinoma. J Natl Cancer Inst 96(11):879–882
46. Saad F, Shore N, Van Poppel H et al (2015) Impact of bone-targeted therapies in chemotherapy-naïve metastatic castration-resistant prostate cancer patients treated with abiraterone acetate: post hoc analysis of study COU-AA-302. Eur Urol 68(4):570–577
47. Santini D, Perrone G, Roato I et al (2011) Expression pattern of receptor activator of NFkB (RANK) in a series of primary solid tumors and related bone metastases. J Cell Physiol 226:780–784
48. Scher HI, Fizazi K, Saad F et al; AFFIRM Investigators (2012) Increased survival with enzalutamide in prostate cancer after chemotherapy. N Engl J Med 367(13):1187–1197
49. Scoletta M, Arduino PG, Reggio L et al (2010) Effect of low-level laser irradiation on bisphosphonate-induced osteonecrosis of the jaws: preliminary results of a prospective study. Photomed Laser Surg 28:179
50. Small EJ, Smith MR, Seaman JJ et al (2003) Combined analysis of two multicenter, randomized, placebo-controlled studies of pamidronate disodium for the palliation of bone pain in men with metastatic prostate cancer. J Clin Oncol 21:4277e–4284e
51. Smith MR, Eastham J, Gleason DM et al (2003) Randomized controlled trial of zoledronic acid to prevent bone loss in men receiving androgen deprivation therapy for nonmetastatic prostate cancer. J Urol 169(6):2008–2012
52. Smith MR, Egerdie B, Hemdezet TN et al (2009) Denosumab in men receiving androgen-deprivation therapy for prostate cancer. N Engl J Med 361:745–755
53. Smith MR, Halabi S, Ryan CJ et al (2014) Randomized controlled trial of early zoledronic acid in men with castration-sensitive prostate cancer and bone metastases: results of CALGB 90202 (Alliance). J Clin Oncol 32(11):1143–1150
54. Smith MR, Saad F, Egerdie B et al (2009) Effects of denosumab on bone mineral density in men receiving androgen deprivation therapy for prostate cancer. J Urol 182:2670–2675
55. Smith MR, Saad F, Oudard S et al (2013) Denosumab and bone metastasis-free survival in men with nonmetastatic castration-resistant prostate cancer: exploratory analyses by baseline prostate-specific antigen doubling time. J Clin Oncol 31(30):3800–3806
56. Van Beek E, Pieterman E, Cohen L et al (1999) Nitrogen-containing bisphosphonates inhibit isopentenyl pyrophosphate isomerase/farnesyl pyrophosphate synthase activity with relative potencies corresponding to their antiresorptive potencies in vitro and in vivo. Biochem Biophys Res Commun 255(2):491
57. Vescovi P, Campisi G, Fusco V et al (2011) Surgery-triggered and non surgery-triggered Bisphosphonates-related Osteonecrosis of the Jaws (BRONJ): a retrospective analysis of 567 cases in an Italian multi center study. Oral Oncol 47(3):191–194
58. Vescovi P, Merigo E, Manfredi M et al (2008) Nd:YAG laser biostimulation in the treatment of bisphosphonate-associated osteonecrosis of the jaw: clinical experience in 28 cases. Photomed Laser Surg 26:37
59. Weitzman R, Sauter N, Eriksen EF et al (2007) Critical review: updated recommendations for the prevention, diagnosis and treatment of osteonecrosis of the jaw in cancer patients. Crit Rev Oncol Hematol 62(2):148–152

16 Bone-Seeking Radionuclide for Therapy

Joe O'Sullivan and Phil Turner

16.1 Introduction

Ionising radiation is utilised in a variety of situations in the management of prostate cancer. Beyond the scope of this book is the use of brachytherapy and external beam radiotherapy (EBRT) as efficacious, radical treatment modalities in the management of localised prostate cancer. Earlier chapters have covered the use of EBRT as a therapeutic option for the treatment of symptomatic bone metastases. This chapter focuses on the place of radionuclide therapy for the management of bone metastases. Recent development of radium-223 dichloride has reinvigorated this field of therapy. Here, analysis is made of the history of radionuclides and their current role in the modern treatment paradigm; the chapter closes by horizon-scanning for the potential future applications of radionuclide therapy, both as part of novel combinations with other agents and in new settings beyond current licensed indications.

Radionuclides are radioactive forms of chemical elements. Chemical elements are composed of atoms, and most chemical elements generally exist in a non-radioactive form. Atoms can be described in terms of two numbers, the atomic number and mass number. The atomic number describes the number of protons in the nucleus. The mass number describes the number of protons plus the number of neutrons in the nucleus. The atomic number defines elements; for example, any atom containing 6 protons will always have an atomic number of 6 and will always be the element carbon. However it is possible for elements to exist in different forms – the atomic number (number of protons) remains constant but the number of neutrons, and therefore the mass number, changes. Stable carbon atoms containing 6 protons and 6 neutrons have a mass number of 12; carbon can also occur as atoms containing 6 protons and 8 neutrons, having a mass number of 14, the so-called carbon-14. These different forms are said to be isotopes of the element. There is an optimal ratio of protons and neutrons, and the isotope with this ratio will exist as the stable form of the element. Deviations from this optimal ratio form unstable isotopes. These unstable isotopes can convert to a more stable form by altering their nuclear configuration of neutrons and protons; the process by which they do this is radioactive decay. This is covered in more detail in Sect. 16.3 below.

16.2 Bone-Seeking Compounds

The physiology of bone metastases has been covered in earlier chapters. To summarise, there is evidence that tumour cells utilise similar

J. O'Sullivan (✉) • P. Turner
Queen's University Belfast,
University Road, Belfast, Ulster BT7 1NN, Ireland
e-mail: joe.osullivan@qub.ac.uk

F. Bertoldo et al. (eds.), *Bone Metastases from Prostate Cancer*,
DOI 10.1007/978-3-319-42327-2_16

mechanisms used by haematopoietic stem cells to home into the haematopoietic stem cell niche [1]. A milieu of signalling pathways are engaged which result in the activation of both osteoclasts and osteoblasts in the complex process of bone remodelling at metastatic sites [2]. It is this process of new bone being laid down that has been exploited by a range of radionuclide compounds that target these sites by virtue of incorporation into this newly formed bone. Thus, in the classical theory of bone-targeted radionuclides, the aim has been to preferentially concentrate radionuclide at sites of metastases by utilising either a radionuclide that has native affinity for newly developing bone matrix or by stably binding a radionuclide to a moiety with such affinity. In this classical description, it is hypothesised that tumour cell death occurs secondary to the radiation emitted at sites of metastases as a consequence of DNA damage from direct and indirect ionisation events, discussed further in Sect. 16.3.2.

The major mineral constituent of bone is hydroxyapatite, largely composed of calcium and phosphate with chemical formula $Ca_{10}(PO_4)_6(OH)_2$. Complex pathways are beginning to be understood about the process by which living bone is mineralised [3]. When sclerotic metastases are forming, an excess of hydroxyapatite is laid down. It is by "hijacking" the pathways that lead to hydroxyapatite formation that allows sequestration of bone-seeking radionuclides within sclerotic metastases. As mentioned previously, two broad options are possible: utilising a radionuclide that has a natural affinity for developing bone matrix or chelating an appropriate radionuclide with another compound which itself has tropism for developing bone. Both these strategies have been used clinically. The clinically utilised radionuclides with natural affinity for bone are elements or compounds that will be processed in a manner analogous to calcium or phosphate. Radioactive isotopes of calcium itself are not used clinically, but radioisotopes of other metals from group 2 of the periodic table including strontium and radium are. Given their chemical resemblance to calcium, it is hypothesised that they are incorporated into developing bone as radium/strontium hydroxyapatite salts. In the case of radioisotopes of phosphorus, this can be administered as phosphate, which, having identical chemistry to phosphate bearing stable phosphorus, is incorporated directly into forming hydroxyapatite.

Radioisotopes of group 2 metals and phosphorus (as phosphate) can be described as having a "natural" tropism for bone. However other radioisotopes can be targeted to a developing bone by binding them to an appropriate carrier molecule. Phosphate groups have provided excellent carrier molecules for this purpose, being relatively easily synthesised and readily absorbed into developing bone. In this case, the phosphate group itself is stable (non-radioactive) but is covalently bound to a radioactive atom and acts to target the radioactive atom to developing bone. Those that have been utilised clinically are ethylenediaminetetramethylenephosphonate (EDTMP) and hydroxyethylidene diphosphonate (HEDP).

16.3 Radioactivity

We have described in the introduction the basic subatomic structure as being a nucleus consisting of protons and neutrons; we have stated that an optimum ratio between the number of protons and neutrons results in stable (non-radioactive) nuclei and that deviations away from this optimum ratio result in unstable nuclei that can become more stable by undergoing radioactive decay. The decay of radioactive nuclei results in the release of energy by one or a combination of the following forms of radiation: alpha, beta and gamma. Detailed analyses of the physics underlying these processes are beyond the scope of this chapter but are readily available in the literature [4, 5]. An appreciation of some fundamental principles of radiation and radiobiology is required; basic concepts reviewed here are forms of radiation, DNA damage, half-life, dose and linear energy transfer (LET).

16.3.1 Forms of Radiation

Alpha particles are energetic particles consisting of 2 protons and 2 neutrons (a helium nucleus). They are relatively massive in atomic terms

(4 amu) and are charged (2+). Alpha particles are released when an unstable atomic nucleus shifts into a more stable form by ejecting 2 protons and 2 neutrons accompanied by kinetic energy. It should be clear from the preceding discussion that the element left behind will have an atomic number reduced by 2 and a mass number reduced by 4 relative to the parent element.

Beta particles are high-energy electrons (or more rarely positrons). They are significantly less massive than alpha particles (1/2000 AMU) and carry a charge (−1 electron or +1 positron). They are released when an unstable nucleus shifts to a more stable configuring in a change that involves a neutron converting into a proton and ejecting an electron (beta minus) or, conversely, a proton converting to a neutron and ejecting a positron (beta positive). For the purposes of this chapter, beta radiation will refer to electron (−1 charge) particles only as there is no current licensed therapeutic agent employing positron radiation.

Both alpha and beta radiation occur when a decaying nucleus releases energy in the form of a high-energy particle. Gamma radiation involves an unstable nucleus simply releasing energy as a photon, part of the electromagnetic spectrum and thus without any mass or charge. Gamma radiation as a process in itself doesn't involve any change in atomic or mass number; however it usually accompanies either alpha or beta decay.

In terms of origin, it should be clear that related, although quite distinct, processes result in the generation of alpha, beta and gamma radiation, respectively. They differ in terms of mass and charge. In terms of biological effect however, they all share a characteristic property: their ability to create ions in material with which they come into contact. They are so-called forms of ionising radiation. It is this ionising ability that confers upon them their unique and profound biological actions, namely, mutagenesis and cytotoxicity.

16.3.2 DNA Damage

There is a large body of evidence [6] supporting the hypothesis that the key process by which any form of ionising radiation generates its biological actions is ionisation resulting in DNA damage. This DNA damage can occur either directly (by radiation directly ionising DNA) or indirectly (by radiation creating aqueous ions which secondarily ionise DNA). Both direct and indirect ionisation of DNA can result in either single-strand or double-strand DNA breakage. The cell has mechanisms for repair of these; however if sufficient DNA damage is induced, it is beyond the limits of repair and cell death ensues [6].

16.3.3 Half-Life

Half-life is an important concept to understand in relation to radionuclide therapy. The SI unit of radioactivity is the Becquerel, where 1 Bq is defined as the amount of radiation resulting from one nucleus decaying per second. In any given sample of material, there are a fixed number of nuclei available to decay and release radiation. The decay of unstable nuclei and corresponding release of radiation is a random process. If all nuclei present have an equal probability of decay, then the overall rate of decay will be greatest at some initial time point. Later, relative to that initial point in time, there will be fewer undecayed nuclei remaining and therefore a reduced rate of overall decay. This type of system, where a quantity decreases at a rate proportional to its current value, is called exponential decay. The half-life is the time taken for the radioactivity present to reduce to a half of its current value. After one half-life, the radioactivity present will be reduced to half its current value, and after a second half-life, it will be reduced by half again, therefore to one-quarter of its current value. Half-lives are constant for a given radionuclide but vary considerably between different radionuclides, ranging from fractions of seconds to thousands of years. This has important implications for the choice of any radionuclide used clinically. Radionuclides with extremely short half-lives will prove very difficult to manufacture, quality assure and administer to a patient before their radioactivity has dropped to a subtherapeutic level. Conversely, radionuclides with extremely long half-lives will pose significant radiation protection issues for

Table 16.1 Comparing types of ionising radiation taken from Turner and O'Sullivan [7]

Type of decay	Particle/photon	Relative mass (AMU)	Charge	Typical LET (kV/μm)
Alpha	Helium nucleus	4	+2	60–300
Beta	Electron (or positron)	1/2000	−1 electron (+1 positron)	0.1–1
Gamma	Photon	0	0	0.3 (LET associated with secondary electrons)

both the patient and wider society, as they will remain radioactive for many years after initial administration to a patient.

16.3.4 Dose and LET

The SI unit for measuring radiation dose delivered is the Gray where 1 Gy = 1 Joule of radiation energy absorbed per kilogram of matter irradiated. This is purely a physical measure of the net energy transfer arising from exposure and takes no account of the biological effects of this irradiation. Irradiation with 1 Gy of each of the different forms of radiation will have significantly different consequences. For both alpha and beta particles, the amount of energy carried varies depending upon the energy with which they are released from their parent radionuclide. Similarly gamma photons can carry a range of energies (within the X-ray portion of the EM spectrum) depending on the precise mass-to-energy change occurring when they are released from their parent isotope. A final important characteristic used to describe any of these forms of radiation and that in part explains their different biological actions is linear energy transfer (LET). LET is a measure of amount of energy deposited per unit length travelled in matter. It varies considerably across different forms of radiation. Alpha particles, being massive and highly charged, interact readily with matter through which they travel. This results in energy being readily given up along their path of travel and therefore a high LET. Beta particles, being significantly lower in mass and charge than alpha particles, stand a much lower chance of interacting with their surrounding atoms per unit length travelled and thus release their energy over a relatively longer path. Further along this spectrum of LET is gamma irradiation. Lacking any mass and charge, it is less likely again to interact with surrounding atoms per unit length travelled and thus generally has the lowest LET of all.

If we take this understanding of LET and apply it to the biological situation of radiation interacting with DNA, we can say that alpha particles will travel over a relatively short range but deposit very large amounts of energy along their path; therefore if this path traverses cell nuclei alpha particles stand a relatively high chance of causing significant DNA damage. Conversely, relative to alpha radiation, gamma radiation will travel further, but a given dose in Gray will tend to result in less DNA damage along the path taken by its constituent photons. Beta radiation exists somewhere between these two extremes, moderately penetrating and with LET typically between that of alpha or gamma irradiation (Table 16.1).

16.4 Clinical Applications of Beta Emitters

16.4.1 Beta Emitters as Single Agents

The early radionuclide compounds used in the modern era were beta emitters. As discussed above, strontium and phosphate have an innate bone-seeking tendency, and radioactive forms of these were used therapeutically, specifically strontium-89 and phosphorus-32 (administered as P-32-phosphate). Additionally, a number of compounds were developed incorporating an appropriate radionuclide with a bone-targeting moiety, specifically samarium-153 EDTMP, rhenium-188 HEDP and rhenium-186 HEDP.

The following Table 16.2 compares the physical properties of each of these.

16.4.1.1 Phosphorus-32

Radioactive phosphorus was one of the first radionuclides used to treat metastatic bone disease dating back to the 1950s [8]. It is rarely used clinically now particularly in the developed world. Medline searches involving "phosphorus" and "neoplasms" or "bone neoplasms" reveal no recent developments. A small study was performed in India in 1999, comparing the palliative efficacy of single-dose P-32 versus single-dose Sr-89, the rationale being that P-32 is apparently cheaper and more readily available in the developing world than imported alternatives. This small study randomised 31 patients with a range of malignancies metastatic to bone, to receive either a single dose of P-32 or Sr-89. The authors found them to broadly equivalent in terms of analgesic benefit with at least 50% pain relief reported by 14 of 15 patients given Sr-89 and 14 of 16 given P-32 [9].

16.4.1.2 Strontium-89

Sr-89 has been extensively studied as a therapeutic radionuclide. In their robust review, Finlay et al. [10] describe 16 prospective clinical observational studies involving Sr-89. These are conglomerate data from various studies using different mechanisms of determining the very subjective experience of "change in intensity of pain" so conclusions are limited. However, "complete response" and "no response" should be consistent across trials – Finlay et al. concluded that complete response of pain to treatment with Sr-89 occurred in between 8 and 77% of patients (mean 32%), whilst no response occurred in between 14 and 52% (mean of 25%). Between these extremes, some response was reported by a mean of 44% of patients, giving a mean overall for "some" or "complete" control of pain of 76%.

Randomised controlled trial evidence is scant. A 1991 study randomised 32 patients with metastatic castration-resistant prostate cancer (mCRPC) to receive 2 injections, 6 weeks apart of either 150 MBq of Sr-89 or stable strontium as placebo [11]. Patients were evaluated across a number of domains including general condition, mobility, analgesia requirements and pain score; these were used to give an overall categorical score between "deteriorated" and "dramatic improvement". In this small trial, there is a trend to improved outcome with the active agent, with all patients in the "dramatic improvement" category and a minority in the "deteriorated" category having received Sr-89. An older again and very small RCT from 1988 randomised 49 patients with metastatic prostate cancer to receive three injections of 75Mbq Sr-89 or saline placebo [12] at monthly intervals. This found no difference in palliation, but 2-year overall survival was improved in the Sr-89 group. However, this trial was underpowered to assess for survival benefit, and these results have not been demonstrated elsewhere. No recent randomised controlled trials have been undertaken examining any disease-modifying or overall survival endpoints with Sr-89 as a single agent.

16.4.1.3 Re-188 HEDP/Re-186 HEDP

As is shown in Table 16.2, two radioisotopes of rhenium have been used clinically as therapeutic radionuclides. Re-186 HEDP decays predominantly via beta decay with the release of a beta particle Emax 1.08 MeV (9% by gamma decay, photon 137 keV); Re-188 HEDP similarly decays predominantly by beta decay with release of beta particle Emax 2.1 MeV (15% by gamma decay, photon 155 keV) [13].

Palmedo et al. conducted a phase I dose escalation study involving Re-188 HEDP [14]. They treated 22 patients with disseminated prostate cancer with single-dose Re-188 HEDP at varying doses (1.3, 2.6, 3.3 and 4.4 GBq). Improvement

Table 16.2 Comparison of commonly used radionuclides

Therapy	Targeting mechanism	T1/2 (days)	Maximum Beta Energy (Mev)	Approximate maximum range in tissue (mm)
P-32	As phosphate	14.3	1.71	8
Sr-89	Calcium mimetic	50.5	1.46	7
Re-188	Via chelation with HEDP	0.7	2.1	11
Re-186	Via chelation with HEDP	3.7	1.08	4.5
Sm-153	Via chelation with EDTMP	1.9	0.81	2.5

in pain occurred in 64 % of patients, lasting on average 7.5 weeks. In the eight patients treated at the highest dose level, 3 of 8 developed grade 3/4 thrombocytopenia and 1 of 8 developed grade 3/4 leucopenia.

O'Sullivan et al. conducted both phase I and phase II trials involving Re-186 HEDP given along with autologous blood stem cell transplantation to abrogate the myelosuppressive effects of the radionuclide. In their phase I trial [15], 25 patients with mCRPC were treated with increasing doses of Re-186 HEDP (2.5–5 GBq) followed by return 14 days later of previously harvested autologous peripheral blood stem cells. Grade III thrombocytopenia lasting >7 days occurred in 2 of 6 patients treated with 5 GBq, making this the maximum tolerated activity. Eight of ten patients with "significant" pain at baseline had reduction in pain by ≥50 % lasting at least 4 weeks. These authors also looked for markers of disease response; 5 of 25 patients had a fall in PSA of ≥50 % lasting for ≥4 weeks.

These authors progressed on to phase II study in which 38 patients with mCRPC were treated with a single dose of 5 GBq of Re-186 HEDP followed 14 days later by autologous peripheral blood stem cell transplantation [16]. Rates of grade 3 thrombocytopenia, leucopenia and anaemia were 21 %, 11 % and 3 %, respectively. Twenty-nine percent of patients had a fall in PSA of ≥50 % sustained for at least 4 weeks. Of patients with pain at baseline, 74 % had a response of at least 1-point reduction on a 5-point pain score.

16.4.1.4 Samarium-153

The most robust phase III RCT evidence for single-agent beta emitters exists for Sm-153 EDTMP. Two relatively recent RCTs have been conducted. Serafini et al. conducted a blinded RCT comparing pain response to Sm-153 EDTMP versus placebo [17]. One hundred and eighteen patients with a range of malignancies metastatic to bone were randomly assigned to receive a single dose of 0.5 mCi/kg (18.5 MBq/kg), 1 mCi/kg (37 MBq/kg) or placebo. The high-dose group showed statistically significant improvements over placebo in both patient-rated and physician-rated pain scores at each of 4 weeks after administration. Analgesia consumption was reduced in the active groups and rose in the placebo group; although this difference was non-significant, it does suggest that the significant improvement in pain scores seen in the high-dose group is not due to changes in analgesia. Thrombocytopenia and leucopenia did occur in treated groups; however this was transient, correcting by week 8. No grade 4 toxicities were reported. A second and more recent phase III trial was undertaken by Sartor et al. [18]. One hundred and fifty-two men with mCRPC were randomised 2 to 1 to receive either a single 37 MBq/kg dose of Sm-153 EDTMP or a non-radioactive Sm-152 EDTMP as placebo. Significant improvements were seen both in subjective measures of patient pain response and analgesia consumption. There was a trend to reduced PSA in the actively treated group with 9 % of patients recording fall in PSA ≥50 versus 2 % in placebo. Sm-153 EDTMP was associated with transient thrombocytopenia and leucopenia, with counts correcting by week 8.

16.4.2 Beta Emitters in Relation to External Beam Radiotherapy

Two small studies have sought to examine the relationship between palliative EBRT to areas of painful bone metastases and radionuclides designed to target the same sites; both utilised Sr-89 as the radionuclide. One examined Sr-89 as adjuvant therapy to EBRT and the other examined Sr-89 versus EBRT. Smeland et al. [19] conducted an RCT in 95 patients with various types of cancer, all of whom had skeletal metastases. Patients all had EBRT to maximum two sites of painful skeletal metastases, treated to a dose of either 30 Gy in 10 fractions or a single 8 Gy fraction. Patients were then randomised to receive either a single dose of Sr-89 chloride at 150 MBq or saline placebo on day 1 of radiotherapy. The primary endpoint was the number of patients with physician-assessed subjective progression (progression being any of increase in pain, increase in analgesia, WHO performance status deterioration and need for additional pain treatment). No difference was found in rates of progression. Maximal haematological toxicity was ≤ grade 2 but occurred more often in patients receiving Sr-89 (≤ grade 2 haematological toxicity in 23 patients vs. 8, $p=0.02$).

Oosterhof et al. conducted an RCT randomising 203 patients with mCRPC to receive either EBRT or a single dose of 150 MBq of Sr-89 chloride [20]. The radiotherapy regimes were by physician preference and ranged widely from 4 Gy in 1 fraction to 43 Gy in 24 fractions. A subjective improvement in pain was seen in 34.7 % of patients treated with Sr-89 and 33.3 % of patients treated with EBRT.

16.4.2.1 Summary of Beta Emitters as Single Agents and in Relation to EBRT

In summary, a number of beta-emitting compounds have been used in a range of metastatic malignancies. Broadly, there is observational evidence of their palliative benefit. More specifically, only for Sm-153 EDTMP is there RCT evidence for a significant palliative benefit over placebo. They are all associated with some degree of toxicity, and their dose-limiting toxicity tends to be haematological. In a single RCT, there appeared to be no palliative benefit gained from the addition of Sr-89 to EBRT. A single RCT also suggests that where disease is encompassable by EBRT, there is no significant difference in rate of improvement in symptoms for EBRT versus Sr-89.

Thus beta emitters may be effective adjuncts to analgesic medication, but for limited disease, they appear to offer little above EBRT. Where the diffuse nature and/or high volume of disease makes adequate coverage with EBRT difficult, beta-emitting radionuclides may offer a more practical and efficacious alternative. However, myelosuppression is a significant toxicity. This problem is compounded by the fact that the more diffuse a patient's disease, the more likely they are to already be relatively myelosuppressed by virtue of the skeletal disease diminishing their bone marrow function. Thus for many patients with diffuse disease and already reduced blood counts, the risk of further myelotoxicity may be so great as to preclude radionuclide therapy with beta agents.

16.4.3 Beta Emitters in Combination with Cytotoxic Agents

The studies above have been single-systemic-agent, bone-targeted therapies in a range of malignancies. In malignancies with a particular predilection (e.g. prostate cancer) for forming bone metastases, several groups have examined the strategy of using a systemic cytotoxic coupled with a bone-targeted radionuclide. Several rationales have been proffered for these strategies. It is possible that a systemic cytotoxic might have disease-modifying action at all sites of disease, with bone-targeting agents then acting as a "consolidation" agent on the bone based metastases. An alternative idea is that the systemic agents might act as a radiosensitiser, compounding the ultimate effect of the bone-targeted agent. A number of trials have examined this concept in beta emitters. These are covered, by radioactive agent, below.

16.4.3.1 Sr-89

A small, early study by Tu et al. [21] treated 103 men with mCRPC using a complicated regime of systemic therapies as "induction" agents (doxorubicin, ketoconazole, vinblastine and estramustine) followed by randomisation into "consolidation" therapy with either doxorubicin alone or doxorubicin + a single dose of Sr-89 (2.035 MBq/kg body weight). The trial was not designed to power any formal hypothesis testing. The authors report an increase in progression-free and overall survival in the Sr-89 arm but concede that these data are non-conclusive and merely generate the hypothesis that this type of regime may confer benefit. This combination was associated with significant toxicity. Neutropenia ($<10^4$/L) occurred in 10 patients during induction, 8 patients during consolidation without Sr-89 and 16 patients during consolidation including Sr-89. Two treatment-related deaths occurred as a result of an MI and an episode of severe neutropenic sepsis; two additional nonfatal MIs occurred. Eleven patients developed DVT.

In a departure from other studies into combination agents that concentrated on bone metastases in mCRPC, a study by Bilen et al. in 2014 examined the concept in hormone-sensitive prostate cancer (HSPC). This is an interesting study as there has been a move towards more aggressive therapy earlier in the course of metastatic prostate cancer (mPC) over recent months. Subsequent to this group publishing their results, phase III data have been published showing a survival benefit for the use of chemotherapy during the hormone-sensitive phase of the illness [22, 23]. This has prompted a shift in practice across most of the developed world to offering docetaxel chemotherapy early in the course of mPC. Bilen et al. [24] treated 79 men with a combination of ADT and two cycles of anthracycline chemotherapy plus six cycles of zoledronic acid; men were randomised to either receive additionally a dose of Sr-89 (148 MBq) or no radionuclide. In contrast to Tu et al. no study-related deaths are reported. Grade 3 bone marrow toxicity occurred in one patient in the control arm and two patients in the Sr-89 arm. No statistically significant difference was seen between PFS or OS in either arm. As the authors note, given the success of ADT, detecting a significant improvement with any additional therapy requires a study powered with very large numbers of patients.

In a final Sr-89 study, Sciuto et al. [25] tested whether or not a sensitising effect was seen by the addition of a cytotoxic to radionuclide treatment versus the radionuclide alone, rather than testing the impact of a radionuclide with a cytotoxic versus cytotoxic alone. They randomised 70 patients with symptomatic mCRPC to receive either 148 MBq of Sr-89 plus 50 mg/m^2 cisplatin or 148 MBq of Sr-89 plus placebo. The cytotoxic effect of cisplatin is mediated by its formation of DNA adducts and cross-links. Its ability to potentiate the anti-neoplastic effects of radiation is well studied, and it is used as an adjunct to radical radiotherapy in multiple forms of squamous cell carcinoma including cervical, anal and head and neck. In this study, the percentage of patients whose pain score improved was significantly higher in the combined treatment group (91 vs. 63 % $p<0.01$). Response scans were performed, and in the 6 months after treatment, radiological progression occurred in 27 % of patients in combined treatment group and 64 % of patients in control group ($p=0.01$). Maximal haematological toxicity was grade 4 anaemia; this affected two patients in combined arm and one patient in placebo arm. No significant differences were found in platelets, leucocytes or haemoglobin in the 3 months after treatment, though there is a trend to reduced leucocytes in the combined treatment arm.

16.4.3.2 Re-186 HEDP and Re-188 HEDP

Both Re-188 HEDP and Re-186 HEDP have been used in combination with cytotoxic agents. Lam et al. [26] conducted a phase 1 dose escalation study of Re-188 HEDP plus capecitabine, an anti-metabolite cytotoxic, in patients with mCRPC in an attempt to find maximum tolerated dose of capecitabine when combined with Re-188 HEDP. This proved to be 2500 mg/m^2 per day of capecitabine when given orally for 14 days followed 2 days later by an infusion of 37 Mbq/kg of Re-188 HEDP. Higher doses of capecitabine resulted in unacceptable bone marrow toxicity. A phase II trial is planned according to the authors.

Taxanes are the only cytotoxic agents for which there is robust, RCT evidence of prolongation in survival in mCRPC [27, 28]. The TAXIUM trial was a phase I trial designed to test the safety of combining a taxane with a radionuclide [29]. A dose escalation schedule was designed consisting of four dose levels of radionuclide with a standard dosage of docetaxel (75 mg/m^2 given at 3 weekly intervals for 6 cycles). Re-186 HEDP was given in increasing activities (1250 up to 2500 MBq) after the third and sixth cycle of docetaxel. Dose-limiting toxicity (DLT) was defined as any grade 4 toxicity lasting more than 7 days or any grade 3 toxicity lasting more than 10 days. Three patients were planned for each dose level expanding to six if a DLT occurred. Grade 3 thrombocytopenia lasting >10 days occurred in one patient treated at dose level three (i.e. after first infusion of Sr-153 2500 Mbq), and treatment was stopped after one further cycle of docetaxel without the patient receiving their second dose of radionuclide. This dose level was expanded to six and a further patient experienced acute renal failure. During the trial, there were production problems with Re-186 HEDP, and the group undertook a phase II trial using a similar regime but with Re-188 HEDP as radionuclide. The TAXIUM 2 trial results are awaited.

Summary of Beta Emitters and Cytotoxics

In summary, there is hypothesis-generating data from small trials that there is a synergistic effect when cytotoxics and bone-targeting radionuclides are used in combination; however this can result in significant toxicity as was seen in the Tu et al. study [21]. Comparing the Tu et al. study with Sciuto et al. [25], Lam et al. [26] and TAXIUM trials [29], there is a suggestion that single-agent cytotoxics in combination with radionuclides are preferable to regimes with multiple cytotoxic agents from a toxicity point of view, as one would expect. A number of phase II trials of combination regimes are planned.

16.5 Alpha Emitters: Radium-223

A combination of both physical characteristics of alpha particle radiation and biological responses to that radiation led researchers to hypothesise that alpha emitters might hold several advantages over beta emitters as radionuclide therapeutics. In terms of physical characteristics, it was postulated that the intense dose deposition over a very short range might concentrate dose within immediate microenvironment of metastases with minimal crossfire into bone marrow compartment, thus limiting myelosuppression. Further, it is known from basic radiobiological studies that high-LET radiation offers a number of tumouricidal advantages over low LET radiation in terms of increased radiobiological effectiveness (RBE) and reduced oxygen enhancement ratio (OER). These concepts are more thoroughly reviewed elsewhere [6, 7]. Recent work has focused on Ra-223; it is a group II metal therefore possessing innate bone-seeking tendency. Its half-life of 11.4 days makes it long-lived enough to be practical to generate and transport to sites of clinical use but not so long-lived as to cause radiation protection concerns.

16.5.1 Preclinical

Early preclinical animal work by Henriksen et al. [30] delivered Ra-223 as the chloride salt by intravenous injection to mice and then calculated activity in a range of tissues with animals sacrificed at various times post-injection. This confirmed that Ra-223 preferentially and quickly concentrated within the skeleton of mice and was retained there, with no statistically significant change in skeletal concentration of dose over initial 14 days following administration – femur-to-blood ratio increased from 118 to 691 within a period of 1 h to 3 days. The post-sacrifice tissue activity data were then used to calculate absorbed dose estimates for a range of tissues again showing significant preferential dose delivery to skeleton.

16.5.2 Phase I

A phase I trial utilising Ra-223 in metastatic cancer patients was conducted by Nilsson et al. [31]. Fifteen prostate and ten breast cancer patients were treated with a single IV injection of 22Ra. Five dose levels were examined with five patients per dose level: 46, 93, 163, 213 and 250 kBq/kg. Maximum CTC grade for haematological toxicity was grade 2 anaemia and grade 1 thrombocytopenia; two patients experienced grade 3 neutropenia. Also, 10 of 25 patients experienced transient diarrhoea. Pharmacokinetic studies showed that blood radioactivity dropped to <1 % initial at 24 h post-infusion, and in six patients who had gamma scintigraphy performed, the small amount of gamma radiation released by daughter nuclides showed that the parent Ra-223 was accumulating preferentially at sites of metastasis as identified previously on 99 m-Tc scans. Finally all patients showed a decline in ALP after

Ra-223 infusion. A detailed phase I pharmacokinetic and biodistribution trial was conducted by Carrasquillo et al. [32]. This treated three patients at 50 kBq/kg, three at 100 kBq/kg and four at 200 kBq/kg. The study did not seek to establish MTD, though adverse events are reported. Leucopenia and diarrhoea were the commonest adverse events with 30 % of patients experiencing grade 3–4 leucopenia and 60 % of patients experiencing grade 1–3 diarrhoea. A drop in PSA was seen in 50 % of patients treated, with a trend to a dose–response relationship; ALP decreased in all treated patients. Dosimetry data are discussed in later dosimetry section.

16.5.3 Phase II

These encouraging phase I data led to three phase II studies in Ra-223 all in mCRPC and summarised in Table 16.3 taken from Turner and O'Sullivan [7]. In an initial dose-response trial, 100 patients with mCRPC were treated with a single infusion of Ra-223 at one of four dose levels: 5, 25, 50 or 100 kBq/kg [33]. The drug was well tolerated at all dose levels, and a dose-dependent improvement in pain was seen. Haematological toxicity was acceptable with grade 3–4 anaemia, neutropenia and thrombocytopenia in 8 %, 3 % and 6 % of treated patients, respectively, and a slight trend to reduced platelet, white cell and neutrophil counts in the two highest dose levels. GI toxicity was more common overall with 43 %, 24 % and 22 % of patients experiencing nausea, vomiting and diarrhoea, respectively, and no differences between dose groups. A randomised, double-blind phase II trial was undertaken by Parker et al. [34]. In this, 122 patients with mCRPC were randomised to receive three infusions of Ra-223 at 6-week intervals at a dose per injection of 25 or 50 or 80 kBq/kg. Its primary endpoint was PSA response and it confirmed a statistically significant dose-response with >50 % PSA reduction for 0 % patients in the 25 kBq/kg group, 6 % patients in the 50 kBq/kg group and 13 % patients in the 80 kBq/kg group. Commonest toxicities were GI and haematological with 21 % of patients experiencing diarrhoea and 16 % experiencing nausea. Grade 3/4 haematological toxicity was seen in 2 of 41 patients in 25 kBq/kg group, 6 of 39 in the 50 kBq/kg group and 7 of 42 in the 80 kBq/kg group. There was no significant difference in haematological toxicity between dose groups. Finally, in a randomised, multicentre, placebo-controlled trial, mCRPC patients undergoing EBRT for pain control were randomised to receive either four injections of Ra-223 at 50 kBq/kg or placebo, given at 4 weekly intervals [35]. Thirty-three patients were assigned to EBRT and Ra-223 and 31 to EBRT and placebo. As in other trials, Ra-223 treatment was acceptable with the only significant toxicity difference between treatment and placebo groups being increased constipation in the treatment group. In the treatment group, constipation was mild to moderate in 11 patients and severe in 1. Median time to PSA progression was 26 weeks (95 % CI 16–39) for Ra-223 compared with 8 weeks (95 % CI 4–12) for placebo ($p=0.048$); significant reduction in ALP was also observed. There was a trend (albeit within this small trial) to improved OS in the treatment group.

16.5.4 Phase III ALSYMPCA

Following the positive phase I and II data in relation to radium, a large, multicentre, placebo-controlled and double-blinded RCT was undertaken with the aim of definitively determining the efficacy of Ra-223 in mCRPC. Men with mCRPC were randomised in a 2:1 fashion to receive either Ra-223 at 50 kBq/kg given at 4 weekly intervals for 6 cycles or placebo given on same time schedule. Overall survival was improved in the Ra-223 treatment group (14.9 vs. 11.3 months HR 0.7 $p<0.001$) [36]. The main secondary endpoint was time to first symptomatic skeletal event. These were defined as any of the following: (i) the first use of external beam radiation therapy to relieve skeletal symptoms, (ii) new symptomatic pathologic vertebral or non-vertebral bone fractures, (iii) spinal cord compression and (iv) tumour-related orthopaedic surgical intervention. Time to first symptomatic skeletal event was prolonged in the Ra-223

Table 16.3 Phase II/III data of 223Ra in mCRPC [7]

Name	Phase	Method	Number	Outcomes
BC-102 [35]	2	4 injections ^{223}Ra of 50 kBq/kg (or placebo) at 4-week intervals Vs. placebo	$N=33$ ^{223}Ra $N=31$ placebo	Significant delay in PSA progression and fall in ALP in ^{223}Ra group Tendency to reduced rate of SRE and improved survival in ^{223}Ra group Well tolerated
BC-103 [33]	2	Single injection ^{223}Ra 5, 25, 50 or 100 kBq/kg	$N=26$@5 kBq/kg $N=25$@25 kBq/kg $N=25$@50 kBq/kg $N=24$@100 kBq/kg	Dose-dependent improvement in pain Well tolerated at all dose levels
BC-104 [34]	2	3 injections ^{223}Ra per subject at 6-week intervals, Either 25,50 or 80 kBq/kg (no dose escalation within groups)	$N=37$@25 kBq/kg $N=36$@50 kBq/kg $N=39$@80 kBq/kg (These N are those treated per protocol and analysed in efficacy calculations. In each group, respectively, 4, 3 and 3 additional patients received 1 or 2 injections and are analysed as part of safety population.)	Dose-dependent fall in PSA and ALP Well tolerated at all dose levels
ALSYMPCA [36]	3	6 injections of 223Ra of 50 kBq/kg (or placebo) at 4-week intervals Vs. placebo Plus best standard of care	$N=614$ ^{223}Ra $N=307$ placebo	^{223}Ra associated with significant improvement in OS (14.9 vs. 11.3 months $p<0.001$) ^{223}Ra associated with significant delay to first SSE (15.6 vs. 9.8 months $p<0.001$) Number of patients experiencing adverse events lower in ^{223}Ra group (all grades) Signal to increased (low grade) diarrhoea in ^{223}Ra group Signal to increased (low grade) myelosuppression in ^{223}Ra group

treatment group (15.6 months vs. 9.8 $p<0.001$). A subsequent detailed analysis of different types of skeletal events in ALSYMPCA revealed the risk of requiring EBRT and of developing spinal cord compression to be reduced in Ra-223 groups, whilst there did not seem to be a significant reduction in the risk of symptomatic pathological bone fracture of need for tumour-related orthopaedic intervention [37]. Times to PSA and ALP increase were both also significantly prolonged by Ra-223 [36]. The authors provide a detailed breakdown of adverse events. The total number of patients experiencing adverse events was lower in the Ra-223 group, and this was true for AE all grades, AE grade 3/4, serious AE and drug discontinuation due to AE. Rates of haematological toxicity were similar between groups with all grades anaemia 31% Ra-223 vs. 31% placebo, all grades thrombocytopenia 12% Ra-223 vs. 6% placebo and all grades neutropenia 5% Ra-223 vs. 1% placebo. There is a signal pointing towards increased, low-grade diarrhoea in Ra-223 treated individuals with 25% of Ra-223 vs. 15% placebo experiencing diarrhoea in all grades, 2 % in each group experiencing grade 3 and none in either group experiencing grades 4 or 5 [36]. In a further, prespecified subgroup analysis of the trial, both the improvement in OS and the improvement in most of the secondary efficacy endpoints were present in Ra-223 group irrespective of previous docetaxel use [38].

16.5.5 Dosimetry

Modern dosimetry techniques in radiotherapy have largely been developed in the realm of EBRT. The process involves calculating electron densities of relevant tissues using CT data. Then detailed knowledge of the behaviour of therapeutic photon beams in material of various electron densities is applied to the data gained from CT scanning. This allows complex models to be developed of dose delivered to different regions of the body being irradiated. It should be clear that an entirely different and more complex modelling set-up is required for dosimetry on the molecular level, and this is an area of intense research currently. A method described above and suitable in preclinical animal experiments involves sacrificing the small animals concerned and performing direct activity analysis on various tissues [30]. This is obviously not feasible in the therapeutic setting and only provides an approximation of doses that may be delivered in humans. A further method that has been attempted is utilising the very small (1.1 %) amount of Ra-223 decay that occurs with the release of gamma photons; these penetrate extracorporeally and can be imaged using a gamma camera; however acquisition times are long and resolution poor. This was performed in Nilsson et al. in the first human trials of Ra-223 in the modern era [31]. This work was qualitative only and allowed the general conclusions to be drawn that Ra-223 accumulated preferentially at sites of metastasis and that clearance was predominantly by the GI tract. Carrasquillo et al. extended this work with their biodistribution paper in 2013 [32]. By acquiring whole-body gamma camera images, they also demonstrated faecal clearance as being the major method of elimination. They quantified gastrointestinal clearance estimating that by day 6–8, a median of 76 % of administered Ra-223 had been excreted. No activity was visualised within the bladder. Analysis was made of energy spectra of gamma emissions being recorded to assess for interorgan translocation of daughter nuclides of parent Ra-223; this suggested equilibrium between parent and daughter and insignificant interorgan translocation. These investigators also acquired serial blood samples post-Ra-223 infusion and assayed for radioactivity. Clearance was rapid and bi-exponential: the total Ra-223 activity had decreased to 0.55 % of infused activity by 24 h, and the half-lives of the fast and slow elimination components were 0.8 and 19 h, respectively.

These data concentrate on pharmacokinetics of Ra-223, rather than actual biodosimetry. Chittenden and colleagues have recently published estimates of organ-level dosimetry [39]. Six patients received two injections of Ra-223 at 100 kBq/kg given 6 weeks apart. Dosimetry estimates were made for bone surfaces, red marrow, kidneys and gut. Their biodistribution measurements were in keeping with previous studies showing administered activity cleared rapidly from blood (1.1 % remaining at 24 h), and most of the administered activity was rapidly sequestered within bone (61 % at 4 h). Estimates of dose delivered to bone surfaces from alpha particles were 2331–13,118 mGy/MBq; doses delivered to red marrow were estimated to be 177–994 and 1–5 mGy/MBQ from activity on bone surfaces and activity in blood, respectively.

16.5.6 Clinical and Future Use of Ra-223

Given the above findings (particularly phase III ALSYMPCA data), Ra-223 has become part of the treatment paradigm in mCRPC. It is now widely used in post-docetaxel chemotherapy and, depending on jurisdiction and reimbursement arrangements, also in the pre-chemotherapy setting. There are a number of potential extensions to the use of Ra-223 in cancer care, and these are being actively explored within a number of trials.

In mCRPC, it has already been mentioned that there are two survival-prolonging cytotoxic agents, docetaxel [27] and cabazitaxel [28]; in addition there is phase III RCT evidence for the survival-prolonging effects of 2 hormonal agents abiraterone acetate [40, 41] and enzalutamide [42, 43]. In earlier chapters, small trial evidence has been presented for a synergistic effect between beta-emitting radionuclides and systemic agents. Overlapping and potentially synergistic toxicity has always been a concern. Given the extremely favourable safety profile of Ra-223, it is possible that it may offer advantageous combination therapy – a systemic agent being used to treat disease in an untargeted fashion with Ra-223 being used to offer consolidation treatment to areas of bone disease (in mCRPC usually the site of highest volume metastatic burden). Trials examining the combination Ra-223 with docetaxel and abiraterone acetate are already recruiting. In the natural history of prostate cancer, bone metastases frequently predate the development of mCRPC, and men may spend months to years with bone metastases in the hormone-sensitive phase of the illness. It is a reasonable hypothesis that providing bone-targeted treatment with Ra-223 earlier in the disease course, during the hormone-sensitive phase, might well provide at least as good or perhaps even better outcomes than waiting until the disease is in a castration-resistant (and more heavily pretreated) form. The idea of utilising Ra-223 in the hormone-sensitive phase of prostate cancer is being tested in the currently recruiting ADRRAD trial (neoadjuvant androgen deprivation therapy, pelvic radiotherapy and radium-223 for new presentation T1–4 N0/1 M1B adenocarcinoma of prostate). This seeks to treat men with hormone-sensitive prostate cancer with hormone therapy and early Ra-223 alongside EBRT to prostate and pelvic lymph node bed in an attempt to target radiation to as many sites of active disease as possible, whilst the disease is responding to hormone therapy. Results from this novel trial are eagerly awaited.

Prostate cancer is only one malignancy with a particular preponderance to metastasise to the skeleton; other common carcinomas with such a phenotype include breast, lung and renal cell. Further, certain malignancies arise within the skeleton including myeloma, plasmacytoma and osteosarcoma. It is an entirely reasonable hypothesis that some of the benefits seen with Ra-223 in mCRPC could also be demonstrated in some or all of these and trials are already underway in breast cancer and osteosarcoma. Finally, and relevant to both prostate and other malignancies, the dosing used in ALSYMPCA has been proven safe but may not be optimal. In phase I and II studies, doses higher than 50 kBq/kg were tolerated [32–34], and it may be that even greater survival or symptomatic benefits can be seen by dose escalation and trials to determine this are underway in prostate cancer.

Bibliography

1. Shiozawa Y, Pedersen EA, Havens AM, Jung Y, Mishra A, Joseph J et al (2011) Human prostate cancer metastases target the hematopoietic stem cell niche to establish footholds in mouse bone marrow. J Clin Invest 121(4):1298–1312
2. Keller ET, Brown J (2004) Prostate cancer bone metastases promote both osteolytic and osteoblastic activity. J Cell Biochem 91(4):718–729
3. Atkins GJ, Findlay DM (2012) Osteocyte regulation of bone mineral: a little give and take. Osteoporos Int 23(8):2067–2079
4. Kassis A, Adelstein SJ (2005) Radiobiologic principles in radionuclide therapy. J Nucl Med 46(no.1 suppl):4s–12s
5. Sofou S (2008) Radionuclide carriers for targeting of cancer. Int J Nanomedicine 3(2):181–199
6. Joiner M, Van Der Kogel A (eds) (2009) Basic clinical radiobiology, 4th edn. Hodder Arnold, London
7. Turner PG, O'Sullivan JM (2015) (223)Ra and other bone-targeting radiopharmaceuticals-the translation of radiation biology into clinical practice. Br J Radiol 88(1050):20140752
8. Friedell HL, Storaasli JP (1950) The use of radioactive phosphorus in the treatment of carcinoma of the breast with widespread metastases to bone. Am J Roentgenol Radium Ther 64(4):559–575
9. Nair N (1999) Relative efficacy of 32P and 89Sr in palliation in skeletal metastases. J Nucl Med 40(2):256–261
10. Finlay IG, Mason MD, Shelley M (2005) Radioisotopes for the palliation of metastatic bone cancer: a systematic review. Lancet Oncol 6(6): 392–400
11. Lewington VJ, McEwan AJ, Ackery DM, Bayly RJ, Keeling DH, Macleod PM et al (1991) A prospective,

randomised double-blind crossover study to examine the efficacy of strontium-89 in pain palliation in patients with advanced prostate cancer metastatic to bone. Eur J Cancer 27(8):954–958
12. Buchali K, Correns HJ, Schuerer M, Schnorr D, Lips H, Sydow K (1988) Results of a double blind study of 89-strontium therapy of skeletal metastases of prostatic carcinoma. Eur J Nucl Med 14(7–8):349–351
13. Russ Knapp FF Jr, Mirzadeh S, Beets AL, O'Doherty M, Blower PJ, Verdera ES et al (1998) Reactor-produced radioisotopes from ORNL for bone pain palliation. Appl Radiat Isot 49(4):309–315
14. Palmedo H, Guhlke S, Bender H, Sartor J, Schoeneich G, Risse J et al (2000) Dose escalation study with rhenium-188 hydroxyethylidene diphosphonate in prostate cancer patients with osseous metastases. Eur J Nucl Med 27(2):123–130
15. O'Sullivan JM, McCready VR, Flux G, Norman AR, Buffa FM, Chittenden S et al (2002) High activity Rhenium-186 HEDP with autologous peripheral blood stem cell rescue: a phase I study in progressive hormone refractory prostate cancer metastatic to bone. Br J Cancer 86(11):1715–1720
16. O'Sullivan JM, Norman AR, McCready VR, Flux G, Buffa FM, Johnson B et al (2006) A phase 2 study of high-activity 186Re-HEDP with autologous peripheral blood stem cell transplant in progressive hormone-refractory prostate cancer metastatic to bone. Eur J Nucl Med Mol Imaging 33(9): 1055–1061
17. Serafini AN, Houston SJ, Resche I, Quick DP, Grund FM, Ell PJ et al (1998) Palliation of pain associated with metastatic bone cancer using samarium-153 lexidronam: a double-blind placebo-controlled clinical trial. J Clin Oncol 16(4):1574–1581
18. Sartor O, Reid RH, Hoskin PJ, Quick DP, Ell PJ, Coleman RE et al (2004) Samarium-153-Lexidronam complex for treatment of painful bone metastases in hormone-refractory prostate cancer. Urology 63(5): 940–945
19. Smeland S, Erikstein B, Aas M, Skovlund E, Hess SL, Fossa SD (2003) Role of strontium-89 as adjuvant to palliative external beam radiotherapy is questionable: results of a double-blind randomized study. Int J Radiat Oncol Biol Phys 56(5):1397–1404
20. Oosterhof GO, Roberts JT, de Reijke TM, Engelholm SA, Horenblas S, von der Maase H et al (2003) Strontium(89) chloride versus palliative local field radiotherapy in patients with hormonal escaped prostate cancer: a phase III study of the European Organisation for Research and Treatment of Cancer Genitourinary Group. Eur Urol 44(5):519–526
21. Tu S, Millikan RE, Mengistu B, Delpassand ES, Amato RJ, Pagliaro LC et al (2001) Bone-targeted therapy for advanced androgen-independent carcinoma of the prostate: a randomised phase II trial. Lancet 357(9253):336–341
22. James ND, Sydes MR, Clarke NW, Mason MD, Dearnaley DP, Spears MR et al (2016) Addition of docetaxel, zoledronic acid, or both to first-line long-term hormone therapy in prostate cancer (STAMPEDE): survival results from an adaptive, multiarm, multistage, platform randomised controlled trial. Lancet 387(10024):1163–1177
23. Sweeney CJ, Chen YH, Carducci M, Liu G, Jarrard DF, Eisenberger M et al (2015) Chemohormonal therapy in metastatic hormone-sensitive prostate cancer. N Engl J Med 373(8):737–746
24. Bilen MA, Johnson MM, Mathew P, Pagliaro LC, Araujo JC, Aparicio A et al (2015) Randomized phase 2 study of bone-targeted therapy containing strontium-89 in advanced castrate-sensitive prostate cancer. Cancer 121(1):69–76
25. Sciuto R, Festa A, Rea S, Pasqualoni R, Bergomi S, Petrilli G et al (2002) Effects of low-dose cisplatin on 89Sr therapy for painful bone metastases from prostate cancer: a randomized clinical trial. J Nuclear Med JNM 43(1):79–86
26. Lam MG, Bosma TB, van Rijk PP, Zonnenberg BA (2009) (188)Re-HEDP combined with capecitabine in hormone-refractory prostate cancer patients with bone metastases: a phase I safety and toxicity study. Eur J Nucl Med Mol Imaging 36(9):1425–1433
27. Tannock IF, de Wit R, Berry WR, Horti J, Pluzanska A, Chi KN et al (2004) Docetaxel plus prednisone or mitoxantrone plus prednisone for advanced prostate cancer. N Engl J Med 351(15):1502–1512
28. de Bono JS, Oudard S, Ozguroglu M, Hansen S, Machiels JP, Kocak I et al (2010) Prednisone plus cabazitaxel or mitoxantrone for metastatic castration-resistant prostate cancer progressing after docetaxel treatment: a randomised open-label trial. Lancet 376(9747):1147–1154
29. van Dodewaard-de Jong JM, de Klerk JM, Bloemendal HJ, van Bezooijen BP, de Haas MJ, Wilson RH et al (2011) A phase I study of combined docetaxel and repeated high activity 186Re-HEDP in castration-resistant prostate cancer (CRPC) metastatic to bone (the TAXIUM trial). Eur J Nucl Med Mol Imaging 38(11):1990–1998
30. Henriksen G, Fisher DR, Roeske JC, Bruland OS, Larsen RH (2003) Targeting of osseous sites with alpha-emitting 223Ra: comparison with the beta-emitter 89Sr in mice. J Nucl Med 44(2):252–259
31. Nilsson S, Larsen RH, Fosså SD, Balteskard L, Borch KW, Westlin J et al (2005) First clinical experience with a-emitting radium-223 in the treatment of skeletal metastases. Clin Cancer Res 11(12):4451–4459
32. Carrasquillo JA, O'Donoghue JA, Pandit-Taskar N, Humm JL, Rathkopf DE, Slovin SF et al (2013) Phase I pharmacokinetic and biodistribution study with escalating doses of (2)(2)(3)Ra-dichloride in men with castration-resistant metastatic prostate cancer. Eur J Nucl Med Mol Imaging 40(9):1384–1393
33. Nilsson S, Strang P, Aksnes AK, Franzèn L, Olivier P, Pecking A et al (2012) A randomized, dose–response, multicenter phase II study of radium-223 chloride for the palliation of painful bone metastases in patients with castration-resistant prostate cancer. Eur J Cancer 48(5):678–686

34. Parker CC, Pascoe S, Chodacki A, O'Sullivan JM, Germá JR, O'Bryan-Tear CG et al (2013) A randomized, double-blind, dose-finding, multicenter, phase 2 study of radium chloride (Ra 223) in patients with bone metastases and castration-resistant prostate cancer. Eur Urol 63(2):189–197
35. Nilsson S, Franzén L, Parker C, Tyrrell C, Blom R, Tennvall J et al (2007) Bone-targeted radium-223 in symptomatic, hormone-refractory prostate cancer: a randomised, multicentre, placebo-controlled phase II study. Lancet Oncol 8(7):587–594
36. Parker C, Nilsson S, Heinrich D, Helle SI, O'Sullivan JM, Fosså SD, et al (2013; 2015) Alpha emitter radium-223 and survival in metastatic prostate cancer. N Engl J Med 369(3):213–223
37. Sartor O, Coleman R, Nilsson S, Heinrich D, Helle SI, O'Sullivan JM et al (2014) Effect of radium-223 dichloride on symptomatic skeletal events in patients with castration-resistant prostate cancer and bone metastases: results from a phase 3, double-blind, randomised trial. Lancet Oncol 15(7):738–746
38. Hoskin P, Sartor O, O'Sullivan JM, Johannessen DC, Helle SI, Logue J et al (2014) Efficacy and safety of radium-223 dichloride in patients with castration-resistant prostate cancer and symptomatic bone metastases, with or without previous docetaxel use: a prespecified subgroup analysis from the randomised, double-blind, phase 3 ALSYMPCA trial. Lancet Oncol 15(12):1397–1406
39. Chittenden SJ, Hindorf C, Parker CC, Lewington VJ, Pratt BE, Johnson B et al (2015) A Phase 1, open-label study of the biodistribution, pharmacokinetics, and dosimetry of 223Ra-dichloride in patients with hormone-refractory prostate cancer and skeletal metastases. J Nucl Med 56(9):1304–1309
40. Ryan CJ, Smith MR, Fizazi K, Saad F, Mulders PFA, Sternberg CN et al (2014) Abiraterone acetate plus prednisone versus placebo plus prednisone in chemotherapy-naive men with metastatic castration-resistant prostate cancer (COU-AA-302): final overall survival analysis of a randomised, double-blind, placebo-controlled phase 3 study. The Lancet Oncology Feb 2015;16(2):152–160
41. de Bono JS, Logothetis CJ, Molina A, Fizazi K, North S, Chu L, et al (2011; 2015) Abiraterone and increased survival in metastatic prostate cancer. N Engl J Med 364(21):1995–2005
42. Scher HI, Fizazi K, Saad F, Taplin M, Sternberg CN, Miller K, et al (2012; 2015) Increased survival with enzalutamide in prostate cancer after chemotherapy. N Engl J Med 367(13):1187–1197
43. Beer TM, Armstrong AJ, Rathkopf DE, Loriot Y, Sternberg CN, Higano CS et al (2014; 2015) Enzalutamide in metastatic prostate cancer before chemotherapy. N Engl J Med 371(5):424–433

17 New Frontiers in Treatment

Sergio Bracarda, Alketa Hamzaj, and Kalliopi Andrikou

In the United States, prostate cancer is the most common cancer in men, with an estimated 220,000 cases diagnosed in 2015 [1]. With a percentage of involvement of more than 80 %, the bone represents the preferential site of metastases for this disease. As a consequence, patients experiencing advanced stage castration-resistant prostate cancer (CRPC) are at increased risk of developing skeletal-related events, including pathologic fractures and spinal cord compression [2].

Despite recent important therapeutic advances in the management of CRPC, there is a continuous medical need to develop further treatment options to overcome the mechanisms of resistance of surviving prostate cancer cells, such as the splice variants of the androgen receptor (AR). All the possible new agents, or combinations, with efficacy data in the area of prostate cancer have been analyzed. Data are presented according to the mechanism of action of the single agents.

S. Bracarda, MD (✉) • A. Hamzaj, MD
K. Andrikou, MD
Medical Oncology, Department of Oncology
Azienda USL Toscana Sud-Est, Istituto Toscano Tumori (ITT), Ospedale San Donato, Arezzo, Italy
e-mail: sergio.bracarda@uslsudest.toscana.it

17.1 Vascular Endothelial Growth Factor (VEGF) Targeting Therapies

In prostate cancer, the VEGF signaling pathway seems to be para-physiological for disease progression: higher levels of VEGF receptor (VEGFR)-2 are observed in high-grade prostate cancer, while patients with metastatic prostate cancer have higher serum VEGF levels and levels of urine and serum VEGF seem to relate with overall survival (OS), in subjects with metastatic CRPC (mCRPC).

VEGFRs are also expressed in human osteoblasts and osteoclasts with the VEGF pathway involved in mechanisms regulating cell migration and survival [3–5]. Moreover, VEGF treatment inhibits the apoptosis of human osteoblasts by increased expression of the Bcl-2, an anti-apoptotic protein, as demonstrated in vitro [5].

All these findings suggest an important role for the VEGF signaling pathway in the processes of prostate cancer progression and bone metastasis.

Several agents targeting angiogenesis have been evaluated in phase III clinical trials in CRPC, but no one demonstrated a clinical benefit in men with CRPC.

17.1.1 Bevacizumab

Bevacizumab is a recombinant, humanized monoclonal antibody blocking VEGF activity. In

F. Bertoldo et al. (eds.), *Bone Metastases from Prostate Cancer*,
DOI 10.1007/978-3-319-42327-2_17

CALGB 90006, a phase II study, 79 patients with chemotherapy-naïve metastatic CRPC received bevacizumab 15 mg/kg combined with docetaxel and estramustine. The progression-free survival (PFS) and median OS were 8 and 24 months, respectively. The observed improvement in OS led to plan a phase III study despite this study did not meet its primary endpoint of PFS [6].

The phase III, double-blind, placebo-controlled study, CALGB 90401, randomized 1050 chemotherapy-naïve mCRPC patients to docetaxel (75 mg/m^2 every 3 weeks) with prednisone (5 mg BID) and either bevacizumab (15 mg/kg IV every 3 weeks) or placebo [7]. The primary endpoint of this trial was OS, while PFS, objective response (OR), and 50% decline in PSA were secondary endpoints. Any statistically significant difference in OS was observed (22.6 months in the bevacizumab group vs. 21.5 months in control group; $p=0.181$) despite an observed improvement in PFS and ORR in the experimental group. Moreover, the addition of bevacizumab was associated with greater treatment-related toxicities (grade ≥3 neutropenia, fatigue, leukopenia, hypertension, gastrointestinal bleeding, and perforation) [7]. As a comment, the OS time of the control group observed in this trial was longer than what reported in other studies (21.5 months vs. 19.2 months observed in TAX 327 study), raising doubts that the study may have been underpowered. Moreover, this trial was not designed to evaluate the role of maintenance of bevacizumab beyond disease progression, which seems to confer a clinical benefit in several types of cancer.

17.1.2 Sunitinib

Sunitinib is an oral multi-tyrosine kinase inhibitor (TKI) of VEGFR-2, PDGFR, FLT-3, and KIT, with a demonstrated activity in two previous phase II studies in patients with mCRPC who failed a previous docetaxel chemotherapy [8, 9].

A randomized, multicenter phase III trial enrolled a total of 873 subjects with progressive mCRPC, after docetaxel chemotherapy. Patients were randomized to sunitinib (37.5 mg daily) or placebo, in a 2:1 ratio. The primary endpoint was OS, with PFS as a secondary endpoint.

While the median OS time was similar in both groups (13.1 vs. 12.8 months, respectively; HR 1.03; 95% CI 0.80–1.32; $p=0.5813$), PFS was significantly longer in the experimental arm (5.6 vs. 4.1 months; $p<0.001$) [10]. The study was stopped on recommendations of the data monitoring committee, after the results of a second interim analysis showing that it was unlikely for the study to meet its primary endpoint.

17.1.3 Lenalidomide

Lenalidomide is an oral immunomodulatory agent which inhibits VEGF signaling and angiogenesis [11]. The MAINSAIL phase III study randomized 1059 chemotherapy-naïve patients with mCRPC to docetaxel (75 mg/m^2, once every 21 days) with prednisone (5 mg BID) and either lenalidomide (25 mg daily, days 1–14) or placebo. Also this study was discontinued on the recommendations of the Data Monitoring Committee, as it was unlikely to meet its primary endpoint (OS). Moreover, patients randomized to experimental arm had higher rates of febrile neutropenia and other non-hematological toxicities [12].

In a phase II trial in patients with mCRPC, a dual anti-angiogenic treatment with *bevacizumab* and *thalidomide* (another oral immunomodulatory agent) was also evaluated in combination with docetaxel. The median OS time (25.9 months) was significantly longer in the experimental arm, but this combination approach resulted also too toxic [13].

17.1.4 Aflibercept

Aflibercept is a recombinant fusion protein consisting of extracellular domains of VEGFR fused to the Fc of a human IgG1 antibody. In the VENICE study, 1224 chemotherapy-naïve patients with metastatic CRPC have been enrolled to receive docetaxel (75 mg/m^2 IV every 3 weeks) and prednisone (10 mg daily) plus aflibercept (6 mg/kg IV, every 3 weeks) or placebo.

No difference in OS was observed between the treatment arms (22.1 months in aflibercept arm vs. 21.2 months in placebo arm, $p = 0.38$), while a statistically significant increase in the number of side effects was reported in the aflibercept arm [14].

17.1.5 Tasquinimod

Tasquinimod is an oral agent with anti-angiogenic activity but an unknown mechanism of action [15]. In a double-blind, placebo-controlled phase II study, 201 patients with mCRPC were randomized in a 2:1 ratio to either tasquinimod or placebo [15]. After an initial double-blind treatment (maximum of 6 months), asymptomatic subjects in the placebo group were allowed to switch to open-label tasquinimod.

The primary endpoint was the proportion of patients who were progression-free at 6 months by RECIST and Prostate Cancer Working Group 2 criteria. This endpoint was superior in the tasquinimod group over placebo (69 % of patients vs. 37 %, $p < 0.001$); also median PFS was longer in the tasquinimod arm over placebo (7.6 vs. 3.3 months, $p = 0.0042$). Of interest, subgroup analyses suggested a clinically relevant impact in PFS for tasquinimod, especially for those with bone metastases (8.8 vs. 3.4 months; $p = 0.019$). Grade 3–4 treatment-related toxicities were more common in the experimental arm (40 % vs. 10 %) [15].

Based on the phase II trial results, a phase III double-blind study was conducted in asymptomatic to mildly symptomatic CRPC patients with bone metastases. In this trial, a total of 1,200 subjects were randomized to tasquinimod or placebo. The primary endpoint was PFS, but the study was powered to detect an improvement in OS as a secondary endpoint. No improvement in OS was observed with tasquinimod (HR = 1.09; CI 95 %, 0.94–1.28), with reasons of this negative result not clear yet [16].

17.2 MET-Targeting Therapies

The HGF/MET pathway plays an important role in various human malignancies, including prostate cancer. A correlation was shown between higher levels of MET expression and higher grade of prostate cancer. Moreover, an increased expression of MET seems to relate with prostate cancer metastasis and the emergence of CRPC [17, 18]. Similarly to VEGF, MET signaling pathway seems also important for osteoblasts and osteoclasts. In prostate cancer, bone metastases are more likely to express MET than soft tissue and lymph node metastases [18].

Thus, an increased expression of MET seems to have an important role in bone metastasis from prostate cancer. Phase two studies specifically enrolling patients with metastatic prostate cancer are ongoing with two MET-targeting agents in development.

17.2.1 Rilotumumab

Rilotumumab (AMG102) is a human monoclonal antibody blocking the binding of HGF to MET. In a recent multicenter, double-blind, phase II study, 142 mCRPC patients progressive after taxane chemotherapy have been randomized (1:1:1), to mitoxantrone (12 mg/m^2, every 21 days) and prednisone (5 mg BID) plus rilotumumab at 15 mg/kg or 7.5 mg/kg or placebo.

Median OS (primary endpoint) was similar among the groups (13.4 vs. 11.6 vs. 11.1 months, respectively). Any difference in PFS or PSA response was also observed among treatment arms [19].

17.2.2 Tivantinib

Tivantinib (ARQ 197) is an oral putative non-ATP competitive inhibitor of the c-MET receptor tyrosine kinase. A phase II study randomized 80 men with chemotherapy-naïve, minimally symptomatic or asymptomatic mCRPC to either tivantinib 360 mg PO BID or placebo. PFS was the primary endpoint of the study. Patients in the tivantinib group had a significantly better PFS in comparison with those in placebo group (medians, 5.6 months vs. 3.8 months, respectively; HR = 0.53, 95 % CI: 0.32–0.89; $p = 0.015$) and a favorable toxicity profile [20].

Other agents targeting the MET pathway are in earlier phases of clinical development, including onartuzumab (MetMab), TAK-701, ficlatuzumab, crizotinib, and JNJ-38877605.

17.3 Dual Inhibition of MET and VEGFR Signaling: Clinical Evidence

MET and VEGFR signaling pathways play an important role in the promotion of tumor cell growth, angiogenesis, invasion, and metastasis and in bone turnover in multiple tumor types including prostate cancer, especially in mCRPC cases with bone metastases.

Resistance to VEGF-targeted therapies may arise from the upregulation of alternative pro-angiogenetic and pro-invasive signaling pathways, including the MET pathway.

Considering the molecular pathophysiology of advanced CRPC, there was a strong rationale for the evaluation of cabozantinib, an orally TKI with potent activity against MET and VEGFR2 in this disease.

In addition, other agents targeting both MET and VEGFR signaling pathways are in development, including foretinib (GSK1363089), golvatinib (E7050), GSK1363089 (XL880), and MGCD265.

17.3.1 Cabozantinib

Cabozantinib is a novel, oral, multiple receptor tyrosine kinase inhibitor with an activity against MET and VEGFR2, as well as RET, KIT, AXL, and FLT [21]. In the initial clinical studies, cabozantinib demonstrated promising results in mCRPC and other malignancies.

After the initial phase I trial evidencing tumor responses in multiple malignancies, a randomized phase II discontinuation study (cabozantinib vs. placebo) was planned.

In the CRPC group of this phase II study, the 87 % of the enrolled patients had bone metastases and 43 % were pretreated with docetaxel.

Cabozantinib was administered at a daily dose of 100 mg during a 12-week lead-in stage. This dosage was associated with frequent side effects, leading to dose reductions in 51 % of subjects by week 12, with 16 % discontinuing therapy due to toxicity prior to week 12. The most common grade 3 toxicities were fatigue (16 %), hand-foot syndrome (6 %), and hypertension (6 %) [22]. A PFS prolongation was observed in the cabozantinib group compared with placebo (23.9 weeks vs. 5.9 weeks, respectively).

In addition, cabozantinib showed a partial/complete response in 99mTc-MDP bone scans in 56 and 19 % of patients, respectively. Among the cases with a present baseline pain, 64 % reported a decrease in pain intensity, with a third of them stopped narcotic pain medication.

Moreover, in the 40 % of treated patients, a discordance was noted between PSA and bone scan response. The high rates of bone scan improvements and the relevant clinical benefit led to a couple of phase III, randomized, double-blind, controlled trials (COMET-1 and COMET-2).

The phase III study COMET-1 [23] randomized 1028 mCRPC patients pretreated with docetaxel, abiraterone, and/or enzalutamide, to receive either cabozantinib (daily dose of 60 mg) or prednisone (10 mg/day) in a 2:1 ratio. Compared to prednisone, cabozantinib improved PFS (5.5 months for cabozantinib vs. 2.8 for prednisone ($p<0.001$)) and bone scan response (41 % for cabozantinib group vs. 3 % for control group ($p<0.001$)) but not significantly increased OS (11 vs. 9.8 months, $p=0.212$)).

Disappointing negative results derived also from the COMET-2 study [24], where cabozantinib was compared with mitoxantrone and prednisone in 119 subjects with symptomatic disease. The primary endpoint, of durable pain response at week 6 (confirmed at week 12) without an increase in narcotic medication, was not achieved in this population with a pain response rates of only 15 % in the cabozantinib arm compared to 17 % in control group ($p=0.773$).

17.4 Dual Androgen Synthesis and Signaling Inhibitor

17.4.1 Galeterone (TOK-001)

Galeterone (TOK-001) is a multifunction oral steroid analog that concomitantly: (1) decreases androgen biosynthesis by inhibiting the enzyme CYP17 (controlling androgen production in the adrenals, testes, and prostate), (2) decreases AR signaling by binding to the AR as a competitive inhibitor of testosterone, and (3) reduces the AR expression in prostate cancer cells by increasing the AR protein degradation and therefore diminishing the cell ability to respond to low levels of androgenic growth signals [25].

More recently, galeterone has been shown to downregulate the levels of constitutively active AR splice variants [26]. As known, these AR variants are upregulated in CRPC cells that have become resistant to CYP17 inhibitors and/or antiandrogens. Galeterone could be effective in CRPC cells expressing AR splice variants such as AR-V7 [27].

In the ARMOR phase I study of chemo-naïve men with CRPC, galeterone (TOK-001) was well tolerated and demonstrated clinical activity. Of 49 patients, 22 % demonstrated a >50 % PSA decline and an additional 26 % had PSA declines of 30–50 % [28].

Based on these preliminary results, a phase II study (ARMOR-2) was started in treatment-naïve cases. The interim data, in nonmetastatic/metastatic treatment-naïve CRPC receiving galeterone (2225 mg/day), showed a maximal reduction in PSA levels of at least 30 % (PSA30) in 8/11 (72.7 %) of the patients; 6/11 (54.5 %) of these patients showed a maximal PSA reduction of at least 50 % (PSA50). In M1 cohorts ($N=39$), PSA30 and PSA50 were, respectively, 85 and 77 %. SD was observed in 72 % of patients with metastatic disease (13 out of 18) and PR in 17 % (3 out of 18).

Galeterone was well tolerated; the most common adverse events were fatigue, increased liver enzymes, gastrointestinal events, and pruritus. Most were mild or moderate in severity and required no action; there were no apparent mineralocorticoid excess (AME) events [29].

Galeterone shares similar MOA with enzalutamide (both drugs inhibit $GABA_A$, which lowers the epileptogenic threshold). The nonclinical data (in vitro) support the clinical observations to date where galeterone has not been associated with an increased seizure risk.

Preliminary data from the ARMOR-2 study showed that six of seven treatment-naïve CRPC patients with high N-terminal AR expression and C-terminal AR loss had PSA reductions of at least 50 %, suggesting that galeterone may have activity in patients with AR splice variant, including AR-V7. According to these data, an open-label phase 3, randomized study (ARMOR-3) is ongoing to evaluate the efficacy and safety of galeterone, compared to enzalutamide, in patients with treatment-naïve metastatic (M1) castration-resistant prostate cancer (CRPC) expressing androgen receptor splice variant-7 mRNA (AR-V7).

17.5 Second-Generation Androgen Receptor Inhibitors

17.5.1 ARN-509

ARN-509 (also referred as *JNJ-56021927*) is an oral small-molecule, nonsteroidal potent and selective antagonist of the AR which acts by inhibiting the action of androgen, nuclear translocation of the AR, and DNA binding to androgen response elements. Unlike bicalutamide, it exhibits no significant agonist activity in AR-overexpressing prostate cancer cells [30]. Like enzalutamide, ARN-509 has been developed to overcome the therapeutic limits of the first-generation antiandrogens.

In a murine xenograft model of mCRPC, ARN-509 showed greater antitumor activity than enzalutamide, for a given dose and plasma concentration. Furthermore, ARN-509 achieved significantly lower steady-state brain levels in respect to enzalutamide, suggesting a lower seizurogenic potential [30].

The ARN-509-001 phase I/II trial enrolled 30 cases with mCRPC and reported a promising activity [31]. At 12 weeks, 42 % of patients displayed a ≥50 % PSA declines with a fluorodihydrotestosterone (FDHT)-PET imaging demonstrating an AR blockade at 4 weeks across multiple doses. JNJ-56021927 (ARN-509) was safe and exhibited linear pharmacokinetics.

The phase II evaluation showed a PSA response at 12 weeks of 91 % in therapy-naïve and 60 % in post-abiraterone acetate mCRPC patients and 89.5 % in nonmetastatic CRPC patients [32, 33]. The phase 3, randomized study ARN-509-003 (SPARTAN) of ADT+ARN-509 compared with ADT + placebo, in patients with high risk (defined as a PSA doubling time ≤10 months) nonmetastatic CRPC, has completed the accrual, and data are not available yet.

According to the distinct mechanism of action of ARN-509 and abiraterone acetate (AA inhibits androgen biosynthesis while ARN-509 targets the AR) and the absence of overlapping clinical toxicities, the combination of both drugs could theoretically delay the emergence of clinical resistance to either drug.

In xenograft models of CRPC, treatment with AA causes a marked suppression of tumor androgen levels which rely with an increased expression of the AR, ligand-independent AR splice variants, and inductions of steroidogenic genes including CYP-17-A1 [34]. The increased expression of several of these genes showed strong correlation with dihydrotestosterone (DHT) levels in recurrent tumors. These data suggest that resistance can potentially be targeted by using combinations with potent AR antagonists such as ARN-509. An ongoing, randomized, double-blinded, placebo-controlled study (56021927PCR3001) is designed to assess the efficacy and safety of ARN-509 in combination with AA + PDN compared with AA + PDN in patients with chemotherapy-naïve mCRPC and will explore mechanisms of resistance that may develop with treatment.

17.5.2 ODM-201

ODM-201 is a novel AR antagonist structurally distinct from all known antiandrogens. In vitro receptor binding studies show that ODM-201 and its major metabolite, ORM-15341, bind with high affinity to wild-type AR inhibitors [35]. In murine castration-resistant VCaP xenograft models, ODM-201 achieves an improved inhibition of tumor growth compared to enzalutamide [35]. ODM-201 also shows an inhibitory activity, without evidence of agonism, against several mutant ARs implicated in resistance to other second-generation AR inhibitors [35]. These include AR F876L, which causes antagonist-to-agonist switching with both enzalutamide and ARN-509 in preclinical models of prostate cancer and which has been identified in plasma DNA from patients with progressive CRPC treated with ARN-509 [35–37]. In contrast to other second-generation AR inhibitors, preclinical studies suggest that the penetrance of ODM-201 and ORM-15341 through the blood–brain barrier after oral administration is negligible.

In the phase I/II ARADES study, ODM-201 was well tolerated and associated with high activity in men with progressive mCRPC, including those previously treated with docetaxel and a CYP17 inhibitor [38]. Overall, 136 patients were accrued. In the phase I study, 24 men with mCRPC received 200, 400, 600, 1000, 1400, or 1800 mg/day of oral ODM-201 in two divided doses. No dose-limiting toxicity was found, while anti-tumor activity was evident with all six doses of ODM-201 tested. A ≥50 % PSA response was observed in 17/21 (81 %) patients who had PSA samples at baseline and week 12.

Twelve patients from phase I entered the phase II part of the trial. In addition to these patients, 112 men were randomized and 110 were treated with 200 mg/day ($n=38$), 400 mg/day ($n=37$), or 1400 mg/day ($n=35$) of ODM-201. Randomization was stratified according to previous treatment that was chemotherapy naïve and CYP17 inhibitor naïve, post-chemotherapy and CYP17 inhibitor naïve, and post-CYP17 inhibitor.

Seventy-eight of 108 (70 %) assessable patients experienced a PSA decline during the first 12 weeks, including a >50 % PSA drop in 44 of 108 (41 %). Dividing patients according to previous treatment, there was an observational trend to higher responses in naïve cases to both chemotherapy and CYP17 inhibitors and in those who had previously received chemotherapy but not CYP17 inhibitors, compared with patients previously treated with CYP17 inhibitors. The highest PSA response was noted with 1400 mg/day of ODM-201 in patients naïve to both chemotherapy and CYP17 inhibitors. There were no clear differences by ODM-201 dose in either soft tissue responses or bone stabilization, although patient numbers were small within each dose group [38, 39].

Another phase I trial (ARAFOR) provides further efficacy data, in men with chemotherapy-naïve and CYP17 inhibitor-naïve CRPC treated with 1200 mg/day of ODM-201 [40]. There was an observed PSA ≥50 % response at week 12, in 25/30 (83 %) patients. A combined analysis of all chemotherapy-naïve and CYP17 inhibitor-naïve patients from the ARADES and ARAFOR trials reported a PSA response rate, of 85 % (33 of 39 patients) after 12 weeks [41]. In most cases, there was a marked and durable decline in PSA levels. ODM-201 has a favorable tolerability profile, and many of the adverse events reported with ODM-201 were considered to be disease related rather than drug related (fatigue or asthenia in 31 %, back pain in 21 %, arthralgia in 16%, and pain in 15 % of patients). ODM-201 has promising antitumor activity in both chemotherapy-naïve and chemotherapy-pretreated patients.

Recently, a randomized, placebo-controlled, double-blind, phase III trial (ARAMIS) has been initiated to test the superiority of ODM-201, 600 mg twice daily versus placebo in men with high-risk nonmetastatic CRPC (those with a PSA doubling time of ≤10 months). The trial has an enrollment target of 1500 patients, who will be treated until confirmed metastasis or death for a total duration of up to 72 months (6 years). The primary trial endpoint is metastasis-free survival, defined as time from randomization until evidence of metastasis or death from any cause, whichever occurs first.

17.5.3 AZD3514

AZD3514 is an oral drug inhibiting the androgen-dependent and androgen-independent AR signaling, by binding to the AR with high affinity, preventing nuclear translocation of the protein and inhibiting ligand-dependent and ligand-independent transcriptional activity (downregulation of androgen receptor levels) [42].

Preclinical studies have shown antitumor activity of AZD3514 in both androgen-sensitive and castration-resistant prostate tumors [43]. In a first-in-man phase I trial, 49 men with CRPC were treated with escalating dose levels of AZD3514 [44]. A PSA decline of ≥30 % and of ≥50 % from baseline was observed, respectively, in 11 of 49 (23 %) and in 7 of 49 (14 %) patients and objective soft tissue responses in 2 of 26 (8 %) patients with measurable disease (RECIST 1.1). Promising antitumor activity was observed, even in patients previously treated with abiraterone acetate. The most common toxicities were nausea and vomiting, almost low-grade toxicity.

17.5.4 EPI-001

EPI-001 is a small-molecule antagonist of AR N-terminal domain (NTD) that inhibits protein-protein interactions necessary for AR transcriptional activity. In xenograft models of CRPC, EPI analogs covalently bound the NTD to block transcriptional activity of AR and its splice variants reducing the prostatic tumor cell growth [45]. Targeting the NTD with this novel agent carries the potential to address constitutively active AR (driven by mutation or splice variants affecting the ligand-binding domain), as well as AR amplification. These mechanisms are known to induce resistance to abiraterone and enzalutamide in preclinical models.

17.5.5 Orteronel

Orteronel (TAK-700) is a novel 17,20-lyase inhibitor. In a phase 3, randomized, double-blind trial comparing orteronel (TAK-700) plus prednisone with placebo plus prednisone in patients with mCRPC progressing on docetaxel therapy, orteronel improved progression-free survival (median 8.3 vs. 5.7 months) compared to placebo but did not improve overall survival (HR 0.886) and pain control as shown in the same settings by abiraterone acetate and enzalutamide [46].

Recently, orteronel has been investigated in chemotherapy-naïve patients with metastatic castration-resistant prostate cancer [47]. In chemotherapy-naïve patients with mCRPC, median radiographic PFS was 13.8 months (95% CI 13.1–14.9) with orteronel plus prednisone and 8.7 months (8.3–10.9) with placebo plus prednisone (hazard ratio [HR] 0.71, 95% CI 0.63–0.80; $p<0.0001$). However, no improvement was achieved in OS, the other primary endpoint (median OS was 31.4 months with orteronel plus prednisone and 29.5 with placebo plus prednisone; HR 0.92, 95% CI 0.79–1.08; $p=0.31$). Orteronel plus prednisone was associated with increased toxic effects compared with placebo plus prednisone. On the basis of these and other data, orteronel is not undergoing further development in mCRPC.

17.6 Immune Checkpoint Inhibitors

In the last few years, promising results have been observed in clinical research studies with the use of checkpoint inhibitors. These treatments work by targeting molecules that serve as checks and balances the regulation of immune responses. By blocking inhibitory molecules or, alternatively, activating stimulatory molecules, these treatments are designed to unleash and/or enhance pre-existing anticancer immune responses. The immune checkpoint inhibitor agents have been investigated in a variety of cancers as monotherapy or combined therapy showing encouraging clinical activity with a tolerable toxicity profile.

17.6.1 Ipilimumab

Ipilimumab is a fully human monoclonal antibody (IgG1) inhibiting CTLA-4 (cytotoxic T-lymphocyte-associated antigen 4), a surface T-cell checkpoint receptor [48, 49]. Ipilimumab has been investigated in various cancers including mCRPC. Along this line, several phase I, II, and III trials have been conducted as single agents or in combination with other therapies (i.e., growth factors, cytotoxic therapy, hormone therapy, radiotherapy) [50–53].

Unfortunately, the phase 3 randomized, double-blind clinical trial (study 043) comparing ipilimumab 10 mg/kg ($n=399$) to placebo ($n=400$) following a single dose of radiotherapy in men with mCRPC who have received prior treatment with docetaxel did not met its primary endpoint of OS (HR=0.85; 95% CI=0.72–1.00; $p=0.053$). However, antitumor activity was observed across some efficacy endpoints, including progression-free survival. As with all potential treatments, there were treatment-related adverse events. These immune-related adverse events (irAEs) were managed using standard ipilimumab-management protocols. The most commonly reported irAEs were gastrointestinal, rash, pruritus, and endocrinopathies, which include adrenal insufficiency, hyper- and hypothyroidism, hypophysitis, and hypopituitarism.

Grade 3 irAEs in the ipilimumab and placebo arms, respectively, were gastrointestinal (GI, 18% vs. 1%), liver (5% vs. 1%), endocrine (2% vs. 1%), and dermatologic (1% vs. 0%). Incidence of drug-related death was 1% [54]. A post hoc analysis suggested that ipilimumab may be more active in mCRPC patients with favorable prognostic factors, including an alkaline phosphatase concentration of less than 1.5 times the upper normal limit, hemoglobin ≥11 g/dL, and no visceral metastases [54]. These data supported the concept of an earlier positioning of immunotherapy in the course of disease to produce better outcomes.

Results from the study 043 support the rationale for using ipilimumab in the ongoing phase III, randomized double-blind CA184-095 study, comparing the efficacy of ipilimumab 10 mg/kg versus placebo in patients with mCRPC who have not received prior cytotoxic treatment chemotherapy. Ipilimumab is now under investigation in various mCRPC settings. A phase II trial is testing *ipilimumab* following sipuleucel-T for patients with chemotherapy-naïve mCRPC (*NCT01804465*). Another ongoing phase II trial is testing *ipilimumab* in patients currently receiving hormone therapy in mCRPC (*NCT02113657*).

17.6.2 Tremelimumab

Tremelimumab is another fully human anti-CTLA-4 monoclonal antibody (IgG2) [55, 56] that has been investigated in prostate cancer both in the neoadjuvant setting and in recurrent disease. In particular, tremelimumab was combined in a phase I dose-escalation trial with short-term ADT in patients with PSA-recurrent prostate cancer (stage D0). The rationale was that short-term ADT would elicit a T-cell anti-PSA immune response that might be potentiated by combining tremelimumab. Eleven patients were treated, and, even though the primary endpoint of the trial was safety, some patients experienced prolongation of the PSA doubling time [57]. Moreover, the immunological analyses performed showed the induction of an antibody-specific immune response against different prostate antigens and cancer testis antigens (SSX-2, PAGE-1, GAGE-2).

17.6.3 Nivolumab

Nivolumab was recently reported in a phase I trial to have activity in several tumor histotypes. In total, 17 patients with CRPC were enrolled in the trial. Even though no objective responses were reported, one patient had a 28 % reduction in measurable lesions. Interestingly, the expression of PD-L1 in two tumor specimens was negative [58].

17.6.3.1 Pembrolizumab

Pembrolizumab, another anti- PD-1 MoAb, is being tested in several tumor histotypes, including CRPC (*NCT02054806*) *such as* other MoAbs directed against different targets. Other recent immune agents include anti- PD-L1, anti-KIR, and anti-LAG-3. Therefore, given the dramatic clinical responses seen in advanced melanoma, combining anti-CTLA-4 and anti-PD-1mAbs, several trials are under way with different immune checkpoint inhibitor combinations (*NCT01772004*, *NCT01714739*, *NCT01968109*).

17.7 Cancer Vaccines

Cancer vaccines have been evaluated in prostate cancer clinical trials. Moreover, the identification of prostate cancer-associated antigens suggests a possible therapeutic role for these agents in the future scenario of this disease.

17.7.1 GVAX

GVAX, deriving from two distinct allogeneic tumor cells producing GM-CSF, is one of the earliest irradiated vaccines tested in prostate cancer [59]. A phase I/II trial evaluated the safety, generation of immune response, OS, radiologic responses, and variation in PSA levels in a mCRPC population. Encouraging results of the study, good tolerability, relationship of OS, and production of antibodies led to plan phase III trials [60].

The first of two phase III trials (VITAL-1) compared GVAX vaccine to docetaxel plus prednisone in asymptomatic patients with mCRPC [61]. The trial was stopped because of a low probability (less than a 30 %) of meet the OS endpoint. The second phase III study (VITAL-2) was planned to compare GVAX plus docetaxel to docetaxel plus prednisone in symptomatic CRPC cases [62]. In August 2008, also this study was stopped, because of a safety review by the IDMC (independent data monitoring committee) showing an imbalance in death rate between the two arms of the study: 67 deaths in the experimental arm and 47 in the standard chemotherapy arm.

17.7.2 Sipuleucel-T

Sipuleucel-T is the only FDA-approved cancer vaccine for prostate cancer. In the phase I study, the PA2024 antigen, composed of human PAP fused to GM-CSF, was demonstrated to be safe without an increased risk of autoimmunity [63].

Two small phase II trials, following the phase I/II studies (D9901 and D9902A) [64, 65], evaluated the ability of this vaccine to treat minimally symptomatic CRPC but failed to meet the primary endpoint of TTP. A later, larger, randomized, double-blind phase III trial (IMPACT study) enrolled 512 patients with asymptomatic or minimally symptomatic metastatic CRPC. This trial met its primary endpoint of OS with a clinical benefit of 4.1 months (25.8 vs. 21.7 months in favor of the experimental arm), leading to the approval of sipuleucel-T by FDA in April 2010.

The observed OS benefit was not associated with differences in time to progression, PSA levels, and effect on measurable disease in the two arms of the study [64–66].

17.7.3 PROSTVAC/TRICOM

PROSTVAC/TRICOM is a pox viral-based vaccine with attenuated vaccinia and fowl pox viral vectors containing the PSA gene and three co-stimulatory proteins: B7-1, LFA-3, and ICAM, tested, after initial preclinical studies, in two small phase I trials [67, 68].

Encouraging results of phase I studies led to a randomized phase II trial which compared TRICOM to placebo in 32 patients with asymptomatic, progressive mCRPC [69]. An observed median OS of 26.6 months was reported in the experimental arm, with no differences in time to progression.

Similar results derived from a second phase II trial evaluated PROSTVAC versus control in 125 minimally symptomatic mCRPC patients. In this trial, a median OS benefit of 8.5 months was observed in cases treated with PROSTVAC (HR = 0.56; 95 % CI = 0.37–0.85; $p = 0.0061$) [70]. These findings led to an international randomized double-blind phase III study in 1298 patients to evaluate the OS benefit for PROSTVAC with or without GM-CSF.

Even if at the moment only a vaccine is approved for prostate cancer, several others are under evaluation in phase III trials suggesting a growing interest for this type of treatment as possible component of the near scenario of prostate cancer treatment.

Conclusions

In recent years, a relevant number of treatment innovations have been introduced in cancer treatment, with the new immuno-oncology (I-O) agents, especially checkpoint inhibitors, frequently representing a new standard of care, because of relevant improvements in OS.

This is not the hypothesized near scenario for mCRPC, where the AR pathway seems to maintain its central role of "driver" for prostate tumoral cells.

As a consequence, innovative molecules able to block the AR, especially in the presence of AR splice variants, seem to be the most promising in this rapidly evolving scenario. Some other agents, able to interfere with emerging pathways, such as AKT, and cancer vaccines may be of future interest, while newly designed clinical trials may modify the situation for I-O agents.

New other options are urgently needed to improve the possibility of disease control in some increasing and "hard-to-treat" clinical situations, such as visceral metastases, after the failure of the cabozantinib study.

References

1. Siegel RL, Miller KD, Jemal A (2015) Cancer statistics, 2015. CA Cancer J Clin 65:5–29
2. Weinfurt KP, Li Y, Castel LD et al (2005) The significance of skeletal related events for the health-related quality of life of patients with metastatic prostate cancer. Ann Oncol 16:579–584
3. Duque JLF, Loughlin KR, Adam RM, Kantoff PW, Zurakowski D, Freeman MR (1999) Plasma levels of vascular endothelial growth factor are increased in patients with metastatic prostate cancer. Urology 54:523–527
4. Bok RA, Halabi S, Fei DT, Rodriquez CR, Hayes DF, Vogelzang NJ, Kantoff P, Shuman MA, Small EJ (2001) Vascular endothelial growth factor and basic fibroblast growth factor urine levels as predictors of outcome in hormone-refractory prostate cancer patients: a cancer and leukemia group B study. Cancer Res 61:2533–2536
5. Street J, Lenehan B (2009) Vascular endothelial growth factor regulates osteoblast survival -evidence for an autocrine feedback mechanism. J Orthop Surg Res 4:19
6. Picus J, Halabi S, Kelly WK, Vogelzang NJ, Whang YE, Kaplan EB, Stadler WM, Small EJ, Cancer and Leukemia Group B (2011) A phase 2 study of estramustine, docetaxel, and bevacizumab in men with castrate-resistant prostate cancer. Cancer 117:526–533
7. Kelly WK, Halabi S, Carducci M, George D, Mahoney JF, Stadler WM, Morris M, Kantoff P, Monk JP, Kaplan E, Vogelzang NJ, Small EJ (2012) Randomized, double-blind, placebo-controlled phase III trial comparing docetaxel and prednisone with or without bevacizumab in Men with metastatic castration-resistant prostate cancer: CALGB 90401. J Clin Oncol 30:1534–1540
8. Sonpavde G, Periman PO, Bernold D, Weckstein D, Fleming MT, Galsky MD, Berry WR, Zhan F, Boehm

KA, Asmar L, Hutson TE (2010) Sunitinib malate for metastatic castration-resistant prostate cancer following docetaxel-based chemotherapy. Ann Oncol 21:319–324

9. Michaelson MD, Regan MM, Oh WK, Kaufman DS, Olivier K, Michaelson SZ, Spicer B, Gurski C, Kantoff PW, Smith MR (2009) Phase II study of sunitinib in men with advanced prostate cancer. Ann Oncol 20:913–920
10. Michaelson MD, Oudard S, Ou Y, Sengelov F, Saad F, Houede N, Ostler PJ, Stenzl A, Daugaard G, Jones RJ, Laestadius F, Bahl A, Castellano DE, Gschwend J, Maurina T, Ye D, Chen I, Wang S, Maneval EC (2011) Randomized, placebo-controlled, phase III trial of sunitinib in combination with prednisone (SU+P) versus prednisone (P) alone in men with progressive metastatic castration resistant prostate cancer (mCRPC). J Clin Oncol 29(Suppl):Abstr 4515
11. Lu L, Payvandi F, Wu L, Zhang L-H, Hariri RJ, Man H-W, Chen RS, Muller GW, Hughes CCW, Stirling DI, Schafer PH, Bartlett JB (2009) The anti-cancer drug lenalidomide inhibits angiogenesis and metastasis via multiple inhibitory effects on endothelial cell function in normoxic and hypoxic conditions. Microvasc Res 77:78–86
12. Petrylak DP, Fizazi K, Sternberg CN, Budnik N, Wit Rd, Wiechno PJ, Bellmunt J, Barton D, Fandi A, Jungnelius U, Li S, Vogelzang NJ, Investigators M (2012) A phase 3 study to evaluate the efficacy and safety of Docetaxel and Prednisone (DP) with or without lenalidomide in patients with Castrate-resistant Prostate Cancer (CRPC): the MAINSAIL trial. ESMO 2012 Congress Abstract LBA24
13. Dahut WL, Gulley JL, Arlen PM, Liu Y, Fedenko KM et al (2004) Randomized phase II trial of docetaxel plus thalidomide in androgen-independent prostate cancer. J Clin Oncol 22:2532–2539
14. Tannock IF, Fizazi K, Ivanov S, Karlsson CT, Fléchon A et al (2013) Aflibercept versus placebo in combination with docetaxel and prednisone for treatment of men with metastatic castration-resistant prostate cancer (VENICE): a phase 3, double-blind randomised trial. Lancet Oncol 14:760–768
15. Pili R, Haggman M, Stadler WM, Gingrich JR, Assikis VJ, Bjork A, Nordle O, Forsberg G, Carducci MA, Armstrong AJ (2011) Phase II randomized, double-blind, placebo-controlled study of tasquinimod in Men with minimally symptomatic metastatic castrate-resistant prostate cancer. J Clin Oncol 29:4022–4028
16. Carducci M, Armstrong A, Pili R, et al. A phase 3, randomized, double-blind, placebo-controlled study of tasquinimod (TASQ) in men with metastatic castrate resistant prostate cancer (mCRPC). Presented at: 2015 European Cancer Congress; Vienna. Abstract 4BA
17. Humphrey PA, Zhu X, Swanson PE, Ratliff TL, Vollmer RT, Day ML (1995) Hepatocyte growth factor and its receptor (c-MET) in prostatic carcinoma. Am J Pathol 147:386–396
18. Knudsen BS, Gmyrek GA, Inra J, Scherr DS, Vaughan ED, Nanus DM, Kattan MW, Gerald WL, Vande Woude GF (2002) High expression of the Met receptor in prostate cancer metastasis to bone. Urology 60:1113–1117
19. Ryan CJ, Rosenthal M, Ng S, Alumkal JJ, Picus J, Gravis G, Fizazi K, Forget F, Machiels J-PH, Zhu M, Jiang J, Dubey S, Loh E, Gerritsen WR (2012) A multicenter, randomized phase II study of rilotumumab (R) (AMG 102) or placebo (Pbo) plus mitoxantrone (M) and prednisone (P) in patients (pts) with previously treated castrate-resistant prostate cancer (CRPC). J Clin Oncol 30(Suppl 5):Abstr 115
20. Monk P, Liu G, Stadler WM, Geyer SM, Sexton JL, Joseph Wright J, Villalona-Calero MA, Wade JL, Szmulewitz RZ et al (2015) Phase II randomized, double-blind, placebo-controlled study of tivantinib in men with asymptomatic or minimally symptomatic metastatic castrate-resistant prostate cancer (mCRPC). J Clin Oncol 33(Suppl 7):Abstr 146
21. Yakes FM, Chen J, Tan J, Yamaguchi K, Shi Y, Yu P, Qian F, Chu F, Bentzien F, Cancilla B, Orf J, You A, Laird AD, Engst S, Lee L, Lesch J, Chou Y-C, Joly AH (2011) Cabozantinib (XL184), a novel MET and VEGFR2 inhibitor, simultaneously suppresses metastasis, angiogenesis, and tumor growth. Mol Cancer Ther 10:2298–2308
22. Smith DC, Smith MR, Sweeney C, Elfiky AA, Logothetis C, Corn PG, Vogelzang NJ, Small EJ, Harzstark AL, Gordon MS, Vaishampayan UN, Haas NB, Spira AI, Lara PN Jr, Lin CC, Srinivas S, Sella A, Schoffski P, Scheffold C, Weitzman A, Hussain M (2013) Cabozantinib for metastatic castration-resistant prostate cancer: results of a Phase II placebo-controlled randomized discontinuation study. J Clin Oncol 31:412–419
23. Smith RM, De Bono JS, Sternberg C, Le Moulec S, Oudard S, De Giorgi U et al (2015) Final analysis of COMET-1: cabozantinib versus prednisone in metastatic castration-resistant prostate cancer (mCRPC) patients previously treated with docetaxel and abiraterone and/or enzalutamide. J Clin Oncol 33(Suppl 7):Abstr 139
24. Basch EM, Scholz MC, De Bono JS, Vogelzang NJ, DeSouza PL, Marx GM et al (2015) Final analysis of COMET-2: cabozantinib versus mitoxantrone/prednisone in metastatic castration-resistant prostate cancer (mCRPC) patients with moderate to severe pain who were previously treated with docetaxel and abiraterone and/or enzalutamide. J Clin Oncol 33(Suppl 7):Abstr 141
25. Vasaitis T, Belosay A, Schayowitz A, Khandelwal A (2008) Androgen receptor inactivation contributes to antitumor efficacy of 17{alpha}-hydroxylase/17,20-lyase inhibitor 3beta-hydroxy-17-(1H-benzimidazole-1-yl)androsta-5,16-diene in prostate cancer. Mol Cancer Ther 7(8):2348–2357. doi:10.1158/1535-7163.MCT-08-0230
26. Purushottamachar P, Godbole AM, Gediya LK, Martin MS, Vasaitis TS, Kwegyir-Afful AK,

Ramalingam S, Ates-Alagoz Z, Njar VC (2013) Systematic structure modifications of multitarget prostate cancer drug candidate galeterone to produce novel androgen receptor down-regulating agents as an approach to treatment of advanced prostate cancer. J Med Chem 56(12):4880–4898. doi:10.1021/jm400048v. Epub 2013 Jun 7
27. Antonarakis ES, Lu C, Wang H (2014) Commentary on "AR-V7 and resistance to enzalutamide and abiraterone in prostate cancer". N Engl J Med 371(11): 1028–1038
28. Montgomery RB, Eisenberger MA, Rettig M et al (2012) Phase I clinical trial of galeterone (TOK-001), a multifunctional antiandrogen and CYP17 inhibitor in castration resistant prostate cancer (CRPC). J Clin Oncol 30(Suppl): Abstr 4665
29. Montgomery B, Eisenberger MA, Rettig MB, Chu F, Pili R, Stephenson JJ, Vogelzang NJ, Koletsky AJ, Nordquist LT, Edenfield WJ, Mamlouk K, Ferrante KJ, Taplin ME (2016) Androgen Receptor Modulation Optimized for Response (ARMOR) phase I and II studies: galeterone for the treatment of castration-resistant prostate cancer. Clin Cancer Res 22(6):1356–1363. doi:10.1158/1078-0432.CCR-15-1432, Epub 2015 Nov 2
30. Clegg NJ, Wongvipat J, Joseph JD et al (2012) Discovery and development of ARN-509: a novel antiandrogen for prostate cancer treatment. Cancer Res 72:1494–1503
31. Rathkopf DE, Morris MJ, Danila DC et al (2012) A phase I study of the androgen signaling inhibitor ARN-509 in patients with metastatic castration-resistant prostate cancer. J Clin Oncol 30(Suppl): Abstr 4548
32. Rathkopf DE, Antonarakis ES, Shore ND et al (2013) ARN-509 in men with metastatic castration-resistant prostate cancer. J Clin Oncol 31:3525–3530
33. Smith MR, Antonarakis ES, Ryan CJ et al (2013) ARN-509 in men with high-risk non-metastatic castration reistant prostate cancer. J Clin Oncol 31(Suppl 6): Abstract 7
34. Efstathiou E, Titus M, Tsavachidou D (2012) Effects of abiraterone acetate on androgen signaling in castrate-resistant prostate cancer in bone. J clin Oncol 30:637–643
35. Moilanen A, Riikonen R, Oksala R et al (2015) Discovery of ODM-201, a new-generation androgen receptor inhibitor targeting resistance mechanisms to androgen signalling-directed prostate cancer therapies. Sci Rep 5:12007
36. Joseph JD, Lu N, Qian J et al (2013) A clinically relevant androgen receptor mutation confers resistance to second-generation antiandrogens enzalutamide and ARN-509. Cancer Discov 3:1020–1029
37. Korpal M, Korn JM, Gao X et al (2013) An F876L mutation in androgen receptor confers genetic and phenotypic resistance to MDV3100 (enzalutamide). Cancer Discov 3:1030–1043
38. Fizazi K, Massard C, Bono P et al (2014) ARADES study group. An open-label, phase I/II safety, pharmacokinetic, and proof-of concept study of ODM-201 in patients with progressive metastatic castration-resistant prostate cancer (CRPC). Lancet Oncol 15(9):975–985
39. Fizazi K, Albiges L, Loriot Y, Massard C (2015) ODM-201: a new-generation androgen receptor inhibitor in castration-resistant prostate cancer. Expert Rev Anticancer Ther 15(9):1007–1017
40. Massard C, Penttinen H, Bono P et al (2015) Pharmacokinetics, activity, and safety of ODM-201 in chemotherapy-naïve patients with metastatic castration-resistant prostate cancer: An open-label phase I trial with long-term extension. J Clin Oncol 33(Suppl 7):Abstr 230
41. Tammela L, Massard C, Bono P et al (2014) European Urology Supplements Safety and efficacy of ODM-201 in chemotherapy and CYP17-inhibitor naïve patients: Analysis of data from the ARADES and the ARAFOR trials (abstract 862). Presented at the 29th Annual European Association of Urology Congress; Stockholm
42. Bradbury RH, Acton DG et al (2013) Discovery of AZD3514, a small-molecule androgen receptor downregulator for treatment of advanced prostate cancer. Bioorg Med Chem Lett 23(7):1945–1948
43. Loddick SA, Ross SJ, Thomason AG et al (2013) AZD3514: a small molecule that modulates androgen receptor signaling and function in vitro and in vivo. Mol Cancer Ther 12:1715–1727
44. Omlin A, Jones RJ, van der Noll R et al (2013) A first-in-human study of the oral selective androgen receptor down-regulating drug (SARD) AZD3514 in patients with castration-resistant prostate cancer (CRPC). J Clin Oncol 31(Suppl): Abstr 4511
45. Myung JK, Banuelos CA, Fernandez JG et al (2013) An androgen receptor N-terminal domain antagonist for treating prostate cancer. J Clin Invest 123:2948–2960. 25(9)
46. Saad F, Fizazi K, Jinga V, Efstathiou E et al; ELM-PC 4 Investigators (2015) Orteronel plus prednisone in patients with chemotherapy-naive metastatic castration-resistant prostate cancer (ELM-PC 4): a double-blind, multicentre, phase 3, randomised, placebo-controlled trial. Lancet Oncol 16(3):338–348. doi:10.1016/S1470-2045(15)70027-6
47. Tanej S et al (2015) Phase III, randomized, double-blind, multicenter trial comparing orteronel (TAK-700) plus prednisone with placebo plus prednisone in patients with metastatic castration-resistant prostate cancer that has progressed during or after docetaxel-based therapy: ELM-PC 5. J Urol 194(4):990
48. Hodi FS, O'Day SJ, McDermott DF et al (2010) Improved survival with ipilimumab in patients with metastatic melanoma. N Engl J Med 363:711–723
49. Bracarda S, Altavilla A, Hamzaj A, Sisani M, Marrocolo F, Del Buono S, Danielli R (2015) Immunologic checkpoints blockade in renal cell, prostate, and urothelial malignancies. Semin Oncol 42(3):495–505
50. Tollefson MK, Karnes RJ, Thompson RH, et al (2010) A randomized phase II study of ipilimumab with

androgen ablation compared with androgen ablation alone in patients with advanced prostate cancer [abstract]. Genitourinary Cancer Symposium (Meeting Abstracts) 168
51. Small E, Higano C, Tchekmedyian N et al (2006) Randomized phase II study comparing 4 monthly doses of ipilimumab (MDX-010) as a single agent or in combination with a single dose of docetaxel in patients with hormone-refractory prostate cance r[abstract]. J Clin Oncol (Meeting Abstracts) 24:4609
52. Harzstark AL, Fong L, Weinberg VK et al (2010) Final results of a phase I study of CTLA-4 blockade in combination with GM-CSF for metastatic castration resistant prostate cancer (mCRPC) [abstract]. J clin Oncol (Meeting Abstracts) 28:4689
53. Fong L, Kwek S, O'Brien S et al (2009) Potentiating endogenous antitumor immunity to prostate cancer through combination immunotherapy with CTLA4 blockade and GM-CSF. Cancer Res 69:609–615
54. Kwon ED, Drake CG, Scher HI et al (2014) Ipilimumab versus placebo after radiotherapy in patients with metastatic castration-resistant prostate cancer that had progressed after docetaxel chemotherapy (CA184-043): a multicentre, randomised, double-blind, phase 3 trial. Lancet Oncol 15(7):700–712
55. Tomillero A, Moral MA (2008) Gateways to clinical trials. Methods Find Exp Clin Pharmacol 30(8): 643–672
56. Poust J et al (2008) Targeting metastatic melanoma. Am J Health Syst Pharm 65(24 Suppl 9):S9–S15
57. McNeel DG, Smith HA, Eickhoff JC et al (2012) Phase I trial of tremelimumab in combination with short-term androgen deprivation in patients with PSA-recurrent prostate cancer. Cancer Immunol Immunother 61:1137–1147
58. Brahmer JR, Tykodi SS, Chow LQ et al (2012) Safety and activity of anti-PD-L1 antibody in patients with advanced cancer. N Engl J Med 366:2455–2465
59. Le DT, Pardoll DM, Jaffee EM (2010) Cellular vaccine approaches. Cancer J 16:304–310
60. Higano C, Corman J, Smith D et al (2008) Phase I/II dose escalation study of a GM-CSF-secreting, allogeneic, cellular immunotherapy for metastatic hormone-refractory prostate cancer. Cancer 113:975–984
61. Higano C, Saad F, Somer B et al (2009) A phase III trial of GVAX immunotherapy for prostate cancer vs. docetaxel plus prednisone in asymptomatic castration-resistant prostate cancer (CRPC). Presented at ASCO GU
62. Small E, Demkow T, Gerritson W et al (2009) A phase III trial of GVAX immunotherapy for prostate cancer in combination with docetaxel vs. docetaxel plus prednisone in symptomatic, castration-resistant prostate cancer (CRPC). GU ASCO
63. Burch PA, Breen JK, Buckner JC, Gastineau DA, Kaur JA, Laus RL et al (2000) Priming tissue-specific cellular immunity in a phase I trial of autologous dendritic cells for prostate cancer. Clin Cancer Res 6:2175–2182
64. Small EJ, Schellhammer PF, Higano CS et al (2006) Placebo-controlled phase III trial of immunologic therapy with sipuleucel T (APC8015) in patients with metastatic, asymptomatic hormone refractory prostate cancer. J Clin Oncol 24(19):3089–3094
65. Higano C, Burch P, Small E et al (2005) Immunotherapy (APC8015) for androgen independent prostate cancer (AIPC): final progression and survival data from a second Phase 3 trial. 13th European Cancer Conference. Paris
66. Kantoff PW, Higano CS, Shore ND et al (2010) Sipuleucel T immunotherapy for castration-resistant prostate cancer. N Engl J Med 363(5):411–422
67. Di Paola RS, Plante M, Kaufman H et al (2006) .A phase I trial of pox PSA vaccines (PROSTVAC) with B7-1, ICAM-1, and LFA-3 co-stimulatory molecules (TRICOM) in patients with prostate cancer. J Translat Med 4, article 1
68. Sanda MG, Smith DC, Charles LG et al (1999) Recombinant vaccinia-PSA (PROSTVAC) can induce a prostate-specific immune response in androgen-modulated human prostate cancer. Urology 53(2):260–266
69. Gulley JL, Arlen PM, Madan RA et al (2010) Immunologic and prognostic factors associated with OS employing a poxviral-based PSA vaccine in metastatic castrate-resistant prostate cancer. Cancer Immunol Immunother 59:663–674
70. Kantoff PW, Schuetz TJ, Blumenstein BA, Glode LM, Bilhartz DL, Wyand M et al (2010) OS analysis of a phase II randomized controlled trial of a Poxviral-based PSA-targeted immunotherapy in metastatic castration-resistant prostate cancer. J Clin Oncol 28(7):1099–1105

18 Approaches for Assessment of Response of Bone Metastases to Therapies

Emilio Bombardieri, Francesco Mungai, Maria Bonomi, Lucia Setti, Eugenio Borsatti, Gianluigi Ciocia, and Laura Evangelista

18.1 Introduction

The recent introduction of new therapeutic agents has proven alternative options in the management of patients with metastatic castration-resistant prostate cancer (mCRPC). Moreover, other novel agents are being studied and developed. Bone represents the most common site of recurrence in mCRPC, occurring in more than 80 % of cases. The evaluation of treatment efficacy in bone metastatic prostate cancer (PC) is mainly focused on the assessment of patient outcomes, but the behavior of bone metastases and their changes due to the therapy are also of great interest. The impressive development of technologies offers today various options for describing the skeletal changes caused by metastases before, during, and after treatments. At present, in clinical practice, the only laboratory test currently used to measure metastatic bone progression remains prostate-specific antigen (PSA). Great importance has been progressively assumed by new modalities of metabolic imaging, such as ^{18}F fluoride, ^{18}F/^{11}C choline, and ^{18}F FDG positron emission tomography (PET)/computed tomography (CT) that are flanking the traditional bone scan (BS) with ^{99m}Tc phosphonates, both with planar acquisition and single-photon emission computed tomography (SPECT). In addition, radiology, besides CT, is proposing the high performance of multimodality magnetic resonance imaging (MRI) that seems to guarantee a very high accuracy in evaluating skeletal involvement.

This chapter overviews the available clinical, biochemical, and diagnostic tools for detecting bone lesions and evaluating their changes as a measure of tumor response or progression during therapy, in mCRPC patients. The most important clinical trials on PC will be analyzed giving more emphasis to the parameters for the evaluation of response. The current guidelines of some international scientific societies on PC will be examined, and their indications about the measurable tools

E. Bombardieri (✉) • L. Setti • G. Ciocia
Nuclear Medicine Department, Humanitas Gavazzeni, Via M. Gavazzeni 21, 24125 Bergamo, Italy
e-mail: emilio.bombardieri@gavazzeni.it

F. Mungai
Department of Diagnostic Imaging, Azienda Ospedaliero Universitaria Careggi, Florence, Italy

M. Bonomi
Medical Oncology Department, Humanitas Gavazzeni, Via M. Gavazzeni 21, 24125 Bergamo, Italy

E. Borsatti
Nuclear Medicine Unit, IRCCS National Cancer Institute (CRO), Aviano, Italy

L. Evangelista
Nuclear Medicine and Molecular Imaging Unit, Veneto Institute of Oncology, IOV – IRCCS, Padua, Italy

F. Bertoldo et al. (eds.), *Bone Metastases from Prostate Cancer*, DOI 10.1007/978-3-319-42327-2_18

able to check the response to treatments will be discussed. Finally, a proposal on possible strategies to evaluate the clinical response to the treatments for skeletal metastases will be formulated.

18.2 Modalities to Evaluate Bone Metastases

18.2.1 Clinical Evaluation

Pain occurs in about 75 % of PC patients with bone metastases and represents the most frequent symptom [1]. Mechanisms involved are different and include spinal compression, nerve root infiltration (neuropathic pain) microfractures, periosteal stretching, increased intraosseous tension (osteopathic pain), and muscle spasms [2]. The evaluation of these complications requires the use of various tools, including clinical, neurophysiological, and imaging investigations. The record of the use of analgesics, timing, and route of administration ("by the mouth, by the clock, by the ladder") and its efficacy is of great importance. The most common clinical approach is the administration of appropriate questioners, such as: the visual analogic scale, the verbal rating scale, the numerical rating scale, and the World Health Organization score [3]. The novel concept of symptomatic skeletal events (SSEs) has become another parameter used to measure bone involvement and consists in a series of events including symptomatic pathologic fracture, irradiation to bone, surgery to bone, or symptomatic spinal cord compression. SSEs were firstly introduced in the trials involving ^{223}Ra and considered as an alternative term/clinical trial end point to describe skeletal morbidity [4–6]. In contrast with skeletal-related events (SREs), the ascertainment of SSEs does not include scheduled radiographic assessments, thus requiring only a clinical assessment.

18.2.2 Markers of Bone Turnover

Bone homeostasis is a result of a continuous remodeling process involving the resorption of old bone by osteoclasts and the formation of new bone by osteoblasts. The maintenance and repair of normal bone depend on the release of enzymes, peptides, and mineral components that have been called "biochemical markers" of bone remodeling. In patients with bone metastases, the physiological balance is disrupted, and the changes of marker levels are a signal of alterations in skeletal homeostasis, with increased rates of osteolysis and/or osteogenesis. For this reason, chemical markers of bone remodeling may potentially be an ideal tool to indicate changes in bone turnover, and these events can be predictive of different events from bone metastasization to the risk of progression, from SREs risk to changes in bone associated with the response to treatment. In Chap. 2 of this book, the most important markers of bone turnover are described and discussed as the amino (N) and carboxy C-terminal cross-linked telopeptide of type I collagen, NTX and CTX procollagen type I N-terminal and C-terminal peptides, or P1NP and P1CP that can reflect the effect of tumor growth on bone turnover. The serum levels of bone-specific alkaline phosphatase (bone ALP) are a good parameter of the osteogenetic activity. In this area, dedicated recommendations by the International Osteoporosis Foundation (IOF) and the International Federation of Clinical Chemistry and Laboratory Medicine (IFCC) suggest that a marker of bone formation (serum procollagen type I N-terminal propeptide, s-PINP) and a marker of bone resorption (serum C-terminal telopeptide of type I collagen, s-CTX) can be adopted in clinical studies as reference analytics for markers of bone turnover [7].

A very important question can be raised on this point. Have the bone turnover markers any role as biochemical parameters of bone metastases? There is a general consensus about the concept that their role is not under discussion in systemic metabolic bone diseases such as osteoporosis, primary hyperparathyroidism, and osteomalacia, where biochemical marker changes are related to the rates of bone resorption and formation. On the contrary, bone marker assessments in "focal" diseases as Paget disease or bone metastasis are not able to give any reliable information related to a single lesion or few localized lesions since their volume is negligible with respect to the mass of the whole skeleton. Besides this, the observed changes in bone marker levels are "specific for bone tissue" but are not "cancer specific" because they are the consequence of alterations in skeletal metabolism that can be caused by any neoplastic or nonneoplastic pathology like age, vitamin D deficiency, and adjuvant hormone therapy [8, 9]. In conclusion, in cancer patients bone turnover markers do not allow to distinguish the contributes of the various components that can cause increase in the marker levels in serum and urine. It's important to stress that the utility of bone markers as biochemical indicators of bone metastatic disease has been extensively studied and validated mainly in the area of diagnosis and prognosis [10–21].

18.2.3 Prostate-Specific Antigen (PSA)

PSA remains today the most reliable circulating marker for PC, as its association with neoplasia is very high, even if its specificity is not absolute. The interpretation of serum levels may be affected by many non-cancer-related factors and also by some medical therapies like hormones or steroid reductase inhibitors (i.e., finasteride and dutasteride) [22]. However, the interpretation of PSA levels showed great clinical usefulness in the diagnosis, in monitoring response to primary treatment, detection of relapses even when not detectable by the current diagnostic imaging (so-called biochemical disease). In Chap. 4, an extensive description of PSA marker has been reported. PSA measurements are fundamental both for the assessment of disease recurrence after primary treatments. PSA is also currently used for the evaluation of response to therapy in metastatic/advanced disease. In patients with evidence of disease and/or in those under treatment with chemotherapy or radiotherapy, the changes of PSA levels in many cases are able to give information on cancer response or progression. Therefore, PSA is generally considered as indicator of response, even if in those patients treated with drugs targeting bone metastases, PSA should be considered more reliable as a marker for tumor but not for bone remodeling. The 50 % decrease in PSA levels with respect to its initial concentrations is currently considered as a predictor of good metabolic response, and this trend is often associated with a better survival [23]. However, in this setting, the changes in PSA value can show unexpected trends. In 20 % of patients considered as stable or responsive (it means that a PSA decrease of 50 % after 4 weeks from the last cycle of chemotherapy) at the end of chemotherapy, a transient increase of PSA (sometimes twofold with respect to the baseline values) can be observed, due to the cytotoxic effects of the therapy and to other metabolic changes. This phenomenon called "PSA surge syndrome" is often seen within the first 8 weeks from the start of treatment [24]. Recent recommendations from the Prostate Cancer Working Group 2 (PCWG2) and PCWG3 define PSA progression, during or after therapy, as the date that a 25 % or greater increase and an absolute increase in 2 ng/mL or more from the nadir is documented, which is confirmed by a second value obtained 3 or more weeks later [25].

18.2.4 Radiology Imaging

18.2.4.1 Conventional Radiology

Radiographs are readily available, cheap, and usually easy for the patient to undergo. Although not particularly sensitive, especially for osteolytic metastases (30–75 % of the trabecular bone must be destroyed before the lesion become visible on conventional radiology), radiographs can give an overview of the status of a particular bone segment and allow the assessment of possible associated fractures. However, evaluation of treatment response of bone metastases by conventional radiology is not currently used in clinical practice because of its low diagnostic accuracy; indeed, radiographic signs of response to therapy of bone lesions (peripheral sclerosis, lesion filling, and condensation) are equivocal and often late [26].

18.2.4.2 Computed Tomography

Computed tomography (CT) allows finer detail assessment of osseous architecture than conventional radiology, detecting much smaller areas of trabecular destruction/invasion; it is also particularly helpful in assessing structures difficult to be imaged by radiographs, such as the sacrum. However, for radioprotection reasons, CT usually focuses on a particular portion of the body and is not usually used for whole-body bone evaluation. Besides, CT presents limited ability in assessing therapeutic response because bone structure rarely normalizes even with completely effective therapy. Consequently, diffuse disease and osteoblastic bone metastases are considered nonevaluable by RECIST (v 1.1) criteria [27, 28]. In particular, the occurrence of new bone sclerotic areas can be erroneously classified as disease progression (CT flare response) by inexperienced radiologists [29].

18.2.4.3 Magnetic Resonance Imaging

Bone metastases become visible on radiographs and CT at a late stage, consequently to the activation of bone cells – osteoblasts and osteoclasts – in response to the presence of tumor cells within the bone marrow. Conversely, magnetic resonance imaging (MRI) allows the direct detection of the tumor tissue replacing the bone marrow, before the osteoclastic/osteoblastic response takes effect, and it is also sensitive to the latter. Furthermore, MRI can be used to provide a whole-body (WB) assessment without any irradiation, contrary to radiographs and CT. It also makes perfect sense to take advantage of this technique for the follow-up of bone metastases [30].

Visual assessment of response to therapy MRI can be done with the use of conventional T1-weighted and STIR (short-tau inversion recovery) acquisitions. Tumor tissue replaces the normal bone marrow fat component (hyperintense on T1w and hypointense on STIR imaging) and appears hypointense on T1w (with equal or lower signal intensity than intervertebral disk and/or muscle) and hyperintense on STIR, at initial phase. When the reactive osteoblastic reaction takes place, the metastatic lesion will develop internal calcified component that appears more hypointense on T1w and hypointense on STIR imaging as well, due to lack of mobile protons.

Possible signs of responding lesion are (Fig. 18.1):

1. Shrinkage or progressive fading of the marrow signal intensity abnormalities
2. Development of "fatty halo sign" (hyperintense on T1w), which represents healing
3. Increasing of the intralesional calcified component within correspondent dimensional stability of the lesion

Conversely, possible signs of evolution and/or persistence of active tumor tissue are (Fig. 18.2):

1. Onset of new marrow signal intensity abnormalities
2. Persistence of noncalcified T1w hypointense and STIR hyperintense foci in a dimensionally stable lesion
3. Development of "cellular halo" (hypointense on T1w and hyperintense on STIR images) at the periphery of a calcified lesion [30]

However, stability in size/appearance of a noncalcified metastasis or dimensional increase of a completely calcified lesion has to be considered as indeterminate signs because they may both be associated with the presence of controlled but still active disease or, on the contrary, "cured" disease with persistence of "scar" tissue [31, 32]. In such cases and when the calcified component is not yet predominant, diffusion-weighted imaging (DWI) will be possibly helping. DWI detects changes in water diffusion that occur when the normal fatty marrow is replaced with highly dense cellularity which restricts normal water movements among cell membranes, so providing morphologic and functional information on lesions. Reconstructed maximum intensity projection (MIP) images of WB-DWI show

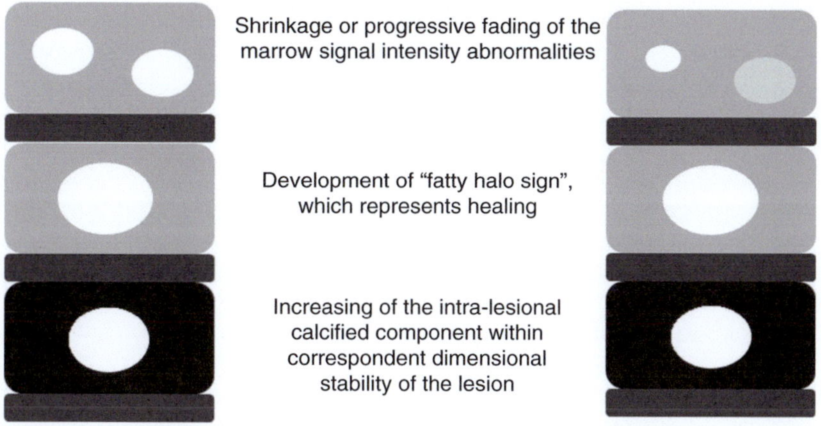

Fig. 18.1 Signs of responding vertebral metastases visible on T1w MR imaging (Modified from Lecouvet et al. [31])

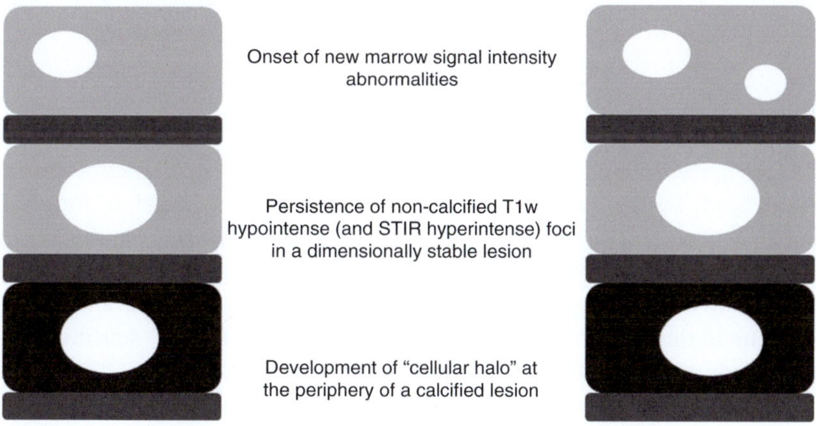

Fig. 18.2 Signs of progressing vertebral metastases visible on T1w MR imaging (Modified from Lecouvet et al. [31])

noncalcified metastatic lesions as high signal intensity foci providing an "at a glance" evaluation of the probably active metastatic involvement [33]. In Table 18.1 are resumed the performances of radiological devices for the detection of bone metastases.

Comparison of consecutive examinations delivers an easy and generally non-ambiguous evaluation of the disease response or progression under therapy (Fig. 18.3).

DWI also allows the calculation of the apparent diffusion coefficient (ADC, units * 10^{-3} mm^2/s) values of the lesions, representing a quantitative analysis used in monitoring over time the response to chemotherapy. It has been in fact shown that ADC values increase within prostate cancer metastases treated with antiandrogen therapy as early as 1 month after treatment initiation [43, 44].

However, both visual and quantitative analysis methods provided by DWI may present pitfalls. In particular, predominantly calcified metastases remain an issue representing false-negative visual findings, and the interpretation of changes in ADC values is indeed complex, mainly because of tumor and response heterogeneity. Newer analysis methods (ADC parametric response or functional diffusion map) taking spatial information and tumor heterogeneity into account and enabling voxel-by-voxel follow-up

Table 18.1 Performances of radiological devices for the detection of bone metastases

	Author (ref)	No. of pts	Sensitivity (%)	Specificity (%)	PPV (%)	NPV (%)	Accuracy (%)
Conventional radiology	Lecouvet et al. [34]	66	63	64	100	70	–
	Ketelsen et al. [35]	14	58.6	–	–	–	–
	Lecouvet et al. [36]	100	86	98	98	87	–
CT	Luboldt et al. [37]	15	67	–	–	–	–
MRI axial skeleton only	Lecouvet et al. [36]	66	100	88	100	100	–
	Luboldt et al. [37]	15	93	–	–	–	–
WB-MRI with DWI	Luboldt et al. [37]	15	100	–	–	–	–
	Ketelsen et al. [35]	14	96.4	–	–	–	–
	Venkitaram et al. [38]	39	70	100	100	–	–
	Wang et al. [39]	49	100	87.2	–	–	–
	Gutzeit et al. [40]	35	91	99	97	97	–
	Mosavi et al. [41]	49	100	98	83	100	98
	Lecouvet et al. [34]	100	98	98	98	98	–
	Stecco et al. [42]	23	80	98.2	–	–	–

of treatment-induced changes seem to overcome these pitfalls [44, 45]; however, further validation by literature is needed. Furthermore, optimization of hardware, sequences and signal analysis, and definite standardization of acquisition method are also necessary to improve the reliability of the results in the future. In Table 18.2 are reassumed the pros and cons of the radiological examinations employed for the detection of bone lesions.

18.2.5 Nuclear Medicine Imaging

Nuclear medicine offers different options for the detection of bone metastases in PC patients: (a) bone scan (BS) as a planar or tomographic imaging (i.e., single-photon emission tomography, SPET) and (b) PET/CT with ^{18}F-fluoride or ^{18}F-fluorodeoxyglucose (FDG) or ^{11}C/^{18}F-choline or ^{11}C-acetate or ^{68}Ga-prostate-specific membrane antigen (PSMA) or ^{18}F-anti-1-amino-3-18F-fluorocyclobutane-1-carboxylic acid (FACBC). Each imaging technique shows a specific mechanism of action to detect bone metastases due to a different uptake and metabolism of the radiopharmaceuticals as extensively reported in Chaps. 7, 8, and 9; therefore, they are associated with different diagnostic performances, mainly based on the type of skeletal lesion (i.e., osteoblastic vs. osteolytic vs. bone marrow invasion) [46–48].

Planar BS using ^{99m}Tc-diphosphonates is the standard technique to detect skeletal metastasis from PC as it is widely available, relatively inexpensive, and highly sensitive. However, the mechanism of uptake of ^{99m}Tc to a suitable phosphonate images the sites of blastic or mixed lesions, missing areas where calcium deposit is missing. This is the reason why BS shows low specificity (falsely positive in case of benign lesions, prior trauma, and arthritis) and flare phenomena. Therefore, an osteoblastic response that occurs as a result of bone healing/flare response during systemic treatments can significantly alter its diagnostic performance and makes very difficult the clinical interpretation of scintigraphic findings. Moreover, in a large retrospective analysis, bone metastases were found in less than 1 % of patients with PSA of <20 ng/mL, therefore yielded a negative predictive of 99.7 % [49]. Although the introduction of tomographic imaging, such as SPET and SPET/CT, has overpassed some limits of BS, these modalities are not able to cover the entire body of patients, and as reported by Hillner et al. [50], SPET/CT is not currently clinical practice. An interesting possibility offered by BS is the calculation of bone

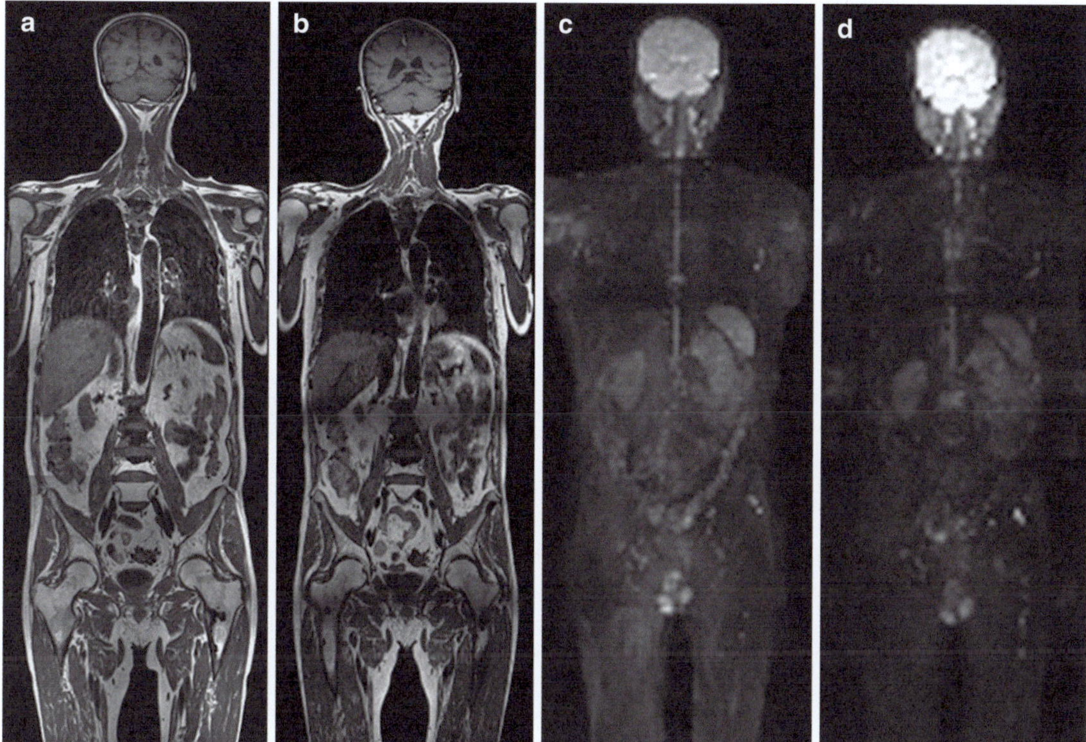

Fig. 18.3 A 6-month follow-up imaging using WB-MRI in 69-year-old man with long-term bone diffuse metastatic disease and new signs of progression during antiandrogenic therapy. (**a**, **b**) Coronal T1w images show long-term calcified metastases as multiple hypointense foci involving vertebrae, ribs, and left femur in (**a**) and appearance of both new bone marrow hypointense foci (femurs and iliac bones) and low-signal intensity tissue adjacent to older ones (e.g., see L2 and left femur in (**b**)). (**c**, **d**) DWI images with 3D radial-MIP (maximum intensity projection) reconstruction identify progression of disease from (**c**) to (**d**) as new appearance of hyperintense bone foci representing tissue with restricted diffusion due to high cellularity (i.e., see left femur, thoracic and lumbar vertebrae). Remaining bone metastases are not clearly seen on DWI, representing false-negative findings due to advanced sclerotic changes inside the lesions

scan index (BSI), than reflecting the extend of metastatic disease [51, 52]. This approach seems to be very interesting, since its measurement can be also automated; nevertheless, this technique was not successful in the clinical routine and remains cumbersome to be adopted [52] (Fig. 18.4).

Even with persisting high costs, PET represents an efficient modality for whole-body scanning in a reasonably short time. With the increasing availability of PET/CT scanners, the possibility of obtaining more detailed and precise CT anatomic localization of PET-directed metabolic abnormalities of tumor lesions, especially in skeletal diseases, has become a clinical reality. Nowadays, a lot of radiopharmaceutical agents are available for PET/CT imaging, especially for the detection of bone metastases. ^{18}F-Fluoride has the desirable characteristics of high and rapid bone uptake accompanied by very rapid blood clearance, which results in a high bone-to-background ratio in a short time. ^{18}F/^{11}C-Choline and ^{11}C-acetate are able to identify the presence of viable PCa tissue and have shown promising results especially for the early detection of bone marrow infiltration. ^{18}F-FDG was mainly used for the definition of osteolytic lesions [52] but seems to be able to identify the presence of viable cells in osteoblastic ones even if the majority of PC displays

Table 18.2 Pros and cons of radiological examinations

	Pros	Cons
Radiography	1. High availability	1. Low diagnostic accuracy
	2. Low cost	2. Not all bones can be screened
	3. Easy for the patient to undergo	3. Equivocal and late response to therapy
	4. Allows assessment of complications (i.e., fractures)	
CT	1. Allows fine bone detail assessment and smaller lesion characterization	1. High radiation dose
	2. Allows evaluation of entire skeleton	2. Limited ability in the assessment of therapy response
MRI with WB and DWI acquisitions	1. Highest diagnostic performance in detection and characterization of bone lesions	1. Advanced diagnostic techniques only available in diagnostic imaging center of excellence
	2. Possible role in the assessment of therapeutic response	2. Longer duration of examination, higher costs

Modified Table 3 from Evangelista et al. [100]
CT computed tomography, *MRI* magnetic resonance imaging, *WB* whole-body, *DWI* diffusion-weighted imaging

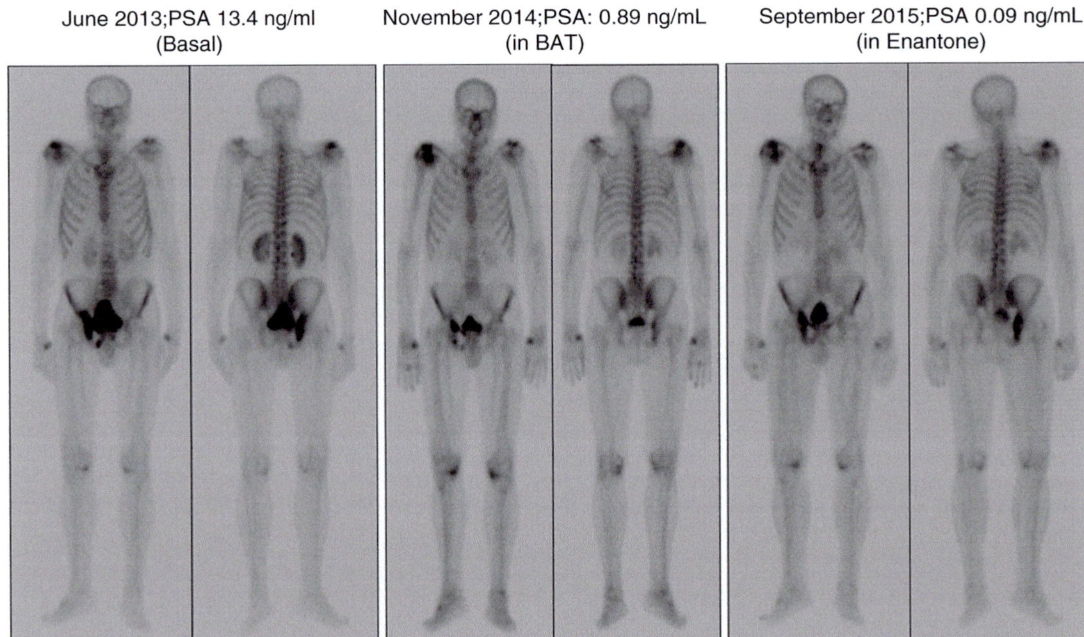

Fig. 18.4 Serial bone scans in patient with prostatic adenocarcinoma (Gleason score, 5+4). (*Left*) First bone scan performed for a biochemical recurrence of disease, after radical treatment. (*Middle*) Second scan, after the administration of bipolar androgen therapy (*BAT*). (*Right*) Third bone scan, after the administration of a further hormonal therapy

a low glycolytic metabolic behavior and does not suggest its current application. In Table 18.3, the performances of nuclear imaging techniques for the detection of bone metastases are reassumed.

The most recent data available in the literature demonstrate a role for radiolabeled choline PET/CT in the assessment of new hormonal therapies, such as enzalutamide [68, 69] or abiraterone acetate [70], and chemotherapy (i.e., docetaxel) [71]

Table 18.3 Performances of nuclear medicine modalities for the detection of skeletal lesions in prostate cancer patients

	Authors (ref)	No. of pts	Sensitivity (%)	Specificity (%)	PPV (%)	NPV (%)	Accuracy (%)
99mTc-phosphonates Bone scan	Garcia et al. [54]	91	65.4	38.5	86.4	15.6	61.5
	Poulsen et al. [55]	50	50.8	82.2	86.4	42.9	60.6
	Even-Sapir et al. [47]	44	57	57	59	55	–
	Iagaru et al. [56]	18	87.5	80	–	–	–
	Damle et al. [57]	72	96.9	41.2	75.6	87.5	77.5
	Palmedo et al. [58]	97	96.4	75.3	98.1	61.4	–
	Withofs et al. [59]	10	66.7	81.6	53.3	88.6	78
	Takesh et al. [60]	37	89.3	–	–	–	–
99mTc-phosphonates SPET	Even-Sapir et al. [47]	44	78	67	72	74	–
	Palmedo et al. [58]	97	96.4	63.7	97.8	51.9	
99mTc-phosphonates SPET/CT	Palmedo et al. [58]	97	96.4	94.2	98.5	87.1	
^{18}F-Fluoride PET/CT	Poulsen et al. [55]	50	93.1	54	81.8	77.9	81
	1. Even-Sapir et al. [47][b]	44	100	62	74	100	–
	Even-Sapir et al. [47][c]	44	100	100	100	100	–
	Beheshti et al. [61]	38	81	93	–	–	86
	Langsteger et al. [62]	42	91	83	–	–	88
	Iagaru et al. [56]	18	100	100	–	–	–
	Damle et al. [57]	72	100	70.6	86.5	100	65.4
	Withofs et al. [59]	10	100	89.5	75	100	92
18F-FDG PET/CT	Iagaru et al. [56]	18	55.6	80	–	–	–
	Damle et al. [57]	72	71.9	100	100	65.4	81.6
^{18}F-Choline PET/CT	Beheshti et al. [63]	70	79	97	84	–	–
	McCarthy et al. [64]	26	96	100	–	–	–
	Poulsen et al. [55]	50	84.7	91.1	95	74.9	86.8
	Beheshti et al. [61]	38	74	99	–	–	88
	Langsteger et al. [62]	42	91	89	–	–	90
	Takesh et al. [60]	37	82.7	–	–	–	–
^{11}C-Choline PET/CT	Fuccio et al. [65]	25	86	100	–	–	–
	Garcia et al. [54]	91	96	92.3	98.7	80	95.6
	Picchio et al. [66]	78	89	98	96	94	95

(continued)

Table 18.3 (continued)

	Authors (ref)	No. of pts	Sensitivity (%)	Specificity (%)	PPV (%)	NPV (%)	Accuracy (%)
^{11}C-Acetate PET/CT	Beheshti et al. [67]	[a]	81.6[a]	98.8[a]	–	–	–

Modified Table 2 from Evangelista et al. [100]
NE not evaluated
[a]Pooled sensitivity and specificity in 394 and 194 patients, respectively
[b]PET
[c]PET/CT

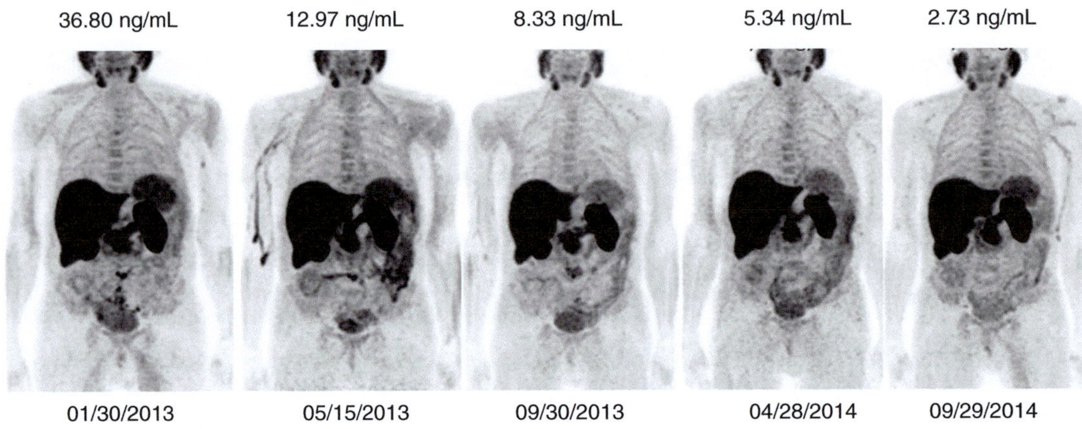

Fig. 18.5 A 73-year-old patient with an advanced prostate cancer underwent serial PET/CT scans before starting and during abiraterone acetate for monitoring the response to therapy. A correlation between metabolic imaging and biochemical values was found

(Figs. 18.5 and 18.6). Choline PET/CT findings agree with PSA changes in the majority of patients with progressive disease, during and after therapy. Conversely, the disappearance of uptake does not always correlate with the disappearance of the cancer lesion since it could be due to the effect of a stable or non-metabolically active focus. Moreover, the appearance of new areas of uptake does not always correlate with certain progression due to the well-known phenomenon of flare reaction, whose correct interpretation in BS has been standardized. This issue is an open area of debate.

18.2.5.1 Flare Phenomenon and Nuclear Medicine Modalities

There some fundamental differences in diagnostic imaging, when they are used to detect cancer lesions and to evaluate changes during any treatment. Nuclear medicine modalities can mainly provide metabolic information and trace some pathologic processes depending on the different employed radiopharmaceuticals, like those for cancer cells, for inflammatory cells, for bone, and for others. This is the reason why, in particular for bone metastases, radiopharmaceuticals have to be differentiated in two main groups: "bone-targeting agents" (^{99m}Tc-phosphonates and 18F-Fluoride) and "cancer-targeting agents" (F18/C11 choline, 18F-FDG, ^{68}Ga-PSMA, 18F-FACBC) (Fig. 18.7), according to the biological processes for their uptake's mechanism. Bone-targeting agents mimic the Ca++ ions path and are able to show the bone remodeling that surrounds bone metastases. On the contrary, cancer-targeting agents enter into the glycolytic metabolism of cancer cells, or

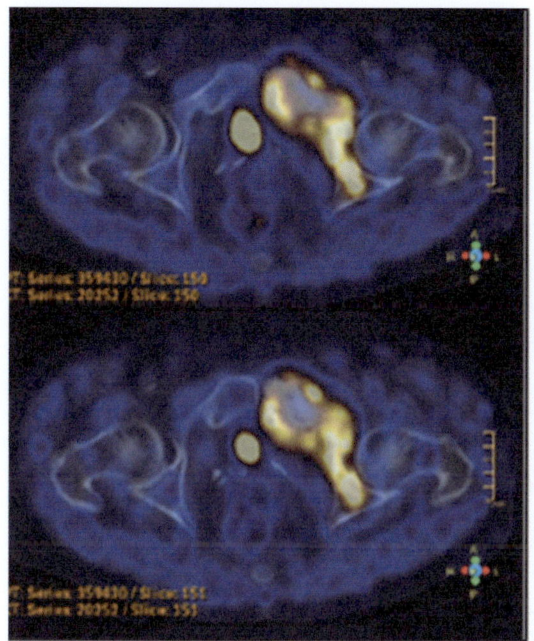

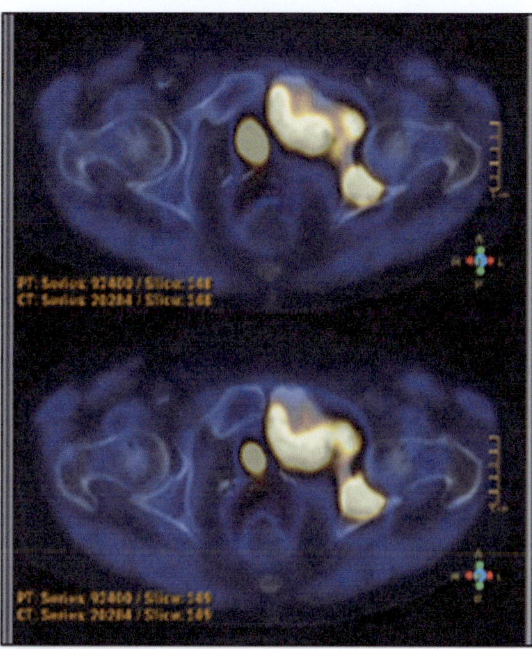

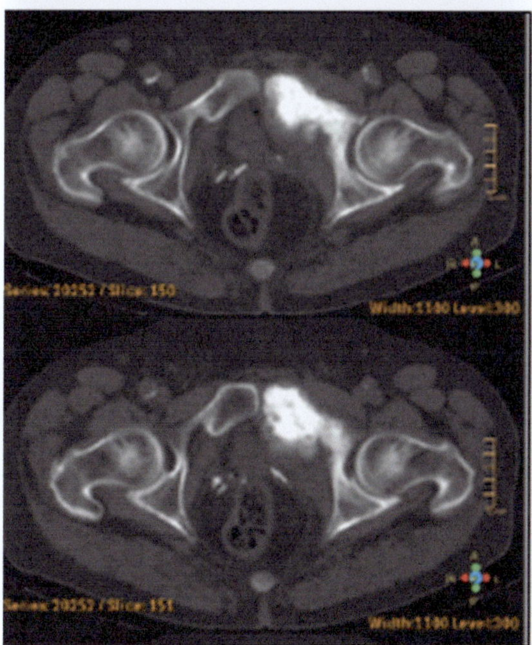

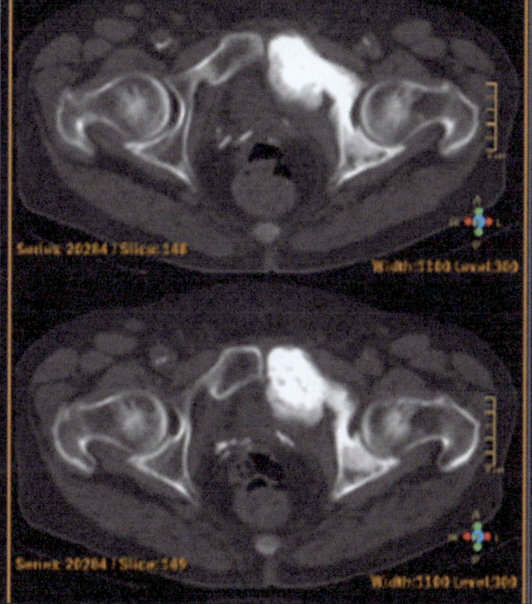

Fig. 18.6 A 65-year-old man, with a prostatic adenocarcinoma (pT2bN0M0; GS 3+4). PET/CT was performed before (*up*) and after (*down*) the administration of docetaxel and zoledronic acid. At the time of the second PET/CT scan, PSA was 6.4 ng/ml. The images revealed an increase of uptake in the pelvis compatible with a progression of disease

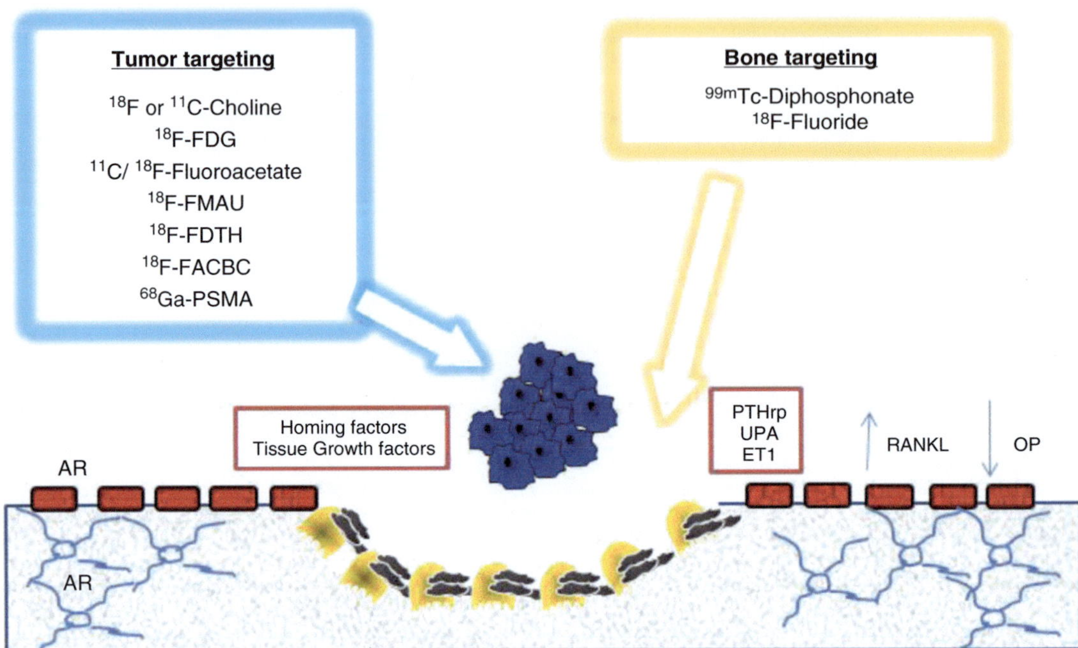

Fig. 18.7 Mechanism of bone metastasis formation and different targets (bone matrix and cancer cells) of the radiopharmaceuticals used in nuclear medicine to image prostate cancer bone metastases. *AR* androgen receptor, *ET1* endothelin 1, *^{18}F-FACBC* ^{18}F-anti-1-amino-3-fluorocyclobutane-1-carboxylic acid, *^{18}F-FDG* 18F-2-deoxy-2-fluoro-D-glucose, *^{18}F-FDTH* ^{18}F-fluoro-5α-dihydrotestosterone, *^{18}F-FMAU* ^{18}F-2'-fluoro-5-methyl-1-β-D-arabinofuranosyluracil, *^{68}Ga-PSMA* ^{68}Ga-labeled prostate-specific membrane antigen, *OP* osteoprotegerin, *PTHrp* parathyroid hormone-related protein, *RANKL* receptor activator of nuclear factor kappa-B ligand, *UPA* urokinase-type plasminogen activator (From Bombardieri et al. [48])

participate to the phospholipid turnover of membranes, or again bind the membrane receptors of kallikrein, androgen, etc.

Prostate cancer bone metastases are imaged by both groups of radiopharmaceutical. However, in accordance with the mechanism of uptake, the behavior of radiopharmaceuticals can be different and therefore is associated with diverse imaging results. Some authors describe an increase of radiopharmaceutical uptake within few weeks after the beginning of the therapy that is correlated with an incorrect interpretation of the imaging and therefore with an erroneous sign of non-response [72, 73]. This "flare" depends on the intense osteoblastic reaction that follows the killing of metastatic localization and determines an increased uptake of radiolabeled phosphonates or fluoride in the crystalline structure of hydroxyapatite. The disappearance of this phenomenon takes usually some months from the start of the drug administration [74]. Based on this metabolic phenomenon, an increased uptake should be interpreted as progression of disease only if new sites of lesion are clearly imaged or a further increase of lesion number is validated by serial scans [75]. The flare phenomenon has been observed in a number of prostate cancer patients under hormonal therapy or treated with chemotherapy [76]. Flare phenomenon has been also observed with cancer-targeting radiopharmaceuticals that are directly incorporated into cancer cells or into the tumor structures [77], particularly for the new class of antihormonal therapies, like abiraterone acetate [70]. Therefore, the biological interpretation should be carefully evaluated because a lot of events can be correlated with the increase of cancer-seeking radiopharmaceutical uptake: (1) inflammatory reaction that follows tumor necrosis and (2) the temporary intensified change of cancer cell metabolism. Again, to overcome these misleading information, it is necessary to evaluate the response to therapy at least after 3 months from the beginning of the treatment, in order to differentiate between disease progression and flare phenomenon. However, some cases of flare phenomenon with ^{18}F-choline PET/CT have been reported in patients undergoing ^{223}Ra dichloride treatment, after the third cycle. In Fig. 18.8, two examples are reported. The mechanisms underlying this process are still unknown; future studies are mandatory.

At present, in prostatic cancer with bone metastases, the evaluation of response to treatment with nuclear medicine imaging gives correct results only if it is performed far from the beginning of the treatments, as it is stated in some recommendations and/or guidelines [43]. Unfortunately, the correlation between the predictive role of response to therapy and the flare reaction has not been confirmed yet. Therefore, these aspects should be extensively investigated with clinical studies, evaluating the relationship between the flare phenomenon and different treatments, like chemotherapy, radiation therapy, and new antihormonal therapies considering that the mechanism of action of these anticancer drugs is significantly different.

In Table 18.4 are reported the main pros and cons of nuclear medicine techniques.

18.3 Parameters of Evaluation Response in Clinical Trials

By examining the most important clinical trials of the last 20 years for the treatment of metastatic PC, it appears that investigators have proposed different biochemical (mainly PSA assessment) and imaging modalities to evaluate the response to treatment (Table 18.5). Even if the modalities to measure response are not exclusively focused on skeletal metastases, the choice of the tools for detection and measurement represents a reliable model for the current clinical practice. As reported in the table, the primary end point of the clinical trials was generally overall survival or progression-free survival (with the exceptions of trials evaluating bone-targeting agents such as zoledronate or denosumab). The prediction of response to therapy with imaging represents a surrogate indicator of survival and although secondary is considered an important issue.

18.4 Indications from Scientific Guidelines

The recommendation for the use of nuclear medicine techniques in accordance with the main international guidelines is reported in Table 18.6. As shown, in the majority of cases, bone scan is strongly recommended, despite the low sensitivity and specificity. On the contrary, the role of ^{18}F-fluoride PET/CT and radiolabeled choline PET/CT is still indeterminate, particularly in the staging phase. Only for the restaging phase, some recommendations have been released for choline PET/CT, but the absence of randomized trials represents the most important hurdle to its application in clinical practice.

18.5 Possible Strategies of Evaluation with Diagnostic Imaging

Based on the available literature evidences, we can reassume them in a flowchart (Fig. 18.9).

In accordance with the site of recurrences, PC patients will be classified as bone-dominant (only skeletal involvement) or no bone-dominant disease (no skeletal, lymph node, visceral, or soft-tissue invasion). The choice of the most appropriate diagnostic tool to visualize BMT would be based on disease grade (i.e., low grade, GS $\leq$7, or high grade, GS 8–10). For example, patients with low-grade PC bone-dominant disease who are candidates to bone-targeted therapies, such as ^{223}Ra, could benefit from techniques targeting bone modalities, like bone scan or SPET with ^{99}mTc-disphosphonate or ^{18}F-fluoride PET/CT. MRI would be used to better characterize the skeletal lesions. Conversely, in patients with bone-dominant disease and a GS $\geq$8, 18F-FDG PET/CT would be added to obtain prognostic and predictive information. Moreover,

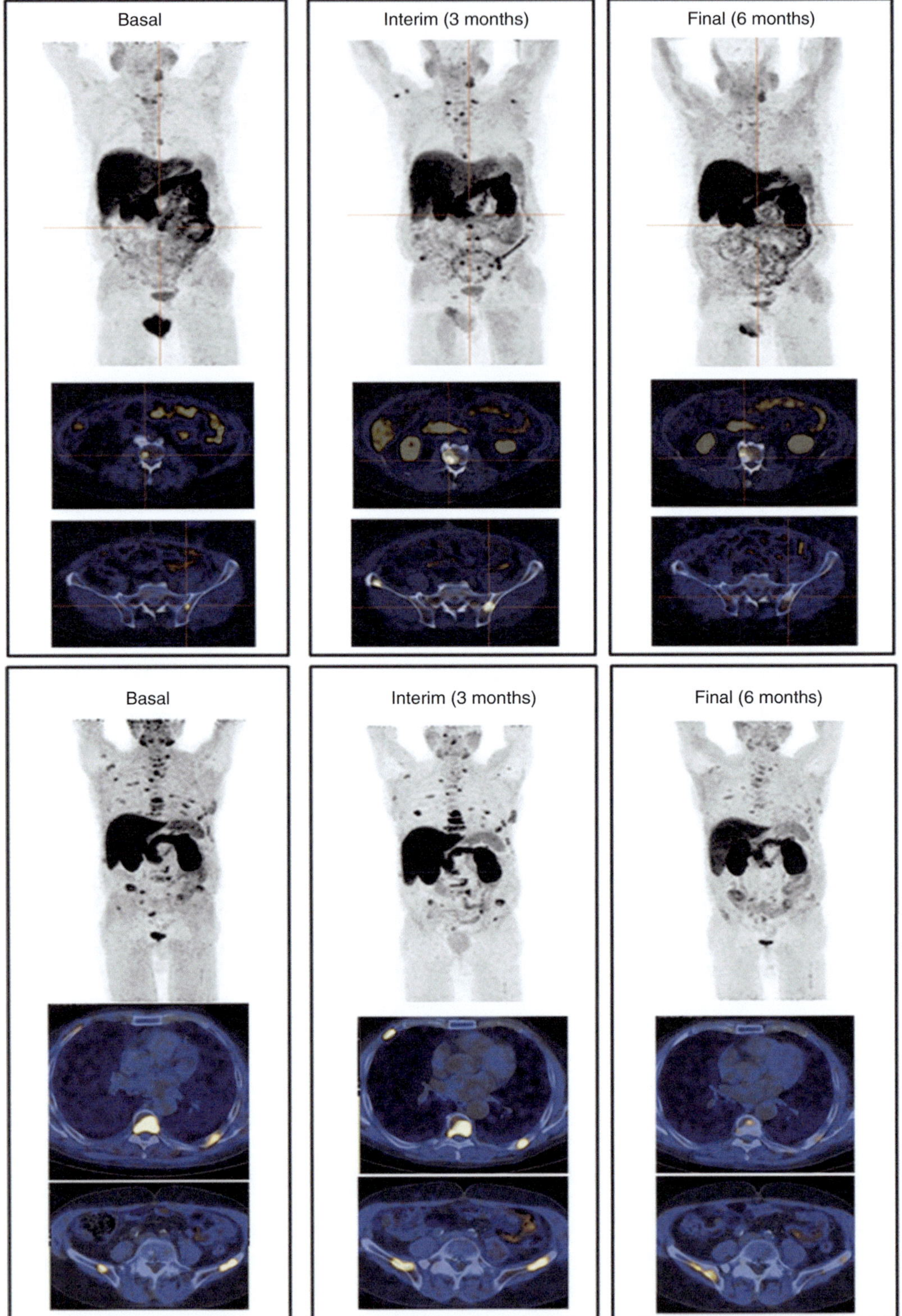

Fig. 18.8 Two examples of patients with flare phenomenon after the administration of ^{223}Ra-dichloride. The flare phenome disappeared after 6 months

Table 18.4 Pros and cons of nuclear imaging techniques for the detection and the evaluation of response to therapies

	Pros	Cons
99mTc-phosphonates Bone scan	1. Low cost [55] 2. High availability [55] 3. Detection of bone metastases several months before they are revealed by planar X-ray	1. Low sensitivity for osteolytic lesions [47] 2. No detection of bone marrow disease 3. Poor sensitivity for osteolytic lesions without bone remodeling 4. Low specificity (false-positive findings in case of degenerative changes, inflammatory processes, trauma, mechanical stress, and Paget disease) [47] 5. Necessity of bone reactive changes to achieve the optimal sensitivity [55] 6. Flare phenomenon due to some systemic treatments (also ^{223}Ra) [80]
99mTc-phosphonates SPET	1. Improves the sensitivity of planar images	1. Limited field of view [47] 2. No improvement in terms of specificity than planar images 3. As bone scan (*see above*) [47]
99mTc-phosphonates SPET/CT	1. Improves the sensitivity of planar images 2. Improves the specificity of planar images [47]	1. Whole-body imaging with this modality is not currently a standard practice 2. Resource implications of increased cost, specialist equipment, and specialist manpower hours 3. Increased radiation dose than BS (from 3 to 5 mSv) 4. As bone scan (*see above*)
^{18}F-Fluoride PET/CT	1. The extraction of fluoride from the blood is rapid. The first pass extraction is 100 % vs 64 % for diphosphonates 2. Superior image quality and therefore high diagnostic accuracy [56] 3. Rapid acquisition protocol (after 15 or 60 min from the injection) 4. As for ^{99m}Tc-diphosphonate is able to identify high bone turnover and remodeling 5. Quantitative and automatic semiquantitative analyses of uptake in the lesions [53]	1. Very sensitive to minimal degenerative changes 2. High costs and increased radiation dose than BS (from 3 to 5–7 mSv) [47] 3. Clinical impact when used to monitor treatment response is uncertain 4. Flare phenomenon due to some systemic treatments (also ^{223}Ra) [79]
^{18}F-FDG PET/CT	1. Can detect bone metastases at early stage of disease (bone marrow involvement) 2. In case of osteolytic lesion and in the presence of aggressive prostatic cancer, the accumulation of tracer is higher for an increase in the glycolytic rate [57] 3. Lack of FDG uptake in the osteoblastic lesion can be associated with the presence of quiescent cells 4. Superior image quality and therefore high diagnostic accuracy 5. Prognostic information [81] 6. Quantitative and automatic semiquantitative analyses of uptake in the lesions [53]	1. Sclerotic metastases can be missed by relatively small amount of viable tumor tissue [78] 2. FDG is limited in moderately or well-differentiated prostate cancer, by the low metabolism of tissue uptake [78] 3. Higher costs and increased radiation dose than BS (from 3 to 5–7 mSv)

(continued)

Table 18.4 (continued)

	Pros	Cons
$^{11}C/^{18}F$-Choline PET/CT	1. More specific for prostate cancer 2. Able to identify three patterns of bone disease (bone marrow involvement, osteoblastic lesions, no active tumor) [63] 3. No uptake in chronic degenerative disease 4. Quantitative and automatic semiquantitative analyses of uptake in the lesions [53]	1. Flare phenomena reported during the administration of abiraterone acetate and GCSF [70] 2. ^{11}C-Choline is not available in centers without on-site cyclotron 3. High costs and increased radiation dose than BS (from 3 to 5–7 mSv)

Modified Table 3 from Evangelista et al. [100]
BS bone scan, *SPET* single-photon emission tomography, *PET* positron emission tomography, *CT* computed tomography, *FDG* fluorodeoxyglucose, *^{223}Ra* radium-223, *GCS*: granulocyte colony-stimulating factor

FDG PET/CT could give supports to other cancer- or receptor-specific radiopharmaceutical agents, such as radiolabeled choline and/or PSMA. Serial imaging acquisition is suggested, according to the PCWG2, particularly at the end of antitumor therapy, but also in interim, if required by the treatment protocol (2–3 months) or by the development of signs or symptoms suggesting tumor progression. In these latter cases, a particular attention should be given to a possible flare reaction. In patients with non-bone-dominant disease, $^{18}F/^{11}C$-choline PET/CT and CT should preferably be used. Additionally, MRI or ^{18}F-fluoride PET/CT can be considered if a more accurate bone evaluation is required. Similarly, those patients with bone disease, the imaging modalities should be repeated every 3 months for the evaluation of disease evolution (progression vs. response). Also in this case a particular attention should be given to a possible flare reaction (as described during abiraterone treatment).

18.6 Authors' Remarks

I. Clinical parameters, like skeletal-related symptoms and pain, are fundamental to evaluate the progression or response during therapy.

II. PSA represents the most common biochemical variable. Although not specific, it is cost-effective.

III. Bone remodeling biomarkers, like bone ALP, are predictive of response to therapy in PC patients with bone metastasis, particularly in those undergoing bone-targeting therapies.

IV. In the radiology field: (a) CT remains the standard of reference, although RECIST criteria are not adapted for the bone; (b) MRI is better than CT due to its morphologic and functional information, but it is characterized by some pitfalls.

V. For nuclear medicine: (a) ^{18}F-Fluoride PET/CT is better than BS, although the costs and the availability of PET is significantly different than scintigraphic examination (higher costs and lower availability for PET). (b) Radiolabeled choline PET/CT represents the commonest cancer-seeking imaging modality. (c) Both bone- and cancer-seeking techniques are characterized by the flare phenomenon, and therefore, a careful analysis of images should be made in case of serial scans, particularly during therapy. (d) However, the predictive and prognostic meaning of flare reaction for these techniques remains still unknown.

Table 18.5 The clinical, biochemical, and imaging approaches for the evaluation of response to treatment, in phase III clinical trials

N	Trial (ref)	N pts	Treatments	Year pub	End points	Markers	Pain scale and clinical data	Imaging technique
1	Zoledronic Acid [82]	214 vs 221 vs 208	Zoledronate (4 mg) *vs* Zoledronate 8 → 4 mg) *vs* Placebo	2002	I, % of pts with SRE[a] II, Time to first SRE, Skeletal morbidity rate[b], time to disease progression, ORR (bone), bone biochemical markers, Qol	ALP, PTH biochem markers[c]	BPI, FACT-G, EURO Qol,	X-ray, bone scan (International Union Against Cancer criteria)
2	TAX 327 [83]	335 vs 334 vs 337	Docetaxel (q21) *vs* Docetaxel (q7) *vs* Mitoxantrone	2004	I, OS II, pain reduction, Qol, PSA response, ORR	PSA	PPI, analgesic intake and FACT-P	WHO criteria (bone scan + CT scan)
3	SWOG 99–16 [84]	338 vs 336	Docetaxel + estramustine *vs* Mitoxantrone + prednisone	2004	I, OS II, PFS (a), ORR, PSA response, toxicity	PSA	None	WHO criteria (bone scan + CT scan)
4	SPARC [85]	635 vs 315	Satraplatin + prednisone *vs* Placebo + prednisone	2009	I, OS, PFS (b) II, TTP Exp: ORR, PSA response, pain response	PSA, (LDH, ALP[e])	PPI	RECIST criteria 1.0 + PCWG2 criteria (CT + bone scan)
5	IMPACT [86]	341 vs 171	Sipuleucel-T *vs* Placebo	2010	I, OS II, time to objective disease progression[d]	(PSA, LDH[f])	Baseline pain score	WHO criteria (bone scan + CT scan)
6	TROPIC [87]	378 vs 377	Cabazitaxel *vs* Mitoxantrone	2010	I, OS II, PFS (c); PSA response, PSA progression, ORR, pain response, TTP	PSA	BPI-SF	RECIST criteria 1.0 (CT + bone scan)
7	Denosumab [88]	950 vs 951	Denosumab *vs* Zoledronate	2011	I, time to first SRE (non-inferiority) II, time to first and subsequent SRE (superiority)	PSA, ALP, biochemical markers[c]	NA	NA

(continued)

Table 18.5 (continued)

N	Trial (ref)	N pts	Treatments	Year pub	End points	Markers	Pain scale and clinical data	Imaging technique
8	COU-AA 301 [89]	797 vs 398	Abiraterone + prednisone *vs* Placebo + prednisone	2012	I, OS II, PSA response; TTPP, rPFS	PSA (LDH, ALP[f])	BPI-SF analgesic intake, FACT-P, time to first SRE	RECIST criteria 1.0 + PCWG2 criteria (CT/MRI + bone scan)
9	AFFIRM [90]	800 vs 399	Enzalutamide *vs* Placebo	2012	I, OS II, rPFS, time to first SRE, QoL, PSA progression; pain palliation, CTC conversion rate; safety; electrocardiographic changes; PK	PSA (LDH[f])	BPI-SF, FACT-P	RECIST criteria 1.1 + PCWG2 criteria (CT/MRI + bone scan)
10	COU-AA-302 [91]	546 vs 542	Abiraterone + prednisone *vs* Placebo + prednisone	2013	I, OS, rPFS II, time to opiate use, time to ChT, time to decline in PS, time to PSA progression	PSA (LDH, ALP[f])	BPI-SF analgesic intake and FACT-P	RECIST criteria 1.0 + PCWG2 criteria (CT/MRI + bone scan)
11	ALSYIMPCA [4]	614 vs 307	^{223}Ra *vs* Placebo	2013	I, OS II, time to increase in ALP, ALP response, time to first SRE, time to ALP normalization, time to PSA progression, safety, QoL	PSA, ALP (LDH)	WHO ladder, FACT-P	Bone scan
12	PREVAIL [92]	872 vs 845	Enzalutamide *vs* Placebo	2014	I, OS, rPFS II, time to ChT, time to first SRE, time to PSA progression, PSA response, soft-tissue response	PSA	BPI-SF, FACT-P	RECIST criteria 1.1 + PCWG2 criteria (CT/MRI + bone scan)

N	Trial (ref)	N pts	Treatments	Year pub	End points	Markers	Pain scale and clinical data	Imaging technique
13	CHARTEED [93]	397 vs 393	ADT + docetaxel *vs* ADT alone	2015	I, OS II, time to CRPC, time to clinical progression, time to PSA response, PSA response % at 6 and 12 ms, toxicity, QoL	PSA	FACT-P	RECIST criteria 1.0 (CT + bone scan)
14	STAMPEDE [94]	1184 vs 593 vs 592 vs 593	ADT *vs* ADT + docetaxel *vs* ADT + zoledronate *vs* ADT + docetaxel + zoledronate	2016 (Ongoing)	I,OS, FFS II, toxicity, QoL, SRE, cost-effectiveness	PSA	EORTC QLQ-C30 + PR25; EuroQoL (EQ-5D)	RECIST criteria 1.0 (CT + bone scan)

SRE skeletal-related event, *ORR* overall response rate, *QoL* quality of life, *ALP* alkaline phosphatase, *PTH* parathormone, *BPI* brief pain inventory, *FACT-G* Functional Assessment of Cancer Therapy – General, *OS* overall survival, *PSA* prostate-specific antigen, *PPI* present pain intensity, *FACT-P* Functional Assessment of Cancer Therapy – Prostate, *WHO* World Health Organization, *CT* computed tomography, *SWOG* Southwest Oncology Group, *PFS* progression-free survival, *SPARC* satraplatin and prednisone against refractory cancer, *TTP* time to pain progression, *LDH* lactate dehydrogenase, *RECIST* Response Evaluation Criteria in Solid Tumors, *PCWG2* Prostate Cancer Working Group 2, *IMPACT* Immunotherapy Prostate Adenocarcinoma Treatment, *BPI-SF* Brief Pain Inventory Short Form, *TTPP* time to PSA progression, *rPFS* radiographic progression-free survival, *AFFIRM* a study evaluating the efficacy and safety of the investigational drug MDV3100, *CTC* cancer tumor cell, *PK* pharmacokinetics, *ChT* chemotherapy, *PS* performance status, *ALSYMPCA* Alpharadin in Symptomatic Prostate Cancer Patients, *CHARTEED* Chemo-hormonal Therapy vs Androgen Ablation Randomized Trial for Extensive Disease in Prostate Cancer, *ADT* androgen deprivation therapy, *CRPC* castration-resistant prostate cancer, *STAMPEDE* Systemic Therapy in Advancing or Metastatic Prostate Cancer: Evaluation of Drug Efficacy, *FFS* failure-free survival, *EORTC* European Organisation for Research and Treatment of Cancer, *QLQ* quality of life questionnaire

PFS (*a*) radiological or biochemical, *PFS* (*b*) death, RECIST PD, two or more new lesion on bone scan, skeletal-related events, symptomatic progression, *PFS* (*c*) tumor progression, PSA progression, pain progression, death

[a]SRE: fracture, radiotherapy, cancer-related surgery to bone, spinal cord compression, initiation of bisphosphonate therapy

[b]Skeletal morbidity rate: N of events/time at risk (years)

[c]N telopeptide, pyridinoline, deoxypyridinoline to creatinine ratio

[d]Time to objective disease progression: WHO criteria PD or two new lesion on bone scan or new pathologic fracture or spinal cord compression

[e]Pre-specified prognostic factors

[f]Used in the Cox regression model to evaluate OS

Table 18.6 International guidelines for the management of prostate cancer patients

Guidelines	Year of pub	Clinical setting	Nuclear medicine imaging		
			Bone scan	^{18}F-Fluoride PET/CT	^{18}F/^{11}C-Choline PET/CT
European Association of Urology (EAU) [95]	2016	Staging	Recommended in intermediate and high-risk pts [LE 2a, GR A]; equivocal findings need to be integrated with other techniques due to low specificity	Indeterminate (similar sensitivity and superior specificity vs BS but less cost-effectiveness; does not detect node metastases)	Indeterminate (higher specificity vs BS, sensitivity still to be determined)
		Restaging/monitoring	After RP or RT only if high baseline PSA (>10 ng/mL) or high PSA kinetics (PSA-DT <6 months or PSA velocity >0.5 ng/mL/month) or in symptomatic pts [LE 3, GR A]	Not mentioned	After RP only if PSA >1 ng/ml [LE 2b, GR A] After RT: recommended to rule out N or M disease in pts fit enough for curative treatment [LE 2b, GR B]
			Refers to St Gallen Consensus for disease monitoring in CRPC		
European Society for Medical Oncology (ESMO) [96]	2015	Staging	Recommended in intermediate high-risk patients [III b]	Not mentioned	Recommended in intermediate high-risk pts (as an alternative to BS + CT or whole-body MRI) [III B]
		Restaging/monitoring	Not specified ("In patients with CRPC on systemic treatment, regular imaging studies should be done to monitor disease response/progression") [V B]		
American Urological Association (AUA) [97]	2015	Staging	Staging/restaging not included in the guidelines		
		Restaging/monitoring			

Guidelines	Year of pub	Clinical setting	Nuclear medicine imaging		
			Bone scan	^{18}F-Fluoride PET/CT	^{18}F/^{11}C-Choline PET/CT
National Comprehensive Cancer Network (NCCN) [98]	V2 2016	Staging	Recommended if intermediate to very high-risk or symptomatic pts	Not recommended (utility limited)	Not mentioned
		Restaging/monitoring	Recommended		To be considered in case of BCF, the best use should be still determined
St. Gallen Consensus Conference for advanced prostate cancer [99]	2015	Staging	Recommended (83 %)[a]	Not recommended (only 47 %)[a]; tracer not specified	
		Restaging/monitoring	Not specified (83%[a] recommended regular monitoring of the treatment apart from clinical and laboratory assessment)		

BS bone scan, *RP* radical prostatectomy, *RT* radiotherapy, *PSA-DT* PSA doubling time, *CRPC* castration-resistant prostate cancer, *CT* computed tomography, *MRI* magnetic resonance imaging, *BCF* biochemical failure

[a]% refers to proportion of panelist

All the abovementioned guidelines report only those modalities supported by a large clinical validation and by a definitive consensus of scientific and clinical communities. Moreover, the accessibility of the diagnostic modalities and the cost/benefit balance are considered. This is the reason why some new imaging/biochemical modalities potentially considered of interest and showing good diagnostic accuracy have not been included as a recommended tool of evaluation

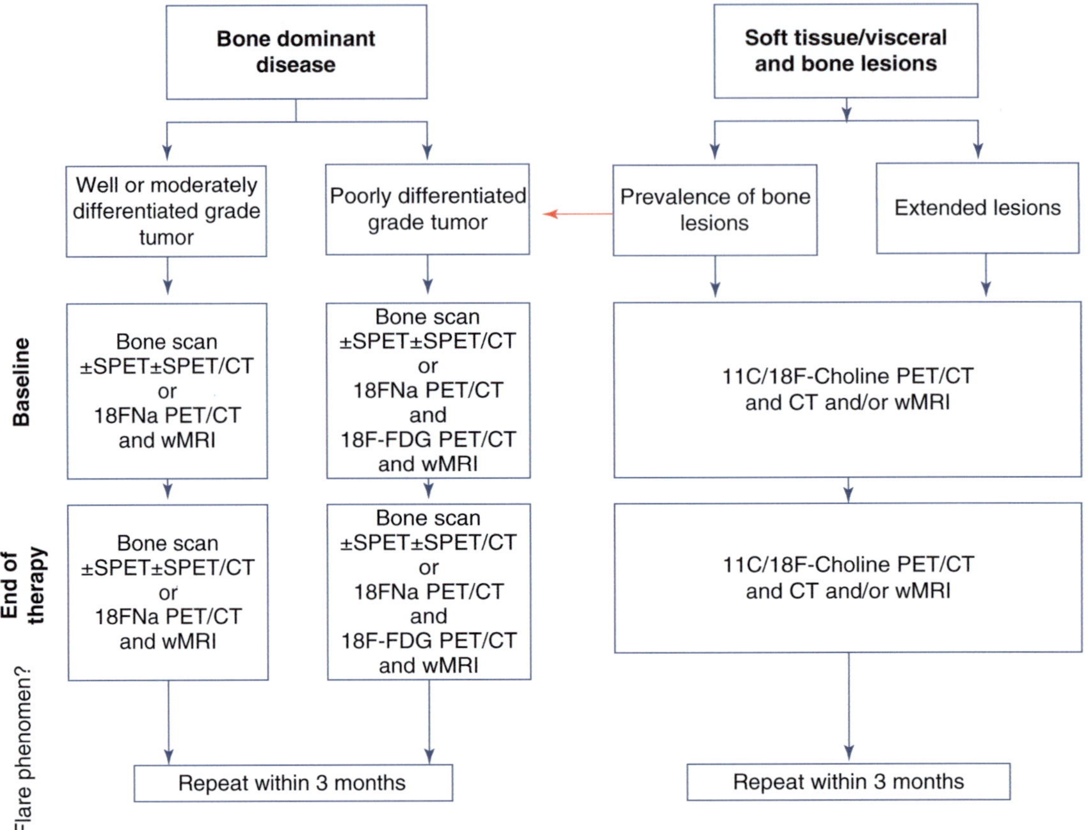

Fig. 18.9 Diagnostic algorithm proposed for assessment of response to therapy in patients with metastatic prostate cancer (From Evangelista et al. [100])

Acknowledgments The authors are grateful to Ms. Annaluisa De Simone Sorrentino for her collaboration in preparing this manuscript.

References

1. Kirby M, Hirst C, Crawford ED (2011) Characterising the castration-resistant prostate cancer population: a systematic review. Int J Clin Pract 65:1180–1192
2. Portenoy RK, Koh M (2010) Cancer pain syndromes. In: Bruera E, Portenoy RK (eds), Cancer pain. Assessment and management, vol 4. Cambridge University Press pp 53–88
3. Van Herk R, van Dijk M, Baar FPM et al (2007) Observational scales for pain assessment in older adults with cognitive impairments or communication difficulties. Nurs Res 56:34–43
4. Parker C, Nilsson S, Heinrich D et al (2013) Alpha emitter radium-223 and survival in metastatic prostate cancer. N Engl J Med 369:213–223
5. Sartor O, Coleman R, Nilsson S et al (2014) Effect of radium-223 dichloride on symptomatic skeletal events in patients with castration-resistant prostate cancer and bone metastases: results from a phase 3, double-blind, randomised trial. Lancet Oncol 15:738–746
6. James ND, Pirrie S, Brown JE et al (2013) Clinical outcomes in patients with castraterefractory prostate cancer (CRPC) metastatic to bone randomized in the factorial TRAPEZE trial to docetaxel (D) with strontium-89 (Sr89), zoledronic acid (ZA), neither, or both (ISRCTN 12808747). J Clin Oncol 31:abstr LBA5000
7. Vasikaran S, Eastell R, Bruyère O, Foldes AJ, Garnero P, Griesmacher A et al (2011) Markers of bone turnover for the prediction of fracture risk and monitoring of osteoporosis treatment: a need for international reference standards. Osteoporos Int 22:391–420
8. Fohr B, Dunstan CR, Seibel MJ (2003) Clinical review 165: markers of bone remodeling in metastatic bone disease. J Clin Endocrinol Metab 88:5059–5075

9. Tamada T, Sone T, Tomomitsu T et al (2001) Biochemical markers for the detection of bone metastasis in patients with prostate cancer, diagnostic efficacy and the effects of hormonal therapy. J Bone Miner Metab 19:45–51
10. Jung K, Lein M (2002) Bone turnover markers in serum and urine as diagnostic, prognostic and monitoring biomarkers of bone metastasis. J Clin Oncol 20:850–856
11. Koizumi M, Yonese J, Fukui I, Ogata E (2001) The serum level of the amino-terminal propeptide of type I procollagen is a sensitive marker for prostate cancer metastasis to bone. BJU Int 87:348–351
12. Zafeirakis AG, Papatheodorou GA, Limouris GS (2010) Clinical and imaging correlations of bone turnover markers in prostate cancer patients with bone only metastases. Nucl Med Commun 31:249–253
13. Koopmans N, de Jong IJ, Breeuwsma AJ, van der Veer E (2007) Serum bone turnover markers (PINP and ICTP) for the early detection of bone metastases in patients with prostate cancer: a longitudinal approach. J Urol 178(3 Pt 1):849–853
14. Zafeirakis AG, Papatheodorou GA, Arhontakis A et al (2010) Predictive implications of bone turnover markers after palliative treatment with (186) Re-HEPD in hormone-refractory prostate cancer with painful osseous metastases. Nucl Med Commun 31:249–253
15. Cook RJ, Coleman R, Brown J, Lipton A, Major P, Hei YJ, Saad F, Smith MR (2006) Markers of bone metabolism and survival in men with hormone-refractory metastatic prostate cancer. Clin Cancer Res 12(1):3361–7.99–100
16. Smith MR, Cook RJ, Coleman R, Brown J, Lipton A, Major P, Hei YJ, Saad F (2007) Predictors of skeletal complications in men with hormone-refractory metastatic prostate cancer. Urology 70(2):315–319
17. Coleman RE, Major P, Lipton A, Brown JE, Lee KA, Smith M, Saad F, Zheng M, Hei YJ, Seaman J, Cook R (2005) Predictive value of bone resorption and formation markers in cancer patients with bone metastases receiving the bisphosphonate zoledronic acid. Clin Oncol 23(22):4925–4935
18. Smith MR, Cook RJ, Coleman R, Brown J, Lipton A, Major P, Hei YJ, Saad F (2007) Predictors of skeletal complications in men with hormone-refractory metastatic prostate cancer. Urology 70(2):315–319)
19. Som A, Tu SM, Liu J, Wang X, Qiao W, Logothetis C, Corn PG (2012) Response in bone turnover markers during therapy predicts overall survival in patients with metastatic prostate cancer: analysis of three clinical trials. Cancer 107(9):1547–1553
20. Metwalli AR, Rosner IL, Cullen J, Chen Y, Brand T, Brassell SA, Lesperance J, Porter C, Sterbis J, McLeod DG (2014) Elevated alkaline phosphatase velocity strongly predicts overall survival and the risk of bone metastases in castrate-resistant prostate cancer. Urol Oncol 32(6):761–768
21. Brasso K, Christensen IJ, Johansen JS, Teisner B, Garnero P, Price PA, Iversen P (2006) Prognostic value of PINP, bone alkaline phosphatase, CTX-I, and YKL-40 in patients with metastatic prostate carcinoma. Prostate 66(5):503–513
22. Payne H, Cornford P (2011) Prostate-specific antigen: an evolving role in diagnosis, monitoring, and treatment evaluation in prostate cancer. Urol Oncol 29:593–601
23. Hillner BE, Siegel BA, Hanna L, Duan F, Quinn B, Shields AF (2015) ^{18}F-fluoride PET used for treatment monitoring of systemic cancer therapy: results from the National Oncologic PET Registry. J Nucl Med 56:222–228
24. Thuret R, Massard C, Gross-Goupil M, Escudier B, Di Palma M, Bossi A, de Crevoisier R, Chauchereau A, Fizazi K (2008) The postchemotherapy PSA surge syndrome. Ann Oncol 19:1308–1311
25. Scher HI, Halabi S, Tannock I, Morris M, Sternberg CN, Carducci MA et al (2008) Design and end points of clinical trials for patients with progressive prostate cancer and castrate levels of testosterone: recommendations of the Prostate Cancer Clinical Trials Working Group. J Clin Oncol 26:1148–1159
26. Galasko CS (1995) Diagnosis of skeletal metastases and assessment of response to treatment. Clin Orthop Relat Res 312:64–75
27. Costelloe CM, Chuang HH, Madewell JE, Ueno NT (2010) Cancer response criteria and bone metastases: RECIST 1.1, MDA and PERCIST. J Cancer Educ 1:80–92
28. Bauerle T, Semmler W (2009) Imaging response to systemic therapy for bone metastases. Eur Radiol 19:2495–2507
29. Messiou C, Cook G, Reid AH et al (2011) The CT flare response of metastatic bone disease in prostate cancer. Acta Radiol 52:557–561
30. Hwang S, Panicek DM (2007) Magnetic resonance imaging of bone marrow in oncology, Part 2. Skeletal Radiol 36:1017–1027
31. Lecouvet FE, Larbi A, Pasoglou V et al (2013) MRI for response assessment in metastatic bone disease. Eur Radiol 23:1986–1997
32. Pasoglou V, Michoux N, Peeters F, Larbi A, Tombal B, Selleslagh T et al (2015) Whole-body 3D T1-weighted MR imaging in patients with prostate cancer: feasibility and evaluation in screening for metastatic disease. Radiology 275:155–166
33. Koh DM, Takahara T, Imai Y, Collins DJ (2007) Practical aspects of assessing tumors using clinical diffusion-weighted imaging in the body. Magn Reson Med Sci 6:211–224
34. Lecouvet FE, Geukens D, Stainier A, Jamar F, Jamart J, d'Othee BJ et al (2007) Magnetic resonance imaging of the axial skeleton for detecting bone metastases in patients with high-risk prostate cancer: diagnostic and cost-effectiveness and

comparison with current detection strategies. J Clin Oncol 25:3281–3287
35. Ketelsen D, Rothke M, Aschoff P, Merseburger AS, Lichy MP, Reimold M et al (2008) Detection of bone metastasis of prostate cancer – comparison of whole-body MRI and bone scintigraphy. Rofo 180:746–752
36. Lecouvet FE, El Mouedden J, Collette L, Coche E, Danse E, Jamar F et al (2012) Can whole-body magnetic resonance imaging with diffusion-weighted imaging replace Tc 99m bone scanning and computed tomography for single-step detection of metastases in patients with high-risk prostate cancer? Eur Urol 62:68–75
37. Luboldt W, Kufer R, Blumstein N, Toussaint TL, Kluge A, Seemann MD et al (2008) Prostate carcinoma: diffusion-weighted imaging as potential alternative to conventional MR and ^{11}C-choline PET/CT for detection of bone metastases. Radiology 249:1017–1025
38. Venkitaraman R, Cook GJ, Dearnaley DP, Parker CC, Khoo V, Eeles R et al (2009) Whole-body magnetic resonance imaging in the detection of skeletal metastases in patients with prostate cancer. J Med Imaging Radiat Oncol 53:241–247
39. Wang X, Zhang C, Jiang X (2009) Prospective study of bone metastasis from prostate cancer: comparison between large field diffusion-weighted imaging and bone scintigraphy. Chinese J Radiol 43:131–135
40. Gutzeit A, Doert A, Froehlich JM, Eckhardt BP, Meili A, Scherr P et al (2010) Comparison of diffusion-weighted whole body MRI and skeletal scintigraphy for the detection of bone metastases in patients with prostate or breast carcinoma. Skeletal Radiol 39:333–343
41. Mosavi F, Johansson S, Sandberg DT, Turesson I, Sorensen J, Ahlstrom H (2012) Whole-body diffusion-weighted MRI compared with (18)F-NaF PET/CT for detection of bone metastases in patients with high-risk prostate carcinoma. AJR Am J Roentgenol 199:1114–1120
42. Stecco A, Lombardi M, Leva L, Brambilla M, Negru E, Delli Passeri S et al (2013) Diagnostic accuracy and agreement between whole-body diffusion MRI and bone scintigraphy in detecting bone metastases. Radiol Med 118:465–475
43. Fitzpatrick JM, Bellmunt J, Fizazi K, Heidenreich A, Sternberg CN, Tombal B et al (2014) Optimal management of metastatic castration-resistant prostate cancer: highlights from a European Expert Consensus Panel. Eur J Cancer 50:1617–1627
44. Reischauer C, Froehlich JM, Koh DM et al (2010) Bone metastases from prostate cancer: assessing treatment response by using diffusion-weighted imaging and functional diffusion maps-initial observations. Radiology 257:523–531
45. Messiou C, Collins DJ, Giles S et al (2011) Assessing response in bone metastases in prostate cancer with diffusion weighted MRI. Eur Radiol 21:2169–2177
46. Afshar-Oromieh A, Zechmann CM, Malcher A, Eder M, Eisenhut M, Linhart HG et al (2014) Comparison of PET imaging with a (68)Ga-labelled PSMA ligand and (18)F-choline-based PET/CT for the diagnosis of recurrent prostate cancer. Eur J Nucl Med Mol Imaging 41:11–20
47. Even-Sapir E, Metser U, Mishani E, Lievshitz G, Lerman H, Leibovitch I (2006) The detection of bone metastases in patients with high-risk prostate cancer: ^{99m}Tc-MDP Planar bone scintigraphy, single- and multi-field-of-view SPECT, ^{18}F-fluoride PET, and ^{18}F-fluoride PET/CT. J Nucl Med 47:287–297
48. Bombardieri E, Bombardieri E, Setti L, Kirienko M, Antunovic L, Guglielmo P et al (2015) Which metabolic imaging, besides bone scan with ^{99m}Tc-phosphonates, for detecting and evaluating bone metastases in prostatic cancer patients? An open discussion. The Quarterly J Nucl Med Mol Imaging 4:381–399
49. Briganti A, Passoni N, Ferrari M, Capitanio U, Suardi N, Gallina A et al (2010) When to perform bone scan in patients with newly diagnosed prostate cancer: external validation of the currently available guidelines and proposal of a novel risk stratification tool. Eur Urol 57:551–558
50. Hillner BE, Siegel BA, Hanna L et al (2015) ^{18}F-fluoride PET used for treatment monitoring of systemic cancer therapy: results from the National Oncologic PET Registry. J Nucl Med 56:222–228
51. Dennis ER, Jia X, Mezheritskiy IS, Stephenson RD, Schoder H, Fox JJ et al (2012) Bone scan index: a quantitative treatment response biomarker for castration-resistant metastatic prostate cancer. J Clin Oncol 30:519–524
52. Ulmert D, Kaboteh R, Fox JJ, Savage C, Evans MJ, Lilja H et al (2012) A novel automated platform for quantifying the extent of skeletal tumour involvement in prostate cancer patients using the Bone Scan Index. Eur Urol 62:78–84
53. Gamez-Cenzano C, Pino-Sorroche F (2014) Standardization and quantification in FDG-PET/CT imaging for staging and restaging of malignant disease. PET Clin 9:117–127
54. Garcia JR, Moreno C, Valls E, Cozar P, Bassa P, Soler M, Alvarez-Moro FJ, Moragas M, Riera E (2015) Diagnostic performance of bone scintigraphy and (11)C-Choline PET/CT in the detection of bone metastases in patients with biochemical recurrence of prostate cancer. Rev Esp Med Nucl Imagen Mol 34:155–161
55. Poulsen MH, Petersen H, Høilund-Carlsen PF, Jakobsen JS, Gerke O, Karstoft J, Steffansen SI, Walter S (2014) Spine metastases in prostate cancer: comparison of technetium-99m-MDP whole-body bone scintigraphy, [(18) F]choline positron emission

tomography(PET)/computed tomography (CT) and [(18) F]NaF PET/CT. BJU Int 114:818–823

56. Iagaru A, Mittra E, Dick DW, Gambhir SS (2012) Prospective evaluation of (99m)Tc MDP scintigraphy, (18)F NaF PET/CT, and (18)F FDG PET/CT for detection of skeletal metastases. Mol Imaging Biol 14:252–259
57. Damle NA, Bal C, Bandopadhyaya GP, Kumar L, Kumar P, Malhotra A, Lata S (2013) The role of ^{18}F-fluoride PET-CT in the detection of bone metastases in patients with breast, lung and prostate carcinoma: a comparison with FDG PET/CT and ^{99}mTc-MDP bone scan. Jpn J Radiol 31:262–269
58. Palmedo H, Marx C, Ebert A, Kreft B, Ko Y, Türler A, Vorreuther R, Göhring U, Schild HH, Gerhardt T, Pöge U, Ezziddin S, Biersack HJ, Ahmadzadehfar H (2014) Whole-body SPECT/CT for bone scintigraphy: diagnostic value and effect on patient management in oncological patients. Eur J Nucl Med Mol Imaging 41:59–67
59. Withofs N, Grayet B, Tancredi T, Rorive A, Mella C, Giacomelli F, Mievis F, Aerts J, Waltregny D, Jerusalem G, Hustinx R (2011) ^{18}F-fluoride PET/CT for assessing bone involvement in prostate and breast cancers. Nucl Med Commun 32:168–176
60. Takesh M, Odat Allh K, Adams S, Zechmann C (2012) Diagnostic role of (18)F-FECH-PET/CT compared with bone scan in evaluating the prostate cancer patients referring with biochemical recurrence. ISRN Oncol 2012:815234
61. Beheshti M, Vali R, Waldenberger P, Fitz F, Nader M, Hammer J, Loidl W, Pirich C, Fogelman I, Langsteger W (2010) The use of F-18 choline PET in the assessment of bone metastases in prostate cancer: correlation with morphological changes on CT. Mol Imaging Biol 12:98–107
62. Langsteger W, Balogova S, Huchet V, Beheshti M, Paycha F, Egrot C, Janetschek G, Loidl W, Nataf V, Kerrou K, Pascal O, Cussenot O, Talbot JN (2011) Fluorocholine (18F) and sodium fluoride (18F) PET/CT in the detection of prostate cancer: prospective comparison of diagnostic performance determined by masked reading. Q J Nucl Med Mol Imaging 55:448–457
63. Beheshti M, Vali R, Waldenberger P, Fitz F, Nader M, Hammer J, Loidl W, Pirich C, Fogelman I, Langsteger W (2009) The use of F-18 choline PET in the assessment of bone metastases in prostate cancer: correlation with morphological changes on CT. Mol Imaging Biol 11:446–454
64. McCarthy M, Siew T, Campbell A, Lenzo N, Spry N, Vivian J, Morandeau L (2011) ^{18}F-Fluoromethylcholine (FCH) PET imaging in patients with castration-resistant prostate cancer: prospective comparison with standard imaging. Eur J Nucl Med Mol Imaging 38:14–22
65. Fuccio C, Castellucci P, Schiavina R, Santi I, Allegri V, Pettinato V, Boschi S, Martorana G, Al-Nahhas A, Rubello D, Fanti S (2010) Role of ^{11}C-choline PET/CT in the restaging of prostate cancer patients showing a single lesion on bone scintigraphy. Ann Nucl Med 24:485–492
66. Picchio M, Spinapolice EG, Fallanca F, Crivellaro C, Giovacchini G, Gianolli L, Messa C (2012) [11C] Choline PET/CT detection of bone metastases in patients with PSA progression after primary treatment for prostate cancer: comparison with bone scintigraphy. Eur J Nucl Med Mol Imaging 39:13–26
67. Mohsen B, Giorgio T, Rasoul ZS, Werner L, Ali GR, Reza DK, Ramin S (2013) Application of C-11-acetate positron-emission tomography (PET) imaging in prostate cancer: systematic review and meta-analysis of the literature. BJU Int 112: 1062–1072
68. Caffo O, Maines F, Donner D, Veccia A, Chierichetti F, Galligioni E (2014) Impact of enzalutamide administration on primary prostate cancer volume: a metabolic evaluation by choline positron emission tomography in castration-resistant prostate cancer patients. Clin Genitourin Cancer 12: 312–316
69. De Giorgi U, Caroli P, Scarpi E, Conteduca V, Burgio SL, Menna C et al (2015) (18)F-Fluorocholine PET/CT for early response assessment in patients with metastatic castration-resistant prostate cancer treated with enzalutamide. Eur J Nucl Med Mol Imaging 2015;42:1276–1283
70. De Giorgi U, Caroli P, Burgio SL, Menna C, Conteduca V, Bianchi E et al (2014) Early outcome prediction on 18F-fluorocholine PET/CT in metastatic castration-resistant prostate cancer patients treated with abiraterone. Oncotarget 5:12448–12458
71. Ceci F, Castellucci P, Graziani T, Schiavina R, Renzi R, Borghesi M et al (2015) C-Choline PET/CT in castration-resistant prostate cancer patients treated with docetaxel. Eur J Nucl Med Mol Imaging
72. Messiou C, Cook G, deSouza MN (2009) Imaging metastatic bone disease from carcinoma of the prostate. Br J Cancer 101:1225–1232
73. Wade AA, Scott JA, Kuter I, Fischman AJ (2006) Flare response in ^{18}F-fluoride ion PET bone scanning. AJR 186:1783–1786
74. Levenson RM, Sauerbrunn BJ, Bates HR, Newman RD, Eddy JL, Ihde DC (1983) Comparative value of bone scintigraphy and radiography in monitoring tumour response in systemically treated prostatic carcinoma. Radiology 146:513–518
75. Pollen JJ, Witztum KF, Ashburn WL (1984) The flare phenomenon on radionuclide bone scan in metastatic prostate cancer. Am J Roentgenol 142: 773–776
76. Mitsui Y, Shiina H, Yamamoto Y, Haramoto M, Arichi N, Yasumoto H, Kitagaki H, Igawa M (2012) Prediction of survival benefit using an automated bone scan index in patients with castration-resistant prostate cancer. BJU Int 110:E628–E6234

77. Shimizu N, Masud H, Yamanaka H, Oriuchi N, Inoue T, Endo K (1999) Fluorodeoxyglucose positron emission tomography scan of prostate cancer bone metastases with flare reaction after endocrine therapy. J Urol 161:608–609
78. Jadvar H (2011) Prostate cancer: PET with 18F-FDG, ^{18}F- or ^{11}C-acetate, and ^{18}F- or ^{11}C-choline. J Nucl Med 52:81–89
79. Wade AA, Scott JA, Kuter I, Fischman AJ (2006) Flare response in ^{18}F-fluoride ion PET bone scanning. AJR Am J Roentgenol 186:1783–1786
80. McNamara MA, George DJ (2015) Pain, PSA flare, and bone scan response in a patient with metastatic castration-resistant prostate cancer treated with radium-223, a case report. BMC Cancer 15:371
81. Jadvar M, Desai B, Si L, Groshen S, Mills J, Murray R et al (2015) Prediction of hormonal resistance in metastatic prostate cancer with FDG PET/CT. J Nucl Med 56:1451
82. Saad F, Gleason DM, Murray R, Tchekmedyian S, Venner P, Lacombe L, Chin JL, Vinholes JJ, Goas JA, Chen B; Zoledronic Acid Prostate Cancer Study Group (2002) A randomized, placebo-controlled trial of zoledronic acid in patients with hormone-refractory metastatic prostate carcinoma. J Natl Cancer Inst 94:1458–1468
83. Tannock IF, de Wit R, Berry WR, Horti J, Pluzanska A, Chi KN, Oudard S, Théodore C, James ND, Turesson I, Rosenthal MA (2004) Eisenberger MA; TAX 327 Investigators. Docetaxel plus prednisone or mitoxantrone plus prednisone for advanced prostate cancer. N Engl J Med 351:1502–1512
84. Petrylak DP, Tangen CM, Hussain MH, Lara PN Jr, Jones JA, Taplin ME, Burch PA, Berry D, Moinpour C, Kohli M, Benson MC, Small EJ, Raghavan D, Crawford ED (2004) Docetaxel and estramustine compared with mitoxantrone and prednisone for advanced refractory prostate cancer. N Engl J Med 351:1513–1520
85. Sternberg CN, Petrylak DP, Sartor O, Witjes JA, Demkow T, Ferrero JM, Eymard JC, Falcon S, Calabrò F, James N, Bodrogi I, Harper P, Wirth M, Berry W, Petrone ME, McKearn TJ, Noursalehi M, George M, Rozencweig M (2009) Multinational, double-blind, phase III study of prednisone and either satraplatin or placebo in patients with castrate-refractory prostate cancer progressing after prior chemotherapy: the SPARC trial. J Clin Oncol 27:5431–5438
86. Kantoff PW, Higano CS, Shore ND, Berger ER, Small EJ, Penson DF, Redfern CH, Ferrari AC, Dreicer R, Sims RB, Frohlich MW, Schellhammer PF (2010) IMPACT Study Investigators. Sipuleucel-T immunotherapy for castration-resistant prostate cancer. N Engl J Med 363:411–422
87. de Bono JS, Oudard S, Ozguroglu M, Hansen S, Machiels JP, Kocak I, Gravis G, Bodrogi I, Mackenzie MJ, Shen L, Roessner M, Gupta S, Sartor AO (2010) TROPIC Investigators. Prednisone plus cabazitaxel or mitoxantrone for metastatic castration-resistant prostate cancer progressing after docetaxel treatment: a randomised open-label trial. Lancet 376:1147–1154
88. Fizazi K, Carducci M, Smith M, Damião R, Brown J, Karsh L, Milecki P, Shore N, Rader M, Wang H, Jiang Q, Tadros S, Dansey R, Goessl C (2011) Denosumab versus zoledronic acid for treatment of bone metastases in men with castration-resistant prostate cancer: a randomised, double-blind study. Lancet 377:813–822
89. Fizazi K, Scher HI, Molina A, Logothetis CJ, Chi KN, Jones RJ, Staffurth JN, North S, Vogelzang NJ, Saad F, Mainwaring P, Harland S, Goodman OB Jr, Sternberg CN, Li JH, Kheoh T, Haqq CM, de Bono JS; COU-AA-301 Investigators (2012) Abiraterone acetate for treatment of metastatic castration-resistant prostate cancer: final overall survival analysis of the COU-AA-301 randomised, double-blind, placebo-controlled phase 3 study. Lancet Oncol 13:983–992
90. Scher HI, Fizazi K, Saad F, Taplin ME, Sternberg CN, Miller K, de Wit R, Mulders P, Chi KN, Shore ND, Armstrong AJ, Flaig TW, Fléchon A, Mainwaring P, Fleming M, Hainsworth JD, Hirmand M, Selby B, Seely L, de Bono JS (2012) AFFIRM Investigators. Increased survival with enzalutamide in prostate cancer after chemotherapy. N Engl J Med 367:1187–1197
91. Ryan CJ, Smith MR, de Bono JS, Molina A, Logothetis CJ, de Souza P, Fizazi K, Mainwaring P, Piulats JM, Ng S, Carles J, Mulders PF, Basch E, Small EJ, Saad F, Schrijvers D, Van Poppel H, Mukherjee SD, Suttmann H, Gerritsen WR, Flaig TW, George DJ, Yu EY, Efstathiou E, Pantuck A, Winquist E, Higano CS, Taplin ME, Park Y, Kheoh T, Griffin T, Scher HI, Rathkopf DE; COU-AA-302 Investigators (2013) Abiraterone in metastatic prostate cancer without previous chemotherapy. N Engl J Med 368:138–148. Erratum in N Engl J Med 368:584
92. Beer TM, Armstrong AJ, Rathkopf DE, Loriot Y, Sternberg CN, Higano CS, Iversen P, Bhattacharya S, Carles J, Chowdhury S, Davis ID, de Bono JS, Evans CP, Fizazi K, Joshua AM, Kim CS, Kimura G, Mainwaring P, Mansbach H, Miller K, Noonberg SB, Perabo F, Phung D, Saad F, Scher HI, Taplin ME, Venner PM, Tombal B; PREVAIL Investigators (2014) Enzalutamide in metastatic prostate cancer before chemotherapy. N Engl J Med 371:424–433
93. Sweeney CJ, Chen YH, Carducci M, Liu G, Jarrard DF, Eisenberger M, Wong YN, Hahn N, Kohli M, Cooney MM, Dreicer R, Vogelzang NJ, Picus J, Shevrin D, Hussain M, Garcia JA, DiPaola RS (2015) Chemohormonal therapy in metastatic hormone-sensitive prostate cancer. N Engl J Med 373:737–746
94. James ND, Sydes MR, Clarke NW, Mason MD, Dearnaley DP, Spears MR, Ritchie AW, Parker CC,

Russell JM, Attard G, de Bono J, Cross W, Jones RJ, Thalmann G, Amos C, Matheson D, Millman R, Alzouebi M, Beesley S, Birtle AJ, Brock S, Cathomas R, Chakraborti P, Chowdhury S, Cook A, Elliott T, Gale J, Gibbs S, Graham JD, Hetherington J, Hughes R, Laing R, McKinna F, McLaren DB, O'Sullivan JM, Parikh O, Peedell C, Protheroe A, Robinson AJ, Srihari N, Srinivasan R, Staffurth J, Sundar S, Tolan S, Tsang D, Wagstaff J, Parmar MK; STAMPEDE investigators (2016) Addition of docetaxel, zoledronic acid, or both to first-line long-term hormone therapy in prostate cancer (STAMPEDE): survival results from an adaptive, multiarm, multistage, platform randomised controlled trial. Lancet 387:1163–1177

95. http://uroweb.org/guideline/prostate-cancer/
96. Parker C, Gillessen S, Heidenreich A, Horwich A; ESMO Guidelines Committee (2015) Cancer of the prostate: ESMO Clinical Practice Guidelines for diagnosis, treatment and follow-up. Ann Oncol 26(Suppl 5):v69–77
97. https://www.auanet.org/common/pdf/education/clinical-guidance/Prostate-Cancer.pdf
98. http://www.nccn.org/professionals/physiciangls/pdf/prostate.pdf
99. Gillessen S, Omlin A, Attard G, de Bono JS, Efstathiou E, Fizazi K, Halabi S, Nelson PS, Sartor O, Smith MR, Soule HR, Akaza H, Beer TM, Beltran H, Chinnaiyan AM, Daugaard G, Davis ID, De Santis M, Drake CG, Eeles RA, Fanti S, Gleave ME, Heidenreich A, Hussain M, James ND, Lecouvet FE, Logothetis CJ, Mastris K, Nilsson S, Oh WK, Olmos D, Padhani AR, Parker C, Rubin MA, Schalken JA, Scher HI, Sella A, Shore ND, Small EJ, Sternberg CN, Suzuki H, Sweeney CJ, Tannock IF, Tombal B (2015) Management of patients with advanced prostate cancer: recommendations of the St Gallen Advanced Prostate Cancer Consensus Conference (APCCC) 2015. Ann Oncol 26:1589–1604
100. Evangelista L, Bertoldo F, Boccardo F, Conti G, Menchi I, Mungai F et al (2016) Diagnostic imaging to detect and evaluate response to therapy in bone metastases from prostate cancer: current modalities and new horizons. Eur J Nucl Med Mol Imaging 2016;43(8):1546–62

Bone Metastases from Prostate Cancer: From Symptom Control to Pain Palliation

19

Augusto Caraceni, Ernesto Zecca, Fabio Formaglio, and Francesca Ricchini

19.1 Pain and Metastatic Prostate Cancer History

Prostate cancer is the second most frequently diagnosed cancer and the fifth leading cause of cancer-related death in men. The majority, around 90 %, of patients with metastatic castration-resistant prostate cancer (mCRPC) have radiological evidence of bone metastases, and bone is the first metastatic site in 80 % of patients [1, 2].

Bone metastases lead to changes in the structural integrity of the bone and manifest as pain and debilitating skeletal-related events (SREs) such as pathological fracture, spinal cord or nerve root compression, hypocalcemia (often asymptomatic), and myelosuppression [3, 4].

As a result of these morbidities, patient quality of life (QOL) — including physical, emotional, and functional well-being — is substantially reduced. Overall skeletal morbidity incurs marked increases in the costs of treating patients with bone metastases. Furthermore, metastasis-associated skeletal morbidities are negative predictors of survival in patients with mCRPC [5–7].

SREs are also associated with reduced survival in prostate cancer patients: in a Danish population-based study, 1-year survival was 87 % in men without bone metastases and 47 % in those with bone metastases but no SREs and 40 % in those with bone metastases and SREs [8].

Debilitating pain is one of the most common morbidities experienced by men with mCRPC, and there is emerging evidence that pain is an important predictor of clinical outcome. Nevertheless, the presence of pain has not been incorporated into prognostic models in this disease state, and only in a few studies of prostate cancer, it has been evaluated [9–11].

For example, in an analysis of 85 patients with mCRPC, Berry et al. identified severe bone pain as predictive of short survival duration. Because of the limited sample size, the analysis was based on a univariate model. More recently, using data from the TAX 327 trial, Armstrong et al. identified pain as a statistically significant prognostic factor of overall survival. The adjusted HR for men who had pain at baseline was 1.48 (95 % CI, 1.23–1.79) and was among the strongest predictors in the multivariable model [12].

In 2008 Halabi et al. combined the data from three randomized phase III multicenter trials conducted by the Cancer and Leukemia Group B from 1992 and 1998 and used seven items from the Brief Pain Inventory (BPI) to assess the impact of pain on a range of daily activities and

A. Caraceni (✉) • E. Zecca • F. Formaglio
F. Ricchini
SC Cure palliative, terapia del dolore e Riabilitazione, Fondazione IRCCS Istituto tumori, Milan, Italy
e-mail: augusto.caraceni@istitutotumori.mi.it

F. Bertoldo et al. (eds.), *Bone Metastases from Prostate Cancer*,
DOI 10.1007/978-3-319-42327-2_19

quality of life, each rated from 0 to 10. The primary end point was overall survival (OS), and the effect of baseline pain interference scores on OS was evaluated. In addition, the effect of baseline pain interference scores on other end points such as progression-free survival (PFS), time to biochemical failure (prostate-specific antigen [PSA] PFS), ≥ 50 % decline in PSA, and objective (bidimensionally measurable) response proportion in men with measurable disease was explored.

In the 599 patient, the median pain interference score was 17 and 38 % of the men had opioid analgesic use at baseline. There was a statistically significant association between pain interference scores and the risk of death. The median survival times were 17.6 months (95 % CI, 16.1–19.1 months) and 10.2 months (95 % CI, 8.6–11.3 months; $p<0.001$) in men with low (<17) and high (>17) pain scores, respectively. Pain was inversely associated with the likelihood of prostate-specific antigen decline, objective response, and time to bone progression [5].

Older data by Turner et al. already suggested that pain was predictor of quality of life independently from other indicators of disease progression such as PSA levels [13]

19.2 Cancer-Induced Bone Pain

19.2.1 Clinical Characteristics

The most common sites for bone metastases in mCRPC are the ribs, spine, and pelvis, although metastases in the skull and long bones have been reported [14–16].

Cancer-induced bone pain (CIBP) is one of the most common types of cancer pain in general, occurring in 28–45 % of patients with bone metastasis [17–19]. Most frequent pain locations are the lower back, overall spine, and lower limbs.

The degree and location of bone metastases do not necessarily correlate with the severity of pain, and not all patients with bone metastases have pain; bone pain was identified in only a third of patients with bone metastases in one large prospective study [17].

It is not yet clear why some bone metastases cause pain and others do not. Cancer-induced bone pain is a complex pain state involving a combination of background, spontaneous, and incident (movement evoked) pain [20].

In the initial presentation, symptomatic bone cancer is usually described as dull pain, constant, and gradually increasing in intensity with time [21]. Often continuous pain is accompanied by a second type of pain known as breakthrough pain or incident pain [22]. Incident or breakthrough pain is also defined as a transitory flare of severe pain superimposed on an otherwise stable pain pattern in patients treated with opioids and can occur spontaneously or on movement or weight bearing [23, 24]. Because breakthrough pain is frequently acute and unpredictable in onset, this pain can be debilitating and difficult to control [22].

Pain is often reported in the body area corresponding to the site of underlying bone lesion; it can also be referred to distant cutaneous area and can be reproduced often by direct stimulation of the soft tissues over the involved bone. Referred pain at distance should be distinguished from irradiated pain due to radiculopathy.

Neurologic dysfunction can be associated with metastatic bone disease, particularly when vertebral metastases encroach on the spinal cord or spinal nerves and nerve roots or when metastatic lesions in the skull impinge on cranial nerves. Neurologic involvement may present as lower or upper extremity pain, weakness, or paresthesias in a radicular pattern.

Metastases of the clivus, for example, may compress the hypoglossal nerve, producing unilateral tongue weakness. Disease in the middle cranial fossa may affect the facial and trigeminal nerves and cause ipsilateral weakness in the upper and lower face or numbness, particularly in the lower lip and jaw area [25]. Unilateral deafness, diplopia, and other visual disturbances may also occur as the result of cranial nerve damage from bony tumors in the anterior part of the skull base (Table 19.1).

Table 19.1 Base of skull syndromes causing pain in prostate cancer

Syndrome	Pain	Cranial nerve involved
Orbital	Retro-supraorbital	II visual loss III, IV, VI diplopia V frontal sensory loss
Cavernous sinus	Supraorbital frontal	III, IV, VI diplopia V sensory loss
Middle cranial fossa	Trigeminal pain, paroxysmal headache	VII, V
Jugular foramen	Mastoid, neck, shoulder	IX, X dysphagia XI trapezoid sternocleidomastoid Weakness XII tongue deviation
Occipital condyle	Unilateral nuchal radiate behind the eye Tenderness of the occipital junction	XII tongue

19.2.2 Pathophysiology of Bone Cancer Pain

The exact mechanism by which tumor in bone produces pain is not completely understood; various postulated mechanisms of bone pain include the role of prostaglandins, local change in bone metabolism and blood flow, and the stimulation of nerve endings by increased intraosseous pressure, cytokines, and locally released neurotransmitters.

Tumors may secrete proteases that cause bone cell lysis, and yet osteoclastic activity is required to break down the mineralized bone matrix; also, tumor cells secrete a number of factors that enhance osteoclastic activity. As the tumor expands outward from the marrow space, it may cause increased intraosseous pressure, particularly if the growth is rapid. This may activate mechanoreceptive nociceptors in bone and stretch the highly innervated periosteum. Edema and inflammation may also contribute to pain, via both increased pressure and secreted mediators, which, in turn, activate pain receptors. Cancer-induced bone pain is a specific pain state with overlapping but distinct features of both inflammatory and specific central and peripheral hyperexcitability mechanism [26]. Cancer cells in the body microenvironment stimulate local inflammatory mediators and create a highly acidic environment, which sensitizes peripheral nerve endings within the bone marrow and bone matrix and thus can explain how resulting pain is associated with a hyperexcitability state within the spinal cord. Peripheral and central hyperexcitability may explain why patients experience constant pain, with severe pain episodes highly sensitive to movement and other innocuous stimuli or initiated by unknown spontaneous mechanism.

Extensive bone disease can also lead to fractures and compression of adjacent nerves, vascular structures, and soft tissue.

19.2.3 Nociceptive and Neuropathic Pain

The participation of somatic bone afferents to the pathophysiology of pain due to bone metastases via the mechanisms briefly summarized above should be regarded as a source of somatic nociceptive pain according to a traditional clinical–pathological classification. The clinical impact of specific mechanisms highlighted in animal experimental models of cancer bone invasion is at the moment unknown. However, patients with pain due to bone metastases can have pain also due to lesions of nerve roots, peripheral nerves of plexus produced by the progression of their bone lesions. These lesions can cause also neuropathic pain. The diagnosis of neuropathic pain requires specific expertise and should be reserved to cases presenting with a neurological lesion associated with sensory and pain related objective symptoms and signs [27]. In all cases, the characteristics of pain should be evaluated in time to identify eventual changes in the pain mechanism as already suggested although bone metastases can cause per se somatic pain for long time periods; the progression to invade other tissue – soft tissue, viscera, and neurological structures – should always be considered.

19.3 Pain Assessment

The initial assessment of pain should include a detailed history, including the location, intensity, frequency, temporal pattern, and specific characteristics of the pain. Knowledge of factors that aggravate and alleviate the pain is also critical to an effective treatment plan. Accurate physical and neurological examination follows a good pain history.

A thorough assessment of pain must also include psychosocial components, such as the patient's attitude toward his diagnosis and treatment, mechanisms for coping with pain and stress, psychological responses to pain (such as anxiety and depression), and attitude regarding controlled substances. These factors often play a role in both the patient's experience of pain and his response to treatment. In addition, information regarding the patient's support system and insurance plans often is crucial to the success of treatment.

To establish the presence of pain, pain severity, and pain relief, consideration must be given to the specific patient population, using instruments with defined psychometric properties.

The literature suggests that clinicians often underreport patients' pain intensity in comparison to the patients' own report of their pain. Therefore, an unfiltered representation of the patient's experience, as measured using a patient-reported outcome, is preferred [28].

Pain intensity must be measured and recorded to help in monitoring therapy results and improve communication with patients on pain by introduction of simple scale measure. Different pain measurement tools have been validated for cancer pain. They can be divided in two main categories: intensity scale and multidimensional questionnaires. Intensity scales are visual analogue scale (VAS), numerical rating scale (NRS), and verbal rating scale (VRS) [29].

NRS seem to have common meaning across cultures while keeping some desirable psychometric properties if compared with VRS [30]. In clinical practice, the pain intensity alone may not be sufficient to evaluate treatment efficacy, and additional clinical information can suggest how much a given pain level bothers the patients, which is the level of pain that the patient considers tolerable, what corresponds to satisfactory pain relief, how the pain interferes with quality of life, and where would the patient place himself along the trade-off between pain relief and side effects.

Several instruments are available for multidimensional evaluation such as the Brief Pain inventory [31], the McGill Pain questionnaire [32], and the Memorial Pain Assessment Card [33]. All of them are valid and reliable and important research tools.

Pain needs to be continually reassessed in the prostate cancer patient since disease progression, response to treatment, and response to pain control maneuvers all influence treatment strategies. The clinician needs to educate both patients and their families and caregivers about pain, its causes and treatments, and their active participation in pain assessment and management. Education should address pain assessment, dose titration, side effect management, and any fears and misconceptions regarding addiction and tolerance.

The steps to be considered when choosing one method for systematic patient assessment are reported in Table 19.2.

19.4 Pain Syndromes in Prostate Cancer Bone Pain

Cancer pain can be described under different clinical domains, etiology, location, and pain mechanism and pain syndromes.

Table 19.2 The steps needed for systematic pain assessment

1.	Choose method of evaluation and frequency
2.	Establish time referral i.e., in example average of last 24 h pain or last week pain. "Pain now" is the most reliable
3.	Pain quality and intensity change in time and episodes of breakthrough should be evaluated aside to baseline pain
4.	A body chart showing different pain sites should be part of the regular assessment
5.	Average and worst pain intensities are considered important clinical variables
6.	Pain intensity measures should be visible in patient's chart and be part of routine evaluation in oncology setting

Cancer pain syndromes can be broadly divided into those that are acute and those that are chronic. Acute pain syndromes usually accompany diagnostic or therapeutic interventions, whereas chronic pain syndromes usually are directly related to the neoplasm itself or to an antineoplastic therapy [34].

In many cases, the presence of symptoms and signs can suggest a specific cancer pain syndrome [34]. The identification of such a syndrome may help to elucidate the etiology of the pain, direct the diagnostic evaluation, clarify the prognosis for the pain or the disease itself, and guide therapeutic intervention.

Caraceni et al. [19] described pain syndrome in a review article "as repeated cluster of symptoms and sign including pain which combined with other relevant information from the history and examination, identify a clinical entity that can be used to define that specific situation."

In a cross-sectional study, 1095 cancer patients with pain were evaluated describing pain mechanism, pain intensity, and pain syndromes. Twenty-two of 51 pain syndrome were prevalent [19].

This survey suggests the existence of disease-related syndrome clusters. A variety of bone pain syndromes were found in prostate cancer and its evolution (Table 19.3).

Patients with prostate cancer were also more likely to experience generalized bone pain and pelvis and long bone pain than other tumor types as shown in Table 19.4.

Table 19.3 Bone pain syndrome in metastatic castration-resistant prostate cancer

Base of skull syndrome
Vertebral syndromes
Diffuse bone pain
Due to multiple bone metastases
Due to bone marrow infiltration/expansion
Focal bone pain
Long bones
Hest wall rib pain
Infiltration of a joint (sacroiliac joint)
Pelvic bony lesions

Table 19.4 Frequency of bone pain syndromes in 65 prostate cancer patients

Base of skull	1.5 %
Vertebral	21.5 %
Pelvis and long bones	26.1 %
Generalized bone pain	40.0 %
Chest wall	4.6 %
Pathological fracture	3.0 %

Modified from Caraceni et al. [19]

19.4.1 Vertebral Pain Syndromes

Vertebral pain syndromes are the most common cause of pain in mCRPC. The thoracic spine is affected in more than two thirds of cases, the lumbosacral spine in 20 %, and cervical spine in 10 %. Tumor usually involves the vertebral body and expands posteriorly. Multiple vertebral lesions are common. Hematogenous spread is the most common route, but tumor can invade the vertebral body from contiguous paraspinal site, pelvic nodes masses. In the assessment of the neck and back, it is necessary to differentiate local pain and referred pain, which are due to stimulation of pain sensitive structures in the spine and its joints and muscles, from radicular and spinal cord-related symptoms. This is important for making for an early diagnosis of epidural spinal cord compression (ESCC) that represents the most important complication. The association of vertebral bone with radiculopathy was described in about 10 % of cases [19].

Local bone pain has a dull, aching, deep quality and can be constant of vertebral metastatic pain, but movement and postures often aggravate it. Pain on activity should be regarded as sign of potential impending bone fracture.

Pain due to vertebral metastases especially when the invasion of the epidural space is already present can be worse when lying down and better when sitting; often pain can be referred to distant body areas from vertebral lesions, though lacking the specific clinical characteristics of radiculopathies in a pseudo-dermatomal fashion (sclerotomes).

The main complications of vertebral lesions are vertebral collapse, radiculopathies, and ESCC.

Collapse of vertebral bodies is particularly frequent in the thoracic spine. They can acutely aggravate the pain syndrome by impingement on the nerve roots and can cause skeletal deformities, implying a higher risk for ESCC or cauda equine compression. Radiculopathies can develop at any level; the pain is felt on the spine, deep in the muscles innervated by the affected root, and in the corresponding dermatome. It is aggravated by position that increases tumor compression on the root, such as lying down. The diagnosis of radiculopathies requires the association of sensory, motor, and reflex findings.

19.4.2 Bony Pain Syndromes: Long Bones, Bony Pelvis, Hip, and Shoulder

Metastases to the pelvis, hip, and femur are common and are associated with incident pain on movement and on weight bearing. There is high propensity of these lesions to fracture. Femur fractures can at time be operated on, but pelvic fractures are not usually operable and severely impact on the patient's ability to move and walk. Shoulder joints and humeri can also be infiltrated by tumors and need to be properly diagnosed to prevent fracture.

19.4.3 Hip–Joint Syndrome

When the acetabulum or the head of the femur are metastatic sites, the characteristic pain is exacerbated by leg movement and weight bearing. The pain often radiates to the knee and thigh. Pain can also be referred only to the knee. This bony lesion can extend into the pelvis and compress the lumbosacral plexus or the sciatic nerve. Lytic lesions of the femoral neck are to be managed with extreme caution even when examining the patient. Pelvic tumor can infiltrate at the same time the lumbosacral plexus and hip bone and sometimes viscera.

19.4.4 Sacroiliac–Joint Syndromes

This syndrome is characterized by local pain at the sacroiliac joint, aggravated electively by weight bearing and manual compression on the joint. The pain can also radiate to the thigh resembling a hip lesion.

19.4.5 Bone Marrow Infiltration or Bone Marrow Expansion Syndrome

Generalized bone pain with symptoms of migrating pain, often fluctuating in intensity in close relationship with therapeutic interventions, is found with diffuse marrow infiltration by solid tumors. The pain is in the limbs, and local bone tenderness is a constant finding especially on the diaphysis of long bones.

19.4.6 Base of the Skull Syndromes

Metastatic lesions to the base of the skull are relatively common during metastatic bone diffusion in prostate cancer.

Headache of moderate to severe intensity at the site of the lesion or referred to the vertex or to the entire affected site of the head is the common pain symptoms. The association of cranial nerve involvement establishes a diagnosis. The base of skull syndromes causing pain is shown in Table 19.1.

19.5 Treatment of Cancer-Induced Bone Pain

The strategies for treatment of CIBP in prostate cancer and/or their complication are reported in Fig. 19.1.

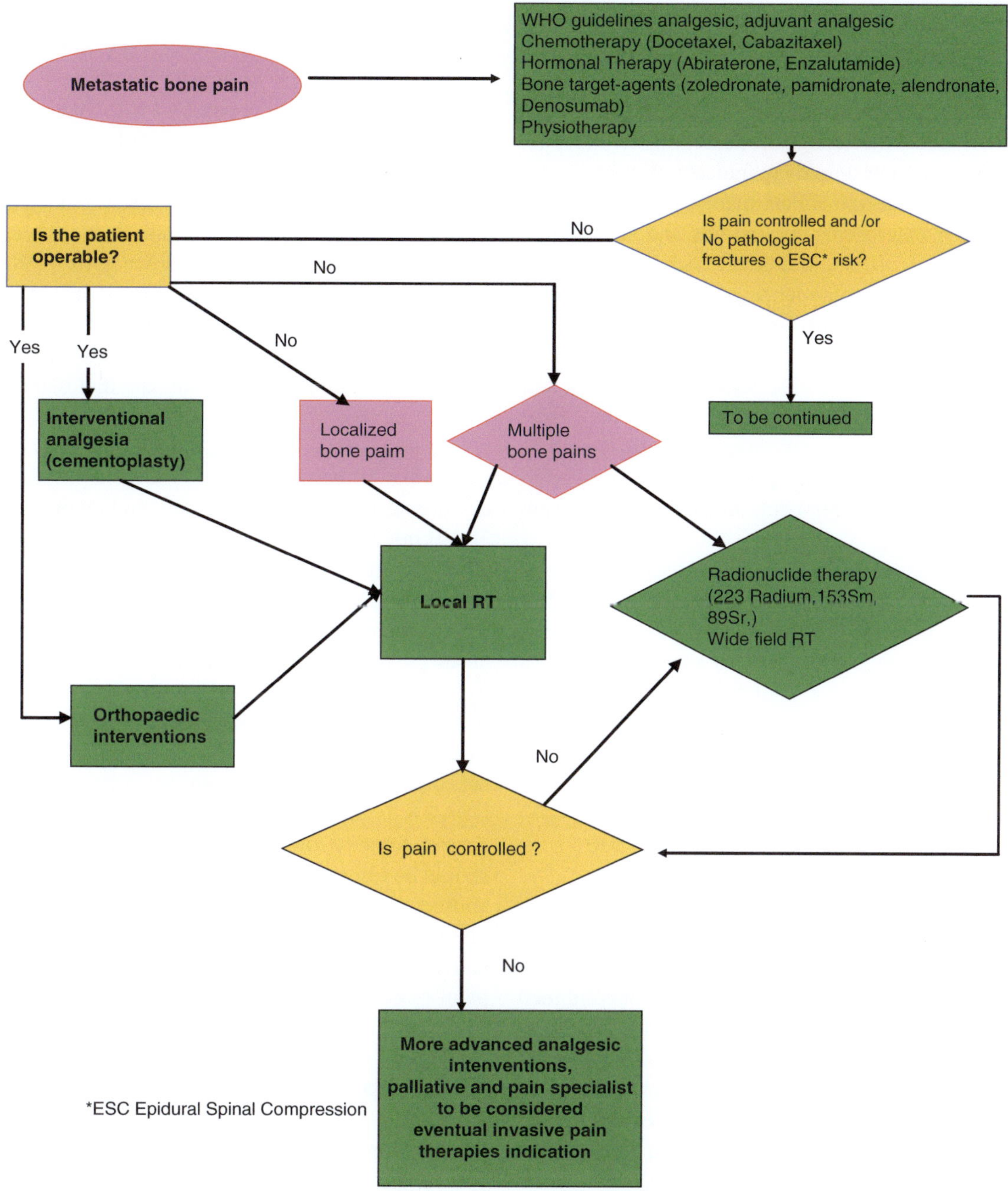

Fig. 19.1 Management of painful skeletal metastases in metastatic castration-resistant prostate cancer

Pharmacological management of CIBP involves the use of analgesic agents such as non-steroidal anti-inflammatory drugs (NSAIDs) and opioid analgesics in combination with adjuvant therapies including bisphosphonates, RANKL antibody, corticosteroids, chemotherapy agents, endocrine therapy radiotherapy, radio metabolic treatment, orthopedic surgery, and rehabilitation.

19.6 Analgesic Pharmacotherapy

Pharmacological treatment of cancer pain is largely based on the World Health Organization analgesic ladder method [35]: drugs should be given "by the clock," rather than "on demand"; preferred way to assume drugs is by the mouth, rather than invasive routes; clinicians should avoid fixed doses of analgesics and adapt drug doses to the individual patient response; and careful management of analgesic unwanted side effects is warranted. This guideline recommends to choose the analgesic according to the pain intensity: non-opioids (paracetamol, aspirin, and nonsteroidal anti-inflammatory drugs) for mild pain management, non-opioids and second-step opioids (codeine, tramadol, and low doses of oxycodone) for moderate pain, and non-opioids and strong opioids for severe pain treatment. Additional – "adjuvants" – drugs should be added at any steps for specific pain syndromes, such as neuropathic pain and pain arising from the cancer bone invasion. A rapid-onset analgesic should be available for the management of pain exacerbations (breakthrough pain, such as pain incident to movements).

This approach is simple to be used also in non-specialist care, inexpensive, and 80% effective [36]. Therefore, it is the mainstay of bone cancer pain treatment. There are no specific guidelines about the management of pain induced by metastases to the bone or from prostate skeletal metastases [37].

19.7 **Non-opioid Analgesic** (See Also Table 19.5)

Paracetamol is largely used as a first-step treatment in cancer pain, as single drug – 500–1000 mg, as needed or every 4–6 h – or combined with opioids. At doses lower than 4000 mg/day, paracetamol toxicity is not clinically relevant. However, it should be considered a weak analgesic. There are insufficient evidences of an improved analgesic efficacy adding paracetamol to a strong opioid [38, 39].

Considering the inflammatory nature of bone cancer pain [40], nonsteroidal anti-inflammatory drugs sound a rationale choice. NSAID efficacy in cancer pain is evidenced by several clinical studies [39, 41]. However, specific analyses of the bone cancer subgroup population are not available. NSAID's gastrotoxicity is well known and increased by a concomitant steroidal therapy. When gastric risk factors are identified, a selective COX-2 NSAID, as etoricoxib, 90 mg once day, is a valid alternative. NSAIDs are contraindicated in severe renal or hepatic insufficiencies, in heart failure, and in patients with bleeding risks. Many clinicians avoid associating NSAIDs to strong opioids when managing severe cancer pain. However, when NSAID's clinical risks are lacking, the association with opioids is advisable, since the augmented analgesic efficacy [38, 39]. Moreover, NSAID collateral effects are not increased by the opioids therapy [38].

Nonsteroidal anti-inflammatory drugs' common choices in palliative care are diclofenac, 50–100 mg BID or TID or – fast-onset release – 50 mg on request; ibuprofen, 600–800 mg TID or as needed; ketoprofen, 50 mg TID or as needed or 200 mg slow release once day; and ketorolac, 10–30 mg, every 6 or 8 h or as needed, only for short periods of treatment. NSAIDs used in cancer pain studies have shown equivalent efficacies, when adjusted to the right dose [41]. Higher doses are more effective on pain; however, toxicity is weakly linked to NSAID's dose and closely dependent from comorbidities and length of the treatment [41]. Intravenous, intramuscular, or subcutaneous injections or suppository route of NSAIDs is equally effective and has the same gastric toxicity of the oral forms; thus, they should be reserved only for patients with unavailability of oral route of administration. Gel or ointment NSAIDs don't penetrate to deep tissues and are considered ineffective in cancer bone pain.

19.8 **Opioids** (See Also Table 19.5)

Opioids are the mainstay in the cancer pain therapy. At the right dose, opioids are very effective in cancer pain, and a skillful use could minimize the relevance of unwanted side effects. In the last years, a surge in US hospital admissions, and even deaths, provoked by opioid overdosage consequences, mainly in patients with chronic non-malignant pain conditions, has pushed authorities to limit long-term opioid therapy eligibility and high dosages of opioid-based schedules [42]. Thus, recent guidelines suggest to refer to

Table 19.5 Analgesic pharmacotherapy in cancer-induced bone pain

Drug class	Drug	Suggested starting dose	Comments
Paracetamol	Paracetamol	500–1000 mg, as needed or every 4–6 h	Maximum dose 4000 mg/day
Nonsteroidal anti-inflammatory drugs Add gastroprotective drugs (as omeprazole, 20 mg tablets, or pantoprazole 20 mg tablets) in elderly and frail patients	Diclofenac	50 mg as needed or every 6 h or 100 mg every 12 h (extended release tablets)	Maximum dose 200 mg/day
	Ketoprofen	50 mg as needed or every 6 h or 100–200 mg once a day (extended-release capsules)	Maximum daily dose 200 mg
	Ibuprofen	600 mg as needed or every 6 h or 800 mg every 12 h (extended-release tablets)	Maximum dose 2400 mg/day
	Ketorolac	10–30 mg as needed or every 6–8 h	Maximum daily dose 120 mg. Consider only for short-period treatments
Opioids Add prophylactic laxatives drug, as macrogol	Codeine (in association with paracetamol 1000 mg)	30–60 mg as needed or every 4–6 h	Maximum paracetamol daily dose 4000 mg
	Tramadol	50 mg as needed or every 6 h or 100 mg every 12 or 24 h (extended-release tablets) up to 400 mg/day	Use lower dosage when other serotoninergic drugs are administered Consider halved dose in parenteral administration Maximal daily dose 400 mg
	Tapentadol	50–100 twice a day up to 500 mg/day	Titrate every 2–3 days from lower dosage. Consider tramadol or other analgesics as rescue drug for episodic pain exacerbations
	Buprenorphine	35–70 mcg/h, 3-day patch	Upper maximum dose 140 mcG/h. Consider other opioids, rather than buprenorphine sublingual tablets, as rescue medication
	Morphine	5–10 mg every 4 h immediate release formulation or 10 every 12 h (slow-release tablets)	Titrate to effect every 24 h increasing of 30–50 % of daily dose
	Oxycodone	5 mg (associated to paracetamol 325 mg) every 4 h 5–10 mg (alone or associated to naloxone), extended release tablets every 12 h Immediate release tablets and solutions can be used starting with 5–10 mg every 4 h	Maximum dose in naloxone-associated tablets, 160 mg/day
	Hydromorphone	1 mg immediate-release tablets should be given every 4 h – 8 mg once a day prolonged release formulation	Use rapid onset morphine or oxycodone–paracetamol as rescue drugs for pain exacerbations
	Fentanyl (transdermal)	12–100 mcg/h 3 days patch	

(continued)

Table 19.5 (continued)

Drug class	Drug	Suggested starting dose	Comments
	Fentanyl (intranasal or transmucosal)	100 mcg intranasal spray or buccal tablet minimum dose (50 mcg are available for intranasal formulation) and higher dosing from 200 to 800 mcg can be used in tolerant patients	Use only for breakthrough cancer pain, in patients on oral morphine or other opioids ATC therapy of at least 60 mg morphine per day or different opioid equivalent doses Maximum 4 doses/day, with a time period of at least 4 h between doses Starting from minimum dose. Titrate to adequate dosage
Steroids	*Prednisone*	5–25 mg once day	
	Desametasone	0,5–4 mg once day	
Neuropathic pain drugs	*Gabapentin*	300 mg three times a day	Maximum dose 3600 mg/day
	Pregabalin	75 mg every 12 h	Maximum dose 600 mg/day

More conservative dose should be considered in frail patients and in combination therapies

specialized pain clinics patients who need dosage above 80–120 mg/day morphine equivalents or who present symptoms of opioid abuse or misuse [42, 43]. Even if there are no analogous warnings in the cancer pain management, a careful conduct is warranted in long survival patients, like in the prostate cancer population.

Codeine is the prototype of the second-step opioid. Suggested schedule of treatment is 30–60 mg as needed or every 4–6 h. In the commonly used associations to paracetamol, this latter maximum dose should not exceed 4000 mg per day. Other opioid drugs with an upper limit of the dose range are the partial mu agonist buprenorphine that is most used as transdermal patches, until a maximum dosage of 140 mcg/h, and the mixed mu agonist and noradrenergic–serotoninergic analgesics tramadol, used until the dose of 400 mg/die by the mouth, and tapentadol that can be prescribed until a maximum dose limit of 500 mg/day [44]. In the last years, the strong opioid oxycodone has been combined to naloxone, in order to reduce its annoying constipating effect, as slow-release tablets, with a maximal dose of 160 mg/day. However, many clinicians are used to prescribe low doses of strong opioids (such as 5 mg of oral morphine every 4 h) also in mild cancer pain treatment, and usefulness to differentiate second-step from third-step categories of analgesics is debated [44–46].

WHO and EAPC guidelines recommend to initiate an opioid therapy using oral drugs, reserving transdermal route to non-naive patients. There are no significant differences in opioid starting therapies based on immediate release and sustained release drugs, taken at the right time [45, 47]. Experts suggest to start with low doses and carefully titrate the opioids every each day or every three days, until adequate pain control is reached [44]. A short-acting opioid (such as oral morphine immediate release) could be prescribed as a rescue analgesic, in association with long-acting opioids, to reach an adequate analgesic level in the titration period [44]. If an opioid treatment doesn't provide an acceptable pain control, or patient experiences non-tolerable side effects, or both, it is advisable to switch toward a different opioids [45]. Transdermal opioids may be effective alternatives in patients unable to swallow [45].

Oral morphine, hydromorphone, and oxycodone have akin analgesic profiles: onset of analgesia in 30–40′ and maximum pain relief after about 1 h, lasting for 3–4 h. All of them are also available as slow-release tablets or capsules, with a 12–24 h enduring analgesia. Their risk–efficacy profiles are comparable, and each of these three drugs could be used as first choice for cancer pain [45]. Transdermal fentanyl or buprenorphine are convenient alternative to oral opioids in some patients [45]. Oral methadone is a first-choice option in the opioid switching practice, but its use is better reserved to experienced clinicians [45].

Episodic pain exacerbations – breakthrough pain – often triggered by movements or weight bearing, are typical features of the cancer-induced bone pain [26]. Fast-acting opioids are the appropriate treatment of the breakthrough cancer pain. Intranasal and oral transmucosal fentanyls have a very quick onset of analgesic activity and should be offered, combined with an around-the-clock opioid treatment, to manage non-volitional episodic cancer pain [48]. Incident pain to movements, when predictable, could be preempted with short-onset oral opioids, taken 1 h before painful events [45].

19.9 Adjuvant Drugs

Steroids have been used extensively in cancer-induced bone pain, largely on the basis of favorable clinical impression [49, 50]. However, literature on the corticosteroids role in cancer pain is very poor and permits to show only a very low evidence of moderate analgesic effect for short-period treatments [51–53]. Clinical studies focused on cancer bone pain are lacking. Steroids are widely prescribed reason of their downregulatory effect on adrenal androgens and androgen receptors. These patients on steroidal therapy may show improvements in several aspects of quality of life and a moderate pain relief. In prostate cancer are commonly used low doses of prednisone or prednisolone, 5–25 mg/day, or dexamethasone, 0,5–4 mg/die [54]. Only one study has specifically examined pain reduction produced by corticosteroids in prostate cancer patients as primary end point [55]. This retrospective study showed a moderate pain improvement, mostly limited to a few month period, in 38 % of the treated patients.

Basic research has documented that cancer may generate pain in bones through neuropathic mechanisms. Several clinicians are used to add neuropathic pain drugs in difficult to treat cancer-induced bone pain patients [56, 57]. Gabapentin, in a range of 900–3600 mg/day dose, and pregabalin, in a 150–600 mg/day dose, are the more often used drugs. However, a recent, robust study on pregabalin analgesic effect in metastatic to the bone cancer failed to show a pain reduction in treated patients [58]. Therefore, at the moment the use of drugs for neuropathic pain should only be recommended in patients with a diagnosis of neuropathic pain due to associated neurological lesions besides bone metastases, such as for compressive radiculopathy, and after consulting a specialist in unclear cases [26, 59, 60].

19.10 When Opioids Do Not Work

Different strategies can be adopted when patients do not respond to first-line analgesic pharmacotherapy. These strategies include more complex pharmacological and non-pharmacological therapies. Opioid responsiveness can be improved by switching to a different opioid [43], or the route of administration can be changed from oral and transdermal to intravenous or spinal. Spinal opioid administration can be proposed for non-opioid analgesics such as ziconotide or for combination of opioid and non-opioid analgesics such as local anesthetics. Invasive procedures for pain relief can be indicated in selected patients. However, all these options require specialist advice in a multidisciplinary setting including specialists in, at least, oncology, radiation therapy palliative care, and pain therapy.

19.11 Pain: Prognosis Implications, Role of Bone-Targeting, and Disease-Modifying Agents

Bone-targeting agents are defined as those compounds in clinical use that act primarily within bone.

A summary of the efficacy of these agents, including end points measuring pain, QOL, and markers of bone turnover, is shown in the Table 19.6 [61].

Several systemic disease-modifying agents also have effects on skeletal outcomes and overall survival in patients with mCRPC as shown in the Table 19.7 [61].

The development of bone target therapies has been largely based on definition of therapy outcome using the concept of SRE and skeletal symptomatic events (SSEs).

Table 19.6 Skeletal outcome and overall survival in randomized studies of bone targeting agents

Agent	Study	Treatment arms	Time to first SRE or SSE Median (months), HR [95 % CI]	Overall survival Median (months), HR [95 % CI]
Zoledronic acid	Saad et al. [68, 69]	Zoledronic acid (214) vs. placebo (208)	16.0 vs. 10.5, 0.677 [0.505–0.908], $p=0.009$	17.9 vs. 15.2, $p=0.091$
Denosumab	Fizazi et al. [70]	Denosumab (950) vs. zoledronic acid (951)	20.7 vs. 17.1, 0.82 [0.71–0.95], $p=0.0002$ for non inferiority, $p=0.008$ for superiority	19.4 vs. 19.8, 1.03 [0.91–1.17], $p=0.65$
^{89}Sr	Porter et al. [71]; Oosterhof et al. [72]. (EORTC-GU group)	^{89}Sr vs. placebo (126 total); Sr (101) vs. local field radiotherapy (102)	Not reported; not reported	6.2 vs. 7.8, $p=0.06$; 7.2 vs. 11, 1.34 [1.01–1.75], $p=0.0457$
^{223}Ra	ALSYMPCA; Parker et al. [62]; Sartor et al. [63]	^{223}Ra vs. placebo	15.6 vs. 9.8, 0.66 [0.52–0.83], $p<0.001$	14.9 vs. 11.3, 070 [0.58–0.83], $p<0.001$

Modified from Body et al. [61]

Table 19.7 Skeletal outcome and overall survival in randomized studies disease modifying agents

Agent	Study	Treatment arms	Time to first SRE or SSE Median (months), HR [95 % CI]	Overall survival Median (months), HR [95 % CI]
Docetaxel	TAX 327; Tannock et al. [73]	Docetaxel q3w + prednisone (335) vs. mitoxantrone q3w + prednisone	Not reported	18.9 vs. 16.5, 0.76 [0.62–0.94], $p=0.009$
	ASCENT; Beer et al. [74]	Docetaxel + calcitriol (125) vs. docetaxel + placebo (125)	13.4 vs. 11.9, 0.78 [0.57–1.074], $p=0.13$	Not assessed vs. 16.4, 0.67 [0.45–0.97], $p=0.04$
Cabazitaxel	TROPIC; de Bono et al. [75]	Cabazitaxel + prednisone (378) vs. mitoxantrone + prednisone (377)	Not reported	15.1 vs. 12.7, 0.70 [0.59–0.83], $p<0.0001$
Abiraterone	COU-AA301; Fizazi et al. [76]; Logothetis et al. [64];	Abiraterone + prednisone (797) vs. placebo + prednisone (398)	25.0 vs. 20.3, 0.615 [0.478–0.791], $p=0.0001$	15.8 vs. 11.2, 0.74 [0.64–0.86], $p<0.001$
	COU-AA302; Ryan et al. [77] .	Abiraterone + prednisone (546) vs. placebo + prednisone (542)	Not reported	Not assessed vs. 27.2, 0.75 [0.61–0.93], $p=0.01$
Enzalutamide	AFFIRM; Scher et al. [78]; Fizazi et al. [65];	Enzalutamide (800) vs. placebo (399)	16.7 vs. 13.3, 0.69 [0.57–0.84], $p<0.001$	18.4 vs. 13.6, 0.63 [0.53–0.75], $p<0.001$
	PREVAIL; Beer et al. [79]	Enzalutamide (626) vs. placebo (532)	31.1 vs. 31.3, 0.72 [0.61–0.84], $p<0.001$	32.4 vs. 30.2, 0.71 [0.60–0.84], $p<0.001$

Modified from Body et al. [61]

The main difference between SREs and SSEs lies in their assessment. SREs have to be radiologically confirmed, while SSEs are assessed on patient symptoms and are therefore identified clinically. SSEs are considered to be more relevant to daily routine clinical care than classical SREs, and not surprisingly, the use of SSEs as an end point is becoming more common in clinical trial design. In 2013 and 2014, time to first SSEs as an end point has been used in trials of bone – targeting agents shown to prolong overall survival [62, 63].

Table 19.8 Changes in pain severity and pain interference from baseline to week 13

	Mean change from baseline (95 % CI)		Treatment difference	*p* value
	Enzalutamide group ($n=591$)	Placebo group ($n=239$)		
Pain severity	−0.15 (−0.28 to −0.02)	0.50 (0.29–0.70)	−0.65 (−0.89 to −0.41)	<0.0001
Pain interference	−0.01 (0.18 to −0.16)	0.74 (0.47–1.00)	−0.74 (−1.06 to −0.43)	<0.0001

Modified from Fizazi et al. [65]

Later in the years, with the introduction of new systemic hormonal therapy such as abiraterone and enzalutamide, the effect of these agents on pain control was explorated. In 2012 Logothetis et al. assessed data collected as part of the randomized phase III COU-AA301 trial of abiraterone acetate plus prednisone versus placebo plus prednisone. They specifically assessed clinically meaningful changes in pain intensity and interference with daily living and found out that abiraterone plus prednisone offers significant benefits compared with prednisone alone in terms of pain relief, delayed pain progression, and prevention of skeletal-related events. In patients with clinically significant pain at baseline, abiraterone acetate and prednisone resulted in significantly more palliation of pain intensity than did prednisone only (45 % vs 28.8 %) [64].

In 2014 Fizazi et al. presented an analyses of secondary end points, including occurrence of skeletal-related events, measures of pain control, and patient-reported health-related quality of life from the AFFIRM trial. They demonstrated that in addition to improving overall survival compared to placebo in patients affected by mCRPC, enzalutamide versus placebo decreases pain severity and pain interference, delays time to pain progression, and improves well-being and QOL. Data regarding changes in pain severity and pain interference are summarized in Table 19.8 [65].

Bisphosphonates and denosumab are well-established therapies to reduce the frequency and severity of skeletal-related events in patients with bone metastasis.

Bisphosphonates operate by inducing osteoclast apoptosis, thereby preventing the development of cancer-induced bone lesions; denosumab acts by binding to and inhibiting receptor activator of nuclear factor kappa B ligand (RANKL), leading to the loss of osteoclasts from bone surfaces [66].

However, the analgesic effect of these medications on bone pain is uncertain. A systematic review has been recently published by Porta Sales et al. Authors analyzed 43 studies enrolling 8595 and 7590 patients, respectively, in bisphosphonate and denosumab trials. Twenty-two (79 %) of the 28 placebo-controlled trials found no analgesic benefit for bisphosphonates. None of the denosumab studies assessed direct pain relief [67].

In conclusion evidence to support an analgesic role for bisphosphonates and denosumab is weak. Bisphosphonates and denosumab appear to be beneficial in preventing pain by delaying the onset of bone pain rather than by producing an analgesic effect per se. In Table 19.9 is summarized the study regarding prostate cancer [67].

Conclusions

Chronic pain is a very significant complication of prostate cancer metastatic to the bones. Pain assessment and treatment is paramount for the quality of life of patients in all phases of the disease and with different prognoses. Careful individualization of symptomatic and palliative interventions and integration with oncological management strategies (chemotherapy hormonal, radiotherapy radionuclide bone target agents, analgesic therapies) requires close collaboration and multidisciplinary settings of care including oncology and palliative care specialists. Continuity of care from diagnosis to the end of life needs that transition of care from active treatment to palliative care is carefully conducted and targeted to individual patient's characteristics.

Table 19.9 Studies with bisphosphonates in prostate cancer patients

Author (year)	Study design	Tumour type	Intervention	Comparator	No. pts enrolled (analysed)	Pain as inclusion criteria	Main outcome measure description	Relative effect estimates	Side-effects	Comments and [risk of bias]Ω
Adami and Milan [80]	RCT Parallel	PC	Clodronate 300 mg/IV/d × 2 wks	Placebo	13 (13)	NO	Main aim: *Bone pain relief* Pain assessment: "VAS 20 cm" "daily analgesic consumption of ketoprofen" at 2 wks	Significant reduction in pain score ($p<0.01$) and analgesic consumption	Not reported	Additional information given of no pain benefit with oral formulation vs. parenteral (at 2 wks) Limitations *not* discussed
Elomaa [81]	RCT Parallel	PC	Clodronate 3.2 g/PO/d × 1 mo. followed by 1.6 g/PO/d.	Placebo	75 (33)	YES	Main aim: *Bone pain relief* Pain assessment: "Presence/absence of bone pain" "Analgesic use" "every mo."	% pts. without pain At 1st mo. CLO 34 % vs. PLA 18 %; NS At 3rd mo. CLO 29 % vs. PLA 4 %; NS At 6th mo. CLO 18 % vs. PLA 15 %; NS	AEs related with PC progression	No. pts at mo. 6; at 1st mo. (63 pts), at 3rd mo. (44 pts) Pain assessed by physician and patient All pts. received ChT Limitations *not* discussed
Kylmälä [82]	RCT Parallel	PC	Clodronate: 300 mg/IV/×5 d followed by 1600 mg/PO/d × 12 months	Placebo	57 (54)	NO	Main aim: *Bone pain relief* Pain assessment: "VAS by patients 5-point scale by doctors"; "Pain reduction at 1,3,6,12 mo. from BL"	Pain reduction was 10 % greater in CLO vs. PLA: NS	More frequent side-effects: N/V 33 %, but NS. No renal impairment observed	All pts. received ChT. Limitations *not* discussed
Smith [83]	RCT Parallel	PC	Group 1: Etidronate 7.5 mg/kg/IV×3 d followed 400 mg/PO/d Group 2: Etidronate 7.5 mg/kg/IV Group 3: Etidronate 400 mg/PO/d	Placebo	57 (50)	YES	Main aim: *Bone pain relief* Pain assessment: "VAS Pain relief at 1 mo from BL" "Analgesic use" "every day"	No effective palliation of bone pain and analgesic use	No serious side-effects reported. Digestive upset was the most common side-effect.	Assessment of pain and analgesic use are not described. Pain assessed by patient and doctor. Limitations *not* discussed

Small [84]	RCT Parallel	PC	Pamidronate 90 mg/IV/q3 wks	Placebo	378 (301)	YES	Main aim: *Bone pain relief* Difference in "Worst pain" to wk 9 from BL	Mean change from BL BPI: PAM −0.86 ± 0.21 vs. PLA −0.69 ± 0.21 $p = 0.576$	Overall, PAM was well tolerated AEs: no difference between PAM and PLA	Polled results of 2 RCT Phase III Pain assessment using BPI worst pain Limitations discussed
Saad [68]	RCT Parallel	PC	Zoledronic 4 mg/IV/q3 w (ZOL4) Zoledronic 8/4/IV/q3w (*a reduction from 8 mg to 4 mg due to renal toxicity*: ZOL8/4)	Placebo	643 (643)	NO	Main aim : *Prevention SRE* Pain assessment: "Mean change pain score at 15 mo. from BL" "every 6 wks"	Mean increase from BL in pain score at 15 mo.: ZOL4 0.58 (0.29; 0.87) vs. Placebo 0.88 (0.61; 1.15); NS ZOL8/4 0.43 (0.16; 0.70) vs. Placebo 0.88 (0.61; 1.15); $p = 0.026$ 95 % CI	In ZOL group fatigue, anaemia, myalgia, fever, and lower-limb oedema occurred ≥ 5 % in at least 5 % more frequent than in PLA group. Few hypo Ca++, increase creatinine and anaemia were reported	Pain was assess using BPI and pain score was a composite of worst pain, least pain, average pain of the last 7 days, and pain right now. Limitations *not* discussed
Weinfurt [85]	RCT parallel Analytic re-analysis	PC	Zoledronic 4 mg/IV/q4 w	Placebo	221 (138)	NO	Main aim: *Re-analysis of bone pain relief* Pain assessment: "% of responders in each arm at 60 wks"	ZOL: 33 % responders PLA: 25 % responders $p = 0.036$ (95 % CI 0.5; 15.6)	Not reported	Re-analyse (Saad [68]) examining the proportions of patients with pain relief. Responders decrease ≥2 points in BPI composite of worst pain, least pain, average pain and current pain Limitations discussed [4, 6]
Mitsiades [86]	RCT Parallel unblinded	PC	Zoledronic 4 mg/IV/4 wks+ DXT 4 mg–1 mg/PO/d+ Octreotide 20 mg/IM/28 d (ZOD)	Zondronate 4 mg/IV/4 wks	38 (38)	NO	Main aim: *Cancer progression* *Survival* *Bone pain relief* Pain assessment: "6-point score combining pain severity and analgesic use" "every 4 wks"	Time to return to basal bone pain. ZOD median >14 months ZOL median 4 months $p < 0.0001$	Three patients developed transient hyperglycaemia in the ZOD arm	ZOL no effect on preventing pain nor analgesic vs. ZDO Limitations *not* discussed

(continued)

Table 19.9 (continued)

Author (year)	Study design	Tumour type	Intervention	Comparator	No. pts enrolled (analysed)	Pain as inclusion criteria	Main outcome measure description	Relative effect estimates	Side-effects	Comments and [risk of bias]Ω
Wang [87]	RCT Parallel unblinded	PC	Zoledronic acid 4 mg/IV/q4 w	Clodronate 1600 mg/ VO/d	137 (137)	NO	Main aims: *Bone progression-free survival (BPFS)* *Bone mineral density (BMD)* *Survival* *SRE* *Pain* *Analgesic use* Pain assessment: "VAS every day to average pain of 3 mo." "Decrease at least 2 points in VAS"	At month 6 (mean pain reduction): ZOL VAS 1.5 (0.7; 2.3) C LO VAS 2.3 (1.8; 2.8); NS At 3 months pain was improved in ZOL 92 % vs. CLO 76 % $p=0.02$ 95 % CI	Most common AEs: ZOL: Renal impair 45 % Gastrointestinal 16 % CLO: Renal impair 34 % Gastrointestinal 31 % Jaw osteonecrosis: 1 patient in ZOL	Mean pain improvement not defined (month 3) Limitations *not* discussed

Modified from Porta-Sales et al. [67]

RCT indicates randomised clinical trial, *PC* prostate cancer, *MX* mixed sample, *SRE* skeletal related events, *N* nausea, *V* vomiting, *PO* per os, *IV* intravenous, *d* day, *mo* month/s, *wks* weeks, *PLA* placebo, *CLO* clodronate, *PAM* pamidronate, *IBAN* ibandronate, *ZOL* zoledronic acid, *DENO* denosomab, *NS* not statistically significant, *BL* baseline, *VAS* visual analogue scale, *MP DMED* daily morphine equivalent dose, *Pts.* patients, *ChT* chemotherapy, *HmT* hormonotherapy, *Δ Control* group that does not receive the treatment being studied nor a placebo to control the treatment arm

References

1. Bubendorf L et al (2000) Metastatic patterns of prostate cancer: an autopsy study of 1,589 patients. Hum Pathol 31:578–583
2. Scher HI, Chung LW (1994) Bone metastases: improving the therapeutic index. Semin Oncol 21:630–656
3. Smith MR et al (2015) Denosumab for the prevention of skeletal complications in metastatic castration-resistant prostate cancer: comparison of skeletal-related events and symptomatic skeletal events. Ann Oncol 26:368–374
4. von Moos R, Sternberg C, Body JJ, Bokemeyer C (2013) Reducing the burden of bone metastases: current concepts and treatment options. Support Care Cancer 21:1773–1783
5. Halabi S, Vogelzang NJ, Kornblith AB, Ou SS, Kantoff PW, Dawson NA, Small EJ (2008) Pain predicts overall survival in men with metastatic castration-refractory prostate cancer. J Clin Oncol 26(15):2544–2549
6. Oefelein MG, Ricchiuti V, Conrad W, Resnick MI (2002) Skeletal fractures negatively correlate with overall survival in men with prostate cancer. J Urol 168(3):1005–1007
7. Depuy V et al (2007) Effects of skeletal morbidities on longitudinal patient-reported outcomes and survival in patients with metastatic prostate cancer. Support Care Cancer 15:869–876
8. Nørgaard M et al (2010) Skeletal related events, bone metastasis and survival of prostate cancer: a population based cohort study in Denmark (1999 to 2007). J Urol 184:162–167
9. Berry WR, Laszlo J, Cox E et al (1979) Prognostic factors in metastatic and hormonally unresponsive carcinoma of the prostate. Cancer 44:763–775
10. Emrich LJ, Priore RL, Murphy GP et al (1985) Prognostic factors in patients with advanced stage prostate cancer. Cancer Res 45:5173–5179
11. Berthold DR, Pond G, De Wit R et al (2006) Association of pain and quality of life (QOL) response with PSA response and survival of patients (pts) with metastatic hormone refractory prostate cancer (mHRPC) treated with docetaxel or mitoxantrone in the TAX-327 study. J Clin Oncol. 24:221s(suppl, abstr 4516)
12. Armstrong A, Garrett-Mayer ES, Ou Yang YC et al (2007) A contemporary prognostic nomogram for men with hormone-refractory metastatic prostate cancer: a TAX 327 study analysis. Clin Cancer Res 13:6396–6403
13. Turner SL, Gruenewald S, Spry N, Gebski V; Metastron Users Group (2001) Less pain does equal better quality of life following strontium-89 therapy for metastatic prostate cancer. Br J Cancer 84(3): 297–302.
14. Wang C, Shen Y (2012) Study on the distribution features of bone metastases in prostate cancer. Nucl Med Commun 33(4):379–383
15. Wang CY, Wu GY, Shen MJ, Cui KW, Shen Y (2013) Comparison of distribution characteristics of metastatic bone lesions between breast and prostate carcinomas. Oncol Lett 5:391–397
16. Conti G et al (2008) Prostate cancer metastases to bone: observational study for the evaluation of clinical presentation, course and treatment patterns. Presentation of the METAURO protocol and of patient baseline features. Arch Ital Urol Androl 80:59–64
17. Grond S, Zeck D, Diefenbach C et al (1996) Assessment of cancer pain: a prospective evaluation in 2266 cancer patients referred to a pain service. Pain 64(1):107–114
18. Banning A, Sjogren P, Henriksen H (1991) Pain causes in 200 patients referred to a multidisciplinary cancer pain clinic. Pain 45(1):45–48
19. Caraceni A, Portenoy RK (1999) An international survey of cancer pain characteristics and syndromes. Pain 82:263–274
20. Middlemiss T, Laird BJ, Fallon MT (2011) Mechanisms of cancer-induced bone pain. Clin Oncol 23:387–392
21. Dy SM, Asch SM, Naeim A, Sanati H, Walling A, Lorenz KA (2008) Evidence-based standards for cancer pain management. J Clin Oncol 26:3879–3885
22. Mercadante S (1997) Malignant bone pain: pathophysiology and treatment. Pain 69:1–18
23. Løhre ET, Klepstad P, Bennett MI, Brunelli C, Caraceni A, Fainsinger RL, Knudsen AK, Mercadante S, Sjøgren P, Kaasa S; European Association for Palliative Care Research Network (2016) From "Breakthrough" to "Episodic" Cancer Pain? A European Association for Palliative Care Research Network Expert Delphi Survey Toward a Common Terminology and Classification of Transient Cancer Pain Exacerbations. J Pain Symptom Manage. pii:S0885-3924(16)00070-1. doi:10.1016/j.jpainsymman.2015.12.329. [Epub ahead of print]
24. Davies A, Buchanan A, Zeppetella G, Porta-Sales J, Likar R, Weismayr W et al (2013) Breakthrough cancer pain: an observational study of 1000 European oncology patients. J Pain Symptom Manage 46:619–628
25. Payne R (1993) Pain management in the patient with prostate cancer. Cancer 71(suppl):1131–1137
26. Falk S, Dickenson AH (2014) Pain and nociception: mechanisms of cancer-induced bone pain. J Clin Oncol 32:1647–1654
27. Brunelli C, Bennett MI, Kaasa S, Fainsinger R, Sjøgren P, Mercadante S, Løhre ET, Caraceni A; European Association for Palliative Care (EAPC) Research Network; International Association for the Study of Pain (IASP) Cancer Pain Special Interest Group (2014) Classification of neuropathic pain in cancer patients: a Delphi expert survey report and EAPC/IASP proposal of an algorithm for diagnostic criteria. Pain. 155(12):2707–2713
28. Basch E (2012) Beyond the FDA PRO guidance: steps toward integrating meaningful patient-reported outcomes into regulatory trials and US drug labels. Value Health 15:401–403

29. Hjermstad MJ, Fayers PM, Haugen DF, Caraceni A, Hanks GW, Loge JH, Fainsinger R, Aass N, Kaasa S; European Palliative Care Research Collaborative (EPCRC) (2011) Studies comparing Numerical Rating S cales, Verbal Rating Scales, and Visual Analogue Scales for assessment of pain intensity in adults: a systematic literature review. J Pain Symptom Manage. 41(6):1073–1093
30. Brunelli C, Zecca E, Martini C, Campa T, Fagnoni E, Bagnasco M, Lanata L, Caraceni A (2010) Comparison of numerical and verbal rating scales to measure pain exacerbations in patients with chronic cancer pain. Health Qual Life Outcomes 8:42
31. Daut RL, Cleeland C, Flanery RC (1983) Development of the Wisconsin Brief Pain Questionnaire to assess pain in cancer and other disease. Pain 17:197–210
32. Melzack R (1975) The McGill Pain questionnaire. Major properties and scoring methods. Pain 1:277–299
33. Fishman B, Pasernak S, Wallenstein SL, Houde R, Holland JC, Foley KM (1987) The Memorial Pain Assessment Card: a valid instrument for the evaluation of cancer pain. Cancer 60:115–118
34. Caraceni A (1996) Clinicopathology correlates of common cancer syndromes. Hematol Oncol Clin North Am 10:57–78
35. World Health Organization (1996) Cancer pain relief, 2nd edn. WHO, Geneva
36. Ventafridda V, Tamburini M, Caraceni A, De Conno F, Naldi F (1987) A validation study of the WHO method for cancer pain relief. Cancer 59:850–856
37. Kane CM, Hoskin P, Bennett MI (2015) Cancer induced bone pain. BMJ 350:h315
38. Nabal M, Librada S, Redondo MJ et al (2012) The role of paracetamol and nonsteroidal anti-inflammatory drugs in addition to WHO step II opioids in the control of pain in advanced cancer. A systemic review of the literature. Palliat Med 26:305–312
39. Vardy J, Agar M (2014) Nonopioid drugs in the treatment of cancer pain. J Clin Oncol 32:1677–1690
40. Mantyh P (2013) Bone cancer pain: causes, consequences, and therapeutic opportunities. Pain 154:S54–S62
41. McNicol E, Strassels SA, Goudas L, Lau J, Carr DB (2005) NSAIDS or paracetamol, alone or combined with opioids, for cancer pain. Cochrane Database Syst Rev (1):CD005180. Review. Update in: Cochrane Database Syst Rev
42. Center for Disease Control and Prevention, U.S. Department of Health and Human Services (2016) CDC Guideline for prescribing opioids for chronic pain – United States, 2016. Morb Mortal Wkly Rep 65:1–49
43. Franklyn GM (2014) Opioids for chronic noncancer pain. A position paper of the American Academy of Neurology. Neurology 83:1277–1284
44. Portenoy RK (2011) Treatment of cancer pain. Lancet 377:2236–2247
45. Caraceni A, Hanks G, Kaasa S et al (2012) Use of opioid analgesics in the treatment of cancer pain: evidence-based recommendations from the EAPC. Lancet Oncol 13:e58–e68
46. Bandieri E, Romero M, Ripamonti CI, Artioli F, Sichetti D, Fanizza C, Santini D, Cavanna L, Melotti B, Conte PF, Roila F, Cascinu S, Bruera E, Tognoni G, Luppi M (2016) Randomized trial of low-dose morphine versus weak opioids in moderate cancer pain. J Clin Oncol 34(5):436–442
47. Klepstad P, Kaasa S, Jystad A et al (2003) Immediate- or sustained-release morphine for dose findings during start of morphine to cancer patients: a randomized, double-blind trial. Pain 101:193–198
48. Caraceni A, Davies A, Poulain P et al (2013) Guidelines for the management of breakthrough pain in patients with cancer. J Natl Compr Canc Netw 11(Suppl 1):S29–S36
49. Shih A, Jackson KC 2nd (2007) Role of corticosteroids in palliative care. J Pain Palliat Care Pharmacother 21(4):69–76, Review
50. Leppert W, Buss T (2012) The role of corticosteroid in the treatment of pain in cancer patients. Curr Pain Headache Rep 16:307–313
51. Paulsen O, Aass N, Kaasa S et al (2013) Do corticosteroid provide analgesic effects in cancer patients? A systematic literature review. J Pain Symptom Manage 46:6–105
52. Paulsen O, Klepstad P, Rosland JH et al (2014) Efficacy of methylprednisolone on pain, fatigue, and appetite loss in patients with advanced cancer using opioids: a randomized, placebo-controlled double-blind trial. J Clin Oncol 32:3221–3228
53. Haywood A, Good P, Khan S et al (2015) Corticosteroids for the management of cancer-related pain in adults (Review). Cochrane Database Syst Rev (4):CD010756
54. De Santis M, Saad F (2016) Practical guidance on the role of corticosteroids in the treatment of metastatic castration-resistant prostate cancer. Urology. pii: S0090-4295(16)00146-1
55. Tannock I, Gospodarowicz M, Meakin W et al (1989) Treatment of metastatic prostatic cancer with low-dose prednisone: evaluation of pain and quality of life as pragmatic indices of response. J Clin Oncol 7:590–597
56. Caraceni A, Zecca E, Martini C et al (2008) Gabapentin for breakthrough pain due to bone metastases. Palliat Med 22:392–393
57. Sjolund KF, Yang R, Lee KH et al (2013) Randomized study of pregabalin in patients with cancer-induced bone pain. Pain Ther 2:37–48
58. Fallon M, Hoskin PJ, Colvin LA et al (2016) Randomized double-blind trial of Pregabalin versus placebo in conjunction with palliative radiotherapy for cancer-induced bone pain. J Clin Oncol 34: 550–556

59. Mulvey MR, Rolke R, Klepstad P, Caraceni A, Fallon M, Colvin L, Laird B, Bennett MI; IASP Cancer Pain SIG and the EAPC Research Network (2014) Confirming neuropathic pain in cancer patients: applying the NeuPSIG grading system in clinical practice and clinical research. Pain 155(5):859–863
60. Boland EG, Mulvey MR, Bennett MI (2015) Classification of neuropathic pain in cancer patients. Curr Opin Support Palliat Care 9:112–115
61. Body JJ, Casimiro S, Costa L (2015) Targeting bone metastases in prostate cancer: improving clinical outcome. Nat Rev Urol 12(6):340–356
62. Parker C et al (2013) Alpha emitter radium-223 and survival in metastatic prostate cancer. N Engl J Med 369:213–223
63. Sartor O et al (2014) Effect of radium-223 dichloride on symptomatic skeletal events in patients with castration-resistant prostate cancer and bone metastases: results from a phase 3, double- blind, randomised trial. Lancet Oncol 15:738–746
64. Logothetis CJ, Basch E, Molina A, Fizazi K, North SA, Chi KN, Jones RJ, Goodman OB, Mainwaring PN, Sternberg CN, Efstathiou E, Gagnon DD, Rothman M, Hao Y, Liu CS, Kheoh TS, Haqq CM, Scher HI, de Bono JS (2012) Effect of abiraterone acetate and prednisone compared with placebo and prednisone on pain control and skeletal-related events in patients with metastatic castration-resistant prostate cancer: exploratory analysis of data from the COU-AA-301 randomised trial. Lancet Oncol 13(12):1210–1217
65. Fizazi K, Scher HI, Miller K, Basch E, Sternberg CN, Cella D, Forer D, Hirmand M, de Bono JS (2014) Effect of enzalutamide on time to first skeletal-related event, pain, and quality of life in men with castration-resistant prostate cancer: results from the randomised, phase 3 AFFIRM trial. Lancet Oncol 15(10): 1147–1156
66. Baron R, Ferrari S, Russel R (2011) Denosumab and bisphosphonates: different mechanism of action and effects. Bone 48:677–692
67. Porta-Sales J, Garzón-Rodríguez C, Llorens-Torromé S, Brunelli C, Pigni A, and Caraceni A (2016) Evidence on the analgesic role of bisphosphonates and denosumab in the treatment of pain due to bone metastases: a systematic review within the European Association for Palliative Care guidelines project. Palliat Med 02692163
68. Saad F et al (2002) A randomized, placebo-controlled trial of zoledronic acid in patients with hormone-refractory metastatic prostate carcinoma. J Natl Cancer Inst 94:1458–1468
69. Saad F et al (2004) Long-term efficacy of zoledronic acid for the prevention of skeletal complications in patients with metastatic hormone-refractory prostate cancer. J Natl Cancer Inst 96:879–882
70. Fizazi K et al (2011) Denosumab versus zoledronic acid for treatment of bone metastases in men with castration-resistant prostate cancer: a randomised, double-blind study. Lancet 377:813–822
71. Porter AT et al (1993) Results of a randomized phase-III trial to evaluate the efficacy of strontium-89 adjuvant to local field external beam irradiation in the management of endocrine resistant metastatic prostate cancer. Int J Radiat Oncol Biol Phys 25:805–813
72. Oosterhof GO et al (2003) Strontium(89) chloride versus palliative local field radiotherapy in patients with hormonal escaped prostate cancer: a phase III study of the European Organisation for Research and Treatment of Cancer, Genitourinary Group. Eur Urol 44:519–526
73. Tannock IF et al (2004) Docetaxel plus prednisone or mitoxantrone plus prednisone for advanced prostate cancer. N Engl J Med 351:1502–1512
74. Beer TM et al (2007) Double-blinded randomized study of high-dose calcitriol plus docetaxel compared with placebo plus docetaxel in androgen-independent prostate cancer: a report from the ASCENT Investigators. J Clin Oncol 25:669–674
75. de Bono JS et al (2010) Prednisone plus cabazitaxel or mitoxantrone for metastatic castration-resistant prostate cancer progressing after docetaxel treatment: a randomised open-label trial. Lancet 376:1147–1154
76. Fizazi K et al (2012) Abiraterone acetate for treatment of metastatic castration-resistant prostate cancer: final overall survival analysis of the COU-AA-301 randomised, double-blind, placebo-controlled phase 3 study. Lancet Oncol 13:983–992
77. Ryan CJ et al (2013) Abiraterone in metastatic prostate cancer without previous chemotherapy. N Engl J Med 368:138–148
78. Scher HI et al (2012) Increased survival with enzalutamide in prostate cancer after chemotherapy. N Engl J Med 367:1187–1197
79. Beer TM et al (2014) Enzalutamide in metastatic prostate cancer before chemotherapy. N Engl J Med 371:424–433
80. Adami S, Mian M (1989) Clodronate therapy of metastatic bone disease in patients with prostatic carcinoma. Recent Results Cancer Res 116:67–72
81. Elomaa I, Kylmälä T, Tammela T et al (1992) Effect of oral clodronate on bone pain: a controlled study in patients with metastatic prostatic cancer. Int Urol Nephro 24:159–166
82. Kylmälä T, Taube T, Tammela TLJ et al (1997) Concomitant i.v. and oral clodronate in the relief of bone pain – a double blind placebo-controlled study in patients with prostate can- cer. Br J Cancer 76:939–942
83. Smith JA (1989) Palliation of painful bone metastases from pros- tate cancer using sodium etidronate: results of a randomized, prospective, double-blind, placebo-controlled study. J Urol 141:85–88

84. Small EJ, Smith MR, Seaman JJ et al (2003) Combined analysis of two multicenter, randomized, placebo-controlled studies of pamidronate disodium for the palliation of bone pain in men with metastatic prostate cancer. J Clin Oncol 21: 4277–4284
85. Weinfurt KP, Anstrom KJ, Castel LD et al (2006) Effect of zole- dronic acid on pain associated with bone metastasis in patients with prostate cancer. Ann Oncol 17:986–989
86. Mitsiades CS, Bogdanos J, Karamanolakis D et al (2006) Randomized controlled clinical trial of a combination of somatostatin analog and dexamethasone plus zoledronate vs. zoledronate in patients with androgen ablation-refrac- tory prostate cancer. Anticancer Res 26:3693–3700
87. Wang F, Chen W, Chen H et al (2013) Comparison between zoledronic acid and clodronate in the treatment of prostate cancer patients with bone metastases. Med Oncol 30:657–663

20 Economic Impact of Prostate Cancer Bone Metastases

Umberto Restelli, Luca Dellavedova, Davide Croce, and Lorenzo Maffioli

With an estimated 1.1 million new diagnoses per year, prostate cancer represents the second most common cancer in men worldwide, accounting for 15 % of all new male cancers. Increased prostate-specific antigen screening has resulted in higher numbers of patients being diagnosed during the early locoregional stages, when the disease is relatively indolent and asymptomatic. Patients with metastatic disease at diagnosis, contrariwise, present with significant symptom burden and have a 5-year survival rate less than 30 %. In these subjects, suppression of serum testosterone with androgen-deprivation therapy (ADT) is usually employed for initial disease control (metastatic hormone-sensitive disease), but the resistance to ADT finally occurs in almost all patients, with a progression to metastatic castration-resistant prostate cancer (mCRPC) that represents the final stage of the disease [1–4]. Advanced prostate cancer preferentially metastasizes to the bone (65–75 % of patients), causing a weakened structural integrity of the skeleton and an increased incidence of skeletal-related events (SREs) such as pathological bone fracture, spinal cord compression, hypercalcemia, and severe bone pain requiring palliative radiation therapy (RT) or surgery.

The impact of metastatic bone disease (MBD) and, thus, of SREs on patients' life is huge [5]. SREs appear to be associated with significant morbidity and are linked to decreased survival. Few years ago, Nørgaard et al. [6] reported the results of a Danish population-based cohort study in which 5-year survival of prostate cancer patients was 56 % without bone metastases, 3 % with bone metastases, and 0.7 % with bone metastases and SREs. Many other trials have reported the significant worsening in quality of life (QOL) of patients with SREs and the benefit on QOL of targeted treatments like radiation therapy [7–9]. Generally speaking, patients with no SREs have higher QOL than those with any SREs, and patients with one SRE have higher QOL than those with multiple SREs (particularly in terms of pain, as measured by standard scales). Similarly, patients with no SREs have better survival than those with one or multiple SREs.

To find proper treatments for bone metastases and SREs, anyway, is crucial not only from a clinical point of view. In the last decade, many countries have faced a reduction of healthcare services' financing due to the current global economic conjuncture: this situation leads to the need to consider also to the economic side of the

U. Restelli • D. Croce
Università Cattaneo LIUC, Crem, Italy

School of Public Health, Faculty of Health Science, University of the Witwatersrand, Johannesburg, South Africa

L. Dellavedova • L. Maffioli (✉)
Nuclear Medicine Department, ASST Ovest Milanese, Legnano, Italy
e-mail: lorenzo.maffioli@ao-legnano.it

F. Bertoldo et al. (eds.), *Bone Metastases from Prostate Cancer*,
DOI 10.1007/978-3-319-42327-2_20

problem, in terms of healthcare resource utilization (HCRU) and related costs.

The economic burden of cancer, although highly variable among subtypes [10], is substantial. In the field of prostate cancer, the significant adverse economic effects of SREs have emerged in all the targeted studies conducted in the last years. Compared with men who have prostate cancer metastatic to the bones and no SREs, men with prostate cancer metastatic to the bones experiencing at least one SRE have not only a twofold increase in the risk of death, but also a twofold increase in the number of emergency department visits and a fourfold increase in the number of hospitalizations, with an additional $ 21,000 in direct medical costs per patient attributed to SREs [11]. Skeletal complications represent a significant public health and health economic burden especially among elderly men with advanced prostate cancer, given the incidence of this disease.

The cost estimates for SREs include costs of treatments provided in the inpatient, outpatient, home health, hospice, and skilled nursing facility settings. They depend on several factors, including the sources of data, healthcare settings, perspective assumed, target population, operationalization of SRE definitions and costs, and length of follow-up [12]. Also the analytical techniques used to estimate costs may influence the results. With this limitation, in the last decade, multiple studies have been conducted to evaluate the economic burden of bone metastatic disease (and its consequences) associated to prostate cancer, in order to better understand where and how we should intervene in order to get both the highest cost-effectiveness ratio, in terms of efficiency in resources allocation, and the highest clinical benefit.

20.1 Direct Health Costs of SREs in Europe

The economic burden of skeletal-related events in patients with bone metastases from solid tumors was investigated in 2013 in a prospective multinational observational study by Hechmati et al. in four European countries: Italy, Germany, Spain, and the UK [13].

The study was conducted on 478 patients enrolled between 2008 and 2010, with age ≥18 years, bone metastases secondary to solid tumors (prostate cancer, breast cancer, lung cancer) or multiple myeloma, an Eastern Cooperative Oncology Group score between 0 and 2, and more than 6 months of life expectancy. A total of 961 skeletal-related events were considered (non-vertebral fractures, vertebral fractures, radiation to bone, spinal cord compression, surgery to bone). The costs per event varied significantly among countries, as reported in the table below.

Skeletal-related event	Mean cost per skeletal-related event (€)			
	Germany	Italy	Spain	UK
Non-vertebral fracture	1,720	2,087	3,209	2254
Vertebral fracture	2,124	2,142	6,968	1,015
Radiation to bone	1,694	2,461	2,378	704
Spinal cord compression	5,,847	4,884	7,903	12,082
Surgery to bone	9,407	3,348	4,263	7,447

In the four countries considered, more than 83 % of costs were due to inpatient stay for spinal cord compression and bone surgery. For non-vertebral fractures in the UK and Spain, more than 88 % of costs were due to inpatient stays, while in Italy and Germany, this proportion was 79 % (19 % for procedures) and 64 % (28 % for procedures), respectively. For vertebral fractures in Italy and Spain, more than 94 % of costs were due to inpatient stays, while in Germany this category of cost covered 83 % of costs (14 % due to procedures) and in the UK 9 % were due to inpatient stays, 37 % to outpatient visits, and 53 % to procedures. The wider difference in terms of costs' proportion among countries was observed also for radiation therapy: in Germany procedures covered 45 % of costs, followed by inpatient stays (42 %) and outpatient visits (13 %); in Italy 78 % of costs were due to procedures, followed by inpatient stays (17 %); in Spain the main cost category was inpatient stays (64 %) followed by outpatient visits (27 %) and procedures

(9 %); and in the UK 50 % of costs were due to outpatient visits and 47 % to procedures.

The highest cost was associated with surgery to bone followed by spinal cord compression in Germany, with spinal cord compression followed by surgery to bone in Italy and the UK, and with spinal cord compression followed by vertebral fracture in Spain, confirming the high regional variability of procedures and cost.

Previous analysis, indeed, had been conducted on the population of single countries. In 2011, Félix et al. [14] conducted a multicenter, retrospective study to assess skeletal-related events' costs in 152 patients with bone metastases in prostate (31 patients) and breast (121 patients) cancers in Portugal. Cost data were estimated according to the Portuguese National Health Service price list, considering activities provided by the hospitals involved in SRE identification and treatment. The estimated mean per capita costs related to skeletal events were 5,711 € (95 CI: 3,467 €–6,052 €) for patients with prostate cancer. In the prostate cancer group, the three main cost categories were hospitalization (38.7 %), medications (31.0 %), and radiotherapy (24.5 %). The mean cost per skeletal-related event in the whole sample is reported in the table below: the highest cost was associated with spinal cord compression, followed by pathologic fracture, hypercalcemia of malignancy, and radiotherapy.

Skeletal-related event	Mean cost per event (€)
Spinal cord compression	13,203
Pathologic fracture	8,730
Hypercalcemia of malignancy	3,008
Radiotherapy	1,485

The year before, Pockett et al. [15] had published a similar article aimed at investigating the hospital burden of SREs associated with bone metastases in prostate cancer, breast cancer, and lung cancer in the Spanish population. Data related to 221 patients with prostate cancer, bone metastases, and SREs with hospital admissions between 2000 and 2006 were considered. The average cost for the first hospital admission of patients with skeletal-related events was 3,585 € (standard deviation: ± 1,538.8 €), while the cost of the first hospital admission of patients with prostate cancer metastatic bone disease but no SREs was equal to 3,180 € (standard deviation: ±2,081.9 €). The impact of SREs on total costs had been demonstrated since 2003 also in the Netherlands, where Groot et al. [16] evaluated the direct medical costs associated with bone metastases in 28 patients with prostate cancer and found a cost per patient equal to 13,051 €, of which 6,983 € were directly due to SREs (more than half of total direct medical costs).

An effort to overcome regional differences and to conduct a wider European analysis on the costs of bone metastases and SREs has been recently made by Pereira et al. [17], with a retrospective multinational study (Austria, the Czech Republic, Finland, Greece, Portugal, Sweden) that investigated the health resource utilization associated with skeletal-related events in patients with bone metastases secondary to prostate, breast, or lung cancer and multiple myeloma. The data sources were hospital charts of 356 patients with >19 years who experienced 744 skeletal-related events. The cost per event (in euros, referred to 2010), calculated assuming the National Health Service perspective, is reported in the table below.

Skeletal-related event	Mean cost per skeletal-related event (€)					
	Austria	Czech Republic	Finland	Greece	Portugal	Sweden
Radiation to bone	14,603	2,258	7,251	9,734	5,144	3,270
Pathologic fracture	10,305	1,858	5,397	4,478	3,676	5,379
Spinal cord compression	22,191	6,140	14,447	7,538	5,739	13,000
Surgery to bone	21,496	6,030	13,343	7,943	7,130	10,666

The mean cost per event among the six countries considered was 7,043 € for radiation to bone, 5,242 € for pathologic fracture, 11,101 € for surgery to bone, and 11,509 € for spinal cord compression. This last event was the most onerous in Austria, the Czech Republic, Finland, and Sweden, followed by surgery to bone. In Greece radiation to bone resulted to be the event with more health resource consumption, followed by surgery to bone, while in Portugal surgery to bone was the most expensive procedure, followed by treatment of spinal cord compression.

20.2 Direct Health Costs of SREs in the USA and Canada

In the last years, several studies have investigated the economic impact of SREs also in the USA and Canada. Taking into account the different features of the health services between these countries and Europe, the results of the analyses were not so dissimilar to European ones since the difference essentially consists in the approach to the problem rather than in the problem itself (higher rate of hospitalization associated with SREs in Europe than in the USA, as well as longer hospital stay; higher rate of outpatient visits and procedures in the USA than in Europe) [18].

The cost of SREs in patients with prostate cancer and bone metastases was first investigated by Lage et al. [19], in a retrospective analysis on 342 patients (from year 2000 to 2005). The per capita mean cost for SRES was 12,469 US$, equally distributed among inpatient (48.7 %) and outpatient (51.3 %) activities. The mean costs per single skeletal-related event are presented in the table below.

Skeletal-related event	Mean cost in US$ (95 % confidence interval)
Therapeutic radiology	5,930 (4,829–7,032)
Pathologic fracture	3,179 (1,745–4,614)
Bone surgery	2,218 (1,059–3,378)
Spinal cord compression	460 (116–803)
Other	681 (316–1,047)

The highest cost was associated with therapeutic radiology (radiation therapy), followed by pathologic fracture, bone surgery, and spinal cord compression.

A following analysis conducted by Barlev et al. [20] assessed the costs from the payer point of view of pathologic fractures, surgery to bone, and spinal cord compression in patients with bone metastases secondary to prostate cancer, breast cancer, or multiple myeloma (data from 2003 to 2009), considering subjects in Medicare and MarketScan databases with a hospitalization due to SREs. A total of 599 hospitalizations with skeletal-related events as primary diagnosis or procedure were identified for patients with prostate cancer with bone metastases: 130 cases of bone surgery (21.7 %), 416 bone fractures (69.4 %), and 53 spinal cord compressions (8.9 %). The mean payer costs for patients with prostate cancer are reported in the table below.

Skeletal-related event	Mean cost in US$ (95 % confidence interval)
Surgery to the bone	42,094 (29,247–54,941)
Pathologic fracture	22,390 (28,417–37,067)
Spinal cord compression	59,788 (41,401–78,176)

A similar analysis was later conducted by Hagiwara and colleagues [21], in a retrospective observational study with data related to 1,237 patients with prostate cancer and bone metastases (from 2002 to 2011, data collected from the Thomson MedStat MarketScan Commercial Claims and Encounters database). Mean per capita costs due to hospital outpatient visits (7,471 US$, SD: ±14,837), physician office visits (5,826 US$, SD: ±11,515), hospitalizations (2,668 US$, SD: ±12,013), emergency department visits (334 US$, SD: ±1,601), lab visits (141 US$, SD: ±461), and home healthcare (119 US$, SD: ±790) were assessed. The costs per SRE were considered both in the inpatient and outpatient settings, as reported in the table below.

Skeletal-related episode	Mean cost in 1,000 of US$ (95 % confidence interval)	
	Inpatient episode	Outpatient episode
Spinal cord compression	54.5 (37.0–71.9)	14.9 (1.4–28.4)
Pathologic fracture	64.1 (48.1–80.2)	11.4 (8.0–14.7)
Surgery to bone	88.8 (64.8–112.9)	4.7 (0.8–8.7)
Radiotherapy	43.0 (35.1–50.9)	11.8 (10.8–12.8)

A further analysis within the US setting was conducted among elderly men (66 years or older) with metastatic prostate cancer by Jayasekera et al. [12]. Patients with incident stage IV prostate cancer between 2000 and 2007 were selected from the Surveillance, Epidemiology, and End Results – Medicare dataset. A total of 1131 metastatic prostate cancer patients with SREs were considered, and their average healthcare utilization was assessed. The annual average cost (2009 US$) for each skeletal-related event is reported in the table below.

Skeletal-related event	Mean cost in US$ (standard deviation)
Any skeletal-related event	53,192 (±44,217)
Spinal cord compression only	50,095 (±44,721)
Pathological fracture only	42,523 (±34,794)
Bone surgery only	60,955 (±45,418)
Pathological fracture with concurrent surgery	56,896 (±39,971)
Spinal cord compression with concurrent surgery	83,681 (±54,098)

The highest healthcare resource utilization was observed for spinal cord compression with concurrent surgery, followed by pre-fracture bone surgery. Considering any skeletal-related event, 51.5 % of the mean total cost was due to inpatient activity, 19.7 % to physicians and non-institutional providers, 12.9 % to skilled nursing facilities, 6.0 % to hospice, 5.0 % to outpatient activities, and 4.9 % to other activities (i.e., home health and durable medical equipment).

Probably, the broadest study in this field (about the US situation) was published by Roghmann and colleagues in 2015 [22]. The authors evaluated hospital charges in a sample of 443,929 patients with prostate cancer and bone metastases from the National Inpatient Database between 1998 and 2010. They assessed a significant (+92 %) increase of the charges associated with hospital visits of patients with bone metastases in the analyzed period, from $ 788,522,108 in 1998 to $ 1,512,449,106 in 2010 (inflation-adjusted values at year 2012). Charges for hospital visits due to SREs rose even more (+94 %), from $ 190,318,566 in 1998 to $ 369,256,799 in 2010. Median charges per visit were higher in patients with SREs compared with patient with prostate cancer and bone metastases not presenting such events, being $ 29,625 per visit vs. $ 17,969 per visit. Moreover, in spite of a decrease of the incidence of SREs and SRE-associated mortality in the study period, health expenditures for SRE-associated hospital visits increased at an alarming rate over the course of the study (370 million dollars in 2010, 24.41 % of the total charges associated with all hospital visits for patients with prostate cancer and bone metastases).

The results of this study have recently been confirmed by another paper by McDougall et al. [11], about the results of a retrospective analysis on the costs of SREs in 3,297 patients with prostate cancer and bone metastases. Cost data were collected from the Surveillance, Epidemiology, and End Results, Medicare database (expressed in 2013 US$), with baseline data referred to the period 2004–2009. For patients with at least one SRE, the mean per capita cost accrued from the date of the first skeletal-related event (≥1) to death was calculated in 72,454 US$ (95 % confidence interval: 67,362–76,958); during the same period, the cost for patients with prostate cancer and bone metastases but free of SREs was 51,263 US$ (95 % confidence interval: 45,439–56,100), with a 21,191 US$ additional cost attributable to SREs.

Data emerged from the US situation are not dissimilar to those concerning Canada, as demonstrated by the results of a retrospective observational open cohort study conducted in the Province of Québec by Perrault et al. and published in 2015 [23]. Data about 626 patients with prostate cancer and metastatic bone disease and 1,671 patients with prostate cancer and no bone metastases (taken as control group) were collected from the Régie de l'Assurance Maladie du Québec database, which contains information on public insurance covered health services, in the interval between 1996 and 2010 (costs expressed in Canadian dollars at December 2012). Patients with ≥2 MBD-related claims or a SRE were compared with the matched control group of patients without MBD. The adjusted annual cost of the healthcare resources used by patients with metastatic bone disease was statistically higher than the cost of those used by the control group in terms of hospitalizations (28,957 $ vs. 10,230 $), emergency room visits (626 $ vs. 324 $), outpatient physician visits (873 $ vs. 517 $), diagnostic procedures (1,449 $ vs. 630 $), and pharmacy (5,099 $ vs. 4,180 $). The total unadjusted annual cost of the healthcare resources used by patients with bone metastases was 37,004 $, of which 11,377 $ were strictly related to metastatic bone disease.

20.3 Costs of Available Treatments

Therapeutic options for mCRPC were primarily palliative until 2004, when clinical trials demonstrated the survival benefit associated with docetaxel therapy. Since then, additional chemotherapeutic agents, immunotherapy, and targeted therapies have emerged and gained approval for the treatment of CRPC and its associated metastatic disease: Abiraterone acetate and enzalutamide (hormone antagonists), cabazitaxel (taxoid), radium-223 dichloride (radiopharmaceutical for bone metastases), and sipuleucel-T (vaccine). With the development of these new agents, together with the emergence of new biomarkers to evaluate treatment efficacy and assess prognosis, the treatment paradigm of prostate cancer is currently being revolutionized [24].

In this setting, not only the analysis of costs related to SREs but also a careful evaluation of the economic impact of these new therapies seems necessary: from the clinical point of view, in fact, all of them have proven to be effective in reducing or delaying SREs and/or increasing survival compared to placebo and best supportive care, while few direct comparative data about their efficacy are available at the moment.

A relatively recent paper (Lew 2013) [25], considering the approved courses of treatment of these latest post-docetaxel agents, has estimated a treatment cost in the USA varying from approximately 47,000 $ for an 8-month course of treatment with abiraterone acetate to approximately 93,000 $ for a standard sipuleucel-T course of three treatments. The costs of cabazitaxel (approximately 50,000 $ for a typical six-cycle treatment), enzalutamide (approximately 60,000 $ for an 8-month course of treatment), and radium-223 dichloride (approximately 70,000–75,000 $ for 6 months) were within the range. These values demonstrate that the overall expense is significant independently from the chosen agent but also that costs differences among them exist. To note, in this kind of analysis not only direct drug costs but also the costs of drug administration, cost of patient monitoring, and also the cost of eventual adverse events and related medications are usually considered. In some papers, instead, the ex factory prices of treatments, which are significantly lower, are reported: about Italy, for example, the cost of these drugs alone (considering the approved courses of treatment) ranges from approximately 26,400 € for cabazitaxel and Ra-223 to approximately 30,800 € for abiraterone (30,200 € for enzalutamide; no data for sipuleucel-T) [26–29]. This may contribute to generate further confusion in a complex analysis in itself.

The results of available cost-effectiveness evaluations are somewhat conflicting. In 2012, the National Centre for Pharmacoeconomics (NCPE) of Ireland stated that abiraterone acetate was not cost-effective for the treatment of patients with mCRPC who have received prior docetaxel-based chemotherapy, since the incremental cost-effectiveness ratio (ICER) values were above the threshold levels of interest of the Irish Health Service Executive (€ 144,485 for quality-adjusted life year (QALY) vs. € 45,000/QALY) [30]. The same applied, 2 years later, to enzalutamide [31]. Also the cost-effectiveness of Ra-223, according to NCPE, is still to be demonstrated [32]. In 2013, two US analyses came to different conclusions, indicating that the reimbursement for abiraterone may have a neutral impact on the health plan budget, given the relatively small size of the eligible prostate cancer population and the expected lower toxicity-related costs as compared with chemotherapy, and thus considering it cost-effective compared to prednisone alone and to the next lowest cost option, mitoxantrone. In this setting, it should be underlined that an intervention is considered cost-effective compared to an alternative intervention if ICER falls below a predetermined threshold. In the USA this threshold is a maximum of $ 100,000 per QALY, significantly higher than European one: negative results in Europe may also be due to this lower acceptable willingness-to-pay (WTP) threshold. Interestingly, cabazitaxel has not been considered cost-effective in any scenarios until now [33, 34]. Recently, the results of a cost-effectiveness analysis of radium-223 in comparison to cabazitaxel, abiraterone, and enzalutamide in Dutch patients with mCRPC previously treated with docetaxel have been published [35]. A Markov model with five health states (from "progression-free survival without symptomatic SREs" to "death") was used, and efficacy, safety, and QALY data were obtained from respective Phase III randomized controlled trials (ALSYMPCA trial2, TROPIC trial3, COU-AA-301 trial4, AFFIRM trial5) by indirect treatment comparisons. The analysis showed that the effectiveness expressed in QALYs was comparable among all the treatments: however, the lifetime costs of mCRPC patients in the Netherlands were lower for Ra-223 treated patients, due to lower drug and symptomatic SREs costs, making Ra-223 a possible cost-saving treatment in this clinical context.

20.4 Final Considerations

The economic impact of prostate cancer bone metastases is significant but difficult to evaluate as a whole. The analysis of the costs related to the disease demands for a targeted intervention on its complications that represent the first item in terms of expenditure. Also the modality of intervention, anyway, should be carefully evaluated from an economic point of view. New available therapies, in fact, do provide clear clinical benefits, but appropriate healthcare utilization and management of associated expenditures is a growing concern, since the costs associated with their use are not negligible. In this setting, direct medical costs associated with their administration, adverse events, monitoring, etc. should be further investigated along with indirect costs, to assess the global expense from the perspective of society. Present data on this topic are still controversial.

A double aim in the choice of the proper treatment for patients affected by prostate cancer with bone metastases emerges, both from the clinical side and from the economical one: first and essential, to find an agent that significantly reduces or delays SREs and then, among available alternatives, to conduct cost-effectiveness evaluations to identify the one leading to the highest efficiency in terms of resources allocation and to investigate the sustainability of its use within national and regional health services.

It is probable that, in the next future, costs of managing patients with mCRPC will arise, considering the possibility that many of these subjects may eventually require treatment with one or more of these new therapies, due to new sequencing or combination of multiple agents. In this setting, the current lack of comparative data for these treatments is problematic and demands further researches. Multidisciplinary collaboration between oncologists, urologists, and various other healthcare professionals will be vital to formulate the best therapeutic strategies and treatment protocols, in order to deliver the most clinically effective and sustainable treatments at the best time, ensuring optimal patient and economic outcomes.

References

1. Ferlay J, Soerjomataram I, Dikshit R et al (2015) Cancer incidence and mortality worldwide: sources, methods and major patterns in GLOBOCAN 2012. Int J Cancer 136:E359–E386
2. Miller DC, Hafez KS, Stewart A et al (2003) Prostate carcinoma presentation, diagnosis, and staging: an

update from the National Cancer Data Base. Cancer 98:1169–1178
3. Mottet N, Bellmunt J, Briers E, et al (2015) Guidelines on prostate cancer. Eur Assoc Urol. Update March 2015. Available at: http://uroweb.org/wp-content/uploads/09-Prostate-Cancer_LR.pdf. Last accessed: 28 March 2016
4. Gartrell BA, Coleman R, Efstathiou E et al (2015) Metastatic prostate cancer and the bone: significance and therapeutic options. Eur Urol. http://dx.doi.org/10.1016/j.eururo.2015.06.039
5. Broder MS, Gutierrez B, Cherepanov D et al (2015) Burden of skeletal-related events in prostate cancer: unmet need in pain improvement. Support Care Cancer 23:237–247
6. Nørgaard M, Jensen A, Jacobsen JB et al (2010) Skeletal related events, bone metastasis and survival of prostate cancer: a population based cohort study in Denmark (1999 to 2007). J Urol 184:162–167
7. DePuy V, Anstrom KJ, Castel LD et al (2007) Effects of skeletal morbidities on longitudinal patientreported outcomes and survival in patients with metastatic prostate cancer. Support Care Cancer 15:869–876
8. Saad F, Gleason DM, Murray R et al (2002) A randomized, placebo controlled trial of zoledronic acid in patients with hormone-refractory metastatic prostate carcinoma. J Natl Cancer Inst 94:1458–1468
9. Weinfurt KP, Li Y, Castel LD et al (2005) The significance of skeletal-related events for the health-related quality of life of patients with metastatic prostate cancer. Ann Oncol 16:579–584
10. Chang S, Long SR, Kutikova L et al (2004) Estimating the cost of cancer: results on the basis of claims data analyses for cancer patients diagnosed with seven types of cancer during 1999 to 2000. J Clin Oncol 22:3524–3530
11. McDougall JA, Bansal A, Goulart BHL et al (2016) The clinical and economic impacts of skeletal-related events among medicare enrollees with prostate cancer metastatic to bone. Oncologist 21:320–326
12. Jayasekera J, Onukwugha E, Bikov K et al (2014) The economic burden of skeletal-related events among elderly men with metastatic prostate cancer. Pharmacoeconomics 32:173–191
13. Hechmati G, Cure S, Gouépo A et al (2013) Cost of skeletal-related events in European patients with solid tumours and bone metastases: data from a prospective multinational observational study. J Med Econ 16(5):691–700
14. Félix J, Andreozzi V, Soares M, et al. (Portuguese Group for the Study of Bone Metastases) (2011) Hospital resource utilization and treatment cost of skeletal-related events in patients with metastatic breast or prostate cancer: estimation for the Portuguese National Health System. Value Health 14(4):499–505
15. Pockett RD, Castellano D, McEwan P et al (2010) The hospital burden of disease associated with bone metastases and skeletal-related events in patients with breast cancer, lung cancer, or prostate cancer in Spain. Eur J Cancer Care 19(6):755–760
16. Groot MT, Boeken Kruger CG et al (2003) Costs of prostate cancer, metastatic to the bone, in the Netherlands. Eur Urol 43(3):226–232
17. Pereira J, Body JJ, Gunther O et al (2016) Cost of skeletal complications from bone metastases in six European countries. J Med Econ 23:1–8
18. Duran I, Fink MG, Bahl A et al (2016) Health resource utilisation associated with skeletal-related events in patients with bone metastases secondary to solid tumours: regional comparisons in an observational study. Eur J Cancer Care. doi:10.1111/ecc.12452
19. Lage MJ, Barber BL, Harrison DJ et al (2008) The cost of treating skeletal-related events in patients with prostate cancer. Am J Manag Care 14(5):317–322
20. Barlev A, Song X, Ivanov B et al (2010) Payer costs for inpatient treatment of pathologic fracture, surgery to bone, and spinal cord compression among patients with multiple myeloma or bone metastasis secondary to prostate or breast cancer. J Manag Care Pharm 16(9):693–702
21. Hagiwara M, Delea TE, Saville MW et al (2013) Healthcare utilization and costs associated with skeletal-related events in prostate cancer patients with bone metastases. Prostate Cancer Prostatic Dis 16(1):23–27
22. Roghmann F, Antczak C, McKay RR et al (2015) The burden of skeletal-related events in patients with prostate cancer and bone metastasis. Urol Oncol 33(1):17.e9–18
23. Perrault L, Fradet V, Lauzon V et al (2015) Burden of illness of bone metastases in prostate cancer patients in Québec, Canada: a population-based analysis. Can Urol Assoc J 9(9-10):307–314
24. Garcia JA, Rini BI (2012) Castration-resistant prostate cancer: many treatments, many options, many challenges ahead. Cancer 118:2583–2593
25. Lew I (2013) Managed care implications in castration-resistant prostate cancer. Am J Manag Care 19:S376–S381
26. Riclassificazione del medicinale per uso umano “Xtandi (enzalutamide)” ai sensi dell’art. 8, comma 10, della legge 24 dicembre 1993, n. 537. (Determina n. 1415/2014), (14A09421). GU Serie Generale n.286 del 10-12-2014
27. Regime di rimborsabilita’ e prezzo, a seguito di nuove indicazioni terapeutiche del medicinale per uso umano “Zytiga” (abiraterone acetato). (Determina n. 927/2014). (14A07107). GU Serie Generale n.214 del 15-9-2014
28. Regime di rimborsabilita’ e prezzo di vendita del medicinale Jevtana (cabazitaxel). (Determinazione/C 2749/2011). GU Serie Generale n. 285 del 7 dicembre 2011
29. Riclassificazione del medicinale per uso umano “Xofigo”, ai sensi dell’articolo 8, comma 10, della legge 24 dicembre 1993, n. 537. (Determina n. 576/2015). (15A03864). GU Serie Generale n.121 del 27-5-2015
30. National Centre for Pharmacoeconomics (Ireland) (2012) Economic evaluation of Abiraterone Acetate

(Zytiga®) for the treatment of patients with metastatic castration-resistant prostate cancer (mCRPC) who have received prior docetaxel-based chemotherapy. May 2012
31. National Centre for Pharmacoeconomics (Ireland) (2014) Cost Effectiveness of enzalutamide (Xtandi®) for the treatment of adults with metastatic castration-resistant prostate cancer whose disease has progressed on or after docetaxel April 2014
32. National Centre for Pharmacoeconomics (Ireland) (2014) Cost Effectiveness of radium-223 (Xofigo®) for castration-resistant prostate cancer with symptomatic bone metastases and no known visceral metastases. Dec 2014
33. Sorensen S, Ellis L, Wu Y et al (2013) Budgetary impact on a U.S. health plan adopting abiraterone acetate plus prednisone for the treatment of patients with metastatic castration-resistant prostate cancer. J Manag Care Pharm 19(9):799–808
34. Zhong L, Pon V, Srinivas S et al (2013) Therapeutic options in docetaxel-refractory metastatic castration-resistant prostate cancer: a cost-effectiveness analysis. PLoS One 8(5):e64275. doi:10.1371/journal.pone.0064275
35. Gaultney JG, Baka A, Leliveld-Kors A, et al (2015) Results of a Dutch cost-effectiveness model of radium-223 in comparison to cabazitaxel, abiraterone, and enzalutamide in patients with metastatic castration resistant prostate cancer previously treated with docetaxel. ISPOR 18th Annual European Congress, Milan

21 Multidisciplinary Approach of Prostate Cancer Patients

Tiziana Magnani, Lara Bellardita, Augusto Caraceni, Filippo de Braud, Giuseppe Procopio, Roberto Salvioni, and Riccardo Valdagni

21.1 The European Partnership for Action Against Cancer

The multidisciplinary management of cancer patients was recognized by the Lisbon roundtable on national cancer plans, cancer registries, and cancer screening programs organized within the Health Strategies in Europe meeting in 2007 as the best way to manage and organize cancer care thanks to the collaboration of all health professionals involved in the diagnostic and therapeutic path [1]. Considering the different levels of organization, implementation, and performance of cancer care in the European countries, though, in 2009, the European Parliament launched the European Partnership for Action Against Cancer (EPAAC) with the aims of collectively addressing the issue of cancer by shared and coordinated prevention and control strategies and offering European health systems some key elements to organize multidisciplinary management of oncologic patients. In the document from the Commission of the European Communities to the European Parliament, the Council, the European Economic and Social Committee, and the Committee of the Regions, great emphasis was placed on the importance of a comprehensive cancer approach and on the central role of the multidisciplinary teams which could ensure more effective care of oncologic patients. Other focuses of interest were patients' quality of life and palliative care, the quality of which dramatically varied between member states and sometimes within the same state [2]. The article "Policy statement on multidisciplinary cancer care" [3] summarized the consensus reached by EPAAC working group after long discussion and literature review. Multidisciplinary team was for the

T. Magnani (✉) • L. Bellardita
Prostate Cancer Program, Fondazione IRCCS Istituto Nazionale dei Tumori, via G. Venezian 1, Milan 20133, Italy
e-mail: tiziana.magnani@istitutotumori.mi.it

A. Caraceni
Division of Palliative Care, Fondazione IRCCS Istituto Nazionale dei Tumori, Milan, Italy

F. de Braud
Department of Medical Oncology, Fondazione IRCCS Istituto Nazionale dei Tumori, Milan, Italy

G. Procopio
Division of Genito-Urinary Medical Oncology, Fondazione IRCCS Istituto Nazionale dei Tumori, Milan, Italy

R. Salvioni
Division of Urologic Surgery, Fondazione IRCCS Istituto Nazionale dei Tumori, Milan, Italy

R. Valdagni
Department of Diagnostic Imaging and Radiotherapy, Università di Milano, Milan, Italy

Division of Radiotherapy, Fondazione IRCCS Istituto Nazionale dei Tumori, Milan, Italy

Prostate Cancer Program, Fondazione IRCCS Istituto Nazionale dei Tumori, Milan, Italy

F. Bertoldo et al. (eds.), *Bone Metastases from Prostate Cancer*, DOI 10.1007/978-3-319-42327-2_21

first time defined as "an alliance of all medical and health-care professionals related to a specific tumor disease whose approach to cancer is guided by their willingness to agree on evidence-based clinical decisions and to coordinate the delivery of care at all stages of the process, encouraging patients in turn to take an active role in their care." According to EPAAC, new and recurrent cancer patients should be managed by the multidisciplinary team early after the diagnosis in order to be proposed the most appropriate treatment upon careful consideration of the pathologic and imaging reports. Palliative care specialists should also participate to guarantee continuity of care and support to patients' needs along the disease trajectory. Patients should be informed of the disease and the treatment options, express their informed consent to the treatment plan, and have access to psychological support and counseling if felt necessary and requested. On the other hand, treatment plan agreed upon by the multidisciplinary team should be evidenced-based and respectful of patients' preferences. Follow-up should regard both the monitoring after treatment and treatment-induced needs (e.g., need for rehabilitation programs) [3].

Table 21.1 reports EPAAC working group's policy statement on the core pillars of multidisciplinary teams. In synthesis, effective multidisciplinary teams should (1) share clear care objectives covering the whole disease trajectory; (2) go through the process of organization by identifying leadership, work flow, actors, and responsibility; (3) set up databases; (4) promote patient empowerment; and (5) seek for policy support. All these actions should facilitate the shift from a disease-focused to a patient-centered approach, thus considering also broader areas of interest, such as the psychosocial aspects, the quality of life, and survivorship [3].

21.2 Experiences in the Literature

Besides the paper by EPAAC working group, several articles highlighted the benefits of managing cancer patients with a multiprofessional approach by a team of trained, skilled, and qualified physicians and health professionals, thus able to deliver the multimodal treatment requested by several oncologic malignancies and ensure quality and continuity of care [4–9]. The interdisciplinary and multiprofessional management of cancer patients reduces the time from diagnosis to completion of necessary pretreatment consultations and to treatment, the number of visits before initiation of care, the duplication of the procedures, and the fragmentation of care; allows the timely detection of disease relapse and treatment-induced complications; applies a personalized medicine, paying particular attention to all the dimensions of the patients, the physical as well as the emotional, social, and spiritual/existential ones; enables to improve care in terms of consistency (i.e., evidenced-base clinical decisions, objective treatment proposals without specialty-driven bias) and continuity (i.e., coordination of therapies); permits to improve communication among health professionals and to share responsibility on complex cases; favors inclusion of patients in trials; offers educational opportunities to the team members to acquire a multidisciplinary knowledge of the disease; and increases patient satisfaction, compliance to treatment, and clinical outcome (Table 21.2) [4–9].

As a result, the involvement of different specialists and health professionals in the care of cancer patients can be considered as the best way to make the shift from operating in silos to team-based care and from individual to shared responsibility. Essential prerequisites for an effective multidisciplinary team working are orchestration and coordination of the activities, and this translates into a few requirements necessary to reach these major goals and to overcome barriers to effective team functioning [6, 8]:

1. The multidisciplinary team needs a leader.
2. Philosophy, dynamics, roles, objectives, and actions need to be made clear and shared within the team.
3. Administrative and cleric support needs to be granted to facilitate organization and coordination of multidisciplinary activities.
4. Health professionals participating in the multidisciplinary team need protected contractual time to attend the multidisciplinary activities.

Table 21.1 EPAAC policy statement to define the core elements of multidisciplinary teams (MDT)

Rationale and definition of MDT	Promotion of MDT considered as an ethical priority, given the benefits of MDT and the imperative to provide all patients with the best possible care
	Fostering MDT considered as imperative to ensuring appropriate clinical decisions
	Multidisciplinary clinical practice guidelines considered as deserving special attention
	Clinical leadership and firm commitment by health-care providers considered as prerequisites to change management and to sustain team structures
	Given the dynamic nature of cancer, networks for knowledge and expertise considered essential
	MDT work considered crucial for future challenges like survivorship
	MDT considered as an alliance of all medical and health-care professionals
Care objectives	Initiation of MDT monitoring immediately after cancer diagnosis
	Need for MDT consensus and patient consent on evidence-based treatment plan
	Decision-making process consistent with evidence-based clinical practice guidelines
	Need for tailoring guidelines to the type of tumor and the conditions of the patient during MDT meeting discussions
	Need for informing the patient on treatment decisions and taking his preferences into account
	Need for offering assess to counseling for psychosocial support and other supportive issues
	Follow-up plan to be integrated with a joint survivorship care plan elaborated by the MDT and shared with the patient
	Follow-up aimed to monitor possible relapse and posttreatment needs including rehabilitation
	In selected cases need for integration between MDT and palliative care team to ensure continuity of care
	Need for involving primary care physicians in the discussion of their patients and in the follow-up management
MDT organization	Need for monitoring all new and recurrent cancer patients
	Need for presenting every case at a tumor board for discussion or assessing adherence of clinical recommendations to evidence and guidelines
	Specialists involved in the MDT formally assigned and ensured protected time to attend multidisciplinary activities
	MDT care protocols to be updated every 2 years
	MDT proactive in promoting educational experiences and quality improvement actions
	Designation of MDT coordinator to ensure efficient discussion within the tumor board, secure professionals' attendance, prepare cases to be discussed, involve specialists necessary for the discussion, and implement decisions taken by the MDT
	Leading position considered as temporary, with clear rules for nomination process and rotation system
	Case management to be provided by an expert nurse or qualified staff member who could be contact person for the patients and the team
Clinical information and assessment	Need for a prospective database with clinical indicators
	Information available for evaluation of outcomes
	Decisions taken and rationale applied considered as important information to be recorded
Patients' rights and empowerment	Need for fluid communication with patients and shared decision-making
	Need for discussing treatment and care preferences with patients before making clinical decisions
	Possibility for patients to have second opinions
	Identification of a responsible physician at every stage of the care process
	Identification of a case manager responsible for communicating with patients
	Improvement of patient experience considered as key element in the quality of care
	Improvement of patients' level of information considered as necessary: on the MDT organization, on the care process, on treatments and treatment-related side effects, on community resources
	Patients and volunteer organizations considered as welcome in cancer centers
Policy support	Need for involving European and national scientific societies and patient associations

Table 21.2 Benefits of multidisciplinary and multiprofessional management of cancer patients

Benefits
Less time from diagnosis to treatment
Fewer consultations before initiation of care
More continuity of care
Timely detection of disease relapse and treatment-induced complications
Application of personalized medicine
Attention to all the dimensions of the patients
Increased consistency in the care: evidence-based clinical decisions, objective treatment proposals without specialty-driven bias
Better communication among health professionals
Shared responsibility on complex cases
Increase in the number of patients included in trials
Educational opportunities to the team members to acquire a multidisciplinary knowledge of the disease
Increase in patient satisfaction, compliance to treatment, and clinical outcome

5. Institutional support should be granted in terms of both funding and organizational issues (meeting room, IT facilities, etc.).
6. The multidisciplinary team needs to learn to work in team, trust each other, and respect the differences in approach.

It is also very important to consider the natural history of the disease to identify the specialists and health professionals who have to be involved in the multidisciplinary management of cancer patients in every phase as well as the multidisciplinary activities which need to be implemented in a particular state of disease. The choice as on whom to involve, and when, enables to optimize resources, efforts, and costs and, at the same time, offer patients the best approach to the disease. For patients with advanced cancers, for example, the multidisciplinary team should also involve the palliative care team in an early stage, as underlined by the EPAAC working group [3], thus implementing the concept of simultaneous care. Indeed innovative treatment modalities and new drugs for many cancers may prolong patients' life, but it is beyond any doubt that, being often affected by an active and symptomatic disease, patients may develop mental and psychosocial distress, functional decline, spiritual issues, and financial problems. It is crucial to identify the needs of this vulnerable population and offer simultaneous care in an early phase of the overall management regimen [10, 11].

21.3 Simultaneous and Palliative Care

Taking care of cancer patients and their quality of life means to offer the best therapeutic options as well as to detect physical, functional, psychological, social, spiritual/existential, and also financial needs [12]. To do that it is necessary to involve different health professionals such as supportive and palliative care experts, physiotherapists, nutritionists, psychologists, social workers, and spiritual counselors. The concept of simultaneous care was developed to address patients' broad array of needs, to focus on the importance of delivering care as well as monitoring and managing pain and symptoms, to improve patient care experience and quality of life, to reduce the use and costs of medical services, to help family caregivers manage the complexity of care, and to facilitate the shift from treatment to palliative care and to end-of-life care [13–17].

According to the World Health Organization (WHO), palliative care is "an approach that improves the quality of life of patients and their families through the prevention and relief of suffering by means of early identification and impeccable assessment and treatment of pain and other problems, physical, psychosocial, and spiritual" [18]. As a result, palliative care should be integrated with standard oncology care, be part of the multidisciplinary team, and thus be offered to all patients with advanced cancer in an early stage. As recommended by the American Society of Clinical Oncology (ASCO) Provisional Clinical Opinion [19] and the European Society of Medical Oncology (ESMO) [20], standard oncology and specialized palliative care should join efforts and work multidisciplinarily early in the disease trajectory for patients with advanced cancer and/or important symptom burden. Data from the literature seem to stress the positive impact of this multiprofessional alliance on

Table 21.3 Barriers to the integration of palliative care in the oncologic care

Education-related barriers	Lack of education and training for medical residents
	Perception of palliative care as pertinent to the end-of-life care by health providers
	Perception of palliative care as pertinent to the end-of-life care by the public
Implementation-related barriers	Inadequate work force
	Difficulty in identifying patients who might benefit from palliative care
	Need for cultural change in the perception of palliative care
Policy-related barriers	Fragmented structures
	Need for greater funding
	Lack of incentives for palliative care personnel

patients' quality of life and cancer experience, on standardization of procedures, in some cases even on better survival rates, on reduced hospitalization and emergency department visits, and on costs [14, 17, 21–33].

At the same time, numerous barriers hinder the integration process, making this indeed one of the biggest challenges in oncology. Different examples are reported in the literature among which are (1) education-related barriers, (2) implementation-related barriers, and (3) policy-related barriers (Table 21.3) [34].

Generally speaking, as smartly observed by Berry et al. [35], "palliative care has a branding problem," and this would explain its underuse in spite of the unquestionable benefits. Palliative care is still perceived by patients, families, and also some physicians as pertaining to the end-of-life issues. Some organizations considered adopting a new name and switched to "supportive care" in some cases. The analysis of 4.701 consecutive patients pointed out an increase in the number of referrals and an anticipation of the referral itself after the name change [36–38]. However, the connection of advanced cancer palliative care with the end of life, in other words with death, is not a semantic one but a fact that should not be denied with nominalistic makeups rather accepted both in the medical community and in society based on an empathic, compassionate, and honest therapeutic ground [39]. The universally accepted terminology of palliative care approach, palliative care speciality, and palliative care services [40] is informing most of the health-care policies in the world and gives also important clinical opportunities. In fact, early referral to palliative care outpatient clinics improved communication and patients' understanding of goals of care and reduced aggressive end-of-life treatments [17, 41]. It is likely that this improvement in communication can also result in increasing patients' autonomy and access to better advanced care directives.

For these reasons, there is a crucial need also for better education about the breadth and scope of palliative care, which must not be confined in end-of-life management and hospice and must embrace relief of suffering, improvement of quality of life, and assistance in dealing with the disease-induced burdens [11]. Education should start at the earliest stage of training and be aimed to address the goals of palliative care as well as improve the physicians' competence [11].

21.4 Organization of Palliative Care Services

Hui and Brera [42] described the most common conceptual models of palliative care with the aim of supporting stakeholders in understanding the rationale for integration. The review addressed the time-based model (i.e., integration is activated on chronological criterion), the provider-based (or palli-centric) model (i.e., primary, secondary, and tertiary care), the issue-based (or onco-centric) model with focus on the solo practice, the congress and the integrated care declinations, and the system (or patient-centric) model (in which referral is automatically triggered by particular clinical events). No matter the model applied, it is fundamental to establish criteria for referral timing and team roles, thus offering patients a continuous process of care without gaps or fragmentation. It is evident that prerequisite to integrated palliative care is to pay particular attention to organization and coordination of care provision, with the aims of merging the different separate components of a system to achieve common goals, optimizing the use of resources and improving the quality of the services offered [43].

Key points for the integration of palliative care in the continuum of cancer care can be summarized as follows:

- Outpatient access to palliative care is fundamental.
- The interdisciplinary nature of palliative care favors the addressing of multidimensional care needs.
- Particular attention has to be paid to the type of patients to be referred and referral time.
- Communication between specialists is mandatory: this could be facilitated by the participation of a member of the palliative care team in tumor boards or, alternatively, by the participation of a medical oncologist in the palliative care team meetings. It must be said, though, that combined tumor boards require effort on both sides and it must be difficult to apply on a routine basis. It is for this reason that protocols ruling referral should be also promoted [44]; several efforts in this direction are already under development [45].

Organization and coordination of care provision become absolute "must have" in oncology where we are assisting at the increase in the number of new diagnoses and, at least for certain malignancies, better survival rates [46]. As a result, more and more patients are treated and monitored with clinics and exams for a very long time. If the multidisciplinary management is recognized as the best approach possible to cancer patients, it becomes crucial to carefully evaluate resources and workload to optimize the process of care. To do so, it is important to avoid generalization and take into consideration the specifics of the different oncologic diseases. The ingredients to activate a multidisciplinary approach to breast cancer [47–50], to colorectal cancer [51, 52], to lung cancer [52, 53], to gynecologic cancer [53], and to prostate cancer [54, 55] substantially differ in terms of health professionals involved, diagnostic and therapeutic paths to be followed, and multidisciplinary activities to be implemented.

21.5 The Case of Prostate Cancer

Prostate cancer, which is the most frequently diagnosed tumor in men with 417,000 new cases every year in Europe [56], is among the malignancies that most benefit from a multidisciplinary and multiprofessional management. The disease is indeed a spectrum of differently behaving forms, from small, clinically insignificant, asymptomatic, indolent tumors to aggressive, rapidly progressing, potentially lethal cancers [57]. The number of diagnoses increased dramatically after the introduction of PSA as a screening tool in the early 1990s. This enabled to detect more and more very low, low, and intermediate cancers [58–60]. With the term of overdiagnosis, the scientific community refers to the phenomenon of detection of a large proportion of indolent prostate cancers that will never evolve and cause symptoms in one's life [61]. Not evolving, these forms do not need to be treated and could be monitored with active surveillance.

Considering that most prostate cancers, although showing very favorable features, undergo treatment, the scientific community refers with "overtreatment" to the phenomenon of treating with curative intent (i.e., with radical prostatectomy, external radiotherapy, or brachytherapy) also those tumors with an indolent behavior that could be spared therapy and therapy-induced side effects all together [62, 63].

The multiple patterns of indolence versus aggressiveness of prostate cancer reflect a difference in the prognosis as well as in the treatment and observational modalities by which the disease can be approached. Depending on the state of the disease, several therapeutic options are actually available: open, laparoscopic, or robot-assisted laparoscopic prostatectomy; conformal, intensity-modulated, or image-guided conventionally fractionated, hypofractionated, or extremely hypofractionated external radiotherapy; low-dose-rate or high-dose-rate brachytherapy; hormonal therapy alone or combined with radical therapies; chemotherapy; radionuclide therapy; observational strategies (active surveillance and watchful waiting); or experimental therapies, e.g., cryotherapy and high-intensity-focused ultrasound [64–73].

Low- and very low-risk tumors with very favorable characteristics can be monitored with active surveillance in alternative to being radically treated, with the possibility of switching to therapy if the initial disease features change in time. On the contrary, prostate cancer with less favorable characteristics, which tend to be more aggressive, needs to be treated often by a multimodal approach with surgery and/or radiotherapy and/or hormonal therapy. In addition, this group of patients has to be tightly followed up after treatment to record treatment-induced side effects as well as disease relapse which would mean the need for administering additional treatment.

Prostate cancer treatments may cause adverse effects that impact on patients' quality of life. Each therapeutic option has a unique profile of adverse effects, with variations depending on the single patient, the disease characteristics, the quality of the procedure performed, and the specialists' expertise. The scenario is complicated by the rapidly evolving highly sophisticated technologies and the launch of promising drugs in different disease settings (i.e., the castration-resistant prostate cancer). A new generation of hormonal agents is being accepted as more effective and less toxic compared with previous molecules. Furthermore, recently discovered chemotherapeutic drugs and radionuclides are showing good results in impacting on survival [65, 68, 70, 72, 73].

It is clear that the synergy among physicians and the sequencing of treatments have become a crucial issue and there is a critical need for interdisciplinary collaboration in order to identify who to treat, when, how, and with what [74].

21.6 Multidisciplinary and Multiprofessional Approach in Prostate Cancer

Considering this complex scenario, the multidisciplinary management of patients with prostate cancer offers the best chance to address the disease by bringing together in a team all the specialists and health professionals involved in the diagnostic-therapeutic path along the disease trajectory as well as in a particular state of the disease [75–90].

There are several physicians and health professionals who have a role in the care of prostate cancer patients: urologic surgeons, radiation oncologists, medical oncologists, experts in nuclear medicine, pathologists, imaging specialists, psychologists, social workers as well as nurses with special training in urologic diseases, experts in rehabilitation, experts in supportive and palliative care, geriatricians, and urologists with special training in sexual rehabilitation [54, 55]. The organization and coordination of these figures are core pillars to a successful multidisciplinary management of prostate cancer patients that, to actively participate in the decision-making process, should receive complete and consistent information about the disease, the therapeutic and observational options, and the therapy-induced side effects [54, 55, 75–90].

Unfortunately this is not the rule. Patients often receive partial, contradictory information from the specialists they contact, thus experiencing decision-making as a difficult and stressful process [91]. What is more, physicians are more likely to recommend the therapy that they are capable of delivering, with urologists opting for radical prostatectomy and radiation oncologists for radiotherapy [92, 93].

21.7 Multidisciplinary and Multiprofessional Approach in Advanced Prostate Cancer

Needless to say, considering the wide range of efficacious treatments now available, sometimes to be delivered by a multimodal approach and often requiring supportive medical pharmacological therapies aimed to monitor side effects and toxicity of anticancer therapies [94–96], it is necessary that urologists, medical oncologists, radiation oncologists together with pathologists, imaging specialists, experts in nuclear medicine, and the palliative care team collaborate closer and build a dynamic and long-lasting relationship [88, 97]. The synergy in this setting is mostly needed to identify the best treatment sequencing and include patients in innovative trials [74]. This means that the multidisciplinary team should share the decision-making on a treatment strategy, monitor safety and efficacy, and opt for new treatments if necessary [98, 99].

Essential ingredients to reach this goal and to overcome the most accredited obstacles such as the late referral to oncologists, the lack of shared follow-up management, and the fear of losing the leadership on some patients are education and training in the other disciplines and in team working [88].

The management by the multiprofessional team is also needed when the patient has an important symptom burden due to the progression of the disease or to therapy-induced side effects. In these cases, the added value of physicians expert in palliative care, nurses, social workers, psychologists, and chaplains in an early phase could enable to focus on symptom management, assess the psychosocial needs, and support patients and families in the decision-making phase throughout the whole disease trajectory [100]. The synergy of the different health professionals could reach the goal of delivering palliative care early and together with life-prolonging treatments [101].

Similarly to what happens in other cancers, there is unfortunately a high level of disparity in the management of this patient population and in the application of the concept of multidisciplinary management. The reasons are related to the difficulty, at least in some countries, to collaborate as a team and to the habit of managing cancer patients in a monodisciplinary setting. At the same time, the integration of palliative or supportive care in an early phase is hindered by the lack of trained personnel and of research, the limited availability of palliative care services, and the limited funding to test interventions able to improve quality of life and reduce pain and symptoms [28, 102–104].

21.8 Prostate Cancer Units: The Key to Improving Organization and Coordination of Resources

A well-organized and coordinated multidisciplinary management of prostate cancer patients is essential to identify the actors to be involved and the activities to be implemented, to protect the time the health professionals dedicate to the disease and to the multidisciplinary activities, to optimize the human and technological resources, to make evidence-based decisions applying guidelines and adhering to diagnostic and therapeutic paths, and to improve patients' care experience (Table 21.4). Multidisciplinary management includes different formats, from the clinical case discussions or tumor boards or multidisciplinary team meetings to the multidisciplinary clinics, the declination and organization of which vary by country and even by institution. The position paper by the European School of Oncology [55], which completed the work of the 2011 discussion paper [54], defined the mandatory and recommended requisites for establishing a Prostate Cancer Unit (PCU), the organizational model that best sets the framework within which

Table 21.4 Benefits of establishing Prostate Cancer Units

Better organization	By identification of the actors to be involved
	By identification of the activities to be implemented
	By contractual time dedicated by health professionals to the disease and the multidisciplinary activities
	By optimization of human and technological resources
Physicians' experience	Agreement on guidelines to be adopted, resulting in evidence-based decisions
	Agreement on diagnostic and therapeutic paths, resulting in adherence to paths of care
	Protected time to attend multidisciplinary activities
Patients' experience	Better care experience

managing prostate cancer patients multiprofessionally, in the attempt of reducing discrepancies in prostate cancer treating centers and in treatment offering and delivery.

The bottom line for Valdagni et al.'s position paper was that prostate cancer patients should be managed by an interdisciplinary and multiprofessional team and receive high quality, standardized, and integrated care throughout Europe. On these premises, the European School of Oncology launched in 2012 the PCU Initiative in Europe and worked, in collaboration with a task force of experts in the field of prostate cancer care (i.e., urologists, radiation oncologists, medical oncologists, psychologists, nurses, cancer center managers, and quality experts), representatives of the main European scientific societies (European Association of Urology, European Association of Urology Nurses, European Board of Urology, European Oncology Nursing Society, European Society for Therapeutic Radiation Oncology, International Psycho-Oncology Society), and patient advocate organizations (Europa Uomo), on the definition of the concept of specialized multiprofessional prostate cancer care to be formalized in PCU. The task force reviewed the minimal requirements described in the discussion paper [54], introduced changes to make them adoptable at a broad European level, and reached a consensus on the minimum standards for quality prostate cancer care applicable in the clinical practice and in the different European health contexts. Patient advocacy representatives were involved in the task force to consider the patient's perspectives on key issues like, for example, the importance of written and electronic information on the disease and treatment options.

The standards, which refer to the macroelements, and the items, which are the specifics to the standards, cover several areas such as general requirements for a PCU; critical mass; personnel distinguished in core team, noncore team, and associated services; clinics; organization; and case management.

Within the concept of multidisciplinary management of newly referred prostate cancer patients, three clinical models are described and accepted. The first is the monodisciplinary clinic performed by the urologist, the radiation oncologist, or the medical oncologist who must refer the case to the multiprofessional team meeting afterward for interdisciplinary evaluation of treatment options. The second is a multidisciplinary clinic in sequence, with the patient seen by the urologist, the radiation oncologist, and the medical oncologist one after the other, possibly with the participation of professionals able to offer psychosocial support and of the nurse providing additional information and support. The third is a synchronous multidisciplinary clinic, with the patient seen together by the urologist, the radiation oncologist, and the medical oncologist, again possibly with the participation of professionals able to offer psychosocial support and of the nurse. Also the patients seen in the multidisciplinary clinics are scheduled in the multiprofessional team meeting, thus promoting interdisciplinary education and quality checks on adherence to clinical guidelines.

The rationale for the position paper was that a well-structured and organized PCU should facilitate and optimize the interdisciplinary collaboration and, as a result, patients' care experience. With this in mind, to better define the organizational structure of the PCU, the task force made efforts to reach a consensus among experts, which is sometimes not evidence based, on several key aspects for a PCU such as the number of urologists, radiation oncologists, medical oncologists, pathologists, imaging specialists, psychologists, nurses, and palliative care specialists, the contractual time for each specialist dedicated to prostate cancer and in some cases to genitourinary tumors, the multidisciplinary activities in which the specialists are involved, and the documented exceptions that can be accepted [55]. The result was a consensus on core criteria which had relevance, feasibility, and applicability to guarantee the largest acceptance and widest spread of PCU in Europe. Considering the emerging innovations in diagnosis and care, one of the most important aspects will be to adapt the model to the rapidly evolving situation with regular updates of the criteria. The concept of PCU needs to be promoted, in some countries along with the shift from monodisciplinary to multidisciplinary approach to prostate cancer patients. To win this challenge, it is of upmost relevance that patients increase their awareness about the opportunity of being treated and followed up in top-quality centers and facilitate the lobbying process by approaching European legislators. Last but by no means least, synergy and networking among PCU should be considered an added value for both professionals and patients [55].

References

1. Gouveia J, Coleman MP, Haward R et al (2007) Improving cancer control in the European Union: conclusion from the Lisbon roundtable under the Portuguese EU presidency. Eur J Cancer 44:1457–1462
2. Commission of the European Communities (2009) Communication from the Commission of the European Communities to the European Parliament, the Council, the European Economic and Social Committee and the Committee of the Regions on Action Against Cancer: European Partnership. Brussels, 24.06.2009 COM(2009) 291/4
3. European Partnership Action Against Cancer consensus group (2014) Policy statement on multidisciplinary cancer care. Eur J Cancer 50:475–480
4. Kagan AR (2005) The multidisciplinary clinic. Int J Radiat Oncol Biol Phys 61:967–968
5. Ruhstaller T, Roe H, Thurlimann B, Nicoll JJ (2006) The multidisciplinary meeting: an indispensable aid to communication between different specialities. Eur J Cancer 42:2459–2462
6. Fleissig A, Jenkins V, Catt S, Fallowfield L (2006) Multidisciplinary teams in cancer care: are they effective in the UK? Lancet Oncol 7:935–943
7. Sidhom MA, Poulsen MG (2006) Multidisciplinary care in oncology: medicolegal implications of group decisions. Lancet Oncol 7:951–954
8. Boyle FM, Robinson E, Dunn SM, Heinrich PC (2005) Multidisciplinary care in cancer: the fellowship of the ring. J Clin Oncol 23:916–920
9. Ko C, Chaudhry S (2002) The need for a multidisciplinary approach to cancer care. J Surg Res 105:53–57
10. Stjernsward J, Foley KM, Ferris FD (2007) The public health strategy for palliative care. J Pain Symptom Manage 33:486–493
11. Von Roenn JH, Voltz R, Serrie A (2013) Barriers and approaches to the successful integration of palliative care and oncology practice. J Natl Compr Canc Netw 11(Suppl 1):S11–S16
12. Zagonel V, Cavanna L, Cetto G et al (2009) The medical oncologist's role in palliative care: AIOM's position. Tumori 95:652–654
13. Bakitas MA, Tosteson TD, Li Z et al (2015) Early versus delayed integration of concurrent palliative oncology care: Patient outcomes in the ENABLE III randomized controlled trial. J Clin Oncol 33: 1438–1445
14. Brumley R, Enguidanos S, Jamison P et al (2007) Increased satisfaction with care and lower costs: results of a randomized trial of in-home palliative care. J Am Geriatr Soc 55:993–1000
15. Gabrielli G, Arena MG (2013) Simultaneous care: integration between medical oncology and supportive care. J Med Pers 11:132–133
16. Parikh RB, Kirch RA, Smith TJ et al (2013) Early specialty palliative care – translating data in oncology into practice. N Engl J Med 369:2347–2351
17. Temel JS, Greer JA, Muzikansky A et al (2010) Early palliative care for patients with metastatic non-small lung cancer. N Engl J Med 363:733–742
18. World Health Organization (WHO) WHO definition of palliative care. www.who.int/cancer/palliative/definition/en/. March 2015
19. Smith TJ, Temin S, Alesi ER et al (2012) American Society of Clinical Oncology Provisional Clinical Opinion: the integration of palliative care into standard oncology care. J Clin Oncol 30:880–887
20. Cherny N, Catane R, Schrijvers D et al (2010) European Society for Medical Oncology (ESMO) Program for the integration of oncology and palliative care: a 5 year review of the designated centers' incentive program. Ann Oncol 21:362–369
21. Gade G, Venohr I, Conner D et al (2008) Impact of an inpatient palliative care team: a randomized control trial. J Palliat Med 11:180–190
22. Meyers FJ, Carducci M, Loscalzo MJ et al (2011) Effects of a problem-solving intervention (COPE) on quality of life for patients with advanced cancer on clinical trials and their caregivers: simultaneous care educational intervention (SCEI) – linking palliation and clinical trials. J Palliat Med 14:465–473
23. Pantilat SZ, O'Riordan DL, Dibble SL et al (2010) Hospital-based palliative medicine consultation: a randomized controlled trial. Arch Intern Med 170:2038–2040
24. Rabow MW, Dibble SL, Pantilat SZ et al (2004) The comprehensive care team: a controlled trial of outpatient palliative medicine consultation. Arch Intern Med 164:83–91
25. Bakitas M, Lyons KD, Hegel MT et al (2009) Effects of a palliative care intervention on clinical outcomes in patients with advanced cancer. The Project ENABLE II randomized controlled trial. JAMA 302:741–749
26. Meyers FJ, Linder J, Beckett L et al (2004) Simultaneous care. A model approach to the perceived conflict between investigational therapy and palliative care. J Pain Symptom Manage 28:548–556
27. El-Jawahri A, Greer JA, Temel JS (2011) Does palliative care improve outcomes for patients with incurable illness? A review of the evidence. J Support Oncol 9:87–94

28. Zimmermann C, Riechelmann R, Krzyzanowska M et al (2008) Effectiveness of specialized care: a systematic review. JAMA 299:1698–1709
29. Penrod J, Morrison RS, Meier DE (2008) Studying the effectiveness of palliative care. Author reply. JAMA 200:1022–1023
30. Bruera E (2008) Studying the effectiveness of palliative care. Author reply. JAMA 200:1022
31. Raftery JP, Addington-Hall JM, MacDonald LD et al (1996) A randomized controlled trial of the cost-effectiveness of a district co-ordinating service for terminally ill cancer patients. Palliat Med 10: 151–161
32. Molassiotis A, Brearley S, Saunders M et al (2009) Effectiveness of a home care nursing program in the symptom management of patients with colorectal and breast cancer receiving oral chemotherapy. A randomized controlled trial. J Clin Oncol 27: 6191–6198
33. Muir JC, Daly F, Davis MS et al (2010) Integrating palliative care into the outpatient private practice oncology setting. J Pain Symptom Manage 40: 126–135
34. Aldridge MD, Hasselaar J, Garralda E et al (2016) Education, implementation and policy barriers to greater integration of palliative care: a literature review. Palliat Med 30(3):224–239
35. Berry LL, Castellani R, Stuart B (2016) The branding of palliative care. J Oncol Pract 12:48–50
36. Fadul N, Elsayem A, Palmer JL et al (2009) Supportive versus palliative care: what's in a name? Survey of medical oncologists and medical providers at a comprehensive cancer center. Cancer 115:2013–2021
37. Dalal S, Palla S, Hui D et al (2011) Association between a name change from palliative to supportive care and the timing of patient referrals at a comprehensive cancer center. Oncologist 16:105–111
38. Rhondall W, Burt S, Wittenberg-Lyles E et al (2013) Medical oncologists' perception of palliative care programs and the impact of name chance to supportive care on communication with patients during the referral process. A qualitative study. Palliat Support Care 11:397–404
39. Parikh RB, Kirch RA, Brawley OW (2015) Advancing a quality-of-life agenda in cancer advocacy: beyond the war metaphor. JAMA Oncol 1:423–424
40. WHO Strengthening of palliative care as a component of integrated treatment within the continuum of care WHO resolution EB134.R7. 2014
41. Jackson VA, Jacobsen J, Greer JA et al (2013) The cultivation of prognostic awareness through the provision of early palliative care in the ambulatory setting: a communication guide. Palliat Med 16:894–900
42. Hui D, Brera E (2015) Models of integration of oncology and palliative care. Ann Palliat Med 4.89–98
43. Kodner DL, Spreeuwenberg C (2002) Integrated care: meaning, logic, applications, and implications--a discussion paper. Int J Integr Care 2:1–6
44. Hui D, Bruera E (2015) Integrating palliative care into the trajectory of cancer care. Nat Rev 13:159–171
45. Bausewein C, Simon ST, Pralong A et al (2015) Palliative care of adult patients with cancer. Dtsch Arztebl Int 112:863–870
46. Partridge AH, Seah DS, King T et al (2014) Developing a service model that integrates palliative care throughout cancer care: the time is now. J Clin Oncol 32(29):3330–3336
47. EUSOMA (2000) The requirements of a specialist breast unit. Eur J Cancer 36:2288–2293
48. Blamey RW, Cataliotti L (2006) EUSOMA accreditation of breast units. Eur J Cancer 42:1331–1337
49. Cataliotti L, De Wolf C, Holland R et al (2007) Guidelines on the standards for the training of specialised health professionals dealing with breast cancer. Eur J Cancer 43:660–675
50. Wilson ARM, Marotti L, Bianchi S (2013) The requirements of a specialist Breast Centre. Eur J Cancer 49:3579–3587
51. Malangone SA, Patel H, Kurtin SE et al (2015) Multidisciplinary management of the patient with metastatic colorectal adenocarcinoma. J Adv Pract Oncol 6:147–152
52. Kehl KL, Landrum MB, Kahn KL et al (2015) Tumor board participation among physicians caring for patients with lung or colorectal cancer. J Oncol Pract 11:e267–e278
53. Horvath LE, Yordan E, Malhotra D et al (2010) Multidisciplinary care in the oncology setting: historical perspective and data from lung and gynecology multidisciplinary clinics. J Oncol Pract 6:e21–e26
54. Valdagni R, Albers P, Bangma C et al (2011) The requirements of a specialist Prostate Cancer Unit: a discussion paper from the European School of Oncology. Eur J Cancer 47:1–7
55. Valdagni R, Van Poppel H, Aichison M et al (2015) Prostate Cancer Unit Initiative in Europe: a position paper by the European School of Oncology. Crit Rev Oncol Hamatol 95:133–143
56. Ferlay J, Steliarova-Foucher E, Lortet-Tieulent J et al (2013) Cancer incidence and mortality patterns in Europe: estimates for 40 countries in2012. Eur J Cancer 49:1374–1403
57. Ahmed HU, Arya M, Freeman A, Emberton M (2012) Do low grade and low volume prostate cancers bear the hallmarks of malignancy? Lancer Oncol 13:e509–e517
58. Caverly TJ, Hayward RA, Reamer E et al (2016) Presentation of benefits and harms in US cancer screening and prevention guidelines: systematic review. J Natl Cancer Inst 108:dJv436
59. Schroeder FH, Hugosson J, Roobol MJ et al (2014) Screening and prostate cancer mortality: results of the European Randomised Study of Screening for Prostate Cancer (ERSPC) at 13 years of follow-up. Lancet 384:2027–2035
60. Duffy MJ (2014) PSA in screening for prostate cancer: more good than harm or more harm than good? Adv Clin Chem 66:1–23

61. Hugosson J, Carlsson S (2014) Overdetection in screening for prostate cancer. Curr Opin Urol 24:256–263
62. Klotz L (2012) Cancer overdiagnosis and overtreatment. Curr Opin Urol 22:203–209
63. Heleno B, Thomsen MF, Rodrigues DS et al (2013) Quantification of harms in cancer screening trials: literature review. BMJ 347:f5334
64. Thompson I, Thrasher JB, Aus G et al (2007) Guideline for the management of clinically localized prostate cancer. American Urological Association (AUA); http://www.auanet.org/education/guidelines/prostate-cancer.cfm_. Reviewed and validity confirmed 2011
65. Cookson MS, Roth BJ, Dahm P et al (2014) Castration-resistant prostate cancer: AUA guideline. American Urological Association (AUA). http://www.auanet.org/education/guidelines/castration-resistant-prostate-cancer.cfm_. Amended 2014
66. Thompson IM, Valicenti R, Albertsen PC et al (2013) Adjuvant and salvage radiotherapy after prostatectomy: ASTRO/AUA guideline. AmericanUrological Association (AUA) and American Society for Radiation Oncology (ASTRO). http://www.auanet.org/education/guidelines/radiation-after-prostatectomy.cfm
67. Mottet N, Bellmunt J, Briers E et al (2015) Guidelines on prostate cancer. Eur Assoc Urol (EAU). http://uroweb.org/guideline/prostate-cancer/
68. Horwich A, Parker C, de Reijke T, Kataja V, on behalf of theESMO Guidelines Working Group (2013) Prostate cancer: ESMO clinical practice guidelines for diagnosis, treatment and follow-up. Ann Oncol 24(S6):vi106–14. http://www.esmo.org/Guidelines/Genitourinary-Cancers/Prostate-Cancer_
69. National Collaborating Centre for Cancer (NICE) (2014) Prostate cancer: diagnosis and treatment. National Collaborating Centre for Can-cer (NICE). https://www.nice.org.uk/guidance/cg175/evidence/cg175-prostate-cancer-full-guideline3
70. National Comprehensive Cancer Network (NCCN) (2015) NCCN clinical practice guidelines in oncology (NCCN guidelines). Prostate cancer. National Comprehensive Cancer Network (NCCN). http://www.nccn.org/professionals/physiciangls/pdf/prostate.pdf_. Vers. 1.2015
71. Bangma CH, Valdagni R, Carroll PR et al (2015) Active surveillance for low-risk prostate cancer: developments to date. Eur Urol 67:646–648
72. Basch E, Loblaw DA, Oliver TK et al (2014) Systemic therapy in men with metastatic castration-resistant prostate cancer: American society of clinical oncology and cancer care Ontario clinical practice guidelines. J Clin Oncol 32:3436–3448
73. European Society for Medical Oncology (ESMO) (2014) Guidelines for the treatment of metastatic castration-resistant prostate cancer. Eur Soc Med Oncol. http://www.esmo.org/Guidelines-Practice/Pocket-Guidelines-Mobile-App. Accesses Oct 2014
74. Renzulli JF, Collins J, Mega A (2015) Radium-223 dichloride: illustrating the benefits of a multidisciplinary approach for patients with metastatic castration-resistant prostate cancer. J Multidiscip Healthc 8:279–286
75. Fitzpatrick JM, Anderson J, Sternberg CN et al (2008) Optimizing treatment for men with advanced prostate cancer: expert recommendations and the multidisciplinary approach. Crit Rev Oncol Hematol 68:S9–S22
76. Bellmunt J, Gelabert A (2007) Medical management of advanced prostate cancer: a multidisciplinary team approach. Expert Rev Anticancer Ther 7:977–979
77. Basler JW, Jenkins C, Swanson G (2005) Multidisciplinary management of prostate malignancy. Curr Urol Rep 6:228–234
78. Carducci MA, Carroll PR (2005) Multidisciplinary management of advanced prostate cancer: changing perspectives on referring patients and enhancing collaboration between oncologists and urologists in clinical trials. Urology 65:18–22
79. Hudak JL, McLeod DG, Brassell SA et al (2007) The design and implementation of a multidisciplinary prostate cancer clinic. Urol Nurs 27:491–498
80. Kurpad R, Kim W, Rathmell WK et al (2011) A multidisciplinary approach to the management of urologic malignancies: does it influence diagnostic and treatment decisions? Urol Oncol 29:378–382
81. Denis L (2011) Prostate Cancer Unit: the patient's perspective. Eur Urol 60:1200–1201
82. Gomella LG (2011) The Prostate Cancer Unit: a multidisciplinary approach for which the time has arrived. Eur Urol 60:1197–1199
83. Valdagni R (2011) Prostate Cancer Units: has the time come to discuss this thorny issue and promote their establishment in Europe? Eur Urol 60:1193–1196
84. Kowalski C, Schulte H, Wesselmann S (2015) Reporting program for cancer care quality indicators. J Oncol Pract 11:158–160
85. Magnani T, Valdagni R, Salvioni R et al (2012) The 6-year attendance of a multidisciplinary prostate cancer clinic in Italy: incidence of management changes. BJU Int 110:998–1003
86. Gomella LG, Lin J, Hoffman-Censits J et al (2010) Enhancing prostate cancer care through the multidisciplinary clinic approach: a 15-year experience. J Oncol Pract 6:e5–e10
87. Korman H, Lanni T Jr, Shah C et al (2013) Impact of a prostate multidisciplinary clinic program on patient treatment decisions and on adherence to NCCN guidelines: the William Beaumont Hospital experience. Am J Clin Oncol 36:121–125
88. Sternberg CN, Krainer M, Oh WK et al (2007) The medical management of prostate cancer: a multidisciplinary team approach. BJU Int 99:22–27
89. Aizer AA, Paly JJ, Zietman AL et al (2012) Multidisciplinary care and pursuit of active surveillance in low-risk prostate cancer. J Clin Oncol 30:3071–3076
90. Aizer AA, Paly JJ, Efstathiou JA (2013) Multidisciplinary care and management selection in prostate cancer. Semin Radiat Oncol 23:157–164

91. Zeliadt SB, Ramsey SD, Penson DF et al (2006) Why do men choose one treatment over another? A review of patient decision making for localized prostate cancer. Cancer 106:1865–1874
92. Fowler FJ, McNaughton Collins M, Albertsen PC et al (2000) Comparison of recommendations by urologists and radiation oncologists for treatment of clinically localized prostate cancer. JAMA 293:3217–3222
93. Moore MJ, O'Sullivan B, Tannock IF (1988) How expert physicians would wish to be treated if they had genitourinary cancer. J Clin Oncol 6:1736–1745
94. Multinational Association for Supportive Care in Cancer, MASCC Guidelines and Assessment Tools. http://www.mascc.org/guidelines-and-tools
95. Ripamonti C, Pessi MA, Boldini S (2012) Supportive care in Cancer Unit at the National Cancer Institute of Milan: a new integrated model of medicine in oncology. Curr Opin Oncol 24:391–396
96. Coleman R, Body JJ, Aapro M, ESMO Guidelines Working Group (2014) Bone health in cancer patients: ESMO Clinical Practice Guidelines. Ann Oncol 25:iii124–iii137
97. Strebel RT, Sulser T, Schmid HP et al (2013) Multidisciplinary care in patients with prostate cancer: room for improvement. Support Care Cancer 21:2327–2333
98. Shore ND (2012) Chemotherapy for prostate cancer: when should a urologist refer a patient to a medical oncologist? Prostate Cancer Prostatic Dis 16:1–6
99. Sartor AO, Fitzpatrick JM (2012) Urologists and oncologists: adapting to a new treatment paradigm in castration-resistant prostate cancer (CRPC). BJU Int 110:328–335
100. National Consensus Project for Quality Palliative Care. Clinical practice guidelines for quality palliative care, 3rd edn. Nationalconsensusproject.org. Assessed May 2013
101. Greer JA, Jackson VA, Meier DE, Temel JS (2013) Early integration of palliative care services with standard oncology care for patients with advanced cancer. CA Cancer J Clin 63:349–363
102. Lupu D, American Academy of Hospice and Palliative Medicine Workforce Task Force (2010) Estimate of current hospice and palliative medicine physician workforce shortage. J Pain Symptom Manage 40:899–911
103. Gelfman LP, Morrison RS (2008) Research funding for palliative medicine. J Palliat Med 11:36–43
104. Hui D, Finlay E, Buss MK et al (2015) Palliative oncologists: specialists in the science and art of patient care. J Clin Oncol 33:2314–2318

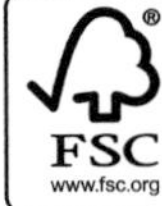

MIX
Papier aus verantwortungsvollen Quellen
Paper from responsible sources
FSC® C105338

If you have any concerns about our products,
you can contact us on
ProductSafety@springernature.com

In case Publisher is established outside the EU,
the EU authorized representative is:
Springer Nature Customer Service Center GmbH
Europaplatz 3, 69115 Heidelberg, Germany

Printed by Libri Plureos GmbH
in Hamburg, Germany